T0321940

RESEARCH IN PSYCHIATRY
ISSUES, STRATEGIES, AND METHODS

CRITICAL ISSUES IN PSYCHIATRY
An Educational Series for Residents and Clinicians

Series Editor: Sherwyn M. Woods, M.D., Ph.D.
University of Southern California School of Medicine
Los Angeles, California

Recent volumes in the series:

CASE STUDIES IN INSOMNIA
Edited by Peter J. Hauri, Ph.D.

CLINICAL DISORDERS OF MEMORY
Aman U. Khan, M.D.

CONTEMPORARY PERSPECTIVES ON PSYCHOTHERAPY WITH
LESBIANS AND GAY MEN
Edited by Terry S. Stein, M.D., and Carol J. Cohen, M.D.

DECIPHERING MOTIVATION IN PSYCHOTHERAPY
David M. Allen, M.D.

DIAGNOSTIC AND LABORATORY TESTING IN PSYCHIATRY
Edited by Mark S. Gold, M.D., and A. L. C. Pottash, M.D.

DRUG AND ALCOHOL ABUSE: A Clinical Guide to Diagnosis
and Treatment, Third Edition
Marc A. Schuckit, M.D.

EMERGENCY PSYCHIATRY: Concepts, Methods, and Practices
Edited by Ellen L. Bassuk, M.D., and Ann W. Birk, Ph.D.

ETHNIC PSYCHIATRY
Edited by Charles B. Wilkinson, M.D.

EVALUATION OF THE PSYCHIATRIC PATIENT: A Primer
Seymour L. Halleck, M.D.

NEUROPSYCHIATRIC FEATURES OF MEDICAL DISORDERS
James W. Jefferson, M.D., and John R. Marshall, M.D.

THE RACE AGAINST TIME: Psychotherapy and Psychoanalysis
in the Second Half of Life
Edited by Robert A. Nemiroff, M.D., and Calvin A. Colarusso, M.D.

RESEARCH IN PSYCHIATRY: Issues, Strategies, and Methods
Edited by L. K. George Hsu, M.D., and Michel Hersen, Ph.D.

STATES OF MIND: Configurational Analysis of Individual
Psychology, Second Edition
Mardi J. Horowitz, M.D.

A Continuation Order Plan is available for this series. A continuation order will
bring delivery of each new volume immediately upon publication. Volumes are
billed only upon actual shipment. For further information please contact the
publisher.

RESEARCH IN PSYCHIATRY
ISSUES, STRATEGIES, AND METHODS

EDITED BY

L. K. GEORGE HSU, M.D.

Western Psychiatric Institute and Clinic
University of Pittsburgh School of Medicine
Pittsburgh, Pennsylvania

AND

MICHEL HERSEN, PH.D.

Center for Psychological Studies
Nova University
Fort Lauderdale, Florida

PLENUM MEDICAL BOOK COMPANY • NEW YORK AND LONDON

Library of Congress Cataloging-in-Publication Data

Research in psychiatry : issues, strategies, and methods / edited by
L.K. George Hsu, and Michel Hersen.
        p.   cm. -- (Critical issues in psychiatry)
    Includes bibliographical references and index.
    ISBN 0-306-44162-4
    1. Psychiatry--Research. 2. Psychiatry--Research--Methodology.
I. Hsu, L. K. George (Lee Keung George) II. Hersen, Michel.
III. Series.
    [DNLM: 1. Psychiatry. 2. Research--methods.   WM 20 R4321]
RC337.R474 1992
616.89'0072--dc20
DNLM/DLC
for Library of Congress   92-14368
                                                           CIP

ISBN 0-306-44162-4

©1992 Plenum Publishing Corporation
233 Spring Street, New York, N.Y. 10013

Plenum Medical Book Company is an imprint of Plenum Publishing Corporation

Printed in the United States of America

Contributors

JACQUES P. BARBER, Center for Psychotherapy Research, Department of Psychiatry, University of Pennsylvania, 3600 Market Street, Philadelphia, Pennsylvania 19104-2648.

CAROLYN BRODBECK, Division of Psychology, Hahnemann University, Philadelphia, Pennsylvania 19102.

KENT F. BURNETT, Counseling Psychology Program and Department of Psychology, University of Miami, Coral Gables, Florida 33124-2040.

DENNIS P. CANTWELL, Department of Psychiatry, University of California at Los Angeles, Los Angeles, California 90024.

DUNCAN B. CLARK, Department of Psychiatry, Western Psychiatric Institute and Clinic, University of Pittsburgh School of Medicine, Pittsburgh, Pennsylvania 15213.

NANCY L. DAY, Western Psychiatric Institute and Clinic, 3811 O'Hara Street, Pittsburgh, Pennsylvania 15213.

AL K. DEROY, Office of Research, University of Pittsburgh, Pittsburgh, Pennsylvania 15260.

JOHN W. DOUARD, Institute for the Medical Humanities, University of Texas Medical Branch, Galveston, Texas 77550.

CARL EISDORFER, Department of Psychiatry and Center for Adult Development and Aging, University of Miami School of Medicine, Miami, Florida 33136.

JEROME A. FLEMING, Harvard Medical School Department of Psychiatry, Psychiatry Service, Brockton/West Roxbury Veterans Administration Medical Center, Harvard School of Public Health, Program in Psychiatric Epidemiology, Brockton, Massachusetts 02401.

SHIRLEY M. GLYNN, Veterans Administration Medical Center of West Los Angeles, Los Angeles, California 90073.

GERALD GOLDSTEIN, Highland Drive, Veterans Administration Hospital, Pittsburgh, Pennsylvania 15206.

DONALD W. GOODWIN, Department of Psychiatry, University of Kansas Medical Center, Kansas City, Kansas 66160.

SILVIA S. GRATZ, Department of Psychiatry, Medical College of Pennsylvania, Eastern Pennsylvania Psychiatric Institute, Philadelphia, Pennsylvania 19129.

JOEL B. GREENHOUSE, Department of Statistics, Carnegie-Mellon University, Pittsburgh, Pennsylvania 15213.

MICHEL HERSEN, Center for Psychological Studies, Nova University, Fort Lauderdale, Florida 33314.

CHUNG-CHENG HSIEH, Harvard Medical School Department of Psychiatry, Psychiatry Service, Brockton/West Roxbury Veterans Administration Medical Center, Harvard School of Public Health, Program in Psychiatric Epidemiology, Brockton, Massachusetts 02401.

GAIL H. IRONSON, Departments of Psychology and Psychiatry, University of Miami, Coral Gables, Florida 33124-2040.

ROLF G. JACOB, Department of Psychiatry, Western Psychiatric Institute and Clinic, University of Pittsburgh School of Medicine, Pittsburgh, Pennsylvania 15213.

BRIAN W. JUNKER, Department of Statistics, Carnegie-Mellon University, Pittsburgh, Pennsylvania 15213.

DAVID J. KUPFER, Western Psychiatric Institute and Clinic, 3811 O'Hara Street, Pittsburgh, Pennsylvania 15213.

DAVID A. LOEWENSTEIN, Department of Psychiatry and Center for Adult Development and Aging, University of Miami School of Medicine, Miami, Florida 33136.

LESTER B. LUBORSKY, Center for Psychotherapy Research, Department of Psychiatry, University of Pennsylvania, 3600 Market Street, Philadelphia, Pennsylvania 19104-2648.

WENDY REICH, Department of Psychiatry, Division of Child Psychiatry, Washington University School of Medicine, St. Louis, Missouri 63110.

STEPHEN D. SAMUELSON, Department of Psychiatry, The University of Texas Health Science Center at San Antonio, San Antonio, Texas 78284-7729.

GEORGE M. SIMPSON, Department of Psychiatry, Medical College of Pennsylvania, Eastern Pennsylvania Psychiatric Institute, Philadelphia, Pennsylvania 19129.

MARK D. SULLIVAN, Department of Psychiatry, University of Washington, Seattle, Washington 98195.

C. BARR TAYLOR, Laboratory for the Study of Behavioral Medicine, Department of Psychiatry, Stanford University School of Medicine, Stanford, California 94305.

JAMES W. THOMPSON, Department of Psychiatry, University of Maryland School of Medicine, Baltimore, Maryland 21201.

MING T. TSUANG, Harvard Medical School Department of Psychiatry, Psychiatry Service, Brockton/West Roxbury Veterans Administration Medical Center, Harvard School of Public Health, Program in Psychiatric Epidemiology, Brockton, Massachusetts 02401.

GARY J. TUCKER, Department of Psychiatry, University of Washington, Seattle, Washington 98195.

A. HUSSAIN TUMA, Western Psychiatric Institute and Clinic, 3811 O'Hara Street, Pittsburgh, Pennsylvania 15213.

GEORGE WINOKUR, Department of Psychiatry, College of Medicine, University of Iowa, Iowa City, Iowa 52242.

WILLIAM J. WINSLADE, Institute for the Medical Humanities, University of Texas Medical Branch, Galveston, Texas 77550.

Preface

This multiauthored textbook is directed to the psychiatric resident and other professionals who are interested in the issues, strategies, and methods of psychiatric research. Although the field of psychiatry has not attained the scientific rigor and clinical sophistication of some of its sister disciplines in the medical arena, considerable progress has been made in the last decade or two, and a full understanding of the types of articles that now appear in such publications as the *American Journal of Psychiatry*, the *Archives of General Psychiatry*, and the *Journal of the American Academy of Child and Adolescent Psychiatry* requires a fair amount of knowledge about research design and strategy. Whereas articles in psychiatric journals 20 years ago dealt mainly with psychodynamic topics and utilized nonexperimental observations, today their counterparts are concerned mostly with psychobiology, clinical features, diagnosis, and treatment, and employ scientific experimental designs. The trend of applying scientific methodology to research in psychiatry is increasing and undoubtedly will continue to do so in the future.

Regrettably, however, only about 1 of every 10 psychiatric residents turns to clinical research as a career. Fewer than half of all the articles that are published in psychiatric journals are first-authored by psychiatrists, and in psychological journals, psychiatrists are first authors of fewer than 5% of the articles. Furthermore, the number of psychiatrists who received Alcohol, Drug Abuse, and Mental Health Administration funding for traditional research project (RO1) grants in fiscal year 1990 was less than half the number of psychologists. It is therefore apparent that the majority of psychiatrists are not clinical researchers, even though all of them are affected by the current emphasis on scientific research in psychiatry and are consumers of the resulting data. Our contention is that whether research is eventually pursued as a career or not, residents should be exposed to its subtleties and nuances, at least so that they will be able to appraise the validity of what is being presented to them in the archival literature. We believe that this volume will enable residents to appreciate research better and perhaps even encourage some of them to participate as active investigators.

The book is divided into six parts that contain a total of 19 chapters. Part I, General Issues, includes two chapters that deal with research in psychiatry as a career and with ethical issues in psychiatric research. Part II, Research Design Strategies, consists of four chapters that deal with the single-case, group comparison, and correlational approaches, and with statistical principles. Part III, Assessment Issues, contains three chapters that consider structured and semi-structured inventories, physiological and behavioral assessment, and biological markers. Part IV, Research Topics, includes six chapters on some of the major areas that are researched by psychiatrists and their mental health colleagues. Part V, Special Populations, includes three chapters that cover research in child and adolescent psychiatry, geriatric research, and the chronically mentally ill. Finally, in Part VI, Epilogue, the future of psychiatric research is discussed.

Many people have contributed their efforts to the publication of this book. First and foremost are our gracious authors, who agreed to share their experiences and expertise with us. Second, we thank Mary Anne Frederick, Beth Fryman, and Mary Newell for their fine technical assistance. Finally, we thank Eliot Werner, Executive Editor at Plenum Press, who agreed with us as to the timeliness of this project.

L. K. GEORGE HSU
Pittsburgh, Pennsylvania
MICHEL HERSEN
Fort Lauderdale, Florida

Contents

CHAPTER 2: ETHICAL ISSUES IN PSYCHIATRIC RESEARCH ....

William J. Winslade and John W. Douard

PART II: RESEARCH DESIGN STRATEGIES

CHAPTER 3: SINGLE-CASE DESIGNS ....

Michel Hersen

CHAPTER 4: GROUP COMPARISON APPROACHES IN PSYCHIATRIC
              RESEARCH 107

Ming T. Tsuang, Chung-Cheng Hsieh, and Jerome A. Fleming

CHAPTER 5: CORRELATIONAL APPROACH 133

Gerald Goldstein

PART III: ASSESSMENT ISSUES

CHAPTER 8: PHYSIOLOGICAL AND BEHAVIORAL ASSESSMENT 195

Rolf G. Jacob, Carolyn Brodbeck, and Duncan B. Clark

CHAPTER 9: BIOLOGICAL MARKERS 235

Stephen D. Samuelson and George Winokur

PART IV: RESEARCH TOPICS

CHAPTER 10:   DIAGNOSTIC ISSUES 265

James W. Thompson

CHAPTER 11:   EPIDEMIOLOGY 293

Nancy L. Day

CHAPTER 12: PSYCHOPHARMACOLOGY 309

Silvia S. Gratz and George M. Simpson

CHAPTER 13: PSYCHOTHERAPY RESEARCH: ISSUES TO CONSIDER IN
                PLANNING A STUDY 331

Jacques P. Barber and Lester B. Luborsky

CHAPTER 14: GENETICS OF ALCOHOLISM

Donald W. Goodwin

CHAPTER 15: BEHAVIORAL MEDICINE

Kent F. Burnett, Gail H. Ironson, and C. Barr Taylor

PART V: SPECIAL POPULATIONS

PART VI: EPILOGUE

PART I

GENERAL ISSUES

CHAPTER 1

Research in Psychiatry as a Career

A. HUSSAIN TUMA, AL K. DEROY, AND DAVID J. KUPFER

INTRODUCTION

The chapters in this volume were chosen to provide an introduction to the development of research skills by psychiatric residents and postdoctoral fellows in psychiatry and to focus on basic research principles and background information with which a trainee in psychiatry should be familiar. Overall, the emphasis is on cognitive skills, such as the development of certain attitudes or ways of thinking about scientific problems, and also on the acquisition of specific technical skills and background knowledge necessary for a critical reading of the literature and the beginning of independent research. In a sense, this volume provides the reader with material relevant to what one might call the *curricular* or formal aspects of training.

In this chapter, we will first highlight issues currently salient to the choice of a research career in psychiatry, discuss existing needs and opportunities in the field of psychiatric research, and allude to determinants of a career choice. Subsequently, we will focus on the needs and functions of the clinical investigator and identify pertinent features of current psychiatric residency training and the training environment. To conclude, we will discuss in depth the sources of

A. Hussain Tuma and David J. Kupfer • Western Psychiatric Institute and Clinic, 3811 O'Hara Street, Pittsburgh, Pennsylvania 15213.   Al K. DeRoy • Office of Research, University of Pittsburgh, Pittsburgh, Pennsylvania 15260.
Research in Psychiatry: Issues, Strategies, and Methods, edited by L. K. George Hsu and Michel Hersen. Plenum Press, New York, 1992.

3

research support in the United States, the considerations involved in the development of a research project, and, finally, the merit criteria typically considered in the review and funding of research proposals.

CHOICE OF A RESEARCH CAREER IN CLINICAL PSYCHIATRY

At the outset, it is useful to remember that in order to determine whether or not to choose a research career in psychiatry, the psychiatric resident should be informed about the kinds of experiences, demands, rewards, and limitations that are typically associated with the profession and life-style of an academic clinical scientist. Given the dearth of valid data in this area, what follows is a brief, anecdotal, but practical description of the specific functions and roles, the incentives and disincentives, that are involved in a clinical research career in psychiatry and, probably, in other health specialties as well.

To begin, we assume that making a career choice or career change entails careful self-appraisal of one's personal and professional development. By the time an individual graduates from medical school, he or she is likely to have achieved a degree of self-understanding that would allow a reasonably realistic assessment of his or her intellectual bent and the psychological, social, and economic values, pressures, and expectations that would make certain occupational roles more or less attractive. A more experienced and informed colleague, a mentor, could certainly help in this process of self- and occupational role appraisal, but the candidate should be able to determine in some general way (at least at the gut level) his or her own inclinations and aptitudes for a career in science.

Experiences that are inherent in the role of a scientist, though generally familiar to those in the field at some level of awareness, may not be readily recognizable or fully appreciated by the young clinical trainee. Nor is the young trainee in a position to appreciate fully both the thrills and frustrations of a career in research as it gradually unfolds. Thus, it is important that the young candidate experience, firsthand if possible, and understand what it means to assume eventually the role of an academic clinical investigator. Again, an experienced, interested, and empathic mentor can help a great deal in clarifying one's goals, pointing out appropriate pathways for accomplishing them, and helping in the development of a realistic perspective or vision of expected career roles.

Research Career Opportunities

For the past four decades, psychiatrists with sound research backgrounds have been in great demand, and will probably remain in demand for years to come. According to some observers, this demand continues to increase and has never been greater than at the present time (Gillin, 1988; Institute of Medicine, 1989; Pincus, Goodwin, Barchas, Cohen, Judd, Meltzer, & Vaillant, 1989; H. A. Pincus, November, 1991 personal communication).

Concern with serious shortages of research personnel in psychiatry dates back to the mid-1940s. Eight years after the establishment of the National Institute of Mental Health (NIMH) in 1946, the Career Investigator Grant Program was initiated (1954), then seven years later the Research Career Development Program (1961), and, soon thereafter, the Research Scientist Development Program (1967)—all in an effort to attenuate the severity of this shortage. John Romano, a distinguished psychiatrist and former member of the NIMH Advisory Council, writing in 1972, provides a historical perspective as follows:

> during the mid 1940s those of us associated with the Research Study Section of NIMH soon became aware of the scarcity of young men and women engaged significantly in psychiatric research. It became clear that the field needed a new type of psychiatrist— namely the research scientist, as contrasted with the teacher-clinician, the practicing psychiatrist, the psychotherapist. (quoted in Boothe, Rosenfeld, & Walker 1974, p. V)

Despite continuing serious efforts during the 1970s, fewer medical school graduates were entering psychiatry compared to those entering other medical specialties, and fewer psychiatrists were receiving postdoctoral research training. For example, in 1982, only 12% of trainees in psychiatry were receiving research training whereas about 35% of the trainees in other medical specialties were receiving such training (Institute of Medicine, 1983). The Research Scientist Development Awards and subsequent programs, such as the Physician Scientist Awards, Clinical Scientist Awards, and, more recently, the First Independent Research Support and Transition (FIRST) Awards, have certainly helped a great deal to increase the number and improve the quality of research personnel in mental health in recent years. Nevertheless, several major reports, including those of the Institute of Medicine, indicate that there are still serious shortages of career investigators in both general psychiatry and child and adolescent psychiatry (Institute of Medicine, 1985, 1989). For example, a report by the National Advisory Mental Health Council to the U.S. Congress characterized the field of child and adolescent psychiatry as suffering from "a lack in the critical mass of researchers and the infusion of fresh talent, resources, and equipment needed to realize its full potential" (National Institute of Mental Health, 1990, p. V).

In an earlier report, the Institute of Medicine (1984) observed that the NIMH then supported fewer research trainees than at any time since 1963. This is in the face of a clear need for career researchers in a number of areas in the biobehavioral sciences. Clearly, this is a complex problem with a variety of interrelated causes and consequences. Nevertheless, symptoms of this chronic shortage of trained research personnel that have been pointed out by several observers (e.g., Burke, Pincus, & Pandes, 1986; Hillman, 1985; NIMH Research Information Source Book, 1989) are manifested in a variety of contexts, including (1) large proportions of teaching faculties of clinical departments with limited or no prior research training or current research involvement; (2) shortages of academically qualified candidates to fill vacant faculty positions in clinical departments; (3) small, and in some instances, decreasing proportions of M.D.s who successfully compete for research grants, National Research Science Awards, Research Scientist Development Awards and (4) relatively small numbers of medical students and residents interested in research as a career; and (5) a decreasing percentage of young investigators among recipients of research grants (e.g., in 1977 well over 25% of all NIMH research grants were awarded to principal investigators under 36 years of age; more recent data show that the percentage has steadily fallen throughout the 1970s and 1980s and is now about 10%, and if we exclude Research Scientist, Small Grant, and FIRST Awards, the percentage drops further to about 5%).

In addition to current shortages in research personnel, rapid evolution in the biomedical and behavioral sciences creates an additional need for new types of specially trained researchers. As we view the field, severe shortages are visible in a wide range of areas of basic and clinical sciences relevant to mental and addictive disorders, especially of children and adolescents. Most compelling are shortages in such newly emerging fields as developmental cognitive neuroscience, developmental neurobiology and neuropsychology, molecular biology and genetics, psychoneuroimmunology and neuropsychopharmacology, and research on nonhuman primate models of major psychiatric and addictive disorders. Needless to say that among current pools of research talent in psychiatry, severe shortages also exist, especially among women and minority researchers. Similar shortages exist among psychiatrists focusing on major mental and addictive disorders of childhood and adolescence.

In the following section, we examine factors that may influence the choice of a research career in psychiatry in the hope of facilitating a rational choice.

Determinants of Career Choice

Most of the literature on factors that influence the selection of research as a career in the health professions has been retrospective and is based, at best, on questionnaires completed after the fact, anecdotal data, and post hoc analysis. Controlled comparative experiments in this area are, to our knowledge, nonexistent. Nevertheless, specific factors and circumstances that are thought to influence the decision to enter a career in clinical research have been identified by several observers over the past decade. For example, following a concise review of the history of the NIH training programs, Wyngaarden (1979) suggested that the following factors have *negative impact* on a physician's decision to enter a research career: increasing societal emphasis in recent years on providing medical care to the disadvantaged; revisions in the medical school curriculum that reduced the amount of research experience; a perceived instability of federal support for biomedical research and research training; lack of acceptance of research training as an appropriate component of residency training by specialty certifying boards; the abolition of the military draft; the relative financial attractiveness of a career in clinical practice; and the negative impact of the "payback provision" of the National Research Science Awards (NRSAs). Other factors not mentioned by Wyngaarden include the extent to which leadership of psychiatry departments and divisions of child and adolescent psychiatry emphasize research training (Dech, Abikoff, & Koplewicz, 1990) and also the extent that the training and clinical programs are integrative in character rather than dichotomous in their approach to scientific and clinical activities (Detre, 1989). This clearly will reflect the favorable or unfavorable attitudes toward research among health professionals in the clinical settings where undergraduate and graduate medical training take place. Finally, there are relatively few centers of excellence in psychiatric research, and those that exist are concentrated in a few geographic locations (as discussed in more detail later). Consequently, the critical mass of outstanding basic and clinical scientists that is necessary to have a significant impact on the department's educational programs and to provide sufficient interaction with young residents and clinical colleagues in their daily activities is simply not available in most Departments of Psychiatry.

Although many of these factors are difficult to study empirically and prospectively, one can, for the present, assume that some of them may play an important role, while there is some research support for the importance of others. For example, in a retrospective survey of 516 successful clinical investigators in internal medicine, Davis and Kelley (1982) focused on, among other issues, the timing of the decision to enter a research career. They found that 21% of their respondents had decided on a research career before entering medical school, 45% while in medical school, and 34% made that decision during residency or fellowship training. Over half of these successful researchers identified a particular person (mentor) or event that most affected their decision to choose a research career. Davis and Kelley also found an inverse relationship between the time the decision was made to enter a research career and the success of an investigator (i.e., the earlier the decision, the more successful the investigator). For the vast majority of the individuals queried, meeting a military obligation was either not relevant or, when relevant, was not felt to have affected their decision to undertake research training. Similarly, the NRSA payback requirement was not perceived to be a major factor. It must be emphasized, however, that for a large proportion of the respondents, some of the questions were hypothetical and/or irrelevant.

Another retrospective study of the careers of 262 physicians in research-oriented positions in England (Wakeford, Evered, Lyon, & Saunders, 1985) found that 41% of the respondents reported a long-standing interest in a research career, 39% had developed such an interest while in a job which was not necessarily research-oriented, and the remaining 20% just happened to learn of an interesting job opportunity in research. The respondents mentioned a total of 10 factors that they perceived as influential in their decision to enter a research career, three of which were considered as "greatly" or "quite a bit" influential by 59% to 85% of the cases. In order of prevalence, these factors were: a desire to find answers to problems; a particular interest in a subject; and the influence of a mentor or teacher. This survey also showed that undergraduate research experience was closely associated with early research career decisions, even though 60% of all the respondents had no research experience as undergraduates.

In a more relevant and recent study, Sledge, Leaf, Fenton, and Chung (1990) examined the subsequent career patterns of 132 graduates of the Advanced Track Program of the Psychiatry Residency Program at Yale University between 1973 and 1982. They found that those who were trained in the University Health Service Track differed significantly from those who trained in the Neurobehavioral Science Track, in that the Health Service graduates spent more hours per week in private office practice and direct clinical service, whereas the Neuroscience Track graduates spent far fewer hours per week in private office practice, spent far more hours per week in research, and had greater scholarly productivity.

Based on these surveys and the weight of anecdotal evidence and experiences of many in this field, it may be concluded that the following factors constitute powerful influences on the choice of research as a career: (1) endowment with a curious, questioning, and probing intellect; (2) early interest, encouragement, and involvement in research in the course of one's educational development, especially in the college and medical school years; (3) the influence of teachers or mentors throughout one's training, particularly during medical school and residency; (4) a work or study environment that promotes independent thinking and scholarship, provides opportunities for research, and rewards academic accomplishment.

In considering a research career, it is useful to have an understanding of the various roles performed by the clinical researcher. These roles are highlighted in the next section.

Interests, Needs, and Functions of the Clinical Researcher

We now describe some of the elements of the researcher's functional role in contemporary academic psychiatry in the hope that those who are considering a research career will be sufficiently stimulated (or provoked) to seek the types of additional and direct experiences that would allow greater familiarity and appreciation of at least some of what constitutes a career in clinical research. In principle, the fundamental issue is that of "goodness of fit" between the intellectual and motivational factors that characterize the trainee in the context of his or her particular life circumstances on the one hand, and the characteristic functions, rewards, challenges, and frustrations associated with the role of the clinical scientist in psychiatry on the other.

Clearly, clinicians and clinical scientists share a number of similar intellectual, motivational, vocational, and socioeconomic interests and attributes; yet there are some major differences in what is more or less important to them. As is true for other types of physicians, the psychiatric clinician probably derives the most satisfaction from diagnosing and treating illness, providing emotional support and guidance for patients and their family members, reducing human suffering, helping restore normal function and a sense of well-being, and, at times, even saving lives. Associated with these inherently "clinical" rewards are, in our contemporary society, high levels of social recognition and financial compensation for the psychiatrist's clinical services. For the clinical scientist, however, identifying important questions concerning the etiology, pathophysiology, epidemiology, prevention or treatment of a psychiatric illness, designing and carrying out studies to answer such questions, and, more broadly, understanding human behavior at a certain organizational level (e.g., molecular, cellular, molar, or clinical), and the prospect of discovering and publishing meaningful results are perhaps the most exciting, motivating, and rewarding aspects of the work. Thus, an intense intellectual curiosity about a clinical puzzle and the enthusiasm needed to solve it are the major motives that drive the researcher to gather data, examine and reexamine issues in new and different ways, and tolerate ambiguity in data with patience, hope, and tenacity. Thus, even though clinicians receive their rewards primarily from the processes and outcomes of their clinical activities, recognition of their direct contributions to the health of specific individuals and families, and also relatively great financial remuneration, the clinical investigator is gratified primarily through the process of discovery, satisfaction of curiosity, and the receipt of peer and social recognition—rewards that are associated primarily with academic pursuits, standards, and values.

By way of a generic, functional role description, one can say that the clinical researcher in psychiatry will typically engage at one or another stage of his or her career in many or all of the following activities (obviously, some of these activities are predominant in earlier phases of the researcher's career while others come later on):

1. Continual pursuit of a series of educational activities (e.g., reading, attending and giving lectures, participating in seminars, workshops, and conferences) with the aim of mastering existing knowledge in a particular research are in both substance and methodology. Moreover, the researcher continually seeks additional knowledge in the basic and clinical sciences that are related to his or her area(s) of interest. Such focused monitoring of a particular field and its value allows the researcher to maintain an expert's level of knowledge of facts, problems, gaps, and promising directions in that field. This, in turn, permits the researcher to develop practical strategies for pursuing new leads to expand current knowledge and discover new findings by formulating new hypotheses, designing laboratory, clinical, or epidemiological investigations, collecting and analyzing data, and writing up and reporting findings to appropriate scientific and professional audiences. Scientists attend to and derive a special pleasure from detailed understanding of things!

2. The search for needed resources, such as space, personnel, and equipment, often involves negotiation with departmental or institutional officials. In addition, the investigator almost always engages in raising external funds to support his or her research program. This entails writing research grant or contract applications and, at times, participating in site visits that may be involved in competitive review of proposals by a public agency or private foundation. (Note that the latter portions of this chapter discuss topics relevant to the pursuit and acquisition of research funding.)

3. Because of the number and nature of developments in science and technology over the past several decades, as well as increased specialization and complexity of research issues, particularly in clinical areas, the conduct of research often entails collaboration with colleagues in several different fields.

4. Training and supervising assistants and junior colleagues in carrying out such research tasks as mastering a laboratory or clinical technique, interviewing patients, administering treatments and evaluating outcomes according to specific protocol requirements, interacting with and assessing the family and other social support systems, ensuring the protection of human subjects from unwarranted risks, and overseeing data acquisition and management are activities in which the clinical investigator typically engages. Clearly, these activities require familiarity with not only the scientific and clinical aspects of the work, but also sensitivity to ethical, administrative, and economic considerations.

5. As a member of the scientific community in psychiatry, the clinical researcher presents and discusses his or her work and that of others in public scientific forums for purposes of disseminating new information and defining the current state-of-the-art and, at times, arriving at a consensus and recommendations regarding the use of research findings in the diagnosis, treatment, or prevention of mental or addictive disorders.

6. As a teacher, supervisor, and mentor, the clinical researcher brings to his or her students and junior colleagues state-of-the-art information, stimulates their thinking and critical questioning of new data or currently accepted practices, facilitates the development and maintenance of an open-minded, questioning, and flexible attitude toward issues of diagnosis and treatment, and counsels them on personal and professional matters.

7. As a member of a peer review group, the established clinical researcher also serves as a referee in research, training, or demonstration proposal competitions, offering informed opinions and comments on the scientific and technical merit of proposals and advising funding source agencies on promising areas and directions of future research. A related and similar role is that of refereeing for scientific journals, serving on editorial boards, and contributing to or making acceptance/rejection decisions regarding manuscripts submitted for publication, and, at times, formulating publication policies.

8. As a consultant, advisor, or counselor to a government or voluntary agency or private-sector firm or foundation, the clinical scientist identifies areas of need and promising research areas for emphasis in future funding initiatives, contributes to the development of research support programs, assists in formulating health goals, standards, and policies, and contributes to public awareness and education.

9. As an expert in a particular clinical area, the clinical scientist serves as a consultant to other health and mental health practitioners on desirable courses of action when faced with difficult diagnostic or treatment problems.

10. As a science administrator, the clinical researcher assumes responsibility for the administration and management of a research program, a laboratory, a university department or school, or a government agency.

11. As a university-based clinician, the investigator maintains a reasonable and necessary degree of involvement in clinical work and other university and outside professional service activities that are either required or are important to, but go beyond, other professional commitments.

12. In order to carry out these functions effectively, an investigator often needs to undertake domestic and international travel and spend a considerable amount of time away from home and family.

13. Yet another consideration worth noting is that a successful clinical scientist, like most other scientists and academicians, can maintain a reasonably comfortable, but not lavish, standard of living.

In general, the functions and role characteristics highlighted here clearly provide the clinical scientist with considerable diversity of roles or variety of life experiences which make such a career both interesting and gratifying. Nevertheless, the psychiatric resident who is considering an academic research career must ascertain the extent to which the type of activities illustrated here match his or her career and personal interests, needs, goals, and expectations. If a research career seems desirable (i.e., the satisfaction to frustration ratio seems acceptable), then the beginning professional must identify and seek out the type of training environment that would facilitate learning more about the various facets of the clinical scientist's roles and their demands, and would allow experiencing some of them firsthand. Once a particular environment is selected, it is vital that one stay in that environment an adequate period of time, say, 5 years, to allow sufficient career growth and mastery to take place before moving on to another setting. Such a tenure may in fact include 1 year of senior residency, 2 years of postdoctoral fellowship, and 1 year or 2 years of junior faculty position.

The "ultimate" career decision, and eventual success and satisfaction, would then hinge on the goodness of fit between these roles and one's personal and professional aptitudes, interests, goals, and expectations. In view of the critical importance of the training environment to the nurturance and development of one's research interests and skills, we highlight in the next section some of the characteristics of desirable training environments.

The Training Environment

Since the primary mission of most residency training programs in psychiatry is to produce well-informed and competent clinical practitioners, the residency curriculum typically focuses on clinical work and on satisfying certification requirements. Moreover, research and research training in mental disorders and substance abuse and dependence are highly concentrated in a few regions of the country. To illustrate, 10 states—New York, California, Pennsylvania, Massachusetts, Maryland, Connecticut, Michigan, Texas, Illinois, and North Carolina—received 68% of Alcohol, Drug Abuse, and Mental Health Administration (ADAMHA) institutes' funds in 1989 (Alcohol, Drug Abuse, and Mental Health Administration, 1989a). Similarly, of the 308 academic institutions that received research, research fellowship, and research training funds from NIMH in 1989, 20 universities, only 6.4% of the total, were awarded 50% of the funds in that year (Alcohol, Drug Abuse, and Mental Health Administration, 1989b). Finally, nine states (Alaska, Idaho, Maine, Montana, Nevada, North Dakota, South Dakota, West Virginia, and Wyoming) received no ADAMHA research grants in 1989. Consequently, owing to this geographic concentration of research and research training opportunities in psychiatry, very few clinical researchers can participate in a significant way in the training of the vast majority of psychiatric residents and serve as role models for them. To the extent that the attending and teaching faculty have not had appropriate research training and have not been engaged in research, it would be reasonable to assume that they tend verbally or by example not to encourage residents to pursue such a course.

A recent Canadian study (Leichner, 1987) reported that while 38% of psychiatric residents expressed a definite interest in full- or part-time research in 1975, only 10% indicated such interest a decade later, and the percentage of those reporting a definite *lack* of interest in research rose sharply during that ten-year period. Although many psychiatric residency training programs aim to equip residents with skills that should enable them to read critically and evaluate the literature relevant to their clinical interests and functions, only a few programs stipulate research experience as a training requirement. Similarly, when clinical researchers distance themselves from regular clinical duties, show little or no enthusiasm for involvement in patient care, and hence gradually lose touch with the clinical staff, they perhaps unwittingly discourage clinically motivated residents from involvement in research. Moreover, in those environments, the relative isolation of research faculty from clinical work and their absence from the clinical scene tend to promote, over time, the development of negative and suspicious attitudes toward research among otherwise dedicated clinical staff and inhibit the development of a positive atmosphere where research is viewed not only as compatible with quality patient care, but perhaps also as important in upgrading and making significant contributions to patient care (Garfinkel, Goldbloom, Kaplan, & Kennedy, 1989; Garfinkel, Kennedy, Kaplan, & Goldbloom, 1989). Thus, a central and continuing involvement of the clinical scientist in patient care and supervision of junior staff is vital not only for the maintenance and improvement of the researcher's own clinical skills and expertise, but also for promoting and maintaining an environment that accepts and encourages scientific pursuits. It behooves the recent medical school graduate who is interested in a clinical research career in psychiatry to investigate the availability of such an environment in the psychiatric settings which he or she seriously considers for training. One will do well to select a university department with a high-quality clinical residency training program *and* a substantial commitment to research. Even though these are few in number, such departments would typically have the critical mass of research faculty to serve as mentors and role models. In addition, for psychiatrists with limited background in research (e.g., those with no prior graduate or Ph.D. training), a minimum of 2 or 3 years in a postresidency research fellowship program would be highly desirable. In fact, a 1988 study in internal medicine showed that those faculty members whose formal research fellowship period was followed by additional years of protected support had the most success in their research careers (Levy, Sherman, Gentile, Hough, Dial, & Jolly, 1988). Such fellowship programs usually include a "hands-on" research apprenticeship and related experiences similar to those outlined earlier. More specifically, elements of such training include some didactic courses either to correct deficiencies in earlier training or to acquire new skills, active participation in ongoing research as a junior partner, participation in regular research seminars and lecture series, identification of a project for independent research, and preparation of an acceptable research protocol. The latter two elements normally entail reviewing the research literature relevant to the problem of interest; conceptualizing the problem and formulating it in terms of specific questions or hypotheses that could be empirically tested; considering and selecting appropriate methods and procedures for gathering and analyzing data; sorting out diagnostic, inclusion, and exclusion criteria for sample selection; consulting with methodologists regarding appropriate sample size, experimental design, and relevant statistical models and methods; developing skills in scientific self-expression and reporting of data to scientific audiences; possibly collaborating with other researchers from different disciplines who share interest in similar problems; becoming sensitized to issues in scientific integrity, including ethical issues concerning research on human and animal subjects and special populations; and, above all, learning and beginning to function as an independent investigator. To function as an independent investigator, one is expected to compete successfully in generating research support. How to generate such support is the topic of succeeding sections.

RESEARCH SUPPORT IN PSYCHIATRY

As a practical guide, we provide some basic information about sources of research support and what is involved in obtaining funds for one's research. More specifically, we will discuss public and private sources of financial support for basic and clinical research, recent data on dollar amounts budgeted and awards made to indicate the magnitude of available research support, key elements in developing a research project, and important points to keep in mind in preparing a grant application. We also briefly discuss the process of applying for funds, what is involved in the assignment, review, and funding of research grant applications, and the scientific, financial, and ethical obligations and responsibilities of investigators and grantee institutions.

Funding Sources

The United States invests heavily in research and development (R&D). In 1990, an estimated $150 billion was expended for R&D (National Science Foundation, June, 1990, Figure 2, p. 3), an amount equivalent to 2.69% of the Gross

National Product in that year (Jankowski, 1990, Table 8-14, p. 55). In Fiscal Year 1990, federal funding for R&D was an estimated $63.805 billion, $8.358 billion (13.1%) of which was for R&D in health (National Science Foundation, April, 1990, p. 2).

There are many sources of research support to which an investigator may apply for funding. These include sources internal to institutions, government agencies, philanthropic and corporate foundations, professional societies, and voluntary organizations and associations. It is important to recognize that each funding source or program has specific priorities, and that these priorities change over time. Therefore, it is advisable to become familiar with the latest information about possible funding sources early on in project development.

Internal Sources

Many universities, hospitals, and research institutes maintain one or more funds that are used to support directly research conducted there. These include, for example, start-up and development funds to support the research of newly independent or recently arrived investigators, faculty recruitment and retention funds, and seed funds (discussed below).

The most common—although an often overlooked—form of internally supported research is termed "unsponsored research." Often this accounts for a significant portion of the research conducted in universities, hospitals, and research institutes. Unsponsored research is *not* supported directly by special funds, but is subsidized by the investigator's institution or organizational unit, such as a university department or academic research center. Most research in the arts and humanities and much research in the social, behavioral, and natural sciences are "unsponsored" by sources external to the institution. Here the costs of research are absorbed by the institutions themselves.

Federal Agencies

Most of the biomedical and behavioral research conducted in the United States is supported by federal funds. The major federal funding sources relevant to research in psychiatry, psychology, and other mental health-relevant disciplines are the Alcohol, Drug Abuse, and Mental Health Administration, National Institutes of Health, National Science Foundation, and the Department of Education.

The *Alcohol, Drug Abuse, and Mental Health Administration* (ADAMHA) is the umbrella agency for the National Institute of Mental Health (NIMH), National Institute on Alcohol Abuse and Alcoholism (NIAAA), National Institute on Drug Abuse (NIDA), and Office of Substance Abuse Prevention (OSAP). In the aggregate, ADAMHA institutes and offices support research, research training, and, to a lesser extent, service demonstrations, clinical training, and public education activities. ADAMHA's primary mission is to support research in mental health, mental illness, alcoholism, and alcohol and drug abuse and dependence. In addition, ADAMHA institutes support studies of psychiatric, psychological, behavioral, and socioenvironmental factors in other diseases, such as AIDS and Alzheimer's disease. The research may have disciplinary or interdisciplinary focus in basic and/or clinical sciences relevant to understanding the etiology, pathophysiology, diagnosis, treatment, epidemiology, and prevention of mental disorders, or of drug and alcohol abuse and dependence, across all age, gender, racial, and ethnic groups. Relevant disciplines include medical, biological, behavioral, social, and physical sciences, such as psychiatry, neurology, radiology, anatomy, genetics, neuroscience, physiology, chemistry, pharmacology, toxicology, endocrinology, immunology, psychology, sociology, anthropology, and economics.

In Fiscal Year 1990, ADAMHA's budget, which included ADAMHA institutes' intramural research, was about $897 million (National Science Foundation, April, 1990, p. 28). This figure included extramural research funding of about $313 million provided through NIMH, $199 million through NIDA, and $113 million through NIAAA (National Science Foundation, April, 1990, p. 28). ADAMHA's extramural research budget in FY 1990 was to support 799 new and competing continuation "research project grants" (RPGs) and 1,470 noncompeting continuation RPGs (National Science Foundation, April, 1990, p. 27). NIMH alone made 1,149 RPGs in FY 1990, 404 new and competing continuation awards, and 745 noncompeting continuations (National Science Foundation, April, 1990, p. 27).

The *National Institutes of Health* (NIH) consists of various bureaus, institutes, and divisions. Obviously, each of the 13 NIH institutes is concerned primarily with understanding, diagnosis, treatment, control, and prevention of the diseases and disorders subsumed under its mission, such as cancer, diabetes, heart disease, or autism. However, there is inevitably some overlap in the specific research programs of the various NIH (and ADAMHA) institutes that are due to such factors as the potential relevance of basic research to several diseases and disorders, and the intricate interrelationships among biological, psychological, and social systems in the development of both normal and abnormal functioning. Those NIH institutes that support basic and clinical research relevant to mental health and behavior and health (behavioral medicine) are the National Institute on Aging (NIA), National Institute of Child Health and Human Development (NICHHD), National Institute of Neurological Disorders and Stroke (NINDS), National Heart, Lung, and Blood Institute (NHLBI), National Institute of General Medical Sciences (NIGMS), National Institute on Deafness and Other Communication Disorders (NIDOCD), National Cancer Institute (NCI), National Center for Human Genome Research (NCHGR), National Institute of Arthritis and Musculoskeletal and Skin diseases (NIAMSD), National Library of Medicine (NLM), and the Office of AIDS Research.

Funding for NIH in Fiscal Year 1990 was an estimated $7.140 billion, the largest amounts of which were earmarked for NCI and NHLBI, estimated at $1.592 billion and $1.023 billion, respectively (National Science Foundation, April, 1990, p. 24). In FY 1990, NIH funded a total of 20,316 research project grants (RPGs), 4,633 new and competing continuation RPGs, and 15,683 non-competing continuation RPGs (National Science Foundation, April, 1990, p. 23). In FY 1989, the average size of traditional research project (R01) grants made by NIH was $163,430, an average of $110,338 of which was for direct costs and $53,092 for indirect costs (National Institutes of Health, August, 1990, p. 21).

ADAMHA and NIH, both major components of the U.S. Public Health Service (PHS), provide various types of funding mechanisms and programs. For example, both ADAMHA and NIH support research training primarily through National Research Service Awards (NRSAs), such as the Institutional Training Grant (T32) Awards and Individual Fellowship Awards. The major purposes of the NRSAs are

> (1) to increase the number of individuals trained for research and teaching in specifically designated biomedical and behavioral areas, and (2) to improve the environment in which the biomedical and behavioral training is conducted. (Alcohol, Drug Abuse, and Mental Health Administration [no date], p. 5)

In FY 1991, stipends made available through the Predoctoral Individual Fellowship (F31) Awards are at the $8,800 per year level, while those for Postdoctoral Individual Fellowship (F32) Awards range from $18,600 to $32,300 per year, depending upon the number of years of postdoctoral research training experience (U.S. Department of Health and Human Services, January 4, 1991, p. 1).

Of particular interest to one who is just beginning his or her career as an independent investigator are the First Independent Research Support and Transition (FIRST) Awards and Small Grant Awards. The *FIRST* (R29) award "is intended to support the first independent investigative efforts of an individual and to provide the transition to traditional types of ADAMHA [or NIH] research project grants" (Alcohol, Drug Abuse, and Mental Health Administration [no date], p. 4). FIRST grants are available for a maximum of 5 years and are not renewable. The FIRST Awards Program was created specifically to assist new investigators. The underlying concept is that those just beginning an independent research career should compete for grants with their peers rather than established investigators. At present, FIRST awards are available through the three ADAMHA institutes and all NIH institutes except NINDS and NIDOCD.

All three ADAMHA institutes, and some NIH institutes, offer *Small Grant* (R03) awards. The ADAMHA Small Grant Program provides up to $50,000 per year for up to 2 years in support of

> research in any scientific area relevant to mental health or drug or alcohol abuse. While proposals may involve a wide variety of biomedical, biobehavioral, or clinical disciplines, relevance to the missions of the ADAMHA institutes must be clear. (U.S. Department of Health and Human Services, November 23, 1990, p. 8)

Priority is given to grant applications from new and "less experienced" investigators, investigators from institutions without a "well-developed research tradition" and adequate resources for research support, for "exploratory studies" proposed by experienced investigators who are changing the focus or direction of their research, and for testing new methods or techniques (U.S. Department of Health and Human Services, November 23, 1990, p. 7).

The most common vehicle for extramural research support provided by ADAMHA and NIH institutes is the "traditional" *Research Project* (R01) award. The research project grant is intended to support "a discrete project related to the investigator's interests and competence" (Alcohol, Drug Abuse, and Mental Health Administration [no date], p. 4). Because competition for R01 grants is considerable, the new investigator who has had little or no prior external research funding should consider applying for a FIRST award. Once the investigator receives an initial award and establishes a research record through publication, he or she is in a better position to compete successfully for an R01 or other federal grant.

A group of related projects, each under the direction of a principal investigator, may be supported by a *Program Project* (P01) grant. A program project grant is designed to support

> a broadly based, multidisciplinary, long-term research program with a particular major objective or theme. [It] involves the organized efforts of groups of investigators who conduct research projects related to the overall program objectives. The grant can also provide support for certain shared resources necessary for the total research effort. (Alcohol, Drug Abuse, and Mental Health Administration [no date], p. 4)

A *Center Grant* (P50) provides support for a center director and "group of collaborating investigators" to engage in a "multidisciplinary, long-term research program with a particular major objective or theme" (Alcohol, Drug Abuse, and Mental Health Administration [no date], p. 4). Such ADAMHA- and NIH-funded centers "are usually developed in response to . . . specific programmatic needs of an Institute" and, in addition to conducting research, "must also serve as regional or national resources for special research purposes" (p. 4).

In addition to the NRSAs, FIRST Awards, and Small Grants, there are other ADAMHA and NIH award mechanisms to enhance investigator competence. These include: the Research Scientist Development (K01) Awards (also called the Special Emphasis Research Career Awards, SERCA) which support scientists who are "committed to research [and] in need of both advanced research training and additional experience"; Research Career Development (K04) Awards, which are intended to "foster the development of young scientists with outstanding research potential for careers of independent research"; Individual Physician Scientist (K11) Awards, which support "newly trained clinicians" in the "development of independent research skills and experience in a fundamental science"; and Physician Scientist (K12) Awards (Program), which support "newly trained clinicians" in the "development of independent research skills and experience in a fundamental science within the framework of an interdisciplinary research and development program" (National Institutes of Health, October, 1990, p. v.).

Another PHS agency that funds research relevant to psychiatry is the

Centers for Disease Control (CDC), whose component subunits and programs sponsor research in epidemiology, international health, chronic disease prevention, health promotion, occupational safety and health, and other areas.

The *National Science Foundation* (NSF) funds research in the physical sciences, life sciences, social sciences, mathematics, and engineering/technology. The components of NSF that support programs relevant to psychiatry are the Directorate for Biological, Behavioral, and Social Sciences, which has programs in cellular biosciences, molecular biosciences, and behavioral and neural sciences, and the Directorate for Computer and Information Science and Engineering, which has programs in intelligent systems and in networking and communications. It is important to note that NSF funds basic research and projects to develop new technologies; it does not fund research focused on health or clinical issues.

NSF provides traditional research awards, research and development (R&D) center awards, and small grant awards. Of particular note is NSF's Small Grants for Exploratory Research (SGER) Program, which

> funds small-scale exploratory work in all fields of science, engineering, and education . . . through brief proposals without the usual external review. Such work includes preliminary research on untested and novel ideas; ventures into emerging research areas; research requiring urgent access to specialized data, facilities, or equipment; or similar exploratory efforts likely to catalyze innovative advances. (National Science Foundation [no date], p. 97)

SGER awards are for up to $50,000 and usually are for 1 year.

In FY 1990, NSF's budget was about $2.499 billion. Of that sum, an estimated $292 million were allocated to the Directorate for Biological, Behavioral, and Social Sciences, and $154 million to the Directorate for Computer and Information Science and Engineering (National Science Foundation, April, 1990, p. 48).

The U.S. *Department of Education* is another major source of support for research in several areas relevant to mental health. Research areas of interest to the department include developmental disabilities and abnormal mental development, learning disabilities, autism, and rehabilitation of persons with cognitive impairments.

Three agencies of the *Department of Defense* (DoD) also provide funding programs relevant to psychiatry. These are: the U.S. Army Medical Research & Development Command, which funds research on combat stress and human factors in the performance of weapons systems; the Office of Naval Research (ONR), which funds research in such areas as artificial intelligence, neuroscience, perception, and behavioral immunology; and the Air Force Office of Scientific Research, which supports research in such areas as visual perception, chronobiology, learning, and cognition.

The *Veterans Health Services and Research Administration*, a part of the Department of Veterans Affairs, does not provide extramural research support to investigators outside the Veterans Administration (VA) system. However, through its many VA Hospitals, it provides facilities, staff, and patient populations that are used as resources by extramural investigators, and it supports intramural research relevant to psychiatry, psychology, and other mental health-relevant disciplines.

Philanthropic Foundations

The 1991 edition of the *Foundation Directory* (Olson, 1990) lists 6,264 independent philanthropic foundations in the United States. In the course of a year, these foundations gave nearly $5.246 billion in the form of grants, fellowships, and other aid (Olson, 1990, Table 1, p. vi). Some of these philanthropic foundations support research in psychiatry and related fields. For example: The John D. and Catherine T. MacArthur Foundation funds research on the psychobiology of depression and other affective disorders, the transition from infancy to early childhood, protective factors in mental disorders, conscious and unconscious mental processes, psychological markers in aging, adolescent development, and mental health law. In 1988 (the latest year for which data are available), the MacArthur Foundation awarded 12 grants in the mental health area; these ranged in size from $20,000 to $3.2 million (Jones, 1990, p. 78). The van Ameringen Foundation supports mental health research and service delivery, except in the areas of mental retardation, alcoholism, and drug abuse. In 1989, the van Ameringen Foundation awarded 13 grants in the mental health field ranging from $20,000 to $250,734 (Jones, 1990, p. 459). The William T. Grant Foundation supports "research projects aimed at improving the mental health of children, adolescents, and youth, with emphasis on enhancing normal development" (W. T. Grant Foundation, January 1990, inside front cover). In 1989, the W. T. Grant Foundation had 113 active research grants of which 30 were awarded in that year (W. T. Grant Foundation [no date], p. 10). These are but three examples of the many philanthropic foundations—large, medium-sized, and small—that fund research and service delivery in psychiatry and related fields.

Private-Sector Firms and Corporation Foundations

Many corporations and corporate foundations fund research relevant to psychiatry. The 1991 edition of the *Foundation Directory* lists 946 corporate foundations in the United States. In the course of a year, these corporate foundations gave more than $1.3 billion in the form of grants, matching gifts, and other aid (Olson, 1990, Table 1, p. vi). Not surprisingly, much of the grant and contract funding from corporate and corporate foundation sources is oriented to the products or "business lines" of the sponsoring firms. Therefore, pharmaceutical firms that produce psychotropic drugs, antidepressants, or anxiolytics, for example, are potential sources of funding for psychopharmacological research. It is important to note, however, that pharmaceutical houses maintain their own intramural research and development capabilities.

The vast majority of research funding they make available to outside investigators is for clinical trials or is in the form of research fellowships.

Professional Societies

Some professional societies, such as the American Psychiatric Association, American Medical Association, and American Psychological Association, provide relatively small amounts of funds for research support, often in the form of fellowships, travel awards, and research prizes.

Voluntary Organizations and Associations

There are various voluntary organizations and associations that fund research in psychiatry and mental health. For example, the Alzheimer's Disease and Related Disorders Association (ADRDA, also known as the Alzheimer's Association) has three external funding programs: Investigator-Initiated Research Grants; Faculty Scholar Awards; and Pilot Research Grants. Investigator-Initiated Research Grants support "biological, clinical, and social/behavioral research relevant to degenerative brain diseases such as Alzheimer's Disease." Faculty Scholar Awards "provide sustained salary support" for junior-level investigators "who are committed to research relevant to Alzheimer's Disease and related disorders . . . [and] have at least two years' post-graduate experience" (Alzheimer's Association [no date]). The Pilot Research Grants program is discussed below under the heading "Seed Funding."

The National Alliance for Research on Schizophrenia and Depression (NARSAD), and the Scottish Rite of Freemasonry for the Northern Masonic Jurisdiction, U.S.A., which sponsors the Scottish Rite Schizophrenia Research Program, are also examples of voluntary associations that support psychiatric and mental health research.

Other Sources

Other sources of research funding include various agencies of state government, local and regional foundations, and state and local chapters of voluntary agencies, associations, and professional societies.

Funding Information Resources

There are a number of sources of information on funding agencies and programs. These include, for example, *ADAMHA Funding Mechanisms for Research Grants & Awards*, *NIH Extramural Programs: Funding for Research and Research Training*, *Annual Register of Grant Support: A Director of Funding Sources*, *Directory of Biomedical and Health Care Grants*, and *Directory of Research Grants*. These and other funding source information resources are listed by agency type in the Appendix to this chapter.

PROJECT DEVELOPMENT

Before seeking funds for a particular project, one must develop the research plan in some detail. Once the study has been designed and, perhaps, "piloted," appropriate sources of potential support are identified and guidelines for proposal preparation are obtained. The request for funding is then made, in accordance with the guidelines, in the form of a proposal, which may be only a brief letter, an expanded "concept paper," a somewhat larger document, or a document of considerable size (several hundred pages), depending on the scope of the effort and funding agency requirements. Thus, there are several steps in project development, which include developing a concept paper, acquiring resources, and assessing feasibility through a pilot project. These steps are discussed next.

The Concept Paper

After one conceives a possible research project, the next step is to produce a concept paper that concisely describes the incipient project. The concept paper may consist of only a paragraph or two, and certainly should not exceed a page or two in length. At minimum it should briefly (1) introduce the research problem(s) to be investigated; (2) outline the purpose, goals, objectives, or specific aims of the project; (3) describe in summary fashion the subjects or materials, any instruments, and methods to be employed; (4) list the expected results, products, or outcomes; and (5) state the significance of the proposed research.

Writing a concept paper aids in clarifying one's ideas. It should serve as the base upon which to construct a proposal for external funding and any other documents describing the project, such as a letter soliciting the interest of a potential sponsor, a letter of intent to submit a proposal, or a proposal to acquire seed funding.

Assessing Feasibility

The next step is to determine, as objectively as possible, whether the project is "doable." This may be done by studying the relevant literature and consulting appropriate others, such as mentors and colleagues. For hands-on objective evaluation of feasibility, one should conduct a pilot or feasibility study.

Seed Funding

Seed funding may be obtained to support, for example, a pilot project, needs assessment, or feasibility study; project planning and development; development or modification of instruments, methods, or techniques; and development and/or preparation of a proposal for external funding. There are various sources of seed funding, including internal sources, such as a "research development fund" maintained by a university, academic department, or research center, and external sources, such as federal agencies, philanthropic foundations, and private-sector firms and corporate foundations.

Many research-oriented universities and other institutions have seed funding programs. One of the advantages of such programs is that proposal review is done locally and turn-around time is relatively short. The University of Pittsburgh, for example, has seed funding programs administered by its Clinical Research Center on Affective Disorders, Center for Neuroscience and Schizophrenia, Adolescent Alcohol Abuse Clinical Research Center, Suicide Clinical Research Center, and Alzheimer's Disease Research Center. The Center for Neuroscience and Schizophrenia, for instance, has a Seed Monies Program that supports "pilot research and encourages the development of innovative research that bridges basic neuroscience concepts and methods with those in clinical and cognitive sciences relevant to the study of schizophrenia" (University of Pittsburgh, 1991, flyer). Those eligible to apply are "postdoctoral fellows (M.D. or Ph.D.) and junior faculty whose interests span both laboratory and clinical sciences" (flyer). Awards are made for up to 1 year, range from $5,000 to $12,000, and are not renewable. Awardees "are encouraged to seek [continuing] support for [the] research through traditional avenues such as NIMH research awards" (flyer). Similarly, the Brain Research Foundation at the University of Chicago's Brain Research Institute has a Seed Grants Program that provides seed funding support for research on methods to "combat the devastating effects of neurological and brain-related disorders."

Among the external sources of seed funding are the three ADAMHA institutes, and some NIH institutes, which offer Small Grant (R03) awards. The ADAMHA Small Grant Program provides up to $50,000 per year for up to 2 years to support "research in any scientific area relevant to mental health or drug or alcohol abuse" (see pp. 15–16 above) (U.S. Department of Health and Human Services, November 23, 1990, p. 8). The Alzheimer's Disease and Related Disorders Association's Pilot Research Grants program

> provide[s] small, one-year grants for worthwhile research proposals, with preference given to investigators new to research into Alzheimer's Disease and related disorders. The objectives of the program are (1) to stimulate interest by new investigators, (2) to enable new and established investigators to test the feasibility of new ideas on a small scale, (3) to enable investigators to generate pilot data to support proposals to NIH, foundations, or the Alzheimer's Association for larger grants. (Alzheimer's Association [no date], flyer)

PROPOSAL DEVELOPMENT

Proposal development is a very labor-intensive and time-consuming process. In most cases, the process requires a minimum of 3 to 6 months, sometimes it requires many more months beyond the minimum, and preliminary work leading up to the proposal may extend back several years.

Types of Proposals

The first time a proposal for external funding is submitted to a funding agency, it is considered to be a "new" proposal by that agency. After an initial award is made, a proposal to fund continuation of a multiyear project or program is a "continuation" proposal, either a "noncompeting" or a "competing" continuation ("renewal") proposal. If, after an award is made, it is found that additional funding is necessary to meet an unanticipated need or unexpected opportunity, a "supplemental" proposal may be submitted. In addition, a proposal may be either "solicited" or "unsolicited" by the funding agency. An *unsolicited proposal* is initiated by the investigator and submitted under an established external funding program, such as those described in *NIH Extramural Programs*, the *NIH Guide for Grants and Contracts*, NSF's *Guide to Programs*, or the *Foundation Directory*. A *solicited proposal*, on the other hand, is submitted in response to a request for proposals (RFP), bid solicitation, or request for applications (RFA), the availability of which is advertised in a publication, such as the *NIH Guide for Grants and Contracts* or *Commerce Business Daily*.

Types of Awards

Grants, contracts, and cooperative agreements are the three primary types of award instruments. A *grant* (i.e., grant in aid) is made to support a project or program undertaken for a specific purpose other than the production and delivery of a specified product or service *per se*. A *contract* is an agreement to procure a product or service as specified by the funding agency. A *cooperative agreement* is similar to a grant, but it provides for substantial scientific and technical involvement of the funding agency in the actual conduct or direction of the research. A grant, contract, or cooperative agreement may include one or more subcontracts. A *subcontract* is a contract for work to be performed at institutions other than that of the principal investigator and is administered by the primary grant or contract awardee (the "prime contractor") rather than the funding source agency.

Another way in which to classify sponsored project awards is by purpose. Among the many purposes for which support may be obtained are: *research*, which may be basic, clinical, applied, or developmental; *instruction*, such as curriculum development or the provision of instruction; *service*, such as the delivery of health care services and service demonstrations; *evaluation* of projects, programs, goods, or services; *scholarships* and *fellowships*; *resource development*; *career development*; and *capital*—for the purchase of equipment or the construction, expansion, or renovation of facilities.

The Preliminary (Pre-)Proposal

A preliminary proposal (often called a preproposal) is, in essence, an expanded and refined concept paper (see p. 21 above). In addition to the elements of the concept paper, a preproposal should include a brief indication of how the project will be administered and an estimated budget.

The funding agency or program may require a preliminary proposal; contingent upon the agency's evaluation of the preproposal, it may then request that a full proposal be submitted. Even if a preproposal is not required, it may be useful for review by mentors and colleagues and then, if feasible, by the program officer.[1] The feedback generated thereby can be useful in preparing a full proposal.

Prerequisites for Proposal Writing

Proposal writing is similar to other types of scientific writing, such as a research paper or dissertation (see Table 1). Thus, before the actual writing is begun, one should be prepared with the concept paper, preproposal (if any), proposal preparation guidelines (see below), literature review, results of any pilot studies, needs assessments and/or feasibility studies, and the instruments, methods, or techniques to be employed. Also, it may be instructive to study and use as models successful proposals written by mentors or colleagues that had been funded by the same funding agency to which one plans to submit.

Proposal Preparation Guidelines and Outlines

Proposal preparation guidelines are usually available from ADAMHA, NIH, and NSF, other federal or state government agencies, and most large and medium-sized philanthropic and corporate foundations. The guidelines should be followed to the letter; proposals that do not conform to the guidelines are normally returned to their authors without further review.

Organization is the key to good writing and makes writing and reading so much easier. Therefore, one should develop and use an outline based on the best available guidelines. In the absence of funding agency guidelines, the outline format shown in Table 1 may be used.[2]

Proposals Submitted on Grant Application Form PHS 398

The PHS 398 application kit is used for all new, competing continuation, and supplemental applications for nearly all types of ADAMHA and NIH awards, including Research Project (R01), Small Grant (R01), FIRST (R29), Program Project (P01), Research Scientist Development (K01), Research Career

---

[1]The program officer is the funding agency staff member who is assigned to receive proposals in a given topic area or for a particular funding program and usually administers the awards made. This individual may participate in the initial review to screen out proposals which clearly do not meet specific program guidelines.

[2]At minimum, with or without agency guidelines, it is suggested that the outline format in Table 1 be used as a checklist to make certain that all essential and desired elements of the proposal are included.

Table 1. Basic Format and Elements of a Resarch Proposal[a]

   I. Title/Signature Page (Cover Sheet)
  II. Abstract (or Executive Summary)
 III. Table of Contents (and Table of Figures and List of Tables)
  IV. Introduction (or Background, or Background and Introduction)
   V. The Problem
      A. Statement of the Problem
      B. Variables
      C. Hypotheses
  VI. Project Goals (and/or Project Objectives, or Purpose or Specific Aims)
 VII. Review of the Literature
VIII. Methods (or Plan, or Plan of Procedure, or Subjects, Methods and Instruments, or Materials
      and Methods)
      [Note that this section may also include data analysis methods, thereby eliminating the need
      for IX. Data Analysis, below.]

IX. Data Analysis (Plan of Analysis)	IX. (Analysis and) Results
X. (Expected Results or Expected Outcomes)	X. Discussion
XI. Significance (and/or Utility and/or Impact)	XI. Conclusion(s)
XII. Resources Available	XII. (Significance)
XIII. (Organization and Administration)	XIII. (Recommendation(s))
XIV. Personnel	
XV. Schedule of Activities (and/or Timetable or Milestone Chart)	
XVI. References	XIV. References
XVII. Budget	
XVIII. Budget Justification	
XIX. (Appendices)	XV. (Appendices)

[a]This is a suggested outline which may be modified. For example, you may want to combine two or more sections (e.g., X. Expected Results/Outcomes and XI. Significance), or you may decide to delete one or more sections.

Those elements listed on the right-hand side of the table below the rule are used in place of those elements listed on the left-hand side when writing a report on the project, or an article, thesis, or dissertation about the project.

Items in parentheses are alternative section headings or optional items to be included only when appropriate.
Note. From A Proposal Writer's Guide by A. K. DeRoy, November, 1990, Pittsburgh: University of Pittsburgh, Office of Research. Copyright 1990 by Al K. DeRoy and University of Pittsburgh. Reprinted by permission.

Development (K04), Clinical Investigator (K08), and Physician Scientist (K11 and K12) awards.[3]

Section 1

The application begins with forms for the cover sheet, abstract, list of key personnel, table of contents, first-year budget, and summary budget. Instructions for completing these forms should be followed to the letter. Assistance

[3]Other PHS application forms include the PHS 2590, which is used for noncompeting continuations of awards for which the original application was made using the PHS 398; the PHS 416-1, sued for new and competing continuations of Individual National Research Service Awards; and the PHS 416-9, used for noncompeting continuations of Individual National Research Service Awards.

with these forms should be available from the administrator of your department, program, unit or laboratory, or your institution's sponsored projects office, budget office, comptroller's office, or other administrative office.

Description

In the PHS 398, the proposal abstract is called the "Description." Whatever it is called—description, abstract, or executive summary—it is one of the most important parts of the proposal, for it is used in preliminary screening and assignment to a peer review committee, and, at times, it is the only portion of the proposal that is read by some reviewers.

In essence, the Description should give the reviewer the highlights of the proposal so as to facilitate and guide the review. As per the PHS 398 instructions, the Description should present "the application's broad, long-term objectives and specific aims, making reference to the health relatedness of the project." It should "[d]escribe concisely the experimental design and methods for achieving goals. . . . [It] is meant to serve as a succinct and accurate description of the proposed work when separated from the application."

Section 2

This section constitutes the project description. Note that PHS 398 applications have page limitations that are *strictly* enforced (with the exceptions noted in the Specific Instructions for Section 2). Make certain to adhere to both the General Instructions and the Specific Instructions for Section 2. As per the Specific Instructions,

> include sufficient information . . . to facilitate effective review without reference to any previous application. Be specific and informative and avoid redundancies. Reviewers often consider brevity and clarify in the presentation to be indicative of a principal investigator's . . . focused approach to a research objective and ability to achieve the specific aims of the project.

The major components of the project description are discussed briefly below.

Introduction

The first portion of the narrative, in revised and supplemental applications *only*, is a one-page introduction. For a revised application, "any substantial additions, deletions, and changes" to the original application should be summarized here. (Note, too, that these changes should be highlighted in the succeeding text "by appropriate bracketing, indenting, or changing of typography.") In a supplemental application, present in summary fashion the major ways in which the supplemental award will alter, amplify, or supplement the original project.

Research Plan

The Research Plan is the heart of the proposal. It consists of nine subsections (A to I), the first four of which must not exceed 20 total pages in length, including any tables or figures. Subsections A through F are discussed below.[4]

In Table 2 are listed sections of the Research Plan as presented and enumerated in the PHS 398 application kit along with comparable sections of the Research Proposal format shown in Table 1. Comparing the two formats may be helpful in developing a proposal to ADAMHA or NIH.

Subsection A. Specific Aims

Specific aims are statements of specific intent that, when taken together, "describe concisely and realistically what the [project] is intended to accomplish and any hypotheses to be tested." It is recommended that this subsection not exceed one page in length. The format used may be a list, narrative, or combination of the two. After stating the specific aims, state the research hypotheses.

In writing specific aims, it may be helpful to begin each with "to" followed by an active verb, such as "identify," "observe," "measure," "compare," "isolate," "characterize." Clarity and conciseness of the study's aims are crucial to understanding and evaluating the relevance and soundness of subsequent components of the proposal.

Subsection B. Background and Significance

The Background and Significance subsection should contain the following elements: a capsule history of the project's development; a review of the pertinent literature cast in the "critical mode"; brief discussion of gaps in existing knowledge that the proposed project will address; the potential significance of the project in relation to its "broad, long-term objectives." In essence, the theoretical and/or clinical rationale and justification for the proposed project is provided here. It is recommended that this subsection be no more than two to three pages in length.

Subsection C. Progress Report

A Progress Report is required for competing continuation and supplemental applications. It presents the progress made "since the project was last reviewed competitively." The elements to be included in this subsection are listed in the Specific Instructions for Section 2.

---

[4]Subsection G pertains to Consultants/Collaborators, subsection H to Consortium/Contractual Arrangements, and subsection I to Literature Cited.

Table 2.   Parallels between the Research Plan in Application for Public Health Service Grant, Grant Application Form PHS 398 and Table 1

Section of the Research Plan in the PHS 398 kit (U.S. Public Health Service: Rev. 10/88)	Section(s) of the Research Proposal format in Table 1
Elements of:	
A. Specific Aims	V. The Problem
	VI. Goals
B. Background and Significance	IV. Background
	VII. Review of the Literature
	XI. Significance
C. Progress Report (only in competing continuation and supplemental applications)	IV. Background
C. Preliminary Studies (optional; only in new applications)	IV. Background
D. Experimental Design and Methods	VIII. Methods (Subjects, Methods and Instruments/Materials and Methods)
	IX. Data analysis
	XV. Schedule of Activities (Timetable)
E. Human Subjects	VIII. Methods (Subjects, Methods and Instruments/Materials and Methods)
F. Vertebrate Animals	VIII. Methods (Subjects, Methods and Instruments/Materials and Methods)
G. Consultants/Collaborators	
H. Consortium/Contractual Arrangements	
I. Literature Cited	XVI. References

Subsection C. Preliminary Studies

This subsection is included *only* in new applications; it is considered to be "useful but optional." In addition to reporting any relevant preliminary work, the information provided should "help to establish the experience and competence of the investigator to pursue the proposed project."

Subsection D. Experimental Design and Methods

The elements to be included in this subsection are listed in the Specific Instructions for Section 2.

Subsection E. Human Subjects

This subsection is included *only* if human subjects will be used. Remember that use of human subjects requires specific protocols and detailed informed consent mechanisms for submission to the appropriate Institutional Review Board for clearance. The elements to be included in this subsection are listed in the Specific Instructions for Section 2.

Subsection F. Vertebrate Animals

This subsection is included *only* if vertebrate animals will be used. The use of vertebrate animals requires clearance from the Institutional Animal Care and Use Committee. The elements to be included in this subsection are listed in the Specific Instructions for Section 2.

Appendix

The Appendix may be used to contain one or more of the following types of items: in new applications, copies of publications pertinent to the background or substance of the proposal; in competing continuation and supplemental applications, copies of any publications resulting from the project to date; highly detailed or otherwise lengthy descriptions of methods, instruments, or materials to be employed in the proposed research; any other relevant materials, such as supplementary graphs, diagrams, tables or charts, and letters of support.

SOME ADVICE ON WRITING PROPOSALS

There are important things to know about proposal writing that typically are not contained in guidelines for proposal preparation and often are learned with experience. Such frequently unrecognized but important ingredients of writing a successful proposal include: addressing explicitly salient program goals of the funding agency and proposal review criteria; getting input from the program officer; working within institutional constraints, working within time constraints; obtaining feedback on the proposal; and clarity of the written presentation.

Characteristics and Goals of the Funding Agency and Proposal Review Criteria

It is important to be knowledgeable about the funding agency and the program to which the proposal will be submitted, including the agency's structure, programmatic interests and priorities, and review criteria and procedures, as well as the research background and interests of the program officer, review committee members, and the review committee's scientific review administrator. Such information may be found in publications of the funding agency (such as program guides, annual reports), for ADAMHA agencies in *ADAMHA Public Advisory Committees* (Alcohol, Drug Abuse, and Mental Health Administration, March, 1990), for NIH in *NIH Advisory Committees* (National Institutes of Health, October, 1990), and for foundations and associations in funding source directories (such as those listed in the Appendix). The program officer, of course, can serve as an excellent source of current and pertinent information about a particular funding program's scope of interest, funding priorities, and review and funding criteria and procedures.

Guidance from the Program Officer

If possible, the program officer should be consulted early in the process when developing the initial concept into a viable project and successful proposal. One could, for example, solicit the program officer's comments on the concept paper, preproposal, or letter of intent. Try to obtain as much relevant information as you can from the program officer, but do not press him or her. Most officers will answer your questions with as much candor as their responsibilities and agencies permit, suggest points to emphasize and those to de-emphasize, help to clarify program/agency interests and priorities, and provide information concerning proposal review criteria and procedures. It may be desirable to have face-to-face meetings with the program officer well before the time the proposal is to be submitted.

Working within Institutional Constraints

Each institution has established policies and procedures that govern proposal preparation and submission. Thus, early on, inform your supervisor (department chairperson, or program, division, or laboratory director) and, if required or beneficial, whoever coordinates the submission of external applications for your institution or organizational unit, about your intention to submit a proposal, its topic, and resources needed for the proposed project. This will help assure that institutional requirements will be met, that any assistance needed in project and proposal development will be provided, and that resources, such as laboratory facilities or patients, will be available.

Working within Time Constraints

As deadlines permit, it is advisable to plan sufficient lead-time to review pertinent literature; conduct a pilot project, needs assessment, or feasibility study; identify, develop, and/or refine instruments, methods, or techniques; write and revise the concept paper, preproposal, full proposal, and other documents; obtain required approvals for the use of human or animal subjects,[5] hazardous materials, or recombinant DNA;[6] have presubmission review of the budget, clearances, and other required forms. Normally, presubmission on review is carried out by grants and contracts officers in your institution's

---

[5]Written clearance for the use of human subjects should be obtained from the appropriate Institutional (Human Subjects) Review Board (IRB) and for use of animal subjects from the Institutional Animal Care and Use Committee (IACUC). These bodies are mandated for institutions that receive federal funding to support research in the psychological, medical, or biological sciences.
[6]Written clearance for the use of hazardous materials and, in some cases, recombinant DNA must be obtained from the appropriate institutional review committee, such as the Institutional Biosafety Committee (IBC).

sponsored projects office and is the last thing done prior to proposal submission. Institutional review can be expedited by going over the budget and required forms with a grants and contracts officer a week or so before the time of submission. Try to allow two working days for the final presubmission review.

Obtaining Feedback on the Proposal

As feasible, it is recommended that you have a presubmission review and critique of a near-final draft of the proposal done by mentors or colleagues (especially those successful with the funding agency), a proposal development specialist, and/or the program officer. Comments and suggestions based on such a review can be invaluable.

It should be noted again that in developing a project, program, or proposal, one should solicit the comments of others, such as the program officer, mentor, and colleagues. However, the beginning investigator should not be intimidated by such feedback. If advice just does not "feel right" or make sense, do not change the focus or nature of your project or proposal in response to that advice. After all, it is your research interests and goals that count, and ultimately you are the one responsible for them.

Clarity of the Written Presentation

Write concisely, in plain English, and avoid the use of jargon. It is very important to pitch the presentation to the reviewers' level of knowledge and comprehension; that is, the proposal should be understood easily by individuals who may not be experts in the specific area of the research, but who are sufficiently knowledgeable in related scientific areas to be reasonably able to evaluate the proposal. Use of highly technical or specialized language is appropriate only if you know for certain that *all* the reviewers are expert in the subject matter(s) discussed in the proposal, which is often not the case.[7] Where highly technical terms are used, it is best to follow the standard practice (i.e., define them where they are first introduced and thereafter as may be necessary or appropriate).

CONCURRENT SUBMISSIONS AND RESUBMISSIONS

Concurrent Submissions

There are two types of concurrent submissions: submission of the "same" proposal to different funding agencies, and submission of proposals pertaining

---

[7] As indicated earlier, information on the membership of ADAMHA peer review groups is to be found in *ADAMHA Public Advisory Committees* and on NIH peer review groups in *NIH Advisory Committees*, available from ADAMHA and NIH, respectively. In many small and medium-sized foundations, proposals are often reviewed by educated laypersons, many of whom may have limited expertise in your area of research.

to different pieces of a project to different agencies. Remember to alter the proposal, or piece, to conform to the guidelines and requirements of the funding source agency and program to which it will be submitted.

Portions of a proposal may be submitted concurrently to different agencies; for example, funding for the laboratory research phase of a project may be requested of one funding source agency, while funding for the clinical research phase may be requested of another.

It is acceptable to submit substantially the same proposal to different agencies concurrently, if none of the agencies involved prohibit it. There are two basic rules in concurrent submission; (1) inform those agencies of the concurrent submission if required to do so; (2) once funding is received from one agency, the others *must be informed as soon as possible* to avoid unnecessary duplication of effort and illegal duplication of funding.

Resubmissions

Initial proposals from beginning investigators may not always be funded after the first submission or resubmission. Even established investigators have proposals rejected. Rejected or unfunded proposals could be, and often are, resubmitted to either the same or a different funding agency or program. In either case, revise the original proposal as necessary and appropriate, incorporating relevant feedback from any written critique, such as the NIH "application review summary statements," mentors and colleagues, the program officer, or others knowledgeable about proposal development. Realism and persistence pay off!

PROPOSAL REVIEW, FUNDING, AND PROGRESS REPORTS

As indicated above, the primary sources of support for research relevant to psychiatry, psychology, and other mental health-relevant disciplines are several components of the U.S. Public Health Service, the National Science Foundation, U.S. Department of Education, and other public, private, voluntary, and philanthropic organizations. In discussing the review, funding, and reporting processes, we focus on those practices and policies that prevail at ADAMHA and NIH. These processes are, in principle, also applicable to the National Science Foundation and other government agencies and, to a lesser extent, to foundations and other nongovernmental funding sources.

Proposal Review

As mentioned earlier, before a proposal is submitted, it must undergo internal institutional review to assure that the proposal conforms to both the institution's and sponsor's policies and that the budget is appropriate and uses the correct rates for fringe benefits, indirect costs, and so forth. Some institutions also require internal review for content, feasibility, and/or significance.

The PHS has three review and funding cycles per year, each with a specific deadline as shown in Table 3. Each cycle begins with an application receipt deadline date, then there is an administrative review, an initial scientific review by a committee of peers, and a second substantive review by a National Advisory Council or Board.

It is critical that a proposal be submitted by the appropriate deadline date. Proposals are usually sent to a central receipt point specified by the funding agency. For all PHS agencies, this is the Division of Research Grants at the National Institutes of Health in Bethesda, Maryland. Once an application is received, it is checked for completeness and compliance with policy and formal administrative guidelines for the type of support requested, including the proposal's format and length, the duration and level of support requested, and status of Institutional Review Board or Institutional Animal Care and Use Committee clearance for the protection of human or animal subjects, respectively. Applications that meet all administrative guidelines and criteria are then assigned by a "referral officer" to an Initial Review Group (IRG) or Study Section for scientific peer review and to a "program unit" for possible eventual funding. It should be noted that for all PHS agencies, the offices and administrators responsible for scientific review of proposals conduct their activities independent of the activities of the offices and staff responsible for program development, funding, and post-award monitoring.

Funding agencies typically organize and maintain review committees, each having expertise and responsibility for evaluating research applications in certain areas of basic, clinical, or applied science relevant to the funding program's mission. Scientists who are actually doing research in these areas are selected to serve on such review committees, typically for a term of 4 years. ADAMHA and NIH review committees normally consist of 12 individuals representing different but relevant research areas. For federal agencies, peer review committee memberships and the areas of research they encompass are a matter of public record and are generally available on request (e.g., see *ADAMHA Public Advisory Committees* and *NIH Review Committees*).

Following receipt of an application by the scientific review administrator of the designated review committee, it is assigned to several of its most appropriate members, who then serve as the primary reviewers. Sometimes the reviewers request information in addition to that provided in the proposal; such additional information is obtained either by the scientific review administrator corresponding with the applicant or through a "site visit" to the applicant and applicant institution. Each proposal is first evaluated by the primary reviewers and then discussed by the full membership of the committee, following which a vote is taken to approve the application, disapprove it, or defer final consideration. If an application is approved, each member privately assigns a score ranging from one to five to reflect the level of scientific merit—the lower the score, the greater the scientific merit. The scientific review administrator then sums the individual scores and converts the result to a priority score that ranges from 100 to 500. As an additional effort at fairness, ADAMHA and NIH institutes use percentile

Table 3. Receipt, Review, and Earliest Funding Dates for Grant Applications to the National Institutes of Health and the Alcohol, Drug Abuse, and Mental Health Administration

Application receipt dates[a]	Initial Review Group dates	National Advisory Council or Board dates	Earliest possible beginning dates
February 1 June 1 October 1	March 1 July 1 November 1	September–October January–February May–June	December 1 April 1 July 1
All new RCDA[c] and research grant applications	Competing continuation, supplemental, and revised research grant and RCDA applications		
All[b] Program Project and Center grant applications			
For all[b] National Research Service Award applications	June–July October–November February–March		
January 10 May 10 September 10			

[a]Unless specified differently in additional instructions, a program announcement, or a request for applications.

[b]Includes new, competing continuation, supplemental, and revised applications.

[c]RCDA = Research Career Development Award.

Note. Unsolicited AIDS applications submitted for expedited review will continue to be received on January 2, May 1, and September 1, including revised applications (NIH Guide, Vol. 17, No. 14, April 15, 1988).

scores to reflect the relative position of an application in the pool of applications recently approved by the same review committees.

After this first level of review, all proposals are sent to a National Advisory Council or Board, which reviews them for conformance with policy and relevance to the mission of the institute. The council or board has the legal power to authorize the awarding of funds for extramural projects and programs. With rare exceptions that are agreed upon in advance, an award cannot be made by a federal agency without prior authorization of the appropriate council or board.

After this two-level review that is typical in PHS agencies, the program staff make the final decision to award the approved funds based on scientific merit (as reflected in the proposal's priority and percentile scores), program priorities, and availability of funds. Each competing application is considered in relation to all other competing applications assigned to a particular program, branch, or division in a particular funding cycle. Thus, for example, applications to NIMH to support research in schizophrenia compete with all others assigned to the Schizophrenia Research Branch in a particular cycle.

Approved applications that are not funded during the cycle in which they were reviewed may be reconsidered in competition with others reviewed subsequently for up to three successive cycles. Reviewers' comments on each application are summarized and sent to the principal investigator in a Summary Statement (the application review summary statements). The principal investigator may then revise the application in view of the critique presented in the Summary Statement and, perhaps, the comments of other colleagues, and then submit it in the next cycle for reconsideration.

Funding and Progress Reports

Awards may be made for periods of up to 5 years, but the actual funds are awarded on a year-to-year basis. At the end of each budget period, the principal investigator is required to submit a progress report, including a financial accounting to the funding agency. The progress report serves as both a vehicle to assure accountability and a means to justify continued funding. The report is usually brief but comprehensive, highlighting the scientific and technical progress made toward accomplishing the project's specific aims and also any shifts in the project's aims, methods, focus or direction since the project was begun or since the period covered in the previous progress report. It also presents and justifies any proposed alterations in the original research plan. For PHS funding agencies, the progress report is incorporated into a continuation application (as defined earlier) along with a budget for the continuation year. If the proposal is a noncompeting continuation proposal, it is reviewed by the program officer and other staff of the bureau, institute, or division to determine if the project should be continued , and if so, at what level of funding for the specified budget period. If the proposal is a competing continuation ("renewal") proposal, then it is reviewed and processed through the two-level review system described earlier.

Given what is said above, it must be recognized that the review and funding processes used and procedures followed by organizations, such as ADAMHA, NIH, and large philanthropic foundations, represent a genuine attempt to provide fair, competent, well-considered, and unbiased proposal review and funding decisions. These processes and procedures require significant investments of time, attention, and expertise on the parts of agency personnel and reviewers.

RESPONSIBILITIES OF PRINCIPAL INVESTIGATORS AND ADMINISTERING INSTITUTIONS

Grant awards are normally made to institutions on behalf of individual investigators. As a result, both awardee institutions and individual principal investigators have responsibilities for administration and both are accountable to the funding agency. More specifically, the institution is responsible for administrating the grant, including monitoring the project's budget and providing timely and accurate accounting reports to the principal investigator and funding agency, and for representing the project and principal investigator to the funding agency in all administrative and fiscal matters. The institution is expected to provide a proper environment for the conduct of research, and to encourage and facilitate research, by providing and maintaining the requisite physical resources, such as libraries, laboratory facilities and office space, and by maintaining an appropriate intellectual climate—one of openness, cooperation, and free inquiry, and a climate in which doing research is rewarded.

Of course, the institution must abide by all applicable laws and regulations. In the present context this involves, for example, establishing and following procedures to handle allegations of fraud or misconduct, maintaining proper fiscal controls, and operating an Institutional Review Board for the protection of human subjects, an Institutional Animal Care and Use Committee for the protection of animal subjects, and an Institutional Biosafety Committee to minimize research risks to the investigator and others. The institution is also responsible for the proper disposition of equipment and making a final financial report to the funding agency following expiration of an award.

The principal investigator is responsible for the scientific substance and conduct of the project, which normally means coordinating and/or overseeing the work of others, such as any co-investigators, research assistants, technicians, and secretarial and clerical personnel, submitting progress and other reports as required and, overall, fulfilling the terms of the award. In addition, the investigator oversees and participates in the implementation of the approved research plan, protection of human or animal subjects, management of the project budget, and the obtaining of necessary clearances and approvals. The principal investigator must, of course, abide by all applicable laws and regulations, and maintain a high standard of ethical conduct; these strictures may entail, for example, assuring the scientific integrity of the project and those involved in it, obtaining subjects' informed consent, and avoiding conflicts of interest. As a scientist, the principal investigator is obligated to report and disseminate the products of research, such as findings and reports on inventions, in such scientific media as peer-reviewed journals, scientific conferences and professional society meetings, workshops, and lectures. (Note that publication of findings in the popular press prior to scientific publication is not in accord with accepted scientific tradition.)

SUMMARY

By way of conclusion we offer several observations which we feel are worthy of consideration:

1. The intellectually gifted young psychiatrist who is interested in a research career will find many attractive and rewarding employment opportunities that combine clinical practice, teaching, and research. The general demand for well-trained academic psychiatrists in the United States, and especially for child and adolescent psychiatrists, is enormous.

2. Psychiatrists with sound research training are consistently successful in competing for a variety of research, research training, and research career awards relevant to mental and addictive disorders. Experienced research psychiatrists in child, adolescent, adult, and aging areas are in constant demand as consultants, and as members of national scientific review or advisory committees and boards of public and private organizations. Often they are involved in developing or influencing national health and mental health policies.

3. Basic and clinical knowledge in medical, psychiatric, biological, and behavioral sciences is expanding at an enormous rate and the potential for effective utilization of this knowledge in solving psychiatric problems is great. However, as the perimeter of our knowledge increases, so does our awareness of what we still do not know about human development, function, and dysfunction.

4. Both the utilization of existing basic knowledge and the conceptualization of clinically relevant new questions and, hence, the design and development of new studies, analysis of data, and formulation of new questions all hinge on the availability and inventiveness of clinical scientists. Basic science is vital, but it is not by itself sufficient to solve clinical problems.

5. The current national climate is fully supportive of the scientific enterprise as the main avenue of solving our health, mental health, and social problems. Moreover, federal support for research and development in the fields of major mental and addictive disorders continues to be substantial and it increases as public and congressional awareness of these problems and their cost to society also increases. Moreover, nongovernmental support is becoming increasingly available, particularly for clinically targeted research.

6. The quality of psychiatric education depends heavily on the research and clinical skills of the faculty. There continues to be an enormous need for well-

trained clinical researchers in general, child, and adolescent psychiatry who can serve as teachers in medical schools and mentors and role models during residency and postresidency fellowship.

7. Progress in psychiatry will depend principally on new developments in its current scientific foundations. This, in turn, rests on the involvement of talented and well-trained young men and women who enter this field during the next few decades. This chapter has attempted to provide some information, guidance, and encouragement for those who have the creative talent and depth of interest to achieve a better understanding of aberrant human behavior and who are resolute enough to find ways and means to better prevent, identify, and treat mental illness. Service to individual patients and their families is a fundamental and noble role in psychiatry, but the efficacy of that service depends on the scientific information and technological tools available to the clinical practitioner, and this is where the contribution of the clinical scientist is paramount.

REFERENCES

Alcohol, Drug Abuse, and Mental Health Administration. (1990, March). *ADAMHA public advisory committees: Authority, structure, function, members.* Rockville, MD: Author.

Alcohol, Drug Abuse, and Mental Health Administration. (no date). *ADAMHA funding mechanisms for research grants and awards.* Rockville, MD: Author.

Alcohol, Drug Abuse, and Mental Health Administration. (1989a). *ADAMHA research grant awards.* Rockville, MD: U.S. Department of Health and Human Services.

Alcohol, Drug Abuse, and Mental Health Administration. (1989b). *ADAMHA research information source book extramural programs.* Rockville, MD: U.S. Department of Health and Human Services.

Alzheimer's Association. (no date). *1991 Grants announcement.* Chicago: Author.

Boothe, B. E., Rosenfeld, A. H., & Walker, E. L. (1974). *Toward a science of psychiatry: Impact of the research development program of the National Institutes of Health.* Belmont, CA: Wadsworth Publishing.

Burke, J. B., Pincus, H. A., & Pardes, H. (1986). The clinician-researcher in psychiatry. *American Journal of Psychiatry, 143,* 968–975.

Davis, W. K., & Kelley, W. N. (1982). Factors influencing decisions to enter careers in clinical investigation. *Journal of Medical Education, 57,* 275–281.

Dech, B., Abikoff, H., & Koplewicz, H. S. (1990). A survey of child and adolescent psychiatry residents: Perceptions of the ideal training program. *Journal of the American Academy of Child and Adolescent Psychiatry, 29,* 946–949.

DeRoy, A. K. (1990, November). *A proposal writer's guide* (2nd ed.). Pittsburgh: University of Pittsburgh, Office of Research.

Detre, T. (1989). Some comments on the future of child and adolescent psychiatry. *Academic Psychiatry, 13,* 189–195.

Garfinkel, P. E., Goldbloom, D. S., Kaplan, A. S., & Kennedy, S. H. (1989). The clinician-investigator interface in psychiatry: I—values and problems. *Canadian Journal of Psychiatry, 34,* 361–363.

Garfinkel, P. E., Kennedy, S. H., Kaplan, A. S., & Goldbloom, D. S. (1989). The clinician-investigator interface in psychiatry: II—the role of the clinical investigation unit. *Canadian Journal of Psychiatry, 34,* 364–368.

Gillin, J. C. (1988). Postresidency research training of psychiatrists. *Psychopharmacology Bulletin, 24,* 291–292.

Hillman, B. J. (1985). The inadequacy in the number and quality of physician researchers: A perspective and approach to the problem. *Investigative Radiology, 20,* 767–771.

Institute of Medicine. (1983). *Personnel needs and training for biomedical and behavioral research.* Washington, DC: National Academy Press.

Institute of Medicine. (1984). *Research on mental illness and addictive disorders: Progress and prospects.* Washington, DC: National Academy Press.

Institute of Medicine. (1985). *Personnel needs and training for biomedical and behavioral research.* Washington, DC: National Academy Press.

Institute of Medicine. (1989). *Research on children and adolescents with mental, behavioral and developmental disorders.* Washington, DC: National Academy Press.

Jankowski, J. E., Jr. (1990). *National patterns of r&d resources: 1990* (NSF 90-316). Surveys of Science Resources Series. Washington, DC: National Science Foundation.

Jones, F. (Ed.). (1990, December). *Source book profiles: An information service on the 1,000 largest U.S. foundations.* New York: The Foundation Center.

Leichner, P. (1987). Postgraduate education in psychiatry: 10 years later. *RCPSC, 20,* 511–517.

Levy, G, Sherman, C., Gentile, N., Hough, L., Dial, T., & Jolly, P. (1988). Postdoctoral research training of full-time faculty in an academic department of medicine. *Annals of Internal Medicine, 109,* 414–418.

National Institute of Mental Health. (1990). *National plan for research on child and adolescent mental disorders: A report requested by the U.S. Congress submitted by the National Advisory Mental Health Council.* Washington, DC: U.S. Government Printing Office.

National Institute of Mental Health Research Information Source Book. (1989). *Extramural program.* Bethesda, MD: Author.

National Institutes of Health, Division of Research Grants. (1990, August). *Extramural Trends, FY 1980–1989.* Bethesda, MD: Author.

National Institutes of Health, Division of Research Grants. (1990, October). *The K awards.* Bethesda, MD: Author.

National Institutes of Health. (1990, October). *NIH advisory committees: Authority, structure, function, members* (NIH Publication No. 91-10). Bethesda, MD: Author.

National Science Foundation, Division of Science Resources Studies. (1990, April). *Federal r&d funding by budget function: Fiscal years 1989–91* (NSF 90-311). Washington, DC: Author.

National Science Foundation, Division of Science Resources Studies. (1990, June). *Science and technology data book* (NSF 90-304). Washington, DC: Author.

National Science Foundation. (no date). *Guide to programs, fiscal year 1991* (NSF 90-25). Washington, DC: Author.

Olson, S. (Ed.). (1990). *The foundation directory, 1991 edition* (13th ed.). New York: The Foundation Center.

Pincus, H. A., Goodwin, F., Barchas, J., Cohen, D., Judd, L., Meltzer, H., & Vaillant, G. (1989). The future of the science of psychiatry. In J. Talbott (Ed.), *Future directions for psychiatry* (pp. 75–106). Washington, DC: American Psychiatry Press.

Sledge, W. H., Leaf, P. J., Fenton, W. S., & Chung, A. M. (1990). Training and career activity: The experience of the Yale advanced track program. *Archives of General Psychiatry, 47,* 82–88.

University of Pittsburgh, Center for Neuroscience. (February 4, 1991). Center for neuroscience and schizophrenia. *Neurotransmitter,* p. 4.

U.S. Department of Health and Human Services. (November 23, 1990). ADAMHA small grant program. *NIH Guide for Grants and Contracts, 19,* 7–11.

U.S. Department of Health and Human Services. (January 4, 1991). National research service award stipend increase. *NIH Guide for Grants and Contracts, 20,* 1.

Wakeford, R., Evered, D., Lyon, J., & Saunders, N. (August, 1985). Where do medically qualified researchers come from? *Lancet,* 262–265.

William T. Grant Foundation. (no date). *Annual report 1989.* New York: Author.

William T. Grant Foundation. (January 1990). *General information brochure.* New York: Author.

Wyngaarden, J. B. (1979). The clinical investigator as an endangered species. *New England Journal of Medicine, 301,* 1254–1259.

APPENDIX: FUNDING SOURCE INFORMATION RESOURCES

Listed below are various directories, program guides, and newsletters that provide information on sources of funding for research, fellowships, service demonstrations, equipment, curriculum development, and other purposes. Those items that are denoted by an asterisk (*) are described in the tables that appear at the end of the Appendix: Table A-1. Coverage of Sponsor Types; Table A-2. Contents; and Table A-3. Indexes. Many of these publications should be available in your institution's library, sponsored projects office, or development office. Also many are available through the numerous regional repositories for The Foundation Center's publications (i.e., The Foundation Center's four Reference Collections and its various Cooperating Collections that together comprise The Foundation Center Cooperating Collections Network).

Computer-Based Funding Source Information

Electronic publications are increasingly available through public and institutional libraries, computer networks such as BITNET and NSFNET, commercial database services, such as DIALOG and BRS, and institutional sponsored project offices. For example, electronic versions of the *NIH Guide for Grants and Contracts* and the *National Science Foundation Bulletin* are available directly from the NIH and the NSF, respectively, in electronic form as well as in hardcopy. Some institutions, such as the University of Pittsburgh, make such electronic information accessible on their mainframe computer systems.

There are also computer-based funding source information database systems that cover funding opportunities relevant to academic research. SPIN, the Sponsored Programs Information Network, provides information on more than 4,100 funding programs, as well as information on funding opportunities published in the *Federal Register* and *Commerce Business Daily*. SPIN is produced and maintained by the Research Foundation of the State University of New York. IRIS, the Illinois Researcher Information System, is similar in concept to SPIN. It has information on more than 5,000 funding programs, but it does not provide information on requests for proposals or other one-time opportunities. IRIS is housed at the University of Illinois at Urbana-Champaign.

Increasing numbers of public and institutional libraries make available an array of on-line and on-disk databases. Most such databases are bibliographic, but there are other types, including funding source information databases, such as the GRANTS Database produced and maintained by Oryx Press, and the Foundation Center Database. The latter is used to produce the Foundation Center's COMSEARCH Printouts series (see description below). If your library does not have a database department, consult the reference librarian.

Contacts and Publishers

Alcohol, Drug Abuse, and Mental Health Administration:
    Office of Extramural Programs
    Alcohol, Drug Abuse, and Mental Health Administration
    5600 Fishers Lane
    Rockville, MD 20857

    (301) 443-4266

National Institutes of Health:
    Office of Extramural Research
    National Institutes of Health
    9000 Rockville Pike
    Bethesda, MD 20892

    (301) 496-1096

National Science Foundation:
    Grants and Contracts Division
    National Science Foundation
    1800 G Street, NW, Room 1140
    Washington, DC 20550

    (202) 357-7547

U.S. Department of Education:
    Grants and Contracts Service
    U.S. Department of Education
    3124 Regional Office Building
    Seventh and D Streets, SW
    Washington, DC 20202

    (202) 708-5514

U.S. Government Documents:
    Superintendent of Documents
    U.S. Government Printing Office
    Washington, DC 20402

    (202) 783-3238

Electronic Databases:
    Illinois Researcher Information System
    Research Services Office
    University of Illinois at Urbana-Champaign
    128 Observatory
    901 South Mathews Avenue
    Urbana, IL 61801

    (217) 333-0284

Sponsored Programs Information Network (SPIN)
   Research Foundation of the State University of New York
   P.O. Box 9
   Albany, NY 12201-0009

   (518) 434-7150

Directories:
   The Foundation Center
   79 Fifth Avenue
   New York, NY 10003

   (212) 620-4230

   Oryx Press
   4041 N. Central at Indian School Road
   Phoenix, AZ 85012-3397

   1-800-279-ORYX (toll free)

   The Taft Group
   12300 Twinbrook Parkway, Suite 450
   Rockville, MD 20852

   (301) 816-0210

   Public Management Institute
   358 Brannan Street
   San Francisco, CA 94107

   (415) 896-1900

Newsletter:
   Office of Research
   American Psychiatric Association
   1400 K Street, NW
   Washington, DC 20005

Federal Government and Independent Agencies

ADAMHA Funding Mechanisms for Research Grants & Awards. Rockville, MD:
Alcohol, Drug Abuse, and Mental Health Administration.

   This publication provides concise descriptions of ADAMHA and its constit-
uent agencies, ADAMHA's grant application receipt and review assignment
procedures, its dual (i.e, two-tiered) review system, and types of awards made
by ADAMHA agencies. Also included is a list of contact addresses and phone
numbers for each of the ADAMHA agencies, and a table for each ADAMHA
agency showing its areas of interest and the types of awards made in each area.

Catalog of Federal Domestic Assistance. Washington, DC: U.S. Government Printing Office.

> The *Catalog of Federal Domestic Assistance* is a government-wide compendium of Federal programs, projects, services, and activities which provide assistance or benefits to the American public. It contains financial and nonfinancial assistance programs administered by departments and establishments of the Federal government.
>
> As the basic reference source of Federal programs, the primary purpose of the Catalog is to assist users in identifying programs which meet specific objectives of the potential applicant, and to obtain general information on Federal assistance programs. In addition, the intent of the Catalog is to improve coordination and communication between the Federal government and State and local governments.
>
> The Catalog provides the user with access to programs administered by Federal departments and agencies in a single publication. Program information is cross referenced by functional classification (Functional Index), subject (Subject Index), applicant (Applicant Index), deadline(s) for program application submission (Deadlines Index), and authorizing legislation (Authorization Index). These are valuable resource tools which, if used carefully, can make it easier to identify specific areas of program interest more efficiently. (Introduction to the 1990 Edition, p. VII).

Commerce Business Daily. Washington, DC: U.S. Department of Commerce.

The *Commerce Business Daily* lists all requests for proposals (RFPs) and bid solicitations available or soon to be made available for all Federal Government agencies. It is published daily (except Saturdays, Sundays, and federal holidays) by the U.S. Department of Commerce.

Federal Register. Washington, DC: U.S. Government Printing Office.

The *Federal Register* is published daily (except Saturdays, Sundays, and federal holidays) by the National Archives and Records Administration and is distributed by the U.S. Government Printing Office. It

> provides a uniform system for making available to the public regulations and legal notices issued by Federal agencies. These include Presidential proclamations and Executive Orders and Federal agency documents having general applicability and legal effect, documents required to be published by act of Congress and other Federal agency documents of public interest. (Issue of February 4, 1991, p. II).

More specifically, the *Federal Register* contains program announcements as well as proposed and final rules and regulations, notices of meetings, and other important notices.

Federal Yellow Book: A Directory of the Federal Departments and Agencies. Washington, DC: Monitor Publishing Company.

Although this is not a directory of federal funding sources *per se*, it may be used to locate the address and phone numbers of any federal agency (or office, bureau, etc.) or name, address, and phone number of any federal program officer. The *Federal Yellow Book* covers the Executive Office of the President, the 14

Executive Departments, all federal independent agencies, and all federal regional offices.

Guide to Department of Education Programs. Washington, DC: U.S. Government Printing Office.

This reference lists all external funding programs sponsored by the U.S. Department of Education by sponsoring unit. Each entry gives the program name and a brief description, information on eligibility to apply, and a contact unit name and phone number.

National Science Foundation Bulletin. Washington, DC: National Science Foundation.

This bulletin is published monthly by the National Science Foundation. It contains program announcements, deadline dates, target dates, and miscellaneous notifications.

National Science Foundation Guide to Programs. Washington, DC: U.S. Government Printing Office.

This directory briefly discusses the NSF's mission and lays out the criteria used in making extramural awards, and then provides a description of each NSF funding program by directorate.

NIH Extramural Programs: Funding for Research and Research Training. Bethesda, MD: National Institutes of Health.

This reference reviews the mission and organizational structure of the National Institutes of Health, describes the various award mechanisms utilized by the NIH, and then, for each Institute and other major organizational or programmatic unit, discusses the mission, structure, and funding programs, and presents a table showing each extramural program and the types of award mechanisms used to provide external funding through that program.

NIH Guide for Grants and Contracts. Bethesda, MD: National Institutes of Health.

Published weekly by the National Institutes of Health, the guide contains program announcements, requests for proposals (RFPs), and miscellaneous notifications for all ADAMHA and NIH institutes.

Office of Naval Research Guide to Programs. Arlington, VA: Office of the Chief of Naval Research.

This directory provides information about the ONR's basic and applied research and research-related programs and priorities. Contact persons' names and addresses are listed with each program description. The directory also contains ONR's guidelines for proposal preparation and submission.

Research Interests of the Air Force Office of Scientific Research. Washington, DC: Bolling Air Force Base, U.S. Air Force Office of Scientific Research.

This publication provides information about the AFOSR's basic and applied research and research-related programs. Contact persons' names and addresses are listed with each program description. The directory also contains AFOSR's guidelines for proposal preparation and submission.

U.S. Army Medical Research & Development Command Broad Agency Announcement. Frederick, MD: Fort Detrick, U.S. Army Medical Research and Development Command.

This publication lists research areas of interest to the U.S. Army Medical Research and Development Command, and provides information and materials needed to apply for grant funding and for contract funding.

Nonfederal Funding Sources

*America's New Foundations. Rockville, MD: The Taft Group.

This reference contains information on "newly established" private, corporate, and community foundations "with assets or total giving of $100,000 or more." (Introduction to the 1991 Edition, p. vi) The book has five indexes: foundations alphabetically by name; foundations by grant type; foundations by recipient type; donors, officers, and trustees alphabetically by name; and grant recipients by location.

*Annual Register of Grant Support: A Directory of Funding Sources. Wilmette, IL: National Register Publishing Company.

> [T]he *Annual Register of Grant Support* has achieved a deserved reputation as an authoritative standard reference source on non-repayable financial support. . . .
> [It] includes details of the grant support programs of government agencies, public and private foundations, corporations, community trusts, unions, educational and professional associations, and special interest organizations. It covers a broad spectrum of interests from academic and scientific research, project development, travel and exchange programs, and publication support to equipment and construction grants, in-service training, and competitive awards and prizes in a variety of fields. (Preface to the 1991 Edition, p. xi)

COMSEARCH Printouts: Broad Topics

> This series indexes and analyzes recent foundation grants in 26 broad subject categories. Each listing contains all grants in the particular subject area reported to the Foundation Center during the preceding year, along with an index listing name and geographic location of organizations which have received grants, a geographic index arranged by state of the recipient organization, and a key word index listing descriptive words and phrases. . . . *Series published annually in September*. (Publications and Services of The Foundation Center: Subject Directories in *The Foundation Directory 1991 Edition*, 1990, p. xxiv)

COMSEARCH Printouts: Geographics

> This series provides customized listings of grants received by organizations in two cities, eleven states, and seven regions. These listings make it easy to see which major foundations have awarded grants in your area, to which nonprofit organizations, and what each grant was intended to accomplish. . . . *Series published annually in September.* (Publications and Services to The Foundation Center: Subject Directories in *The Foundation Directory 1991 Edition*, 1990, p. xxiv)

COMSEARCH Printouts: Special Topics

> These are three of the most frequently requested special listings from the Center's computer databases. The three special listings are: [t]he 1,000 Largest U.S. Foundations by Asset Size; [t]he 1,000 Largest U.S. Foundations by Annual Grants Total; [t]he over 2,000 Operating Foundations which Administer their Own Projects or Programs. . . . *Series published annually in September.* (Publications and Services of The Foundation Center: Subject Directors in *The Foundation Directory 1991 Edition*, 1990, pp. xxiv–xxv)

COMSEARCH Printouts: Subjects

> This series includes 28 specially focused subject listings of grants reported to the Foundation Center during the preceding year. Listings are arranged by the state where the foundation is located and then by foundation name, and include complete information on the name and location of the grant recipient, the amount awarded, and the purpose of the grant. . . . *Series published annually in September.* (Publications and Services of The Foundation Center: Subject Directories in *The Foundation Directory 1991 Edition*, 1990, p. xxiv)

Corporate 500: The Directory of Corporate Philanthropy. San Francisco: Public Management Institute.

Despite its title, this reference provides information on nearly 600 corporations. A typical entry lists the contact person, principal business of the corporation, subsidiary companies, types of activities supported, organizational eligibility, restrictions, geographic areas where most or all of the corporation's giving is concentrated, a descriptive analysis of the corporation and its giving, the corporation's areas of funding interest, officers and directors of the corporation and/or corporate foundation, a "contributions profile," information on the application process, and a sample of recent grants (including names and locations of the recipients and the amounts given or awarded).

Corporate Foundation Profiles. New York: The Foundation Center.

"Corporate foundation profiles are reproduced from reports originally published in quarterly editions of *Source Book Profiles* [see description below] over the previous two-year period" (Introduction to the 1990 Edition, p. vii).

Directory of Biomedical and Health Care Grants. Phoenix, AZ: Oryx Press.

This reference provides information on more than 3,000 funding programs for biomedical research and health care delivery of the Federal Government, state and local governments, corporations, corporate foundations, private and community philanthropic foundations, and professional associations. Each program description includes information on the nature of the program, program restrictions, eligibility requirements, grant size, submission deadline dates, contact address and phone number, and *Catalog of Federal Domestic Assistance* program number for federal programs.

*Directory of International Corporate Giving in America. Rockville, MD: The Taft Group.

> [T]he *Directory of International Corporate Giving in America* (ICGA) is a unique source of information on the charitable giving activities in the United States of foreign-owned firms. . . . [I]ncluded [are] firms that have a minimum 10 percent investment by a non-U.S. headquartered company. More than three-fourths of the profiles cover direct giving programs, providing valuable leads to corporate charitable and discretionary budgets. (About This [1991] Edition, p. vii)

*Directory of International Grants and Fellowships in the Health Sciences. Bethesda, MD: National Institutes of Health, John E. Fogarty International Center for Advanced Study in the Health Sciences.

> This directory was compiled to help U.S. and non-U.S. biomedical and behavioral scientists locate fellowships for training outside their home country as well as grants for research projects within their home country. It was prepared in response to increasing numbers of requests for information about international fellowships in the biomedical sciences. The directory provides a convenient listing of over 180 organizations and agencies that support fellowships and research grants. (p. iii)

*Directory of International Opportunities in Biomedical and Behavioral Sciences. Bethesda, MD: National Institutes of Health, John E. Fogarty International Center for Advanced Study in the Health Sciences.

> This directory provides a convenient listing of organizations and agencies that support fellowships for research in the biomedical and behavioral sciences. It was prepared primarily for U.S. postdoctoral scientists seeking opportunities in foreign countries. Organizations that do not limit their support to U.S. citizens are included in this listing. Thus, the directory should also be helpful to foreign scientists. (p. i)

*Directory of New and Emerging Foundations. New York: The Foundation Center.

> The *Directory of New and Emerging Foundations* is intended to provide as comprehensive a view as possible of recently formed foundations, and to serve as a convenient tool for grantseekers interested in potential new sources of funding. . . . The *Directory* includes only those organizations which meet the Foundation Center's definition of a community or private grantmaking foundation and which held assets of $1 million or more or gave $100,000 or more in the latest year of record." (Introduction to the 1991 Edition, p. v)

Directory of Research Fellowship Opportunities in Psychiatry. Washington, DC: Office of Research, American Psychiatry Association.

This directory lists research fellowship opportunities in psychiatry in the United States and Canada. Each entry includes the title of the program, the name, address and telephone number of the fellowship director, a brief discussion of the subject-matter areas covered, the names and area(s) of expertise of participating faculty members, the length of the fellowship, and the amount of the stipend. The entries are listed alphabetically by state/province and institution.

Directory of Research Grants. Phoenix, AZ: Oryx Press.

> The *Directory of Research Grants* . . . is a tool for individuals and institutions in search of support for research. The Directory contains more than 5800 grant programs which are arranged alphabetically by grant title. Each program includes a description, deadline date, *Catalog of Federal Domestic Assistance* program number for federal programs, restrictions or requirements, contact names and addresses, telephone numbers, and funding amounts. (Introduction to the 1991 Edition, p. vii)

The Foundation Center Source Book Profiles: An Information Service on the 1,000 Largest U.S. Foundations. New York: The Foundation Center.

> *Source Book Profiles* provides grantseekers with the facts they need to identify, research, and contact appropriate funding sources among the nation's 1,000 largest foundations. These foundations account for approximately 60 percent of all foundation grant dollars awarded in a given year. However, they represent less than five percent of the total number of active grantmaking foundations in the U.S., and because they are among the most visible of all foundations, competition for their grants is especially keen. . . . (Introduction to the January–December 1990 Edition, p. xix)

The Foundation Directory. New York: The Foundation Center.

> *The Foundation Directory* is the standard reference work for information about private and community grantmaking foundations in the United States. It is used by fundseekers, foundation and government officials, scholars, journalists, and others generally interested in foundation giving in this country. (Introduction to the 1991 Edition, p. v)
>
> *The Foundation Directory* is one of the first tools grantseekers should consult to identify foundations that might be interested in funding their project or organization. It provides basic descriptions of the giving interests and current fiscal data for the nation's largest foundations—those with assets of $1 million or more or annual giving of at least $100,000. Indexes help grantseekers to quickly identify foundations which have expressed an interest in a particular subject field or geographic area or which provide the specific type of support needed. (Introduction to the 1991 Edition, p. xiii)

The Foundation Directory, Part 2: A Guide to Grant Programs $25,000–$100,000. New York: The Foundation Center.

> *The Foundation Directory, Part 2* . . . [provides] complete descriptive information on the second tier of U.S. grantmaking . . . private and community foundations making grants of $25,000 to $99,999 annually and holding assets of less than $1 million. It is designed as a companion volume to *The Foundation Directory*, which reports on foundations with assets of at least $1 million or total annual giving of at least $100,000.
>
> *The Foundation Directory, Part 2* can also stand alone as a guide to smaller but significant grantmakers whose giving often supports local organizations. (Introduction to the 1991–1992 Edition, p. vii)

Foundation Grants to Individuals. New York: The Foundation Center.

> *Foundation Grants to Individuals* is the most comprehensive listing available of
> private U.S. foundations which provide financial assistance to individuals. [It] con-
> tains those . . . active private grantmaking U.S. foundations . . . that The Foundation
> Center has identified as conducting ongoing grantmaking programs for individuals. It
> describes giving for a variety of purposes including scholarships, student loans,
> fellowships, foreign recipients, travel internships, residencies, arts and cultural proj-
> ects, and general welfare. . . .
>
> For inclusion in *Foundation Grants to Individuals* a foundation must meet three
> criteria: 1. It must make grant awards to or for individuals of at least $2,000 a year. . . .
> 2. It must select recipients of its grants by its governing board or an independent
> selection committee. [3.] It must accept applications from individuals directly or
> through an intermediary. The one exception to this requirement is a special category,
> "Awards, Prizes, and Grants by Nomination," where information is given on awards
> programs sponsored by foundations and programs which require nominations from
> sources other than the individuals themselves, such as institutions or organizations
> affiliated with the foundation. (Introduction to the 7th Edition, pp. v–vi)

The International Foundation Directory. London, U.K.: Europa Publications Limited.

This book provides information on more than 750 foundations worldwide,
listed by countries in which they are located and indexed by name and by "main
activities." The criteria for inclusion of an organization in the book are:

> they must have some capital endowment, they must operate independently and at
> discretion, they must engage in international activity, and, in particular, they must not
> be adjuncts of other institutions of a different class, such as government departments
> or universities. (Introduction to the First Edition, p. xv)

Also included are

> foundations of such wealth that although they may be restricted to regional or national
> boundaries their activities are on so great a scale as to have an international impact,
> through their example, their prestige, the work of the scholars they endow or the
> institutions they support, or otherwise. . . . [and] national and international organiza-
> tions serving the common purposes of institutions which themselves may figure in the
> list: bodies like the Council on Foundations and the Foundation Center in the United
> States, the National Council of Social Service in Britain, or the International Council of
> Voluntary Agencies in Geneva (Introduction to the First Edition, p. xv)

*National Data Book of Foundations: A Comprehensive Guide to Grantmaking Founda-
tions*. New York: The Foundation Center.

This reference lists nearly all private and community grantmaking foundations in the United States. The entries contain information from each foundation's IRS Form 990-PF, the informational federal tax return filed by each private
and community foundation, as required by law. The information provided is
very basic—foundation name, contact name, address, financial data, and IRS
number, unlike the detailed listings in other directories published by The
Foundation Center.

National Directory of Corporate Giving: A Guide to Corporate Giving Programs and Corporate Foundations. New York: The Foundation Center.

This reference contains information on more than 1,500 corporations that make grants and/or other types of contributions to nonprofit organizations. Included is information on corporate giving programs, corporate foundations, and "unorganized" corporate giving. The corporations profiled "vary from those with specific interests and structured formal giving mechanisms to those with broad purposes and unstructured, informal contributions programs." (Introduction to the 1989 Edition, p. v)

National Guide to Foundation Funding in Higher Education. New York: The Foundation Center.

This reference contains information on more than 2,900 foundation funding sources for institutions of higher education and activities carried out by or in such institutions. The foundations listed each gave $10,000 or more to higher education. Included in each entry is information on: foundation name, address, and telephone number; year and place of incorporation; the name(s) of the donor(s); assets and expenditures; areas of funding interest; types of support provided; restrictions; application and review; contact person; names of the officers and directors of the foundation; foundation staff; recent gifts and grants made to higher education.

Psychiatric Research Report. Washington, DC: American Psychiatric Association.

Psychiatric Research Report is a quarterly newsletter that contains information about research fellowships and research funding opportunities, as well as feature articles and other information. It is published by the Office of Research of the American Psychiatric Association.

Taft Corporate Giving Directory: Comprehensive Profiles of America's Major Corporate Foundations and Corporate Charitable Giving Programs. Rockville, MD: The Taft Group.

> the . . . *Taft Corporate Giving Directory (TCGD)* is a unique, single-volume source providing detailed descriptive profiles of 500 of the largest and most important corporate charitable giving programs in the United States. Each company profiled makes contributions of at least $500,000 annually. Significantly more than two-thirds of these profiles cover direct giving programs, detailing difficult-to-gather information not available from IRS Form 990s, corporate annual reports, or in directories limiting their coverage to foundation philanthropy. (About This [1990] Edition, p. ix)

Taft Foundation Reporter: Comprehensive Profiles and Giving Analyses of America's Major Private Foundations. Rockville, MD: The Taft Group.

This reference contains information on more than 500 foundations. There are seven indexes to maximize utility and make the information highly

Table A-1. Coverage of Sponsor Types

Resource	Federal government and independent agencies	Voluntary and/or professional organizations	Philanthropic foundations	Corporations/corporate foundations
America's New Foundations			Yes	Yes
Annual Register of Grant Support: A Directory of Funding Sources	Yes	Yes	Yes	Yes
Corporate 500: The Directory of Corporate Philanthropy				Yes
Corporate Foundation Profiles				Yes
Directory of Biomedical and Health Care Grants	Yes	Yes	Yes	Yes
Directory of International Corporate Giving in America				Yes
Directory of International Grants and Fellowships in the Health Sciences	Yes	Yes	Yes	Yes
Directory of International Opportunities in Biomedical and Behavioral Sciences	Yes	Yes	Yes	Yes
Directory of New and Emerging Foundations			Yes	Yes
Directory of Research Grants	Yes	Yes	Yes	Yes
The Foundation Center Source Book Profiles: An Information Service on the 1,000 Largest U.S. Foundations			Yes	Yes
The Foundation Directory			Yes	Yes
The Foundation Directory, Part 2: A Guide to Grant Programs $25,000–$100,000			Yes	Yes
Foundation Grants to Individuals		Yes	Yes	
The International Foundation Directory		Yes	Yes	
National Data Book of Foundations: A Comprehensive Guide to Grantmaking Foundations			Yes	Yes
National Directory of Corporate Giving: A Guide to Corporate Giving Programs and Corporate Foundations				Yes
National Guide to Foundation Funding in Higher Education			Yes	Yes
Taft Corporate Giving Directory: Comprehensive Profiles of America's Major Corporate Foundations and Corporate Charitable Giving Programs				Yes
Taft Foundation Reporter: Comprehensive Profiles and Giving Analyses of America's Major Private Foundations			Yes	

Table A-2.   Contents

Resource	Sponsor name, address, telephone	Contact person(s) name, [address], telephone	Sponsor area(s) of interest/ program topic area(s)	Eligibility requirements	Application procedures	Recent awards	Other information
America's New Foundations	Yes		Yes	Yes	Yes	Yes	Yes
Annual Register of Grant Support: A Directory of Funding Sources	Yes	Yes	Yes	Yes	Yes	Yes	Yes
Corporate 500: The Directory of Corporate Philanthropy	Yes	Yes	Yes	Yes	Yes	Yes	Yes
Corporate Foundation Profiles	Yes	Yes	Yes	Yes	Yes	Yes	Yes
Directory of Biomedical and Health Care Grants	Yes	Yes	Yes	Yes			Yes
Directory of New and Emerging Foundations	Yes		Yes	Yes	Yes	Yes	Yes
Directory of International Corporate Giving in America	Yes	Yes	Yes		Yes	In some cases	Yes
Directory of International Grants and Fellowships in the Health Sciences	Yes		Yes	Yes			Yes
Directory of International Opportunities in Biomedical and Behavioral Sciences	Yes		Yes	Yes			Yes
Directory of Research Grants	Yes	Yes	Yes	Yes			Yes

The Foundation Center Source Book Profiles: An Information Service on the 1,000 Largest U.S. Foundations	Yes	Yes	Yes	Yes	Yes	Yes
The Foundation Directory	Yes	Yes	In some cases	In some cases		Yes
The Foundation Directory, Part 2: A Guide to Grant Programs $25,000–100,000	Yes	Yes	In some cases	In some cases		Yes
Foundation Grants to Individuals	Yes	Yes	Yes	Yes	Yes	Yes
The International Foundation Directory	Yes	Yes	In many cases	In many cases		Yes
National Data Book of Foundations: A Comprehensive Guide to Grantmaking Foundations	Name and address only	Name and address only				Yes
National Directory of Corporate Giving; A Guide to Corporate Giving Programs and Corporate Foundations	Yes	In some cases	In some cases	In many cases	Yes	Yes
National Guide to Foundation Funding in Higher Education	Yes	Yes	Yes	Yes	Yes	Yes
Taft Corporate Giving Directory: Comprehensive Profiles of America's Major Corporate Foundations and Corporate Charitable Giving Programs	Yes	Yes	Yes		Yes	Yes
Taft Foundation Reporter: Comprehensive Profiles and Giving Analyses of America's Major Private Foundations	Yes	Yes	Yes	Yes	Yes	Yes

Table A-3.   Indexes

Resource	By sponsor name	By sponsor area(s) of interest/program topic area(s)	By geographic location of sponsor	By types of awards made	Other
America's New Foundations	Yes	Yes		Yes	Yes
Annual Register of Grant Support: A Directory of Funding Sources	Yes	Yes	Yes		Yes
Corporate 500: the Directory of Corporate Philanthropy	Yes	Yes	Yes	Yes	Yes
Corporate Foundation Profiles		Yes	Yes	Yes	
Directory of Biomedical and Health Care Grants	Yes	Yes			Yes
Directory of International Corporate Giving in America	Yes	Yes	Yes	Yes	Yes
Directory of International Grants and Fellowships in the Health Sciences		Yes	Yes		
Directory of International Opportunities in Biomedical and Behavioral Sciences				Yes	
Directory of New and Emerging Foundations	Yes	Yes			
Directory of Research Grants	Yes	Yes			Yes
The Foundation Center Source Book Profiles: An Information Service on the 1,000 Largest U.S. Foundations	Yes	Yes	Yes	Yes	Yes
The Foundation Directory	Yes	Yes	Yes	Yes	Yes
The Foundation Directory, Part 2: A Guide to Grant Programs $25,000–$100,000	Yes	Yes	Yes	Yes	Yes
Foundation Grants to Individuals	Yes	Yes	Yes	Yes	Yes
The International Foundation Directory	Yes	Yes			
National Data Book of Foundations: A Comprehensive Guide to Grantmaking Foundations			Yes		
National Directory of Corporate Giving: A Guide to Corporate Giving Programs and Corporate Foundations	Yes	Yes	Yes	Yes	Yes
National Guide to Foundation Funding in Higher Education	Yes		Yes	Yes	Yes
Taft Corporate Giving Directory: Comprehensive Profiles of America's Major Corporate Foundations and Corporate Charitable Giving Programs	Yes	Yes	Yes	Yes	Yes
Taft Foundation Reporter: Comprehensive Profiles and Giving Analyses of America's Major Private Foundations		Yes	Yes	Yes	Yes

accessible—indexes to foundations by field of interest, by types of grants made, by state, and by location of recent grant recipients, and indexes to foundation donors, officers, and key staff by name, by state of birth, and by alma mater. A typical entry includes contact name, address and phone number, a "fiscal summary," type of foundation, funding interests, types of grants made, information about the donor(s) to the foundation, the foundation's "philosophy," "contributions analysis," types of grant recipients, list of officers and directors along with their affiliations, a summary of "application and review procedures," "grants analysis," and a list of recent grants made and recipients thereof.

CHAPTER 2

Ethical Issues
in Psychiatric Research

WILLIAM J. WINSLADE AND JOHN W. DOUARD

INTRODUCTION

The primary goal of psychiatric research is to increase scientific knowledge about human psychology and behavior. Other chapters in this book treat the methodologies for achieving this goal as well as special topics and areas about which knowledge is sought. In this chapter, we consider ethical issues that arise in the course of formulating and conducting psychiatric research.

By "ethical issues," we mean those issues that concern the duties of researchers to their subjects and the rights of research subjects. We also consider some ethical aspects of research design and methodology. Finally, we discuss some specific problems that often arise in psychiatric research.

Our approach to ethical issues is to provide an overview of issues that should be considered by anyone who designs and implements a psychiatric research project. Our primary aim is to identify and clarify these issues rather than to analyze them in detail. A large body of literature on the ethics of human subject research in general, and psychiatric research in particular, is readily available. Before the beginning researcher can profitably consult such literature,

William J. Winslade and John W. Douard • Institute for the Medical Humanities, University of Texas Medical Branch, Galveston, Texas 77550.

Research in Psychiatry: Issues, Strategies, and Methods, edited by L. K. George Hsu and Michel Hersen. Plenum Press, New York, 1992.

however, it is necessary to have a clear grasp of potential ethical problems. Thus, we pose general ethical questions and set the stage for the analysis of particular problems that might be present in a specific research project.

The following are three ethical principles to which we shall refer throughout this chapter:

1. Persons have a right to the greatest possible degree of autonomy (literally: self-rule) compatible with similar autonomy for others.
2. Benefits and burdens of social life ought to be distributed fairly throughout society.
3. Burdens of a social practice that individuals are expected to bear by society must be small relative to the benefits to society the practice provides.

The first two are principles of justice; the third is a principle of social utility, which cannot be invoked to override principle 1 and/or principle 2. In other words, principle 1 and principle 2 must be satisfied before principle 3 can be applied to a social situation. Although here we are stating these principles in a general and abstract form, we will apply them concretely to ethical issues of clinical research.

ETHICAL ASPECTS OF RESEARCH DESIGN

The first question that arises about the ethics of research design is whether the knowledge sought is worth acquiring. Do the expected benefits of the research (i.e., the new knowledge gained) outweigh the costs (i.e., the time, effort, and money invested or the risks to research subjects)? Obviously trivial or useless information obtained at great economic or emotional cost is of little value. Similarly, one must justify as very important any research that puts research subjects at considerable risk of physical harm. That justification includes the review of all clinical research involving human subjects by an Institutional Review Board (IRB). According to the Department of Health and Human Services regulations, every institution receiving federal funds that engages in human subject research is required to establish at least one IRB to review the research protocols. Each IRB must have at least five members "with varying backgrounds" who have both ethical and professional competence. No IRB can be composed entirely of men or entirely of women, or be restricted to members of one profession. Each IRB must have at least one member whose primary interests are in nonscientific areas, and at least one member who is not affiliated with the institution and is not related to someone affiliated with the institution. Also, no participating member may be conducting research under review. Over the past 30 years, evolution of the IRB has been driven in part by the need to discourage and prevent pointless or harmful research. Thus, IRBs require that a proposed research project not only demonstrate that it is designed to yield scientific knowledge, but also that the benefits of the knowledge gained outweigh the costs and risks.

Most current psychiatric research projects do not place research subjects at significant risk of physical harm. For example, comparative drug trials or studies of the effectiveness of treatment programs may reveal which drugs or treatment programs offer greater benefits, although neither program puts subjects at significant risk of being harmed. In psychiatric research, however, this has not always been the case. Experiments involving lobotomy, psychosurgery, convulsive therapies, or early drug trials that were conducted in the 1930s and 1940s prior to institutional regulation or government oversight probably did cause harm to vulnerable psychiatric patients.

Undoubtedly, the IRB review process discourages researchers from submitting clearly pointless or dangerous proposals for research. It also requires a researcher to demonstrate and document the value of the research as well as the plan for carrying out such research. The IRB review process, however, is an administrative procedure that examines only written documents. Although an IRB actually has the authority to monitor the research it approves, rarely is such authority exercised in practice. Furthermore, studies of IRB approval rates suggest that most protocols actually submitted to these review boards eventually are approved. This may mean that all protocols are meritorious, or it may reflect the bias of peer reviewers in favor of the value of research. In any event, IRB review of human subject research is well established and fully bureaucratized at all institutions that receive federal funds for research. Thus, psychiatric researchers must submit proposed research to an IRB for review and satisfy the demands for documentation and justification imposed by the IRB.

The specific ethical issues that IRBs consider important are the following:

1. Are prospective subjects likely to be *capable* of providing adequately informed consent?
2. Is the language of the written informed consent form clear and intelligible to prospective subjects?
3. Will prospective subjects be adequately informed about the risks and benefits that may result from their participation in the research?
4. Does the content of the written consent form contain any *coercive* elements?
5. What are the criteria for allowing institutionalized persons to be clinical research subjects?
6. In a double-blind study, in which an experimental treatment is compared with either a placebo or a standard treatment, do expected benefits to subjects outweigh risks?

IRBs confront these questions whenever a research proposal is reviewed. They are not the only questions that arise, but they are central ethical issues that must be resolved before a research protocol can legitimately be approved. In the next section, we shall discuss these issues in somewhat more detail.

INFORMED CONSENT

On the ground that all persons have a right to autonomy, every clinical research protocol, if it is to be federally funded, is required to obtain "adequately informed consent" from all legally competent subjects. If a prospective subject is not legally competent, but is expected to benefit and suffer negligible or no harm from the experiment, then she or he must have a legal guardian provide informed consent. Every research protocol reviewed by an IRB includes a subject consent form which contains several elements:

1. A statement that the study involves research. A description of the research, including its goals and procedures, written in language subjects can understand.
2. The basis of subject selection.
3. A description of reasonably foreseeable benefits *to the subject* (if any), and a description of the expected risks and discomforts *to the subject* (if any).
4. Disclosure of alternative therapies.
5. Confidentiality assurances.
6. An offer to answer questions.
7. A statement that subjects are free to consult an advisor.
8. A statement of the possibility of compensation if the subject is injured, and a description of financial remuneration for participation (if any).
9. A statement that participation is voluntary and that the subject may discontinue participation at any time without penalty or prejudice.

Historically, the doctrine of informed consent rests on a principle articulated most directly in the Nuremberg Code:

> The person . . . [involved as a subject in research] . . . should be so situated as to be able to exercise free power of choice without the intervention of any element of force, fraud, deceit, duress, over-reaching or other ulterior form of constraint or coercion. (Levine, 1986, p. 425)

Generally, IRBs have the authority to monitor the process of acquiring adequately informed consent to ensure satisfaction of this principle, but most IRBs in fact just review the consent form for its completeness with respect to items 1 to 9 outlined above. The integrity of an IRB depends to a large extent on the seriousness and detail with which it reviews the subject consent form, especially since it is not usually practical for it to monitor the consent process itself.

One of the most pressing problems IRBs must address is the language in which the subject consent form is expressed. If it is in language that is too technical, it may not be comprehended by prospective subjects, even though they may sign the form. At the same time, the details of the experiment cannot be washed out by eliminating technical considerations altogether. Clearly, it is largely the responsibility of the research team and/or the subject's attending physician to ensure that the subject understands the nature, methods, and purpose of the experiment. The role of the IRB is to determine if the written consent strikes the best balance possible between comprehensibility to lay persons and a sufficiently accurate account of the experiment. In this respect, one virtue of IRB review is that such committees are made up of members of the scientific community *and* lay representatives.

Standards for assessing the risk/benefit ratio of a protocol vary somewhat with the seriousness of the illness with which subjects suffer. If the illness is terminal (e.g., AIDS), and there is either no standard treatment or the standard treatment carries risks at least as great as the experimental treatment, then it is morally permissible even in the absence of foreseeable benefits to test the experimental treatment on human subjects. Indeed, it may be ethically wrong *not* to test new experimental treatments on terminally ill patients. It is true, of course, that a well-designed experimental treatment should, in this case, have yielded some positive results in animal experiments. Otherwise, there would be no reason to experiment on human subjects. Nonetheless, in the initial experiments on human subjects, it is often the case that no benefits can be promised in the consent form, and it would be unethical to do so.

If there are standard treatments that can either cure or ameliorate an illness, an IRB will generally approve a research protocol only if the experimental treatment is tested against the standard treatments. (This can be done either as a double-blind or an "open-label" experiment. We consider special ethical issues raised by the former below.) The most widely accepted ethical standard for assessing comparative research protocols is that the standard and experimental treatments be in "equipoise"; that is, it ought reasonably to be expected that the risks and benefits of the two treatments will be very close to equal. Therefore, it is unethical to continue testing experimental treatments on human subjects that are clearly inferior or superior to standard treatments.

WHAT IS COERCIVE?

It is important to understand that IRBs have the responsibility to examine research protocols for subtle as well as overtly coercive measures that tend to undermine a prospective research subject's *free* and informed consent. We may not want to call these measures "coercive," but they can undermine a subject's right to autonomy.

For example, some protocols offer subjects financial inducements for volunteering, and federal regulations specify that no "undue inducements" be offered. That restriction is a vague guideline, and IRBs need to exercise moral judgment in assessing any financial inducements offered with a protocol. *Some* inducement is often deemed necessary, since a well-designed experiment needs a subject population large enough to yield statistically significant results.

One standard is that financial inducements may only be as great as the amount of money a "normal, healthy" volunteer would lose in work and travel time. This sort of remuneration, it can be argued, does not mask the significant risks of harm or discomfort a subject is likely to endure. But what about financial rewards over and above compensation for time, travel, and "labor" that are *intended* to offset the risks from the subject's point of view? First, if expected benefits are great enough and risks low enough, such rewards are not necessary, and persons who would volunteer only if paid money in this case are not truly volunteers. Hence that would be unethical. If expected risks and benefits are relatively insignificant and the illness is treatable, then financial incentives may be ethical if they are not so great that they undermine the voluntary nature of the experiment. Finally, if risks are high and benefits low, or if the illness is terminal and currently untreatable, financial inducements are probably unethical. In the first case, they mask the risks, and in the second case subjects are so vulnerable that financial incentives, in addition to being unkind, are inherently manipulative. (A similar point holds for prisoners and other patients who are confined for long periods in an institution, such as some psychiatric patients.)

Another point that needs to be mentioned is that "significance" with respect to risks and benefits is not well defined. It is a matter of both clinical and ethical judgment, on the one hand, and *community* standards, on the other, whether or not risks and benefits are significant. An IRB, acting as representatives of a community, is likely to be a better judge of significance than an individual scientist.

We have been reluctant to assert definitely that financial incentives are or are not ethically permissible. The reason is that to some people, a certain increment of money may seem like nothing more than compensation for time, work, and travel expenses; to others, the same increment may be the only income they have at the time. However, the IRB cannot assess the economic standing of subjects who are being recruited for a protocol. This problem, we feel, cannot be resolved except by eliminating financial rewards altogether, and scientists are inclined to think that monetary incentives are required to ensure a sufficiently large number of subjects for their research. It ought to be kept in mind, however, that setting monetary incentives too low may yield a preponderance of subjects from a lower socioeconomic class, thus violating the principle that benefits and burdens ought to be distributed equitably across society. Setting them too high may count as an undue inducement and may therefore border on coercion.

One final point is worth emphasizing. Financial incentives ought not to be listed among the benefits that subjects are expected to receive from their participation in an experiment. Expected benefits are best thought of as *medical* benefits only. Although not all IRBs accept this view, placing monetary incentives in the consent form under benefits of research can be considered an undue inducement (Macklin, 1989).

PRISONERS AND OTHER INSTITUTIONALIZED PATIENTS

There are special Department of Health and Human Services (DHHS) regulations that constrain recruitment of prisoners for research protocols. First, each IRB must have at least one prisoner or prisoner's representative (i.e., someone who *primarily* represents the interests of prisoners), and the majority of IRB members are not allowed to be associated with a prison, apart from their membership on the IRB. Second, the research must not promise advantages to the prisoner that impair her or his capacity reasonably to weigh the risks of the research (e.g., special privileges or early release). Third, risks associated with the research must be approximately the same for prisoners and nonprisoners. Selection procedures must be fair, so that prisoners do not bear an inequitable burden of participation. Fourth, prisoners must be expected to be available for follow-up care, and must be informed of this fact. Finally, parole cannot be affected by participation in research, and prisoners must be so informed.

Clearly, all these provisions are intended to protect prisoners from any undue inducement and to provide them with a fair social distribution of the benefits and burdens of the research. The reason prisoners are singled out is particularly relevant to psychiatric research. Prisoners are a relatively distinct class of especially vulnerable persons vis-à-vis clinical research. They are socially stigmatized and are therefore prime candidates for discriminatory subject-selection processes. Prisoners are stigmatized by virtue of being prisoners, and because they are predominantly poor and nonwhite. Furthermore, as prisoners, they are held in closed institutions against their will, and their survival depends on the good will of authorities. Hence their right to autonomy is diminished and they are potentially manipulable.

Although in the last two decades the rights of psychiatric inpatients have been protected to a greater extent than in earlier periods, psychiatric patients are still stigmatized to some extent and are held in closed institutions against their will. Furthermore, the patients in state psychiatric facilities are largely poor and are often members of minority groups. Like prisoners, these patients are more vulnerable to coercion and manipulation than other persons. Nonetheless, there are no special guidelines designed to provide protection to institutionalized psychiatric patients over and above the regulations that guide all human subject research. Hence it might be argued that IRBs are morally responsible for exercising special precautions with respect to psychiatric inpatients. Our view is that IRBs ought to exercise their best moral and clinical judgment in assessing *all* research protocols. The moral burden for assessing the vulnerability of particular subjects falls primarily on the shoulders of clinical research scientists themselves, since they are in a position to know the details of subjects' personal histories (this point is discussed in more detail below). But it is worth noting that IRBs are, because of their structure and place in the medical bureaucracy, limited in scope.

ETHICS AND RESEARCH METHODS

We shall conclude our discussion of the role and responsibilities of the IRB system by examining briefly some methodological issues that have ethical implications. On the one hand, research methods must, for ethical and scientific reasons, be expected to yield statistically significant results. On the other hand, methodological rigor must also be ethically correct. What follows is, to some extent, a simplification of the methodological issues, but it is not, we hope, misleadingly simple.

Some clinical experiments have only one "arm": that is, they test a single experimental treatment on a population of patients, without a control group. Other experiments have two or more arms (we shall consider only the case of experiments with two arms). In two-armed research programs, an experimental treatment is tested against either a placebo (an inert intervention), or it is tested against a standard treatment. Within the class of two-armed experiments, either the subject, or the investigator and the subject, may not know whether or not the subject is receiving the experimental treatment (called *single* and *double-blind* experiments, respectively). Another possibility within this class of experiments is that subject and investigator may both know whether or not the subject is receiving the experimental treatment. "Open-label" experiments, as they are called, are used only in two-armed experiments in which an experimental treatment is tested against a standard treatment. In double-armed, double-blind experiments, subjects are randomly assigned to the arms. These experiments are called *randomized clinical trials* (RCTs).

In principle, RCTs are intended to correct for bias that may contaminate an experiment if the investigator, the subject, or both know to which arm the subject has been assigned. Neither single-arm nor open-label experiments, for example, can eliminate the possibility that mere knowledge that the subject has about her or his treatment may affect the treatment. Other ways of correcting for bias have been proposed, and some have been used. But because RCTs are still considered the "gold standard" of unbiased research, we limit our discussion to this method. However, single-arm experiments are ethically required when they are used to test treatment for diseases that are terminal and for which there is no treatment. The reason should be obvious: if there is even presumptive evidence from animal studies that, in this sort of case, an experimental treatment is effective, it would be ethically irresponsible to design a placebo-controlled experiment, since by definition placebos are inert.

Ethical analysis of RCTs is somewhat more complicated, and, at this point, we shall only mention several issues with which IRBs may be concerned. The first requirement is that when standard and experimental treatments are being used, there ought to be no reason to believe that the treatments will be significantly differentially effective. They ought to be in equipoise. Clearly, if either treatment is better than the other, it ought to be used to treat patients: to do otherwise would be to violate the principle that physicians ought to do no harm. (In placebo-controlled trials, this requirement is relaxed; that is, partly because RCTs are expensive to perform, and partly because the principle of utility justifies testing an experimental agent.)

During the course of an RCT, if either therapy begins to prove superior and the illness is severe, patients ought to be removed from the study and offered the therapy they prefer. This holds true even if, in the case of an experimental therapy, no statistically significant result has been achieved. This happened during the first controlled experiments with AZT, now a standard therapy for some AIDS-related diseases.

The final point we will consider is that participation in an RCT may be considered a burden in itself because it undermines the traditional doctor–patient relationship. That relationship involves the expectation by the patient that she or he is the primary concern of the physician. This is particularly problematic for patients who are members of a disadvantaged class, as would be the case of patients committed to a state psychiatric facility. Later, we will discuss steps that may be taken to minimize this problem. Here we note only that assessing benefits and burdens, which is a function of IRBs as well as research scientists, entails value judgments. Since the values of members of an IRB, investigators, and subjects often vary, it would seem to be in keeping with the principle of autonomy to allow prospective subjects to choose for themselves whether or not to participate in an otherwise appropriate RCT (Veatch, 1987).

We have been examining ethical issues of clinical research from the point of view of IRBs in securing ethically appropriate and legally correct clinical research protocols. In the remainder of the chapter, we shall examine ethical issues of research from the point of view of the physician's responsibilities to patients. At this point, a few concluding remarks about IRBs are in order.

For practical, including political and legal, reasons IRBs are limited in scope. An IRB represents the interests of its institution in securing government funding for clinical research programs. IRBs are not, therefore, in a position to change regulatory law. If there is something wrong with the law from a moral point of view, changes will have to be initiated from other quarters. However, an IRB *can* (1) ensure that protocols *at least* satisfy the ethical standards embodied in law, and (2) can *interpret* the law to some (usually minimal) extent. As an example of (2), recall that some, but not all, IRBs require that financial incentives be listed separately from benefits in the subject consent form. This is an interpretation that is not spelled out explicitly in the law.

ETHICAL ASPECTS OF
THE RESEARCHER–SUBJECT RELATIONSHIP

Once a research protocol has been approved by an IRB and a study is initiated, ethical issues may arise in the process of carrying out the research. In this section, we identify typical ethical problems for psychiatric researchers arising out of features of the special relationship between researcher and subject. These issues include the familiar topics of subject competence, informed consent, and confidentiality. In addition, we discuss less frequently examined issues, such as researcher's zeal, therapeutic misconceptions, the use of economic incentives, and other external pressures on the researcher–subject relationship.

When a patient consults a therapist for treatment, it is because the patient feels a need for help. The patient enters into a treatment relationship and authorizes treatment by giving an informed consent. The therapist incurs a duty of personal care by accepting the patient and agreeing to treat the patient in an appropriate professional manner. The researcher–subject relationship is structured differently. The researcher seeks to acquire knowledge and needs the subject to participate as part of the study. The fact that much psychiatric (and other medical research) is *also* therapeutic should not obscure the fact that the primary goal of research is the acquisition of knowledge. A researcher–therapist not only has dual loyalties, but also may have conflicting duties. As a researcher, one seeks to carry out the research protocol; as a therapist, one must seek to maximize a patient's health. The demands of the research may conflict with the clinical duties of personal care. For example, the situation is more clear in the case of nontherapeutic research. The researcher has no duty of personal care to the subject apart from that arising out of the research project itself. The researcher not only *needs* the subject for the sake of the research, but also has special *duties* to the subject in the context of the research. We have already reviewed the duties of researchers to subjects imposed by federal guidelines and implemented by IRBs. Here we want to stress the moral implications of the researchers' dependence upon and need for the subject's participation in the research. In general, because subjects are expected to submit to procedures that may inconvenience them or pose risks for the sake of the research goals, it is particularly important that researchers respect the rights and respond to the vulnerabilities of their subjects.

Competence and Informed Consent

As we previously discussed in connection with the IRB, respect for the personal autonomy of research subjects is manifested by the informed consent requirement. Whereas the IRB reviews the disclosure of information in the consent form, further ethical issues may arise in the actual process of obtaining consent from research subjects. Although the IRB has the legal authority to monitor the informed consent process, in practice it is rarely, if ever, done. Thus, researchers self-regulate the implementation of their research projects.

When a prospective subject is invited to participate in a psychiatric research project, the researcher must first assess the subject's competence to consent to be a research subject. Essentially, *competence* refers to the subject's ability to take in and assess information about the nature of the research as well as its risks and benefits. Subjects who have delusional beliefs about the research or who are disorganized in their thinking may not be competent. Subjects who are depressed or anxious may nevertheless sufficiently understand a particular research project to be deemed competent. It is the researcher's responsibility to make sure that the subjects who are enrolled in a study are competent.

For researchers who desire to enroll subjects in their studies, it may be tempting to resolve doubts about subjects' competency in favor of finding them competent. But researchers must avoid allowing their vested interest in pursuing research goals to distort competency determinations. For example, if a prospective subject suffers from a "therapeutic misconception" (i.e., that the proposed research is primarily therapy when it is not), it would be unethical for the researcher to rationalize enrolling such an incompetent subject on the grounds that the research is valuable and the risks are minimal. Understandably, a researcher who is eager to pursue a project may be inclined to enroll needed subjects even if their competence is doubtful. But the researchers' zeal should not obscure their obligation to enroll only competent subjects in the research.

Although it is the researchers' duty to seek only competent research subjects, it should not be assumed that mental illness precludes competence to consent to research. Empirical research on informed consent in psychiatric research has shown that some mental patients are competent and others are incompetent to consent to research. It is the task of the ethical researcher to select subjects from those who are competent. For subjects who are incompetent, consent for participation in research should be sought from a legally authorized representative (Benson, Roth, & Winslade, 1985).

Even if a subject is competent to consent or refuse to participate, it is also required that her or his consent be adequately informed and voluntary. It may be tempting to gloss over the appropriate information if a subject seems willing to participate, say, because of a good therapeutic relationship with the researcher or because the subject is eager to please the researcher. Or the subject may consent to the research because of real or imagined benefits extrinsic to the research that may result from participation. Once again, the researcher must guard against gaining consent in ways or for reasons the researcher suspects or knows are unethical. One example commonly offered by researchers for enrolling subjects whose competence or consent may be questionable is that research subjects get more and closer attention for their personal and other health needs. This favored status toward research subjects on grounds unrelated to research is exploitative of them and discriminating toward other patients. Thus, it is doubly unethical.

It may be a *consequence* of participation in research that subjects are monitored more closely and thereby receive benefits. The benefit is a good thing, but the promise of or potential for such an extrinsic benefit is not a relevant moral reason for enrolling a research subject in a study.

Incentives for Participating in Research

Some subjects are motivated to participate in research because they endorse or share investigators' goals of acquiring new knowledge about human behavior and mental disorder. Others are willing to participate if asked, but may have no special interest in the goals of research. Still others are willing to participate because of the incentives that are offered, usually monetary compensation or its equivalent in privileges. Are such incentives morally appropriate?

We believe that the use of monetary incentives that directly benefit subjects are not objectionable in principle. If a subject receives a benefit that would otherwise not be provided and to which the subject is not entitled, then it is not unethical to offer it, especially if few or minimal risks are taken to gain the benefit. As we argued earlier, however, this is not a benefit of the research as such, but a result of the carrying out of the research project. Compensation for inconvenience or risk is not inherently unethical. It is the exploitation of the incompetent, the uninformed, or the involuntary subject that is wrong.

A practice that we find more questionable than direct monetary benefits to research subjects is the payment of fees to well-situated recruiters, such as physicians, nurses, or other professionals, for referrals. Although we acknowledge the pragmatic value of such practices, we wonder if the subtle influence on prospective subjects from professionals not engaged in the research is appropriate. The idea of direct payment to subjects seems both more beneficial to the subjects and more directly responsive to their preferences.

Financial incentives to research subjects may be appropriate, especially if the subject does not share the goals of the researcher. We commonly accept this means of recruiting subjects for nontherapeutic research. It should be no less permissible in situations of psychiatric research when a therapeutic relationship may also be present. To deny financial rewards to a subject because of a therapeutic relationship seems implicitly to exploit the therapeutic relationship for purposes of research. If research is conducted more as an arms-length commercial transaction to benefit subjects economically while advancing the goals of research, the process may be a Pareto optimum for all parties (i.e., everyone is better off and no one is worse off). As we argued earlier, however, the line between a legitimate incentive and a subtle coercion may be hard to draw.

Confidentiality

It is generally agreed that confidentiality of personal information about research subjects should be protected as fully as possible. Psychiatric research records are particularly sensitive documents. The fact that a person is a psychiatric patient at all may be embarrassing or may threaten employment or personal relationships. Psychiatric research may deal with intimate feelings or unusual conduct. Some research, such as drug and alcohol or violence studies, concern socially or legally unacceptable behavior. Here special federal privacy protections are available to protect subjects and facilitate research. Even psychiatric research that poses no special risks about confidentiality deserves careful protection because of respect for subjects' personal rights.

The promise of confidentiality should be supported in practice by records that are kept in a secure place, free from the likelihood of disclosure to unauthorized persons. Research records, unlike medical records, are not routinely subject to review or release to insurance companies, government agencies, or other authorized third parties. Thus, research records should in practice be kept separate as much as possible from a subject's medical records. In the case of therapeutic research, this may not always be feasible. In any case, research records that may contain sensitive personal information not directly related to the research should not be revealed to anyone other than those with a legitimate need to have access to the records.

As with all medical records containing personal information, efforts must be made to prevent gossip about research subjects' past history or present behavior. By their attitudes and practices, researchers convey to their colleagues and their subjects their respect for the dignity of their subjects. Ensuring the privacy and confidentiality of research subjects' personal information, even if disclosure would not be perceived as harmful, is one way that professionals show respect for the personal autonomy and rights of their subjects.

THE RIGHT TO PARTICIPATE IN RESEARCH

Thus far, we have emphasized the duties of researchers to protect the rights and interests of psychiatric patients who may be cognitively or emotionally impaired. We have also stressed that IRBs must anticipate and prevent exploitation of vulnerable patients and patient populations. As our discussion of economic incentives for participating in research indicates, research subjects are subject to external pressures. They are also subject to institutional forces as well as transference relationships with their therapists who may also be researchers. We should not overlook the fact that research subjects may not be incompetent, vulnerable, or easily influenced. Furthermore, if we really take informed consent seriously, we must keep in mind that the right to consent to research presupposes a right to participate in research. If regulation of research becomes overloaded by bureaucratic rules, subjects may be discouraged from participating and researchers may disregard the rules. It is critical that regulation of research does not become overly paternalistic toward either researchers or subjects.

In addition to the formalities required by the informed consent process, it is important to keep in mind the ethical values which underlie it. The increased emphasis on informed consent in research grows out of an appreciation of the personal rights of research subjects and the professional responsibilities of researchers. But this appreciation, in turn, rests upon respect for the individuals involved and the integrity of their relationship in a research context. The informed consent requirement is based upon the reciprocity that provides moral support for the relationship.

Reciprocity is not satisfied, however, merely by going through the motions of signing consent forms. Researchers must make a serious effort to communicate effectively with their subjects. Just as therapists owe a duty of personal care to their patients, researchers owe a duty of personal communication with their subjects. Such communication may even require education of psychiatric research subjects: for example, to dispel therapeutic misconceptions or relieve conscious or unconscious anxieties about being a research subject. Thorough

communication with potential subjects allows those who are willing to participate in research to overcome their doubts and those who desire to refuse to be
adequately informed (Fried, 1974).

We want to emphasize that,in addition to the information provided to
research subjects, the manner in which it is presented is of ethical importance.
Researchers who respect their subjects as persons will seek to present proposed
research to subjects in a way that recognizes a subject's particular personal
capacities, vulnerabilities, and sensitivities. For example, with a subject who is
passive, it may be necessary to encourage that person to ask questions or explore
feelings. With a subject who is distrustful of the researcher, it may be desirable
to give the subject time to think over and reread information about the research.
Therapists who are also researchers may want to utilize third parties to seek
consent from the therapists' patients. Even though such a practice may not be
legally required, it may be ethically preferable.

Special attention to the manner in which research subjects are approached
when asked to participate in research has two ethical dimensions. First, the
manner in which a prospective subject is treated may show not only respect for
the subject's personal feelings, but also for the integrity of the researcher–
subject relationship. Second, the manner in which subjects are approached can
also enhance the appearance of propriety of the research project. Psychiatric
research is subject to professional, legal, and public scrutiny. If all aspects of it
are conducted in a manner that provides evidence of respect for subjects as well
as for scientific validity, the search for knowledge will be reinforced by high
standards of professional ethics.

REFERENCES

Benson, P., Roth, L., & Winslade, W. J. (1985). Informed consent in psychiatric research: Preliminary
    findings from an ongoing investigation. *Social Science and Medicine, 20*, 1331–1341.
Fried, C. (1974). *Medical experimentation: Personal integrity and social policy.* New York: American
    Elsevier Publishing.
Levine, R. (1986). *Ethics and regulation of clinical research* (2nd ed.). Baltimore: Urban & Schwarzen-
    berg.
Macklin, R. (1989). The paradoxical case of payment as benefit to research subjects. *IRB: A Review of
    Human Subject Research, 11*(6), 1–3.
Veatch, R. (1987). *The patient as partner.* Bloomington and Indianapolis: Indiana University Press.

PART II

RESEARCH DESIGN
STRATEGIES

CHAPTER 3

Single-Case Designs

MICHEL HERSEN

INTRODUCTION

The evaluation of the single case has had a long and varied history, ranging from the case study method of psychoanalysis to the careful experimental analysis of behavior from the laboratories of operantly oriented psychologists. As an experimental method, single-case designs were first applied to clinical problems by Shapiro (1966) and then were received with great favor by the behavior therapists, who used them to evaluate the efficacy of their newly developed therapeutic strategies (Barlow & Hersen, 1973; Barlow, Blanchard, Hayes, & Epstein, 1977; Hersen, 1990; Hersen & Barlow, 1976; Martin & Epstein, 1976; Risley & Wolf, 1972; Thoresen, 1972; Thomas, 1978; Yates, 1970). First categorized for use in psychiatric research by Barlow and Hersen (1973), single-case experimental designs (in which the patient serves as his or her own control) were described as an "alternative approach" to the more costly and time-consuming group designs, in which experimental and control conditions (using carefully matched patients) are contrasted.

In their 1973 article in the *Archives of General Psychiatry*, Barlow and Hersen, aside from underscoring the issue of cost in large-scale outcome research, pointed out the ethical dilemma in withholding treatment or providing only placebo treatment for control patients in group comparison studies. Several other disadvantages of the group comparison method and advantages of the single-

Michel Hersen • Center for Psychological Studies, Nova University, Fort Lauderdale, Florida 33314.
Research in Psychiatry: Issues, Strategies, and Methods, edited by L. K. George Hsu and Michel Hersen. Plenum Press, New York, 1992.

case strategy were outlined in that paper. The first is concerned with *masked* findings, in which some patients in an experimental group improve as a function of treatment whereas other patients worsen, thus statistically canceling out the overall effect. Indeed, this is the clearest illustration of the group comparison design's not allowing for the specific evaluation of unique patient characteristics correlated with improvement or deterioration. By contrast, in the single-case experimental design, such uniqueness of response becomes the object of the analysis. In instances where treatment fails, innovation involving application of novel approaches is evaluated experimentally in the single-case approach.

The second issue concerns statistical versus clinical change. In the single-case design, the experimenter is intent on maximizing therapeutic application and in evincing large clinical changes that have impact on the patient's condition. By contrast, often in group-controlled studies, if the N is sufficiently large, small but basically therapeutically insignificant changes will attain statistical significance. This, of course, has only limited value to the practicing clinician, who must bring about *major* improvements in patients. On the other hand, the single-case experimental analysis permits the experimenter to vary therapeutic conditions (e.g., successively adding treatments) so that clinical significance is attained.

The third issue relates to the mechanisms of therapeutic change. Given its flexibility in adding and subtracting therapeutic strategies from a composite treatment approach, single-case designs are therefore most useful in identifying the "therapeutically active ingredients" of a multicomponent therapy (Barlow & Hersen, 1973, p. 320).

The fourth consideration is the patient's variable response pattern typically seen during the course of treatment. In this instance, there are advantages in using single-case methodology, given that repeated measurements are taken throughout baseline and treatment phases of study. By contrast, in the usual application of group comparison methodology, assessments are limited to pretreatment, midpoint, termination, and follow-up. Thus, the vicissitudes of the therapeutic process are not reflected with complete accuracy in group comparison designs.

There are a number of additional features of the single-case approach that make it a useful tool in the armamentarium of the clinical researcher operating in the psychiatric setting. Given the close relationship between treatment and assessment in the varied single-case strategies, the experimenter is able to determine the ability of a given treatment to exert control over the dependent measures. By introducing, removing, and then reintroducing treatment, the short-term strength of its application can be readily determined. Also, for rare disorders, where the small N would preclude matching experimentals and controls, the single-case approach proves to be invaluable. The same holds true for unusual variants of more standard diagnostic categories where a similar small N exists.

Related to the aforementioned is the complementary use of single-case and group comparison designs. I should point out to the reader that there are specific occasions when the two approaches can be used in tandem. Consider the case where two novel treatment approaches have been developed for a specific disorder. Rather than rushing off to carry out a 3- to 5-year, long-term, group outcome study that will literally cost the National Institute of Mental Health (NIMH) a million dollars, it behooves the methodical clinical researcher to first document the controlling effects of the two treatments in single-case analyses. In so doing, the therapeutic procedures (be they pharmacological or psychological) can be refined, with some of their limitations and possibly side effects identified. At that point, when good therapeutic control over dependent measures has been documented and a treatment manual developed, a contrast between the two approaches in a group-controlled study would be warranted. Indeed, given the pilot work carried out using single-case methodology, the clinical researcher is more likely to be testing two *viable treatments*, thus enhancing the probability of uncovering clinically and statistically important information for the scientific community.

In the sections that follow, the mechanics and general procedures of single-case research will be presented. Included are discussions of Repeated Measurement, Choosing a Baseline, Changing One Variable at a Time, Length of Phases, and Evaluating Irreversible Procedures. Next to be considered are some of the design strategies typically used in single-case research: A-B-A-B Design, Interaction Designs, Multiple-Baseline Designs, the Changing-Criterion Design, and Other Design Options. This is followed by an analysis of the particular issues faced in carrying out drug treatment using single-case evaluations. For most of the designs outlined and described, published examples originating from the psychiatric setting serve as illustrations. The chapter concludes with an examination of the case against and for statistical analysis and a discussion of replication in single-case research.

REPEATED MEASUREMENT

A unique aspect of single-case research is that measurements are taken repeatedly during baseline and treatment phases, thus permitting an analysis of trends in the data. Included, of course, are the observation of motoric behavior (e.g., out-of-seat for an attention deficit-hyperactivity child), physiological functioning (e.g., heart rate in a phobic individual when confronted with the fear-inducing object), and the evaluation of the cognitive-attitudinal state of the patient (e.g., the score on a self-report inventory of depression).

Whatever the measurement system being used,

> the operations involved in obtaining such measurements . . . must be clearly specified, observable, public, and replicable in all respects. . . . Secondly, measurements taken repeatedly, especially over extended periods of time must be done under exacting and totally standardized conditions with respect to measurement devices used, personnel involved, time or times of day . . . instructions to the subject, and the specific environmental conditions (e.g., location) where the measurement session occurs. (Hersen & Barlow, 1976, p. 71)

As noted by Hersen (1982),

Each of the measurement systems poses some unique challenges to the single-case
researcher. When motoric measures are taken and human observers are used, independent reliability checks are required. These reliability checks can be expressed
either as a percentage of agreement for interval data (with 80% considered minimally
acceptable) or as a correlation for continuous data (with $r = .80$ considered minimally
acceptable). (p. 92)

For comprehensive surveys of behavioral assessment strategies, the reader is
referred to Bellack and Hersen (1988) and Hersen and Bellack (1988).

Special problems are posed when physiological measures are repeatedly
taken. Hersen (1990) has underscored that, as part of standardization, not only
must the clinical researcher be concerned with appropriate functioning of the
equipment, but he or she must be attuned to the patient's adaptation to such
equipment. Fatigability can become a major confound, if the intertrial interval is
too short. This can be a particularly vexing problem when male sexual arousal is
being assessed. Decreased sexual responsivity may not necessarily reflect
therapeutic amelioration but simply may be a function of fatigue. Here the
clinical researcher must exert care to avoid arriving at erroneous conclusions.

On the other hand, the use of self-report data in single-case research is
fraught with other problems, such as responding in a fashion perceived by the
patient to be consistent with clinical expectation. However, by using alternate
forms of a scale or correlating self-report data with the motoric and physiological
channels, some of the problems can be avoided. Nonetheless, the clinical
researcher must keep in mind the data in the behavioral literature that show
general desynchrony among the motoric, physiological, and cognitive channels
(Hersen, 1973, 1978). Irrespective of desynchrony among the three channels,
how the patient feels must always be given credence (Hersen, 1978). Indeed, if
improvements were to occur only in the motoric and physiological channels, it is
questionable if treatment could be considered totally successful.

Finally, there is a specific problem faced by clinical researchers who conduct
single-case research in the inpatient psychiatric setting that affects standardization of the data collected. Given the change of shifts and the significant
differences in composition and attitude of the day, afternoon, evening, and
weekend personnel, the precision of data collection times and the consistency of
data collectors are of enormous import; otherwise, confounds in the data are
likely to appear.

CHOOSING A BASELINE

In most single-case experimental designs the initial period of observation
involves the natural frequency of occurrence of the behavior of interest and is
referred to as the *baseline phase* (labeled A). The A phase serves as the standard
by which subsequent treatment phases are contrasted. Ideally, assessment of
baseline results in a stable pattern of data, thus facilitating the interpretation of

treatment effects in the B phase. Frequently, however, stability of data is not the pattern that emerges.

In contrast to researchers who use animals, the clinical researcher will find that the ability to develop or select a baseline is considerably more constricted. Indeed, the clinical researcher does not have the luxury of "creating" ideal baseline conditions and must accept the baseline pattern that is found. Since the clinical researcher is frequently under time constraints (especially in the inpatient setting), there are fewer opportunities to experimentally evaluate reasons for such baseline variability. As noted by Hersen (1982) "sometimes adjustment in the measurement scale being used may reduce extensive variability. That is, at times, the measurement interval may not be appropriate for the behavior under study and therefore leads to extraneous variability" (p. 93).

Let us now consider the most frequently encountered baseline patterns, originally identified by Hersen and Barlow (1976). Although the patterns listed in Table 1 are representative, other possibilities, of course, do exist.

The first issue in selecting a baseline concerns the number of data points required to identify a trend. The minimum acceptable number, by convention, is three (Barlow & Hersen, 1973). However, at times, when the pattern is highly variable or extreme, more points are indicated. On the other hand, when institution of treatment may be emergent (e.g., severe head banging, suicidality), for obvious reasons the exigencies of therapeutics will supersede the elegance of experimental purity, and baseline assessment will be minimized.

With three successively increasing points, an upward trend in the data is established. Conversely, of course, three successively decreasing points represents a decreased trend in the data. In addition to trend, the single-case researcher is interested in the slope of the curve, with the steeper slopes indicating greater power. Although statistical strategies for evaluating slopes have been developed (see Kazdin, 1984), the vast majority of single-case researchers rely on visual inspection (cf. Huitema, 1985; Jones, Vaught, & Weinrott, 1977; Wampold & Worsham, 1986) to analyze their results.

Table 1. Baseline Pattern

1. Stable baseline
2. Increasing baseline (target behavior worsening)
3. Decreasing baseline (target behavior improving)
4. Variable baseline
5. Variable-stable baseline
6. Increasing-decreasing baseline
7. Decreasing-increasing baseline
8. Unstable baseline

Note. From "Single-Case Experimental Designs" by M. Hersen in *International Handbook of Behavior Modification and Therapy*, edited by A. S. Bellack, M. Herson, and A. E. Kazdin, 1982, Table 1. New York: Plenum Press. Copyright 1982 by Plenum Press. Reprinted by permission.

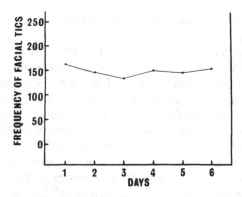

Figure 1.   The stable baseline. Hypothetical data for mean numbers of facial tics averaged over three daily 15-min videotaped sessions. From *Single-Case Experimental Designs* (Fig. 3-1, p. 77) by M. Hersen and D. H. Barlow, 1976, New York: Pergamon Press. Copyright 1976 by Pergamon Press. Reprinted by permission.

A quintessential example of the stable baseline is seen in Figure 1. Given that there is little variability (i.e., no upward or downward trend), institution of treatment after this pattern should lead to a clear interpretation: no change in improvement or worsening.

The second baseline trend listed in Table 1 is the increasing baseline in which there is worsening of the target behavior (e.g., tics increasing in rate). With this pattern, if treatment is successful, a reversal of the trend will be noted, allowing for a clear interpretation of the data. On the other hand, if treatment has no effect, then the slope of the curve will remain the same. The most problematic case occurs when it is difficult from the resulting data to determine whether there is a mere continuation of the trend begun in baseline or whether the trend represents a deterioration induced by the treatment. If there is a marked change in the slope of the curve from baseline to treatment, the interpretation of deterioration because of treatment would be justified.

The third pattern, in which the baseline is decreasing and the target behavior is improving, presents problems for immediate interpretation. Is it simply a continuation of the trend seen in baseline? Here treatment would have to be removed and reinstated to fully evaluate its controlling effects on the target behavior. On the other hand, if treatment that follows the decreasing baseline makes the patient worse, a clear reversed trend in the data will be apparent, and an unambiguous interpretation is possible.

The fourth pattern, the variable baseline, is depicted in Figure 2. Examination of the figure reveals a tic frequency that ranges from 24 to 255, with a pattern, often seen in clinical research, of alternating low- and high-data points. One strategy for dealing with this pattern, at least cosmetically, is to "block" the data by averaging tic frequency across two day periods. Although visually improved, the basic pattern remains, making interpretation of subsequently

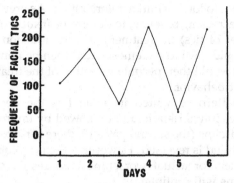

Figure 2. The variable baseline. Hypothetical data for mean number of facial tics averaged over three 15-min videotaped sessions. From *Single-Case Experimental Designs* (Fig. 3-4, p. 79) by M. Hersen and D. H. Barlow, 1976, New York: Pergamon Press. Copyright 1976 by Pergamon Press. Reprinted by permission.

applied treatment difficult unless there is a massive reduction of both variability and tic frequency. With this pattern, the possibility exists that the wrong measurement strategy is in place and that perhaps it should be replaced.

The fifth pattern, as presented in Table 1, is referred to as the variable-stable baseline. Having initial variability, the clinical researcher continues baseline assessment until stability appears. At that point, treatment can be initiated and a meaningful interpretation of its effects can be determined. However, the problem here is that in inpatient settings such extension may not be possible for ethical, pragmatic (i.e., the time factor), or clinical considerations (self-injurious or aggressive behaviors).

The sixth pattern that appears in Figure 3 (increasing then decreasing)

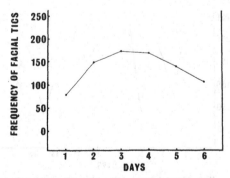

Figure 3. The increasing-decreasing baseline. Hypothetical data for mean number of facial tics averaged over three daily 15-min videotaped sessions. From *Single-Case Experimental Designs* (Fig. 3-6, p. 81) by M. Hersen and D. H. Barlow, 1976, New York: Pergamon Press. Copyright 1976 by Pergamon Press. Reprinted by permission.

involves improvement following initial deterioration. As previously described in the section on the decreasing baseline, to determine if subsequent improvement (diminished number of tics) in treatment is a continuation of the decreasing trend, treatment would have to be removed and then be reinstated. The resulting A-B-A-B design would then permit evaluation of the treatment's controlling effects on the target behavior.

The seventh pattern presented in Table 1 is the decreasing-increasing baseline and involves initial deterioration followed by improvement. As noted for the increasing baseline (the second pattern), there is no problem if treatment is effective and the trend is reversed. However, there is a problem when there is no effect of treatment or actual worsening as a result, since the trend of worsening symptoms will continue.

The unstable baseline, which is depicted in Figure 4, is the final pattern that we will consider. As the reader will note, the baseline in this instance has been extended with the hope that variability would diminish. However, this has not happened, and unless subsequent treatment is very powerful and significantly decreases variability, the ensuing experimental analysis will not confirm the controlling effects of treatment.

CHANGING ONE VARIABLE AT A TIME

In single-case research, only one variable is altered from one phase to the succeeding one (Hersen, 1990; Hersen & Barlow, 1976). This basic tenet holds whether the first, middle, or last phase is being evaluated. It should be clear that if two variables (i.e., treatments) were to be introduced simultaneously from baseline to treatment, it would not be possible to determine which of the two contributes most or is responsible for change in the target measure.

The one variable rule is best exemplified by the A-B-A-B design, in which

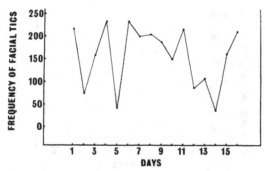

Figure 4. The unstable baseline. Hypothetical data for mean number of facial tics averaged over three daily 15-min videotaped sessions. From *Single-Case Experimental Designs* (Fig. 3-8, p. 82) by M. Hersen and D. H. Barlow, 1976, New York: Pergamon Press. Copyright 1976 by Pergamon Press. Reprinted by permission.

only one variable is manipulated from one phase to the next (baseline, followed by treatment, treatment removed, treatment reinstated). At times, the B phase consists of a compound treatment involving several therapeutic techniques. Therefore, in the A-B-A-B design that evaluates a compound treatment, the unique contribution of each of the components cannot be ascertained. But in the A-B-A-B-BC-B design, where A is baseline, B is one treatment component, and C is a second treatment component, the separate effects of B and the additive effects of C over B can be determined without violating the one variable rule.

The most frequently encountered examples of the violation of the one variable rule are found in the A-B-A-C design and in the A-B-A-BC design. In the former example, the investigator incorrectly assumes that differential effects of A and C can be determined but fails to take into account the possible sequencing effects of the two treatments. In the latter example, the investigator incorrectly assumes that the addition of C over B in the BC phase can be contrasted with the B phase. But here, too, the possible sequencing effects of B and BC are ignored. In general, failure to adhere to the one variable tenet occurs at the end of the experimental analysis.

It should be underscored that the one variable rule has special implications for drug evaluations. In this instance, if the investigator were to follow baseline (A) with active drug treatment (B), the intermediary step of placebo (A') is omitted, thus altering two variables at a time. The more appropriate sequence, however, would involve baseline assessment (A), placebo (A'), active drug (B), a return to placebo (A'), and the reinstatement of the active drug (B).

LENGTH OF THE PHASES

In the ideal single-case analysis, the number of data points per phase is relatively equal. Otherwise, if for example data points in treatment far exceed those obtained in the preceding baseline, it is possible that changes seen are due to the extended time factor and not to the treatment itself. However, additional factors contribute to the actual lengths of phases, such as staff reactions, ethical and treatment considerations, time limitations, and the relative length of adjacent phases. It should be obvious that when evaluated behaviors include aggression and self-injury, baseline measurements will by necessity be shortened, as contrasted to the longer treatment phases. Here, clinical considerations are of greater concern than experimental elegance. Conversely, in some single-case studies, where the short-term effects of treatments are evaluated, intervention phases (B) will be shortened so that treatment effects do not become permanent and baseline (A)responding can be recovered (e.g., the second A phase in the A-B-A-B design).

An excellent and ideal example of the length of adjacent phases is seen in Figure 5. In this A-B-A-B study (Miller, 1973), retention control training (a behavioral treatment strategy) was applied to a child suffering from secondary enuresis. The number of enuretic episodes and the frequency of daily urination

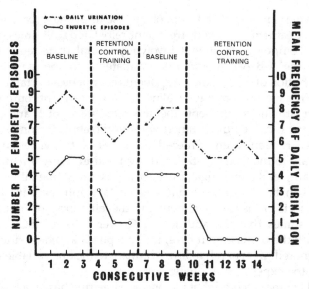

Figure 5. Number of enuretic episodes per week and mean number of daily urinations per week for Subject 1. From "An Experimental Analysis of Retention Control Training in the Treatment of Nocturnal Enuresis in Two Institutionalized Adolescents" by P. M. Miller, 1973, *Behavior Therapy*, 4, p. 291, Fig. 1. Copyright 1973 by Academic Press. Reprinted by permission.

served as the target measures. From the relatively stable baseline (A), the reader will note the marked effects of treatment (B), and then a worsening of symptoms when baseline procedures were reinstated (the second A phase). However, when treatment (B) was reinstated, this last phase was extended from 3 to 5 data points (i.e., weeks) to ensure the subsequent permanence of the effect. Such extension is a common practice for obvious reasons in the second B phase of the A-B-A-B design. Nonetheless, Miller's study nicely illustrates the equivalence of phases in the A-B-A portion of the study.

EVALUATING IRREVERSIBLE PROCEDURES

In single-case research, the majority of therapeutic strategies that are implemented (e.g., feedback, social reinforcement, punishment techniques, short-acting pharmacological agents) can be withdrawn and reinstated repeatedly, thus permitting such analyses as the A-B-A-B design. However, in the technical sense, instructional sets cannot be withdrawn, since they remain part of the patient's cognitive set. Thus, discontinuation of instructions is not analogous to the removal of some kind of reinforcement or the short-acting drug, methylphenidate. However, instructional sets can be evaluated in alternative single-case strategies, such as in the multiple-baseline design (cf. Hersen &

Bellack, 1976), and as a constant across phases of a variety of single-case analyses (e.g., Kallman, Hersen, & O'Toole, 1975). In addition, the manipulation of an instructional set from a positive to a negative expectation has been evaluated in a variant of the basic A-B-A-B design (Barlow, Agras, Leitenberg, Callahan, & Moore, 1972).

A-B-A-B DESIGN

The A-B-A-B design is a simple albeit powerful single-case strategy that can be used to document the controlling effects of treatment over the target(s) selected for modification. (I have briefly presented an illustration of the design [Miller, 1973] in the section on Length of Phases.) Let us now consider the specific logic underlying the use of the A-B-A-B design. In the A-B-A-B design, the natural frequency of the behavior under consideration is first evaluated in baseline (A), followed by implementation of treatment in B. If improvement in B is noted, removal of treatment in the second A phase serves to confirm experimental control over the targeted measure. Then, when B is reinstated and improvement once again occurs, there is the second opportunity to show the controlling effects of treatment over the dependent measure.

Lombardo and Turner (1979) used an A-B-A-B design to examine the effects of thought stopping in a 26-year-old male psychiatric inpatient whose severe obsessions focused on "imaginal relationships" he had with other patients on the ward during previous hospitalizations. Despite the patient's attempts to control obsessive ruminations via distraction, he failed to reduce the intensity of his symptoms.

Throughout the study, the patient was instructed to note the beginning and ending times of each obsessive episode. This permitted determination of the rate of ruminations and the total time per day spent ruminating. Baseline involved a 6-day observation period followed by introduction of thought stopping on Day 7. Thought stopping consisted of the patient's raising his right index finger whenever he had obtained a vivid obsessive image. Then the therapist shouted, "Stop," and the patient lowered his finger. To fade the "Stop" intensity, the therapist first shouted "Stop," then said it loudly, subsequently used a normal speaking voice, then said it softly, and finally whispered it. The patient subsequently verbalized "Stop" covertly. "Depending upon how rapidly the patient gained control, four to six repetitions of stopping were used at each voice intensity" (Lombardo & Turner, 1979, p. 269). Treatment was discontinued on Day 18 and was reinstated on Day 28. Also, a 6-week follow-up evaluation was included in this single-case analysis.

Results of the Lombardo and Turner A-B-A-B design are presented in Figure 6. With the exception of Day 5, baseline (A) was completely stable (modal response = 40 min). Introduction of thought stopping in B led to a marked diminution of obsessiveness. Removal of treatment in the second baseline (A) led to renewed obsessiveness, indeed, above the levels seen in the initial baseline

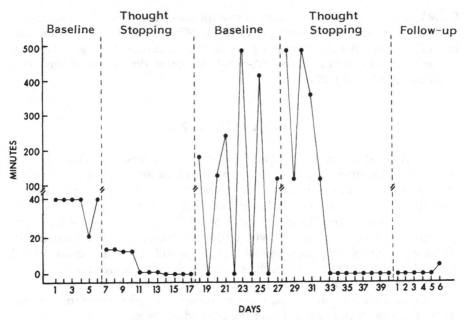

Figure 6. Duration of obsessive ruminations during baseline, treatment, and 6-week follow up. From "Thought-Stopping in the Control of Obsessive Ruminations" by T. W. Lombardo and S. M. Turner, 1979, *Behavior Modification*, 3, p. 271, Fig. 1. Copyright 1979 by Sage Publications. Reprinted by permission.

although considerably more unstable. On Day 27, thought stopping was reinstated and once more led to dramatic improvements to a 0-level on Days 33 to 40. Zero-level obsessiveness was maintained throughout the first few weeks of the follow-up but rose slightly during Week 6.

Despite the apparent dramatic success of thought-stopping treatment with this patient, the results are tempered by the fact that there were no controls implemented for the effects of instructions and patient and therapist expectancies. Of course, given the use of self-report data, such extraneous variables are more likely to have an effect, as contrasted to when motoric and physiological measures are employed.

INTERACTION DESIGNS

The vast majority of psychological treatments contain several components and, given the constraints of the one variable rule across phases, the possible additive effects of such components can be evaluated in interaction designs. In one such single-case analysis, Kallman *et al.* (1975) examined the effects of reinforcing standing (B phase), reinforcing standing and walking (BC phase), and reinforcing standing and walking with the aid of a walker (BCD phase) in a patient whose conversion reaction took the form of not being able to walk. The resulting design included six phases, with only one variable manipulated from one phase to the next: (1) B, (2) BC, (3) B, (4) BC, (5) BCD, and (6) BC. The reader will note that the addition of C over B in Phase 2, its subsequent removal in Phase 3, and its reintroduction in Phase 4 permit an evaluation of its additional controlling effects. Similarly, in Phase 5, the addition of D over BC and removal in Phase 6 allow for an evaluation of its controlling effects.

Numerous permutations of the interaction design exist, including the following illustration of an A-B-BC-B-BC design that evaluated the effects of reinforcement (B) and feedback (C) in the eating behavior of an anorexia nervosa patient (Agras, Barlow, Chapin, Abel, & Leitenberg, 1974). During the course of this single-case analysis, the patient was presented with four, 1,500 calorie meals a day. In the reinforcement condition, the patient was accorded privileges contingent on weight gain. In feedback, the patient was given information about her weight, caloric intake, and mouthfuls actually consumed.

Results of the interaction design appear in Figure 7, indicating a slight weight increase during baseline but a diminished caloric intake. With introduction of reinforcement, there was decreased weight and caloric intake. By contrast, with the addition of feedback to reinforcement in Phase 3, a substantial

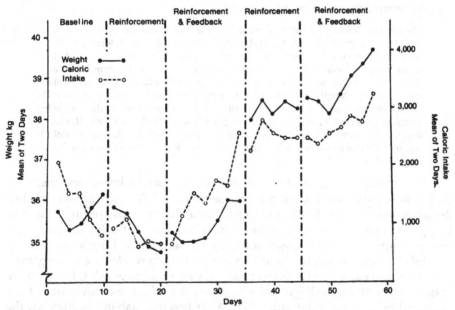

Figure 7. Data from an experiment examining the effect of feedback on the eating behavior of a patient with anorexia nervosa. From "Behavior Modification of Anorexia Nervosa" by W. S. Agras et al., 1974, *Archives of General Psychiatry, 30*, p. 283, Fig. 4. Copyright 1974 by the American Medical Association. Reprinted by permission.

increase in weight and caloric intake was noted. But this leveled off when feedback was removed in Phase 4. Finally, in Phase 5, feedback was reinstated and resulted in another marked increase in weight and caloric intake. To summarize, results of this interaction design confirm the controlling effects of feedback on caloric intake and weight gain, but do not provide confirmation of the effects of reinforcement.

MULTIPLE-BASELINE DESIGNS

Multiple-baseline designs can be used to evaluate psychological treatments that are not subject to clear discontinuation, such as in the case of instructions, or where several targets independent of each other are selected for modification. First described in 1968 by Baer, Risley, and Wolf,

> In the multiple-baseline technique, a number of responses are identified and meas-
> ured over time to provide baselines against which changes can be evaluated. With
> these baselines established, the experimenter then applies an experimental variable to
> one of the behaviors, produces a change in it, and perhaps notes little or no change
> in the other baselines. (p. 94)

Subsequently the investigator applies the same treatment to the next target and continues treatment until a preset criterion has been attained. Treatment is only applied to the independent targets when there is general baseline stability.

As previously noted by Hersen (1982),

> The strategy described above is referred to as the *multiple-baseline design across behav-*
> *iors.* An assumption, of course, is that the targeted behaviors are independent of one
> another. Otherwise, treatment for one may lead to covariation in a second, thus
> obfuscating the controlling effects of the treatment. In essence, the multiple-baseline
> design across behaviors is a series of A-B designs, with every succeeding A phase
> applied to one targeted behavior until treatment has finally been applied to each.
> Treatment effects are inferred from the untreated baselines. That is, the controlling
> effects of treatment on dependent measures are documented if, and only if, change
> occurs when treatment is directly applied. In this respect, the design certainly is
> weaker than that in the A-B-A-B design, where the effects of controlling variables are
> directly shown. (p. 108)

In addition to the multiple-baseline design across behaviors, there are (1) the multiple-baseline design across settings and (2) the multiple-baseline design across subjects. In the multiple-baseline design across settings, the *same behavior* is targeted for modification across two or more settings, with the same treatment applied in time-lagged fashion in the second and third setting. In the multiple-baseline design across subjects (actually not a single-case strategy in its strictest sense since several subjects are treated simultaneously), two or more patients with identical diagnoses and exposed to the same environment are evaluated in baseline at the same time. After baseline stability is attained, the first patient is treated. Then, in time-lagged fashion, after baseline assessment has been extended for the second patient, that individual is accorded the identical treatment. Such sequencing continues until all patients have been treated. The logic of this design is the same as the multiple-baseline design across behaviors, in that treatment effects are inferred from the untreated baselines: in this instance, the untreated patient.

An excellent example of a multiple-baseline design across behaviors appears in a study by Goldstein and Malec (1989). In this investigation, the subjects were six chronic alcoholics who suffered from "alcohol amnesic syndrome." Here we will focus on Subject 6 whose baseline performance on five orientation items (Doctor's Name, Hospital's Name, Head Nurse's Name, Canteen Location, and Trainer's Name) was *incorrect* in each instance. After five sessions of baseline data collection, memory training was instituted in Session 6 for the "Doctor's Name." memory training involved providing this patient with the correct response to the question followed by his repeating the correct answer 20 times, with a 2-minute rest after 10 repetitions. The criterion to move onto the second item was the correct recall on 4 of 5 consecutive days during probe sessions or the completion of 10 days of training.

Results of the multiple-baseline analysis, depicted in Figure 8, clearly indicate that when treatment was directly applied to the specific target, only then was improvement in memory noted. Indeed, training on one item (e.g., Doctor's Name) did not yield concurrent improvement on the next item (Hospital's Name) until that item was specifically targeted with memory training. Therefore, the results confirm the controlling effects of memory training when specifically applied to each of the five items.

I will not present an example of the multiple-baseline design across settings since it is quite similar to the multiple-baseline design across behaviors, with the exception that there is one target that is treated sequentially and cumulatively across the several settings. However, I will illustrate use of the multiple-baseline design across subjects, since this strategy obviously represents a moderate departure from using only one subject. In a recent study, Morin, Kowatch, and Wade (1989) used the multiple-baseline design across subjects to evaluate the efficacy of behavioral procedures to reduce total "awake time" in three patients who were suffering from insomnia, secondary to work-related lower and upper back pain. Patient 1 was a 46-year-old African-American female with a 5-year history of low back pain and sleep-maintenance insomnia for more than 1 year. Patient 2 was a 35-year-old while male with a 1½-year history of neck, back, and shoulder pain and onset and sleep-maintenance insomnia of more than 1 year. Patient 3 was a 46-year-old African-American male with a 1-year history of back pain with concurrent sleep-maintenance insomnia. These three patients had been referred by a medically oriented pain clinic to the authors. Treatment for insomnia consisted of stimulus control instructions and a sleep restriction procedure conducted in 6 weekly 1-hour sessions. "The goals of this combined intervention were to regulate wake/sleep schedules, reassociate bed/bedroom with sleep, and consolidate sleep over a shorter period of time spent in bed" Morin *et al.* (1989, p. 297). The three patients, who were treated simultaneously, maintained sleep diaries that were corroborated by all-night polysomnography.

Results of this study are presented in Figure 9. Inspection of Figure 9

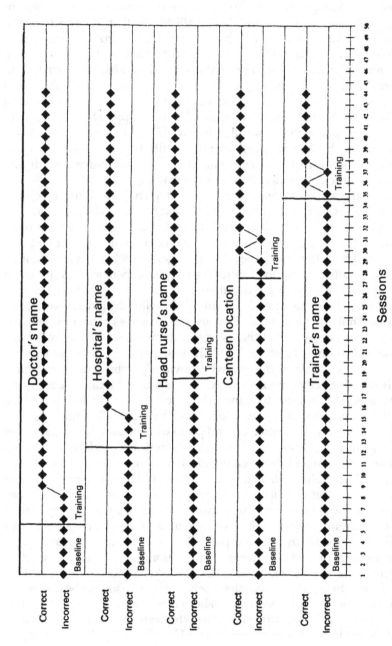

Figure 8. Training data for recall by Subject 6, used only as a criterion for correctness. From "Memory Training for Severely Amnesic Patients" by G. Goldstein and E. A. Malec, 1989, *Neuropsychology*, 3, p. 15, Fig. 6. Copyright 1989 by the Philadelphia Neuropsychology Society. Reprinted by permission.

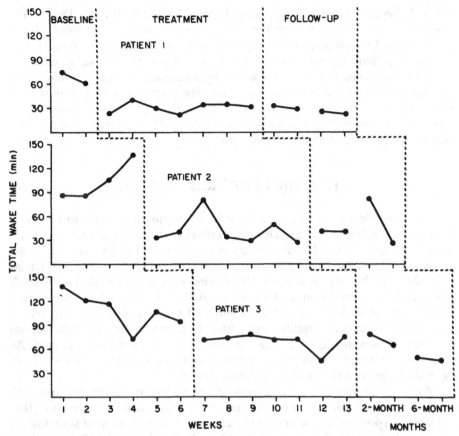

Figure 9. Weekly changes of total wake time per night across patients. From "Behavioral Management of Sleep Disturbances Secondary to Chronic Pain" by C. M. Morin, R. A. Kowatch, and J. B. Wade, 1989, *Journal of Behavior Therapy and Experimental Psychiatry*, 20, p. 298, Fig. 1. Copyright 1989 by Pergamon Press. Reprinted by permission.

indicates that for Patient 1 dramatic improvements were noted after introduction of treatment, which were maintained during the follow-up period. Similarly, for Patient 2, only when treatment was applied to him did his total wake time decrease. His gains were generally maintained during follow-up, with the exception of Month 4. Finally, when treatment was applied to Patient 3, moderate improvement was noted, with gains maintained during follow-up. However, the reader will note the downward trend during baseline, which appears to continue in treatment. Therefore, the controlling effects of treatment for Patient 3 are not completely established.

Although the Morin *et al.* (1989) study represents a nice illustration of the multiple-baseline design across subjects, there are a few minor design problems. First, it would have been better if there were three points in baseline for

Patient 1. Second, baseline might have been extended further for Patient 3 in order to obtain greater stability (i.e., no downward trend). And third, use of data accrued through polysomnography would have been more preferable than relying on patient reports of wakefulness, since these can be exaggerated.

I should point out that of the multiple-baseline designs available, the strategy across subjects is the weakest since the effects of treating one subject are inferred from the untreated subject who is awaiting treatment. Basically, we have here little more than a series of A-B designs, with each succeeding treated subject being exposed to a longer baseline.

CHANGING-CRITERION DESIGN

The most ideally suited design to evaluate shaping treatments to accelerate or decelerate behaviors is the changing-criterion design (Hartmann & Hall, 1976). The logic of this design strategy is simple and first involves a baseline assessment. Then, treatment is instituted until a preset criterion level is attained and stability at that level is achieved. Next, a more stringent criterion is selected, and treatment is applied and continued until stability at the new level is met. Changes in the second criterion are contrasted with the first criterion, which now serves as a new baseline. Treatment then progresses through several increasingly more stringent criteria until the end point criterion is attained. As the reader can see, the changing criterion design bears some similarity to both the A-B design and the multiple-baseline design.

As an illustration of the changing-criterion design, Hartmann and Hall (1976) documented deceleration of cigarette smoking using a procedure that combined response cost and reinforcement. Baseline evaluation of smoking for one subject appears in Panel A of Figure 10, and ranged from 40 to 51 cigarettes a day. In Panel B, the first treatment phase, the criterion was set at 46 cigarettes a day (a 5% decrease). If the subject smoked an additional cigarette, the response-cost assessment was $1.00 and then $2.00 for the 48th cigarette. Thus, an escalating response cost was established. Concurrently, if fewer cigarettes were smoked, then the set criterion, an increasing bonus of $0.10 per cigarette, was awarded to the subject.

A careful evaluation of the data in Figure 10 shows that each succeedingly more difficult criterion was met, thus yielding six replications of the treatment's controlling effects.

OTHER DESIGN OPTIONS

Before going on to a discussion of the evaluation of pharmacological approaches with single-case strategies, I will briefly consider some of the formulations of the multiple-baseline designs and the simultaneous treatment design.

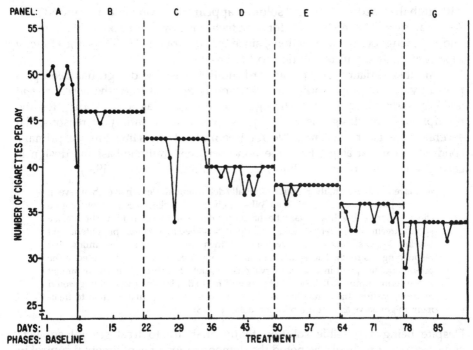

Figure 10. Data from a smoking-reduction program used to illustrate the stepwise criterion-change design. The solid horizontal lines indicate the criterion for each treatment phase. From "The Changing Criterion Design" by D. P. Hartmann and R. V. Hall, 1976, *Journal of Applied Behavior Analysis, 9*, p. 529, Fig. 2. Copyright 1976 by the Society for the Experimental Analysis of Behavior. Reprinted by permission.

Variations in Multiple-Baseline Designs

First, let us consider the case in the multiple-baseline design across behaviors, where the target behaviors may not be independent of one another and modification in the first leads to concurrent modification in the second. Following the logic of this design, then, the applied clinical researcher *has not* documented the controlling effects of treatment. However, rather than discarding such an analysis, Kazdin and Kopel (1975) argued that,

> In case of ambiguity with the effects of a multiple-baseline design, it often is possible to include a partial reversal in the design for one of the behaviors. The reversal phase, or return to baseline, need not be employed for all of the behaviors (i.e., baselines) for which data are collected. Indeed, one of the reasons for using a multiple-baseline design is to avoid the A-B-A-B design and its temporary removal of treatment. However, when the specific effect of the intervention is not evident in a multiple-baseline design, one may have to resort to a temporary withdrawal of the intervention for one of the baselines to determine the effect of the intervention. (p. 607)

Although the Kazdin and Kopel solution appears to be valuable, the added A-B-A-B strategy will be most useful for such techniques as feedback, reinforcement, and modeling, but not instructions, since they are *irreversible*. Thus, the strategy represents only a partial solution to the problem.

Another variation of the standard multiple-baseline design has been proposed by Watson and Workman (1981) and is referred to as the *nonconcurrent multiple-baseline design*. This strategy was designed as a substitute for the multiple-baseline design across subjects, when, for a variety of reasons, the several subjects are not available for treatment at the same time, a primary condition of the strategy. How the nonconcurrent multiple-baseline design is carried out is described as follows by Watson and Workman (1981):

> In this research design, the researcher initially determines the length of each of several baseline phases (e.g., 5, 10, 15 days). When a given subject becomes available (e.g., a client is referred who has the target behavior of interest and is amenable to the use of a specific treatment of interest), (s)he is randomly assigned to one of the pre-determined baseline lengths. Baseline observations are then carried out; and assuming that responding has reached acceptable stability criteria, treatment is implemented at the pre-determined point in time. Observations are continued throughout the treatment phase, as in a simple A-B design. Subjects who fail to display stable responding would be dropped from the formal investigation; however, their eventual reaction to treatment might serve as useful replication data. (p. 258)

Despite being a possible solution to the inability to treat several subjects simultaneously, it should be noted the demonstration of experimental control in the nonconcurrent multiple-baseline design is weaker than the already weak experimental control documented in the standard multiple-baseline design across subjects. Indeed, what we have here are separate A-B designs (albeit replicated) with initial baseline lengths predetermined for each subject.

Our next variation of the multiple-baseline procedure is referred to as the *multiple-probe technique* and is a recommended procedure when repeated assessment is not possible because of subject reactivity. In this instance, Horner and Baer (1978) recommended that assessment be interspersed, thereby resulting in fewer points on the graph. An example (hypothetical) of probes obtained every five days is contrasted with reported data in Figure 11. As the reader can see, hypothetical probes (solid triangles) represent quite excellent approximations of the reported data (open circles) in this illustration, lending support to the variation. However, it is unclear whether probes can always be good approximations, especially when data are more variable and/or unstable.

Simultaneous Treatment Design

Consistent with the one variable rule highlighted in an earlier section of this chapter, I have argued that the single-case strategy is best suited for evaluating specific techniques or the addition of one technique over another (e.g., the interaction design). However, there is a strategy referred to as the *simultaneous treatment design*, in which it is possible to compare two or more

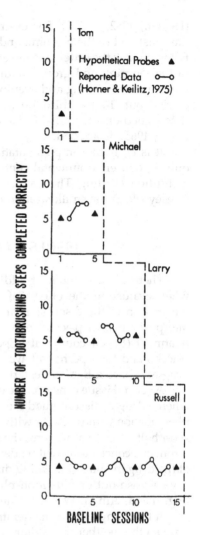

Figure 11. Number of toothbrushing steps conforming to the definition of a correct response across 4 subjects. From "Multiple-Probe Technique: A Variation of the Multiple Baseline" by R. D. Horner and D. M. Baer, 1978, *Journal of Applied Behavior Analysis, 11*, p. 194, Fig. 2. Copyright 1978 by the Society for the Experimental Analysis of Behavior. Reprinted by permission.

treatments with a single individual (Kazdin & Geesey, 1977; Kazdin & Hartmann, 1978). Unfortunately, this design is difficult to carry out pragmatically, given the particular circumstances required. A minimal requirement is the possibility of evaluating two stimulus dimensions, such as treatment agents (i.e., therapists), locations, or times of day.

In baseline, for the simultaneous treatment design, the targeted behavior is evaluated for each of the stimulus dimensions (e.g., morning and evening). Then two or more interventions (e.g., group versus individual contingencies) are assessed in both the morning and evening. The design is implemented in counterbalanced fashion to avoid a "treatment-stimulus dimension confound"

(Hersen, 1982, p. 112). For example, after baseline, group contingencies are administered in the morning and individual contingencies in the evening. The following day the order is reversed, with individual contingencies administered in the morning and group contingencies in the evening. Alternation of treatments in the morning and evening is continued until a sufficient trial has been carried out. In the third phase of the study, the most effective treatment, determined on the basis of visual analysis or Latin square statistics (see Benjamin, 1965), is applied.

It is clear that implementation of the simultaneous treatment design requires good environmental control, such as an inpatient unit or other similar institutional setting. The reader is referred to the excellent study by Kazdin and Geesey (1977) for an illustration of the design.

ISSUES IN DRUG EVALUATIONS

There are a number of additional issues faced by the clinical researcher when evaluating the effects of drugs in single-case designs. The first was touched on in the discussion of changing one variable at a time: namely, the interposition of a placebo phase (A') between baseline (A) and active drug treatment (B). Of course, it is possible to begin the single-case design with placebo and then perhaps have an A'-B-A'-B design, or begin with an active drug and have a B-A'-B design.

A second issue concerns the carryover effects from adjacent phases, such as when a drug is discontinued but its effects persist into the placebo phase. This phenomenon is more likely with long-acting drugs as contrasted to those with short half-lives. In any event, the investigator must exercise caution; otherwise, erroneous conclusions will be derived from data reflecting the persistent effect of the drug in spite of its being discontinued. One solution to the problem is to have a wash-out or transition phase in which drug dosage can be decreased (e.g., Field, Aman, White, & Vaithianathan, 1986).

A third important consideration involves the use of the double-blind procedure so that neither the patient nor the assessor is aware of whether a drug or placebo condition is in force. Even more difficult to implement in single-case research is the triple-blind, in which the prescribing physician also is unaware of the condition in force. This would require a cooperative hospital pharmacy and preset strategies, with preset lengths of phases in which several patients with the same disorder are treated with the same drug and are assigned randomly to single-case designs (e.g., A'-B-A'-B; B-A'-B-A').

Problems in implementing double-blinds in single-case research have been addressed by Hersen and Barlow (1976):

> A major difficulty in obtaining a "true" double-blind trial in single case research is related to the experimental monitoring of data (i.e., making decisions as to when baseline observation is to be concluded and when various phases are to be introduced and withdrawn) throughout the course of investigation. It is possible to program

phase lengths on an *à priori* basis, but then one of the major advantages of the single case strategy (i.e., its flexibility) is lost. However, even though the experimenter is fully aware of treatment changes, the spirit of the double-blind trial can be maintained by keeping the observer . . . unaware of drug and placebo changes. . . . We might note here additionally that despite the use of the double-blind procedure, the side effects of drugs in some cases . . . and the marked changes in behavior resulting from removal of active drug therapy in other cases often betray to nursing personnel whether a placebo or drug condition is currently in operation. (p. 206)

Despite the complexities inherent in evaluating pharmacological agents in single-case strategies, the recent literature has a good number of such examples. Included are evaluation of behavioral procedures while the drug is taken consistently across experimental phases (Wells, Turner, Bellack, & Hersen, 1978), the addition of pharmacotherapy to behavior therapy (Payton, Burkhart, Hersen, & Helsel, 1989; Turner, Hersen, & Alford, 1974; Turner, Hersen, Bellack, & Wells, 1979; Turner, Hersen, Bellack, Andrasik, & Capparell, 1980) and the primary effect of the drug itself (Field *et al.*, 1986; Helsel, Hersen, Lubetsky, Fultz, Sisson, & Harlovic, 1989; Ryan, Helsel, Lubetsky, Miewald, Hersen, & Bridge, 1989; Williamson, Calpin, DiLorenzo, Garris, & Petti, 1981).

Possible design options assessing the effects of pharmacological agents are listed in Table 2, but others not indicated are feasible as well. Designs 4 to 15 are experimental in nature, in that the controlling effects of the drug can be documented. Listed in Table 2 as well is whether no blind, a single blind, or a double-blind can be carried out with the given strategy.

I will now consider an excellent published example of Design No. 13. In their study, Liberman, Davis, Moon, and Moore (1973) contrasted the effects of

Table 2. Single-Case Experimental Drug Strategies

Number	Design	Type	Blind possible
1.	A-A'	Quasi-experimental	None
2.	A-B	Quasi-experimental	None
3.	A'-B	Quasi-experimental	Single or double
4.	A-A'-A	Experimental	None
5.	A-B-A	Experimental	None
6.	A'-B-A'	Experimental	Single or double
7.	A'-A-A'	Experimental	Single or double
8.	B-A-B	Experimental	None
9.	B-A'-B	Experimental	Single or double
10.	A-A'-A-A'	Experimental	Single or double
11.	A-B-A-B	Experimental	None
12.	A'-B-A'-B	Experimental	Single or double
13.	A-A'-B-A'-B	Experimental	Single or double
14.	A-A'-A-A'-BA'-A	Experimental	Single or double
15.	A'-B-A'-C-A'-C	Experimental	Single or double

[a]A = no drug; A' = placebo; B = drug 1; C = drug 2.
Notes. From *Single-Case Experimental Designs: Strategies for Studying Behavior Change* (Table 6.1.) by M. Hersen and D. H. Barlow, 1976, New York: Pergamon Press. Copyright 1976 by Pergamon Press. Reprinted by permission.

placebo and Stelazine in a 21-year-old chronic schizophrenic male using an A-A'-B-A'-B strategy. The target was social interaction, evaluated by recording the patient's willingness to engage in 18 daily half-minute chats with nursing personnel on the inpatient unit. When he refused such chats, the response was labeled "asocial."

During the baseline phase (A), all medication was removed. Examination of Figure 12 indicates that this resulted in an increase in asocial behavior. In A' placebo was introduced, first resulting in improvement and then a return of asocial behavior. In the next phase (B), introduction of Stelazine yielded considerable improvement, which then reversed in the next phase (A') when placebo replaced the drug. Removal of the active drug in A' documents the controlling effects of Stelazine over the target behavior. And, when Stelazine was reintroduced in the second B phase, improvement again was quite dramatic, once more documenting the powerful controlling effects of the drug.

The effects of imipramine were carefully evaluated by Field *et al.* (1986) in a more recent single-case analysis using an A-B-A'-B-A'-B design. Changeover phases were interposed between A and B when imipramine was increased and on two occasions between B and A' when it was reduced to 0. The patient was a 22-year-old woman suffering from moderate mental retardation, deafness, and visual impairment in one eye as a consequence of congenital rubella. She had

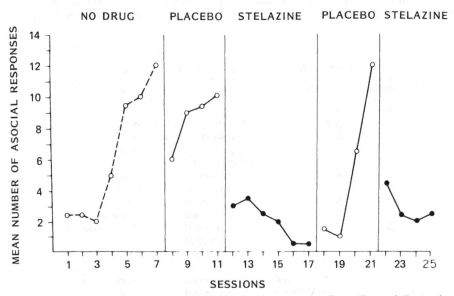

Figure 12. Average number of refusals to engage in a brief conversation. From "Research Design for Analyzing Drug-Environment-Behavior Interactions" by R. P. Liberman *et al.*, 1973, *Journal of Nervous and Mental Disease, 156*, p. 435, Fig. 2. Copyright 1973 by the Williams & Wilkins Company. Reprinted by permission.

very limited communication skills and had been institutionalized for 11 years. Prior to the imipramine drug trial, this patient had evinced crying, poor appetite, and screaming outbursts.

Percentage of time crying, percentage of meals consumed, and number of screaming outbursts were assessed twice a week for 30 minutes in the ward dayroom by two of the nursing personnel in 10-sec intervals. Inspection of Figure 13 indicates that percentage of time crying was low in baseline and in the first imipramine phase, higher although variable in the placebo phase, low in the second imipramine phase, increased in the second placebo phase, and low once again in the third imipramine phase. Nonetheless, it is not completely clear whether crying increased in placebo as a result of imipramine withdrawal, if one considers the low rate of that behavior in the initial baseline (A) phase.

By contrast, data for percentage of meals consumed (58.7% on placebo; 71.0% on imipramine) and screaming outbursts (7.5 per week on placebo; 2.4 per week on imipramine) clearly document the controlling effects of the tricyclic antidepressant.

From a design standpoint, use of a changeover phase of a week, in which there is an increase or decrease of the drug, represents an attractive feature. However, there are two minor weaknesses in the design: (1) skipping from baseline (A) to active drug (B) without the intermediacy placebo (A') phase, and (2) having only two data points in some of the phases.

Our final example of a pharmacological evaluation was conducted by Payton *et al.* (1989) and involved the effects of placebo and dextroamphetamine (Dexedrine) on the excessive movements of a 7.8-year-old boy (IQ of 66) with microcephaly and attention deficit-hyperactivity disorder. The patient had been referred to an inpatient unit for dually diagnosed mentally retarded children for noncompliance, physical intrusiveness, and aggression.

An A-A'-B-B'-A'B-B' design was carried out, with A as baseline, A' as placebo, B consisting of 5 mg b.i.d. of Dexedrine, B' consisting of 10 mg b.i.d. of Dexedrine, A' as placebo, B consisting of 5 mg of Dexedrine b.i.d., and B' consisting of 10 mg of Dexedrine b.i.d. Data in Figure 14 were collected in a classroom setting 90 minutes after the morning dose of medication. Observations during structured classroom activities were made every 10 seconds for 50 such intervals. Movement (the target behavior) referred to out of seat, tapping fingers, swinging feet, and body rocking.

Examination of Figure 14 shows a high rate of movement in baseline (A) and little improvement in the placebo (A') phase. However, in the Dexedrine phases (B and B'), there was marked improvement which reversed in the second placebo phase (A'). Finally, when Dexedrine was reintroduced (B and B'), excessive movement again was reduced to manageable levels. Dexedrine 10 mg b.i.d. was slightly better than Dexedrine 5 mg b.i.d., in that there was less variability of response. In summary, this single-case analysis documents the controlling effects of Dexedrine over placebo and baseline with respect to significantly reducing excessive movement in a child suffering from attention deficit-hyperactivity disorder.

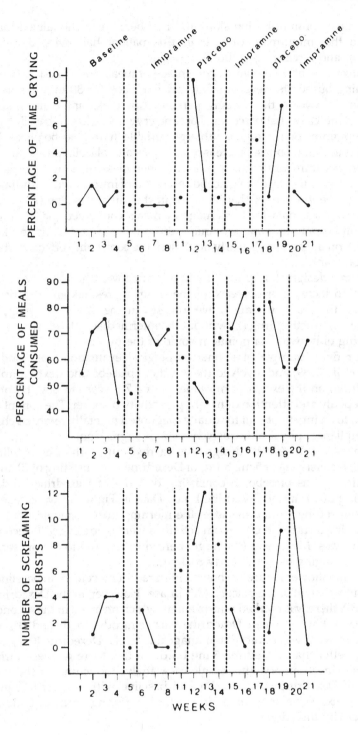

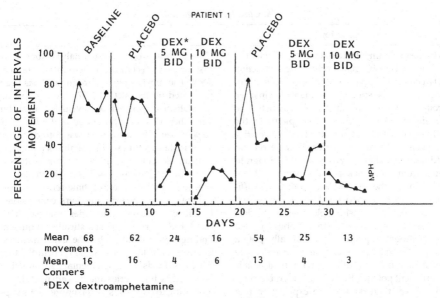

Figure 14. Percentage of intervals of movement across all phases, mean percentage of movement per phase, and mean Conners scale scores per phase for Patient 1. From "Treatment of ADDH in Mentally Retarded Children: A Preliminary Study" by J. B. Payton, J. E. Burkhart, M. Hersen, and W. J. Helsel, 1989, *Journal of the American Academy of Child and Adolescent Psychiatry, 28*, p. 763, Fig. 1. Copyright 1989 by American Academy of Child and Adolescent Psychiatry. Reprinted by permission.

CASE AGAINST AND FOR STATISTICAL ANALYSIS

Probably the most controversial issue in single-case research is whether statistical procedures are of value to the investigator (cf. Baer, 1977; Hartmann, 1974; Huitema, 1985; Jones *et al.*, 1977; Kazdin, 1984; Keselman & Leventhal, 1974; Kratochwill, Alden, Demuth, Dawson, Panicucci, Arnston, McMurray, Hempstead, & Levin, 1974; Michael, 1974a,b; Suen, 1987; Suen & Ary, 1987; Wampold & Worsham, 1986). Rather than rehashing at length what has appeared so many times in the literature, the basic arguments are presented in abbreviated form in Table 3. Despite the fact that the material is almost one

---

Figure 13. Percentage of time crying, percentage of meals consumed, and number of screaming outbursts during baseline, imipramine, and placebo periods. There was a 1-week transition phase, providing for dosage changes, between most drug phases of the experiment. From "A Single-Subject Study of Imipramine in a Mentally Retarded Woman with Depressive Symptoms" by C. J. Field, M. G. Aman, A. J. White, and C. Vaithianathan, 1986, *Journal of Mental Deficiency Research, 30*, p. 194, Fig. 1. Copyright 1986 by Blackwell Scientific Publications. Reprinted by permission.

Table 3.   The Case for and against Statistics

Case for	Case against
"The basic argument against the use of statistics in single-case research involves the distinction between *clinical* and *statistical* significance. Indeed, one of the specific arguments against the group comparison method is that statistics do not give the experimenter a 'true' picture of the individual pattern of results. That is, positive and negative treatment effects cancel out; in addition, statistics may possibly yield significance from very weak overall treatment strategies. Thus, if the effect of treatment is not sufficiently substantial to be detected by visual inspection (i.e., considerable overlap of data between baseline and treatment phases), then the treatment applied is not clinically potent and its controlling effects have not been clearly documented. On the other hand, if treatment is of sufficient potency to yield considerable clinical change, then there is the expectation that such change may approach the social norm (i.e., social rather than statistical validation) (see Kazdin, 1977.) This being the case statistical analysis should prove superfluous" (Hersen, 1982, p. 176).	"The advocates of statistical analyses for single-case research recommend them for several reasons. The most persuasive argument has been presented by Jones *et al.* (1977). In contrasting the statistical approach with visual analysis for a number of studies published in the *Journal of Applied Behavior Analysis*, it was found that in some instances, time-series analyses (cf. Glass, Willson, & Gottman, 1974) confirmed the experimenters' conclusions based on visual inspection. In other instances, time-series analyses did not confirm the experimenters' conclusions. In still other cases, time-series analyses indicated the presence of statistically significant findings not identified by the experimenters. Consequently, Jones *et al.* (1977) concluded that 'All three kinds of supplementary information provided by time-series analysis are useful. It is rewarding to have one's visual impressions supported by statistical analysis. It is humbling and/or educational to have other impressions not supported. And it is clearly beneficial to have unseen changes in the data detected by a supplementary method of analysis. It is difficult to see how operant researchers can lose in the application of time-series anlysis to their data (p. 166)'" (Hersen, 1982, p. 196).

decade old, there has been no change in the arguments of the antagonists and the protagonists.

In considering the above arguments about the use of statistics in single-case research, Kazdin (1976) has cogently argued that such analyses may prove to be of value when (1) there is little baseline stability and much overlap between baseline and treatment phases; (2) in newer areas of research where treatment strategies, not yet fully refined, fail to yield large clinical differences; and (3) in uncontrolled ("natural") research settings where again implementation of the treatment does not yield changes of large *clinical* magnitude. In short, it would appear that the arguments for using statistics are for instances when visual inspection does not detect changes. But if this is the case, is a weak treatment worth pursuing further for purposes of refinement? I would argue to the contrary. Indeed, the major value of the single-case approach from my perspective is its flexibility and potential for documenting *initially large clinical changes* that can then be subjected to more careful scrutiny in group-controlled research (i.e., the factorial design). In such group-controlled research, statistics are of paramount importance to *document the superiority of one technique over another*. The reader will recall, however, that the unique feature of single-case research is to document the *controlling effects* of the treatment over the targeted behavior. If one has difficulty in showing the controlling effects of a treatment and must resort to complicated statistical procedures to do so, perhaps the strategy in question is not sufficiently powerful to warrant a subsequent comparative investigation—*caveat emptor*!

REPLICATION

In the first edition of our book on single-case designs (Hersen & Barlow, 1976), we acknowledged the importance of replication, arguing that

> Replication is at the heart of any science. In all science, replication serves at least two purposes: First, to establish the reliability of previous findings and, second, to determine the generality of these findings under differing conditions. These goals, of course, are intrinsically interrelated. Each time that certain results are replicated under different conditions, this not only established generality of findings, but also increases confidence in the reliability of these findings. (p. 317)

Indeed, replication in single-case research has particular importance, given criticisms of the work of applied behavioral researchers for reporting "chance findings" in such designs, despite clear documentation of experimental control over targeted measures. The issue here, of course, is not experimental control, but believability. The implicit question is how many times must similar experimental control be documented before the scientific community is willing to categorize the finding from one "chance" to that of "scientifically replicable?"

In considering the issue of replication, the reader must keep in mind the three types of replication that have been identified in the literature (Barlow & Hersen, 1984; Hersen & Barlow, 1976; Sidman, 1960): direct replication, clinical replication, systematic replication. Let us first define these three types of replication and then see how they apply to problems dealt with in the psychiatric setting.

As defined by Sidman (1960), *direct replication* is the "repetition of a given experiment by the same investigator" (p. 72). Direct replication could be documented with the same subject or, better yet, across different subjects with similar characteristics. To rule out extraneous factors, the clinical researcher must ensure that the identical procedure has been implemented with each subject. Originally, Hersen and Barlow (1976) argued for three successful replications of an original effect. But how many replications truly are needed before the scientific community is satisfied that it is an "audience variable?" If results are mixed in a direct replication series, it behooves the investigator to ascertain sources of variation (e.g., subtle patient characteristics), which then begin to delimit the generality of the treatment under study. Also, mixed results often lead to a refinement of the therapeutic strategy so as to enhance its effectiveness across slightly different patients.

Clinical replication has been defined by Hersen and Barlow (1976) as the

> administration of a treatment package containing two or more distinct treatment
> procedures by the same investigator or group of investigators. These procedures would
> be administered in a specific setting to a series of clients presenting similar combina-
> tions of multiple behavioral and emotional problems, which cluster together. (p. 336)

Hersen and Barlow then go on to point out that the utility of such replication

> depends to some extent on the consistency or reliability of the diagnostic category. If
> the clustering of the target behaviors is inconsistent, then the patients within the series
> would be so heterogeneous that the same treatment package could not be applied to
> successive patients. For this reason, and because of the advanced nature of the
> research effort, clinical replications are presently not common in the literature. (p. 336)

Guidelines for carrying out clinical replication are basically similar to those in
the case of direct replication. However, because of intersubject variability, the
length of the replication series by necessity will be longer.

Finally, we consider *systematic replication*, defined by Hersen and Barlow
(1976) as

> any attempt to replicate findings from a direct replication series, varying settings,
> behavior change agents, behavior disorders, or any combination thereof. It would
> appear that any successful systematic replication series in which one or more of the
> above-mentioned factors is varied also provides further information on generality of
> findings across clients since new clients are usually included in these efforts. (p. 339)

The word *systematic*, however, may be a misnomer, since the research effort is
decentralized and typically conducted in several settings. What emerges over
time as research findings are adduced are the very specific limitations of given
therapeutic procedures, either with respect to therapists (in the case of psychological treatments), settings, or patients. Thus, systematic replications will help
to determine the so-called exceptions to the rule: that is, when does a specific
treatment fail to be effective for a particular patient or in the hands of a specific
therapist? Systematic replication clearly defines the upper limits of the treatment, which then forestalls the rote application of such an approach.

SUMMARY

The single-case approach to treatment has been depicted as a viable
alternative to group-controlled research, but also as a research strategy that
dovetails with the comparative evaluation of treatments in such group-controlled
studies. In examining single-case research, some of the unique attributes of this
approach have been emphasized, including repeated measurement, choosing a
baseline, changing one variable at a time, length of phases, and evaluating
irreversible procedures. This was followed by descriptions of some of the major
design strategies, illustrated with examples found in the psychiatric literature.
Included were the following: A-B-A-B Design, Interaction Designs, Multiple-
Baseline Designs, Changing Criterion Design, and Other Design Options. Spe-

cial consideration was then given to issues in drug evaluations, followed by discussion of the case against and for statistical analysis and the issues involved in the three types of replication procedures.

REFERENCES

Agras, W. S., Barlow, D. H., Chapin, H. N., Abel, G. G., & Leitenberg, H. (1974). Behavior modification of anorexia nervosa. *Archives of General Psychiatry, 39,* 279–286.

Baer, D. M. (1977). Perhaps it would be better not to know everything. *Journal of Applied Behavior Analysis, 10,* 167–172.

Baer, D. M., Wolf, M. M., & Risley, T. R. (1968). Some current dimensions of applied behavior analysis. *Journal of Applied Behavior Analysis, 1,* 91–97.

Barlow, D. H., & Hersen, M. (1973). Single-case experimental designs: Uses in applied clinical research. *Archives of General Psychiatry, 29,* 319–325.

Barlow, D. H., & Hersen, M. (1984). *Single-case experimental designs: Strategies for studying behavior change (2nd ed.).* New York: Pergamon Press.

Barlow, D. H., Agras, W. S., Leitenberg, H., Callahan, E. J., & Moore, R. C. (1972). The contribution of therapeutic instruction to covert sensitization. *Behaviour Research and Therapy, 10,* 411–415.

Barlow, D. H., Blanchard, D. B., Hayes, S. C., & Epstein, L. H. (1977). Single case designs and clinical biofeedback experimentation. *Biofeedback and Self-Regulation, 2,* 221–236.

Bellack, A. S., & Hersen, M. (Eds.). (1988). *Behavioral assessment: A practical handbook* (3rd ed.). New York: Pergamon Press.

Benjamin, L. S. (1965). A special latin square for use of each subject "as his own control." *Psychometrika, 30,* 499–513.

Field, C. J., Aman, M. G., White, A. J., & Vaithianathan, C. (1986). A single-subject study of imipramine in a mentally retarded woman with depressive symptoms. *Journal of Mental Deficiency Research, 30,* 191–198.

Glass, G. V., Willson, V. L., & Gottman, J. M. (1974). *Design and analysis of time series experiments.* Boulder: Colorado Associated University Press.

Goldstein, G., & Malec, E. A. (1989). Memory training for severely amnesic patients. *Neuropsychology, 3,* 9–16.

Hartmann, D. P. (1974). Forcing square pegs into roundholes: Some comments on "an analysis-of-variance model for the intrasubject replication design." *Journal of Applied Behavior Analysis, 7,* 635–638.

Hartmann, D. P., & Hall, R. V. (1976). The changing criterion design. *Journal of Applied Behavior Analysis, 9,* 527–532.

Helsel, W. J., Hersen, M., Lubetsky, M. J., Fultz, S. A., Sisson, L., & Harlovic H. (1989). Stimulant drug treatment of four multihandicapped children using a randomized single-case design. *Journal of the Multihandicapped Person, 2,* 139–154.

Hersen, M. (1973). Self-assessment of fear. *Behavior Therapy, 4,* 241–257.

Hersen, M. (1978). Do behavior therapists use self-reports as major criteria? *Behavioral Analysis and Modification, 2,* 328–334.

Hersen, M. (1982). Single-case experimental designs. In A. S. Bellack, M. Hersen, & A. E. Kazdin (Eds.), *International handbook of behavior modification and therapy* (pp. 167–203). New York: Plenum Press.

Hersen, M. (1990). Single-case experimental designs. In A. S. Bellack, M. Hersen, & A. E. Kazdin (Eds.), *International handbook of behavior modification and therapy* (2nd ed., pp. 175–210). New York: Plenum Press.

Hersen, M., & Barlow, D. H. (1976). *Single-case experimental designs: Strategies for studying behavior change.* New York: Pergamon Press.

Hersen, M., & Bellack, A. S. (Eds.). (1976). *Behavioral assessment: A practical handbook*. New York: Pergamon Press.

Hersen, M., & Bellack, A. S. (1988). DSM-III and behavioral assessment. In A. S. Bellack & M. Hersen (Eds.), *Behavioral assessment: A practical handbook* (3rd ed., pp. 67–84). New York: Pergamon Press.

Horner, R. D., & Baer, D. M. (1978). Multiple-probe techniques. A variation of the multiple baseline. *Journal of Applied Behavior Analysis, 11*, 189–196.

Huitema, B. E. (1985). Autocorrelation in applied behavior analysis: A Myth. *Behavioral Assessment, 7*, 107–118.

Jones, R. R., Vaught, R. S., & Weinrott, M. R. (1977). Time-series analysis in operant research. *Journal of Applied Behavior Analysis, 10*, 151–167.

Kallman, W. M., Hersen, M., & O'Toole, D. H. (1975). The use of social reinforcement in a case of conversion reaction. *Behavior Therapy, 6*, 411–413.

Kazdin, A. E. (1976). Statistical analysis for single-case experimental designs. In M. Hersen & D. H. Barlow (Eds.), *Single-case experimental designs: Strategies for studying behavior change* (pp. 265–316). New York: Pergamon Press.

Kazdin, A. E. (1984). Statistical analysis for single-case experimental designs. In D. H. Barlow & M. Hersen (Eds.), *Single-case experimental designs: Strategies for studying behavior change* (pp. 285–234). New York: Pergamon Press.

Kazdin, A. E. (1985). *Behavior modification in applied settings* (3rd ed.). Homewood, IL: Dorsey Press.

Kazdin, A. E., & Geesey, S. (1977). Simultaneous-treatment design comparisons of the effects of earning reinforcers for one's peers versus for oneself. *Behavior Therapy, 8*, 682–693.

Kazdin, A. E., & Hartmann, D. P. (1978). The simultaneous-treatment design. *Behavior Therapy, 9*, 912–922.

Kazdin, A. E., & Kopel, S. A. (1975). On resolving ambiguities of the multiple-baseline design: Problems and recommendations. *Behavior Therapy, 6*, 601–608.

Keselman, H. J., & Leventhal, L. (1974). Concerning the statistical procedures enumerated by Gentile et al.: Another perspective. *Journal of Applied Behavior Analysis, 7*, 643–645.

Kratochwill, T., Alden, K., Demuth, D., Dawson D., Panicucci, C., Arnston, P., McMurray, N., Hempstead, J., & Levin, J. (1974). A further consideration in the application of an analysis-of-variance model for the intrasubject replication design. *Journal of Applied Behavior Analysis, 7*, 629–633.

Liberman, R. P., Davis, J., Moon, W., & Moore, J. (1973). Research design for analyzing drug-environment-behavior interactions. *Journal of Nervous and Mental Disease, 156*, 432–439.

Lombardo, T. W., & Turner, S. M. (1979). Thought-stopping in the control of obsessive ruminations. *Behavior Modification, 3*, 267–272.

Martin, J. E., & Epstein, L. H. (1976). Evaluating treatment effectiveness in cerebral palsy: Single subject designs. *Physical Therapy, 56*, 385–394.

Michael, J. (1974a). Statistical inference for individual organism research: Mixed blessings or curse? *Journal of Applied Behavior Analysis, 7*, 647–653.

Michael, J. (1974b). Statistical inference for individual organism research: Some reactions to a suggestion by Gentile, Roden, & Klein. *Journal of Applied Behavior Analysis, 7*, 627–628.

Miller, P. M. (1973). An experimental analysis of retention control training in the treatment of nocturnal enuresis in two institutionalized adolescents. *Behavior Therapy, 4*, 288–294.

Morin, C. M., Kowatch, R. A., & Wade, J. B. (1989). Behavioral management of sleep disturbances secondary to chronic pain. *Journal of Behavior Therapy and Experimental Psychiatry, 20*, 295–302.

Payton, J. B., Burkhart, J. E., Hersen, M., & Helsel, W. J. (1989). Treatment of attention deficit disorder with hyperactivity in mentally retarded children: A preliminary study. *Journal of the Academy of Child and Adolescent Psychiatry, 28*, 761–767.

Risley, T. R., & Wolf, M. M. (1972). Strategies for analyzing behavioral change over time. In J. Nesselroade & H. Reese (Eds.), *Life-span developmental psychology: Methodological issues* (pp. 175–183). New York: Academic Press.

Ryan, E. P., Helsel, W. J., Lubetsky, M. J., Miewald, B. K., Hersen, M., & Bridge, J. (1989). Use of

Naltrexone in reducing self-injurious behavior: A single case analysis. *Journal of the Multihandicapped Person, 2,* 295–309.

Shapiro, M. B. (1966). The single case in clinical-psychological research. *Journal of General Psychology, 74,* 3–23.

Sidman, M. (1960). *Tactics of scientific research: Evaluating experimental data in psychology.* New York: Basic Books.

Suen, H. K. (1987). On the epistemology of autocorrelation in applied behavior analysis. *Behavioral Assessment, 9,* 113–124.

Suen, H. K., & Ary, D. (1987). Autocorrelation in applied behavior analysis: Myth or reality? *Behavioral Assessment, 9,* 125–130.

Thomas, E. J. (1978). Research and service in single-case experimentation: Conflicts and choices. *Social Work Research and Abstracts, 14,* 20–31.

Thoresen, C. E. (1972, April). *The intensive design: An intimate approach to counseling research.* Paper presented at the meeting of the American Educational Research Association, Chicago.

Turner, S. M., Hersen, M., & Alford, H. (1974). Effects of massed practice and meprobamate on spasmodic torticollis: An experimental analysis. *Behaviour Research and Therapy, 12,* 259–260.

Turner, S. M., Hersen, M., Bellack, A. S., & Wells, K. C. (1979). Behavioral treatment of obsessive-compulsive neurosis. *Behaviour Research and Therapy, 17,* 95–106.

Turner, S. M., Hersen, M., Bellack, A. S., Andrasik, F., & Capparell, H. V. (1980). Behavioral and pharmacologic treatment of obsessive-compulsive disorders. *Journal of Nervous and Mental Disease, 168,* 651–657.

Wampold, B. E., & Worsham, N. L. (1986). Randomization tests for multiple-baseline designs. *Behavioral Assessment, 8,* 135–143.

Watson, P. J., & Workman, E. A. (1981). The non-concurrent multiple baseline across-individuals design: An extension of the traditional multiple baseline design. *Journal of Behavior Therapy and Experimental Psychiatry, 12,* 257–259.

Wells, K. C., Turner, S. M., Bellack, A. S., & Hersen, M. (1978). Effects of cue-controlled relaxation on psychomotor seizures: An experimental analysis. *Behaviour Research and Therapy, 16,* 51–53.

Williamson, D. A., Calpin, J. P., DiLorenzo, T. M., Garris, R. P., & Petti, T. (1981). Combining dexedrine (dextro-amphetamine) and activity feedback for the treatment of hyperactivity. *Behavior Modification, 5,* 399–416.

Yates, A. J. (1970). *Behavior therapy.* New York: Wiley.

CHAPTER 4

Group Comparison Approaches in Psychiatric Research

MING T. TSUANG, CHUNG-CHENG HSIEH, AND JEROME A. FLEMING

INTRODUCTION

Comparative population psychiatric research, regardless of the complexity of the methodology, involves studying the relationship between a risk determinant and a health outcome. A *risk determinant* is also referred to as an "independent variable," "risk factor," "exposure," or "treatment" in a typical comparative study. Simply put, the outcome experience of a group of people who have been exposed to a risk determinant is compared to that of another group who have not been so exposed, and the relation between exposure and outcome is evaluated empirically. In psychiatry, the risk determinant or exposure may be whether the individual has a certain disorder (i.e., schizophrenia or affective disorder) or some combination of psychiatric symptomatology. The outcome might be measured as long-term functioning, mortality rates, morbidity rates, or familial psychopathology.

The application of design principles and statistical methods in comparison studies (Anderson, Auquier, Hauck, Oakes, Vandaele, & Weisberg, 1980; Camp-

Ming T. Tsuang, Chung-Cheng Hsieh, and Jerome A. Fleming • Harvard Medical School Department of Psychiatry, Psychiatry Service, Brockton/West Roxbury Veterans Administration Medical Center, Harvard School of Public Health, Program in Psychiatric Epidemiology, Brockton, Massachusetts 02401.

Research in Psychiatry: Issues, Strategies, and Methods, edited by L. K. George Hsu and Michel Hersen. Plenum Press, New York, 1992.

bell and Stanley, 1963) to psychiatry deserves special consideration. Because of the nature of many psychiatric disorders in terms of chronicity and changing symptoms over time, the comparison of specific disorders to each other and to normals becomes much more difficult. Therefore, our goal in this chapter is to describe general group comparison approaches and how they apply specifically to psychiatric research and its unique problems.

In the following sections, we will describe facets of the group comparison approach in psychiatry: measures of outcome occurrence, measures of relation or association, types of group comparison studies (including examples), and considerations of validity. Classification of comparison studies, which can include both experimental and nonexperimental designs (cross-sectional and longitudinal), will be explained and clarified. Application of principles of validity to questions concerning group comparison studies will also be addressed. And finally, various examples of comparative psychiatric family studies will be used to elucidate the nature of a comparative study.

MEASURES OF OUTCOME OCCURRENCE AND ASSOCIATION IN POPULATIONS

The frequency of outcome occurrence in a population can be measured in several ways. The two most commonly used parameters are the *proportion* (prevalence) and the *density* (incidence) measurements. Kramer (1957) previously compared and contrasted these two types of measurements in the setting of psychiatric research. The first measurement, prevalence, is simply the proportion of people in a population who have a particular health condition at a given point in time. An example of this would be the percentage of 16-year-old high school students who have an affective disorder. As a proportion, a prevalence rate is a dimensionless quantity. The second measurement, incidence, refers to new outcome events occurring over time among members of the population who are candidates for such events. Incidence density quantifies the number of outcome events occurring per unit population per unit time. It is, therefore, not dimensionless since there is a time element associated with the measurement. For example, in a group of 2,000 schizophrenic patients followed for an average of 3 years, 18 deaths (the outcome event) occurred during the follow-up period. The incidence density of death (the "mortality rate") would be 3 per 1,000 persons per year (18/[3 years × 2,000] = 6 per 2,000 per year = 3 per 1,000 per year).

A density measure is often called a *rate* (Elandt-Johnson, 1975). In everyday usage, however, a rate can be used synonymously with proportion: for example, unemployment rates, tax rates, prevalence rates, and survival rates. To avoid confusion, it is important to know in what context and in which sense rate is being used.

Other measures of frequency of outcome that are related to prevalence and incidence measures are encountered frequently in comparative psychiatric research. Risk and cumulative incidence are estimates of the probability of an outcome event occurring over a specified period of time. The prediction of the likelihood of a particular outcome event for an individual is typically called a *risk*. *Cumulative incidence* is used to describe the probability of an outcome occurrence among a population group. Survival rate is the complement of a cumulative incidence of death for a population group. These measures are dimensionless.

Cumulative incidence can be either an *observed probability* or a *derived estimate* from the incidence rate. The observed cumulative incidence can be compromised by the loss of subjects from the candidate population that are due to events other than the one under study. For example, an observed 5-year survival rate for a group of schizophrenic patients can be distorted by the number of patients who are lost to follow-up, even if those lost to follow-up had the same probability of survival. That is, outcomes occurring among the missing would not be included in the numerator of the calculation, but the denominator of the observed cumulative incidence would still use the same number of candidates from the population as at the beginning of the observation period.

Thus, the 5-year survival rate that would typically be reported in the psychiatric literature is not an observed value. Instead, it is a theoretical value, the complement of a theoretical cumulative incidence which is derived from the observed incidence density (Chiang, 1968). In the situation where those lost to follow-up have the same likelihood of dying, the estimate of the observed incidence density is not affected by the competing causes of subject removal (e.g., lost to follow-up) from the candidate population since those who were removed would no longer be among the candidates for the occurrence of the next outcome event. For the prognosis of an individual patient, one minus the probability of surviving 5 years can be referred to as "the risk of dying in 5 years."

If there is an association between the risk determinant and outcome, the frequency of the outcome event's occurring would be different for the "exposed" group and the "not exposed" group. Therefore, the measure of the association is obtained by contrasting the measures of outcome occurrence between the compared groups. The contrast between these two measures of frequency of outcome occurrence can be expressed as a *difference* or a *ratio*. The magnitude of the difference or ratio summarizes the degree of difference in the frequency of outcome between the two groups and expresses the strength of association between the determinant and outcome. In comparative psychiatric research, a ratio is most often used to express the strength of an association. The ratio contrast between two proportions or between two densities is commonly known as the *relative risk*. Relative risk is thus a general term which can represent cumulative incidence ratio, risk ratio, or incidence density ratio. It is important, therefore, to know in what context the term "relative risk" is being used. For example, suppose the mortality rate among patients with schizophrenia is 3 per 1,000 persons per year, and among those with major depression it is 1 per 1,000 persons per year; the relative risk of dying ("relative force of mortality") between schizophrenic patients and depressive patients is 3 (relative risk = 3/1). Relative risk here refers to an incidence density ratio (incidence rate ratio).

GROUP COMPARISON STUDY DESIGNS

Even though the focus of group comparison psychiatric research is the relative magnitude of the rates of an outcome occurrence between two groups, there can be enormous variation in approaches and designs depending on the postulated time relation between the determinant and outcome, the timing of data collection, the types of populations, and the sampling methods used (Miettinen, 1985a). Hence a host of group comparison approaches can be encountered in actual practice. We will describe the following research paradigms and their applications in psychiatric research: experimental, cross-sectional, prospective cohort, retrospective cohort, and case–control studies.

Experimental Studies

In an *experimental study*, the investigator has complete control over the experiment and can randomly assign study subjects to each comparison group. Observations of outcome events of interest (e.g., recurrence of a psychiatric illness or the occurrence of death) are recorded for all study subjects. Clinical trials and intervention studies are the most common forms of experimental studies conducted with humans. To ensure comparability between groups and obtain valid results, a researcher conducting an experimental study applies three basic research strategies: *randomization*, the *use of placebos*, and *blinding*.

With *randomization*, group assignment is determined by chance and the groups are likely to be similar in all respects other than the exposure under study. For example, in a treatment trial, the outcome rates for the comparison groups are likely to be the same in the absence of any treatment effect. However, if, by chance, randomization does not achieve a balanced distribution of factors which are known to influence the outcome, the investigator needs to take the imbalance into consideration through the use of appropriate statistical methods in the analysis. Alternatively, study subjects can first be matched on these factors, before being randomly assigned to comparison groups, to establish a balanced distribution. When the number of study subjects is sufficiently large, randomization is assumed to achieve a balanced distribution of factors which may influence outcome but are unknown and unmeasured.

By using a *placebo* or "sham treatment," the difference in outcome between groups can be attributed to the effects of the drug or treatment *per se*, rather than the effects of other aspects of the procedure, activity, or environment associated with the administration of the drug or treatment being studied. The effects of extraneous aspects of the treatment procedure are sometimes known as the *placebo effect*.

The method of *blinding* can eliminate the influence of an investigator's bias for or against a medication in the handling, treatment, and observation of patients in a clinical trial. Greater standardization is achieved when both the investigator and the patient are unaware of the treatment assignment ("double-blinding"). This technique ensures that, during the experiment, the environmental conditions of the groups are similar and that the same study procedures are applied to each and every study subject.

Even though use of the experimental method is recognized in many fields as the *sine qua non* of empirical research, it has several important limitations in population studies. Ethical considerations dictate that experiments involving human subjects can only study exposures (treatments or medications) which are designed to be potentially beneficial. It is unethical to expose human subjects to harmful or potentially harmful treatment conditions or environmental agents. In addition, constitutional characteristics (such as inherited or congenital traits) cannot be randomized; therefore, many human traits and disorders cannot be evaluated by experimental study. Finally, in the assessment of a treatment, if the follow-up period necessary for the ascertainment of outcome events is long, the treatment assessed may be obsolete by the time the results are available (Elwood, 1988).

Two examples of experimental studies in psychiatric research will be presented. One study illustrates a clinical treatment trial for testing the effectiveness of a specific treatment drug and the second example presents a description of an intervention study.

Recent literature suggests that sodium valproate (Depakote) is effective in treating bipolar disorder patients. In order to test this hypothesis, an experimental clinical trial was conducted. Patients consecutively admitted to the hospital, who met the selection criteria for the study (i.e., diagnostic criteria for bipolar disorder), were randomly assigned to a Depakote treatment group or to another treatment group (lithium). The design called for the assignment of 35 patients to each of the two treatment groups. To make sure that there were no biases in the selection of the 35 patients for each treatment group, they were randomly assigned. The first step in this process is to generate from the set of numbers (1, 2, 3, . . . 70) 35 random numbers to be assigned to the experimental group (Depakote). The remaining 35 numbers are assigned to the comparison group (lithium). This can be done using the computer or by using published tables of random numbers which generally are contained in many statistical text books. For instance, computer-generated numbers could be obtained by simply requesting that 35 numbers, falling in between 1–70, be selected randomly. There are specific computer programs available which are used for generating random numbers based on ones' particular design requirements. In this case, the random numbers chosen corresponded to the order of admission to the hospital. So, for example, if the random numbers 1, 5, 28 were chosen for the Depakote treatment, then the first, fifth, and twenty-eighth patients admitted to the hospital were assigned to the Depakote group until there were 35 randomly selected subjects in the group. The same process was completed for the lithium group. If a patient admitted to the hospital was not eligible for the study, the next admission was substituted for that slot and the random selection process was continued.

After a specified treatment period, the levels of bipolar symptomatology were compared statistically. Raters of a bipolar assessment scale were blind to the patients' group membership. Using this design, the differences in outcome, as measured on a bipolar rating scale, can be attributed to the effects of the drugs under study. This study met the requirements of an experimental design because of randomization and the application of blinding procedures. Owing to this design, if the 35 patients assigned to the Depakote treatment group had significantly better scores on the bipolar rating scale than the 35 patients who were not given Depakote, the difference can be attributed to the effects of the drug.

Currently, we are conducting a study, using an experimental design, to evaluate a new program for deinstitutionalizing chronic psychiatric patients and maintaining them in the community (intervention study). The purpose of this study is to measure the effects of various psychosocial rehabilitation approaches on the patients' discharge and maintenance in the community. The design of this study calls for pairs of patients to be matched on the basis of diagnosis, age, length of current admission, and life-time days in mental health facilities. The matching procedure ensures that the groups of interest will be similar on all factors except the variable being studied. One patient from each pair is randomly assigned to a treatment ward and the other patient is assigned to a nontreatment ward. This process is similar to flipping a coin, where, if it is heads, patient 1 is assigned to the treatment ward and patient 2 is assigned to the nontreatment ward. The opposite would occur if tails appear. Following the completion of the experimental treatment (rehabilitation program) on the specialized treatment ward, patients are randomly assigned to one of three residential aftercare programs. A predetermined system is in place which specifies which program a patient, coming off the treatment ward, is assigned. This system is based on the same random number assignment principles discussed above. Data on patient functioning and satisfaction with care will be analyzed across the three residential programs and the nontreatment ward program. If those patients in the rehabilitation program have a significantly better aftercare level of functioning versus those patients with no intervention treatment, the difference is likely to be due to the effects of treatment and aftercare programs. In addition, the three aftercare residential programs can also be compared.

Nonexperimental Studies

In a nonexperimental study, the investigator has no control over the group designation of each study subject. Generally, the investigator selects subjects for different exposure conditions from already existing groups. With this design, an investigator can only observe the subjects; hence nonexperimental studies are often called *observational studies*. Several types of nonexperimental comparative studies that are used in psychiatric research are described below.

Cross-Sectional Studies

In a *cross-sectional study*, data on exposure and outcome for a defined population are collected at the same point in time. Outcome status of those with and without the exposure, expressed as prevalence rates, is compared. This design is useful for describing the health status and health care needs in different populations. For diseases of slow onset and long duration, as is the case for many psychiatric disorders, an accurate measurement of incidence may be difficult to achieve given the uncertainty as to the exact point in time of the outcome occurrence. In these cases, only the prevalence can be reliably measured. Since the measurements of exposure and disease are made at the same point in time in a cross-sectional study, it may be impossible to determine whether the exposure preceded or resulted from the disease or was merely concomitant with the disease with no causal implication.

A cross-sectional design could be used to compare various social and psychiatric functioning measurements across diagnostic classifications. For example, a researcher might select 100 schizophrenics, 100 manics, and 100 depressives from consecutive admissions to a psychiatric hospital based on specific diagnostic criteria and one hundred normal subjects for the purposes of comparison. In this case, the diagnostic categories would be considered exposure groups. Functioning at the time of selection could be measured in terms of such factors as marital status, occupational status, and severity of psychiatric symptoms and could be rated good, fair, or poor. The prevalence of poor functioning (outcome) would then be statistically compared across the four exposure groups (schizophrenia, mania, depression, and normals). This study is cross-sectional because the data determining diagnoses (exposure) and functioning (outcome) were collected at and referred to the same point in time.

Longitudinal Studies

Unlike a cross-sectional study, in a *longitudinal study* the time sequence between the exposure and the outcome can be determined. The effect of the exposure, which precedes the occurrence of outcome, is the object of study. Cohort and case-control studies are the two main categories of nonexperimental longitudinal studies.

Cohort Studies. In a *cohort study*, individuals free from the outcome event, who are candidates for such an event, are selected to form the comparison groups (together they constitute a cohort) based on the presence or absence of an exposure. Cohort members are followed over time to determine the frequency of new outcome events in each group. Depending on the timing of data collection in relation to an outcome occurrence, the experience of a cohort can be studied prospectively or retrospectively.

In a *prospective cohort study*, the exposed and nonexposed groups are defined on the basis of current characteristics and are then followed over time to ascertain outcome events. This design is similar to that of an experimental study, except the investigator has no control over the group assignment of each study subject.

In a *retrospective cohort study*, the outcome has already occurred at the time the exposed and nonexposed groups are defined. Exposure status is based on subject characteristics at work in the distant past, and the subsequent outcome is reconstructed up to some later point in time (which can be the present, the recent past, or the future). Three specific examples of cohort studies will be described below.

The first study is a follow-up and family study of major psychoses, and takes a retrospective cohort approach. That is, the study groups were formed and outcome was assessed in the 1970s, which was approximately 30 to 40 years after index hospitalization of those patients who comprised the various exposure groups. Study subjects were selected from among the 3,800 patients admitted to a psychiatric hospital between 1934 and 1945. Of these cases, 525 subjects met research criteria (Feighner, Robins, Guze, Woodruff, Winokur, & Munoz, 1972) for schizophrenia ($n = 200$), mania ($n = 100$), and depression ($n = 225$). In addition, there were 310 subjects who had an initial clinical diagnosis of schizophrenia but subsequently did not meet research criteria for schizophrenia for a number of reasons and were labeled *atypical schizophrenia* (Tsuang & Dempsey, 1979). These subjects were selected in 1972, based on a close examination of detailed hospital records from the late 1930s and early 1940s (Morrison, Clancy, Crowe, & Winokur, 1972). A nonpsychiatric surgical group (normal proband group) was also selected, matched to the psychiatric groups for sex, socioeconomic status, and age range, all of whom had been admitted to the surgical department during the same period of time for appendectomy or herniorrhaphy.

The goal of this study was to conduct, 30 to 40 years after their hospitalizations, personal but blind interviews with as many of these patients and controls, and as many of their first-degree relatives as possible. These interviews took place between 1975 and 1979. The interviews were blind in that the interviewer did not know whether the subjects were former psychiatric patients, formal surgical patients, or relatives. The interview assessed schizophrenic, affective, and neurotic symptomatology along with physical and psychiatric treatment history. Long-term outcome was evaluate in terms of marital, occupational, residential, and psychiatric status. These outcome measures, along with family data, were then compared statistically among the exposure cohort groups (psychiatric and normal) 30 to 40 years after index admission (Tsuang, Woolson, & Fleming, 1979; Tsuang, Winokur, & Crowe, 1980). It is interesting to note that since the subjects for this study were selected in 1972, based on 1930–1940 information, but then followed through 1979, this particular design has in the past been referred to as a *historical prospective* study.

The second project, which has been proposed, is an example of a prospective follow-up and family study of major psychoses. The design of this particular prospective study required the selection of a cohort of 400 patients with undiagnosed psychoses, and comparison groups of 200 schizophrenics, 200 bipolar disorder patients, and 200 patients with major depression. These subjects were identified through a structured psychiatric interview—the Schedule for Affective Disorders and Schizophrenia (SADS). In addition, extensive baseline data concerning demographics, psychosocial functioning, premorbid functioning, clinical history, and family history were collected for all subjects and controls. In this prospective design, the study subjects would be reinterviewed after 2 years to reevaluate symptomatology and psychosocial adjustment. Comparisons will then be made between diagnostic groups to describe the comparative course and outcome of the undiagnosed psychoses. This information, along with family data, will lead to the identification of prognostic indicators and to the development of diagnostic criteria for homogeneous subtypes of undiagnosed psychosis. This study illustrates a classic prospective design: the outcome of interest (follow-up information) has yet to occur at the time the exposed (undiagnosed psychosis) and nonexposed groups (schizophrenia, bipolar disorder, and major depression) are defined.

A more extensive longitudinal study, conducted on the national level, was the epidemiologic catchment area (ECA) program (Eaton & Kessler, 1985; Eaton, Holzer, Van Korff, Anthony, Helzer, George, Burnam, Boyd, Kessler, & Locke, 1984; Regier, Myers, Kramer, Robins, Blazer, Hough, Eaton, & Locke, 1984). The purpose of this project was to use a longitudinal design to obtain incidence and mental health service use data for the DSM-III psychiatric disorders. Over 17,000 community residents in five sites (Baltimore, New Haven, North Carolina, St. Louis, and Los Angeles) were interviewed with the Diagnostic Interview Schedule (DIS) and reinterviewed a year later using the same instrument. The longitudinal prospective follow-up design for this project was crucial for collecting the data necessary to meet the goals of the study. One goal was to compare the distribution of psychiatric diagnoses between the initial interview and the reinterview to determine remission rates and recurrence rates. Another goal was to evaluate the use of mental health services over the period of a year by those subjects who had psychiatric disorders. This study is a good example of how data collected prospectively can be used to calculate incidence rates.

Because of the length of time between exposure and outcome, prospective cohort studies can be very costly. For this reason, retrospective cohort studies, in which the outcome has already occurred, are very appealing. Mortality studies are a good example of retrospective cohort analysis. For instance, two comparison groups of schizophrenics and psychiatrically symptom-free normals could be selected on the basis of psychiatric and medical hospital records from the 1930s. These two groups could, of course, be matched for age at admission and sex. Overall mortality rates as well as specific causes of death, measured at the present time, could then be compared between the two groups. More sophisticated statistical comparisons of survival functions could also be performed. This would be a simple retrospective cohort study in which the exposed (schizophrenic) and nonexposed (normal) groups have been defined and the outcome (death) has already occurred. It is clear that the time, effort, and expense involved in a prospective mortality study would be much more extensive and costly.

Case–Control Studies. In a case–control study, individuals are chosen on the basis of existing outcome (illness or no illness). Subjects with the outcome are cases and those without the outcome are controls. The proportion of cases and the proportion of controls who have been exposed to the risk determinant are identified and compared.

Conceptually, this design can be thought of as one means of sampling two population groups under comparison (Miettinen, 1985a). Cases are members of the population who have developed the outcome event, and controls are a sample drawn from the population from which all possible cases arise and have been enrolled. The controls provide information on the relative size of the comparison groups according to the exposure status.

To illustrate, suppose our population was a community comprised of 2,000 people with an affective disorder, and 50,000 without an affective disorder, all of whom were observed for an average of 3 years. During the period of observation, a total of 32 deaths occurred. From an examination of their medical records, 12 had a history of affective disorder and 20 did not. Therefore, based on the total population, the relative risk of dying between the two groups was 15 (12/2,000 ÷ 20/50,000). Let us say that available resources did not allow the investigator to determine the mental health status of each and every one of the 52,000 residents in the community. Using a case–control sampling approach, the cases would be the 32 subjects with the outcome event (death), and the controls would be a sample of the 52,000 residents who were candidates for the outcome event. Now suppose time and money dictated that only 1% of the residents could be sampled and examined, hence we would have 520 subjects as controls. By definition, taking a random sample of the population, the distribution of affective disorders among these 520 controls would be proportional to the distribution among the total population. Therefore, 20 controls would be expected to have an affective disorder and 500 would not. It is highly unlikely in psychiatric research that measurements can be made on the basis of the total population. Therefore, methods such as the case–control study are used to estimate such population measurements as relative risk.

Table 1 displays a crosstabulation of the outcome and exposure status for this sampling design. The odds of exposure (affective disorder) among the cases (12/20) is contrasted with the odds of exposure among the controls (20/500). The ratio between the two odds is (12/20) ÷ (20/500) or 15, which is exactly what would have been obtained had all the residents been included in the analysis. Thus, the odds ratio obtained in a case–control study is an estimate of the

Table 1.   Results of a Case–Control Study
of Relative Risk of Dying

Exposure status	Cases (deaths)	Controls (population sample)
With affective disorder	12	20
Without affective disorder	20	500
Total	32	520

relative risk of an event outcome's occurring in the total population between two comparison groups. This illustrates the basic principle of sampling. Measurements made on a random sample of the population should closely estimate the *true* value of the measurement if one could assess the total population.

If the population is closed (i.e., without in-migration or out-migration), and the controls are samples of the candidate population (including both cases and noncases), then the odds ratio is an estimate of relative risk (more specifically, cumulative incidence ratio or risk ratio). In practice, many investigators select samples from those who were alive at the end of the observation period (noncases) as the controls. Strictly speaking, the odds ratio obtained by comparing cases with samples of noncases approximates the relative risk only if the outcome is an infrequent event in the population. The relative risk obtained would represent cumulative incidence odds ratio or risk odds ratio. In the above example, with a 1% sample of noncases (52,000 − 32 = 51,968) resulting in a sample of 519 as the control group (still about 520), the odds ratio obtained would still approximate the relative risk. Here having only 32 deaths out of 52,000 qualifies as a rare event, and thus selecting the controls from the noncases (n = 51,968) versus all subjects (n = 52,000) has little effect on the estimation of the relative risks.

If, on the other hand, the population is dynamic (with in- and out-migration) and is in a steady state (in-migrations equals out-migrations, and dead subjects are replenished by living subjects with similar characteristics), the candidates would be the total 52,000 subjects living in the community ("noncases") at any time. The exposure odds ratio obtained from the cases and noncase controls in a dynamic population is, therefore, a direct estimate of the relative risk without the rare-event assumption (Miettinen, 1985a). Here, the odds ratio would be a direct estimate of incidence density ratio or incidence rate ratio. For a more detailed discussion of the interpretation of the odds ratio in a case-control study, interested readers are referred to the Appendix of this chapter.

Even though the case–control design is only now receiving greater attention in psychiatric research, its advantages in terms of studying uncommon illnesses over other types of group comparison approaches (particularly the advantage of efficiency), will ensure its expanded application in the future. But, as will be discussed later in this chapter, this design is also prone to some research biases.

VALIDITY CONSIDERATIONS IN GROUP COMPARISONS

When comparing two groups, the relative risk obtained for the relation between a determinant and an outcome can be distorted by factors which compromise the validity of the comparison. These factors include noncomparability of the population composition in the two groups, noncomparability of the information collected between groups, and noncomparability of the two groups in terms of extraneous attributes included in the formation of the contrast (Miettinen, 1985a). All forms of noncomparability result in a biased estimate of relative risk. Biased relative risk measures either over- or underestimate the true relation between the risk determinant and outcome. Frequently encountered biases in comparative studies are: *selection bias, information bias,* and *confounding bias* (Monson, 1990).

Selection bias is most likely to occur in studies where the outcome status is already known, such as retrospective cohort or case–control studies. In a retrospective cohort study, if identification and enrollment of exposed and nonexposed individuals is influenced by the development of the outcome of interest, selection bias can occur. For example, in a study of the relation between occupational exposure to solvents and the development of Alzheimer's disease in an occupation cohort, if the files of the employees who developed the disease have been removed from the current company roster, been kept in a separate location (perhaps for processing of worker's compensation), and not been available to the investigator, then enrollment into the study would be affected by the outcome status and the experience based on this partial cohort could be biased.

In a case–control study, the controls should be a representative sample of the candidate population in terms of the distribution of the exposure. However, this sample may be systematically nonrepresentative for many reasons (Lewis & Pelosi, 1990). For example, individuals may refuse to cooperate in interviews and this noncooperation may be systematically associated with the exposure under study. In a hospital-based case–control study, admission to a hospital may be determined by factors related to the exposure. This source of error has been described by Berkson (1946).

The selection of controls in a case–control study has been a controversial issue (Miettinen, 1985b). Nevertheless, theoretical and practical principles of selecting valid controls have been proposed in epidemiologic literature (Miettinen, 1985a). As described before, controls are to be representative of the population from which the cases arise in terms of the distribution of the exposure. In practice, this translates into three guiding principles: (1) the controls and the cases should come from a shared population source; (2) the selection of controls should be independent of the exposure; and (3) exclusion criteria should be applied symmetrically to cases and controls regarding incidental, secondary diagnoses (Miettinen, 1985a), or co-morbid conditions (Schwartz & Link, 1989).

Using theoretical examples, Schwartz and Link (1989) showed that nonsymmetric exclusion of co-morbid conditions between cases and controls can lead to biased relative risk estimates. Nonsymmetric exclusion occurs when controls are screened not only for the disorder of interest but also for any other psychiatric disorders or for high scores on scales of psychiatric symptoms. If cases that have other psychiatric disorders or that are high on symptom scores are included, and if exposures have effects on the development of these other disorders or symptoms, using a screened control group makes it difficult to separate the effects of exposures on other disorders or symptoms from the effects of exposures on the disorder under study (Schwartz & Link, 1989).

It should be noted that the concept and criteria of screening will be different when outcomes in family members, rather than in index subjects, are under study. For comparisons involving family members, a design other than the case–control study is required. The probands (index cases and "controls") in a family study can be screened to a different degree to form the desired contrasts in the comparison (see the section on comparative family studies).

Information bias occurs when noncomparable methods are used to collect data on the comparison groups ("observation bias"). Observation bias can occur when subjects are lost to follow-up in a cohort study. If subjects lost to follow-up have a different outcome experience from the other study participants, and the rate of loss is different between the comparison groups, biased comparisons can result. Information bias can also occur in a case–control study when members of comparison groups provide information with varying degrees of accuracy ("recall bias"). For example, mothers who gave birth to mentally retarded children might recall medications using during pregnancy with a different degree of accuracy than mothers who gave birth to healthy children. Information bias can also occur from interviewer bias. This error refers to any systematic differences in the soliciting, recording, or interpreting of information from study participants by the investigator or co-workers and can affect every type of design.

Confounding bias occurs when the populations of the comparison groups have an imbalanced distribution of characteristics which are independent determinants of outcome. These characteristics are said to be associated with both the exposure (because their distribution in the two groups is imbalanced) and the outcome (because they are predictors of the outcome). Table 2 illustrates a situation in which confounding bias might occur in a psychiatric research setting.

In Table 2, it can be seen that age is a predictor of outcome (mortality density is higher among older subjects) and that age is unevenly distributed between the comparison groups (the schizophrenic group has more "person-years" contributed by younger subjects). Even though the mortality density should be threefold when schizophrenia is compared with major depression, the relative risk estimated among all subjects was only 1.5. Hence, if age is not considered in the above comparison, a biased relative risk results.

The *placebo effect* commonly attributed to experimental studies, and described previously, can also occur in nonexperimental studies. For example, in a

Table 2. Confounding Bias in a Comparative Study
of the Mortality Rate (Density) for Major Psychosis

Sample	Deaths	Person-years	Mortality rate (per 1,000 person-years)
Younger subjects (<65 years of age)			
Schizophrenia	9	3,000	3.0
Major depression	1	1,000	1.0
Relative risk = 3.0			
Older subjects (65+ years of age)			
Schizophrenia	15	1,000	15.0
Major depression	15	3,000	5.0
Relative risk = 3.0			
All subjects			
Schizophrenia	24	4,000	6.0
Major depression	16	4,000	4.0
Relative risk = 1.5			

prospective cohort study of physical exercise and mental well-being in the elderly, the nonexercise group must receive exposure to the same social environment as the exercise group, otherwise the difference in mental well-being observed between the two groups could be due to the additional social interaction the exercise group would have from contact with care personnel and other participants. The contrast obtained would be "exercise plus additional social interaction" versus "no exercise plus no social interaction," with the difference in mental well-being observed between the two groups not being attributed to exercise alone. If comparable extraneous attributes cannot be achieved in a comparative study, one needs to be cautious concerning study inferences.

Even though the methods used in experimental studies to increase validity cannot, in general, be used in nonexperimental studies, considerations of validity, to avoid biases, still need to be addressed. In experimental studies, comparability of effect between groups is achieved by use of a placebo, comparability of populations is achieved by randomization, matching, and statistical adjustment, and comparability of data collection is achieved by blinds or double-blinds. In nonexperimental studies, these goals are achieved by careful study design, standardization of study protocol and execution, the use of blinds whenever possible, matching of population characteristics in study design, and by stratification or modeling of other risk determinants in the statistical analysis (Anderson et al., 1980; Hennekens and Buring, 1987). Although the effects of some biases can be mitigated (at least partially) in the data analysis, the consequences of other biases (such as selection and information bias) may be impossible to rectify once they have occurred. Consequently, prevention of bias in the design and execution of an investigation is crucial to the validity of its findings.

The choice of study population can minimize potential biases in several ways. Selection of hospitalized controls (such as surgical patients) in a case–control study may increase comparability with the cases in terms of the subjects' willingness to participate and the similarity in the referral pattern or selective factors that influenced the subjects' choice of a particular hospital. The environment under which the interviews were conducted would also be similar for cases and controls. All those factors decrease the likelihood of nonresponse and avoid selection and recall biases. However, the investigator must constantly assess whether the controls are selected independently of exposure so that the exposure distribution of these controls is representative of the population experience from which the cases arise.

If it is known that all the cases included in a study are drawn from a particular geographical area, then the control population can be selected from the same area (i.e., neighborhood controls) to increase representativeness. For cohort studies and clinical trials in which loss to follow-up or nonresponse must be minimized, the investigator might want to choose populations that are well defined with respect to occupation, place of employment, area of residence, or to belonging to special groups, such as college alumni, U.S. veterans, or members of health maintenance organizations. Individuals at high risk of developing the outcome event under study are more likely to participate in a study (Hennekens and Buring, 1987).

In the data-collection stage, the following procedures are used to maximize validity: (1) the standardization and calibration of specific instruments, including questionnaires, interviews, physical examinations, and forms for abstracting data from records; and (2) the standardization of study protocols, the training and supervising of study personnel, and the use of blinds in the administration of all instruments by study personnel.

Confounding variables can be dealt with by matching in the design stage or using conditioned methods in the analysis stage. That confounding variables can bias relative risk estimates has been shown in Table 2. *Conditional analysis* may be conducted by combining relative risk estimates from each stratum defined by the confounding variables (stratified analysis) or by developing a model for computing relative risk as a function of the confounding variables (multivariate regression analysis) (Anderson *et al.*, 1980). However, these conditional analytic procedures will be of limited value if the data collection procedures preclude subsequent analytic stratification. Consider the following extreme example: in a prospective cohort study, all exposed individuals were male and all nonexposed individuals were female. Because exposure is wholly conditional on sex, each stratum lacks information from one of the two exposure categories. With such data, the exposure is completely confounded with sex, and no analytic method can separate the effect of exposure from that of sex.

Matching, which can be considered a stratified sampling design, is commonly used to avoid this problem. In a cohort study, exposed and nonexposed subjects are matched in terms of the confounding variable(s) prior to their enrollment in the study. This way both exposed and nonexposed subjects are included in each stratum as defined by the confounding variable or variables. Adjusted relative risk can then be obtained by pooling the strata-specific relative risk estimates by some weighted average procedure. The examples described in the section on prospective cohort design employed this matching strategy. In a case–control sampling design, stratified sampling is accomplished by matching controls (who are, in fact, samples of the candidate population) and cases with regard to the confounding variables. Subsequently, each case and its matched controls constitute a stratum. This ensures that within the stratum defined by the confounding variables, there will always be both cases and controls for analysis. Matching on confounding variables in a case–control study makes the distribution of these variables in controls artificially similar to that in cases. Since confounding variables are correlated with the exposure, the distribution of exposure among the controls is representative of that among the candidate population only in terms of the matched variables. Therefore, to obtain accurate, adjusted, relative risk estimates in case–control studies, conditional analyses, based on a matched design, need to be performed (Schlesselman, 1982).

COMPARATIVE FAMILY STUDIES IN PSYCHIATRIC RESEARCH

In general, the purpose of a *comparative family study* is to investigate whether there is a tendency for a disorder to occur among genetically related family members (i.e., the familiarity of a disorder). The typical family study examines the risk of a particular disorder (i.e., schizophrenia) in the relatives of cases with the disorder versus the risk in relatives of a normal comparison group. It is the selection of the comparison group that is usually at issue in family studies. In this section, several issues regarding family studies in psychiatric research are discussed: (1) the choice of the general population as the comparison group in a family study; (2) the variety of epidemiological designs used to conduct family studies; and (3) options in the choice of comparison groups in family studies.

The problems of using the general population as the comparison group in family studies have been discussed in a series of letters to the editor which appeared in the *Archives of General Psychiatry* (Baldessarini, 1984; Gershon, 1984; Weissman, Kidd, & Prusoff, 1984). These letters were prompted by an earlier publication in which rates of affective disorder in relatives of depressed and normal proband groups were compared. The authors of that earlier paper (Weissman, Kidd, & Prusoff, 1982) characterized their investigation as a "case–control" study. Their "control" group, selected from the community, had "no evidence of psychiatric disorder or treatment" (p. 1398). Baldessarini (1984), however, argued that the risk of psychiatric disorders in relatives of these normal probands is, in fact, not representative of the risk in the general population, since the general population would contain subjects meeting criteria for various psychiatric disorders (including affective disorder). The key issue in this debate is whether the "risk in the general population" should serve as the referent in family studies. There seem to be two choices. If interest is in measuring the lifetime prevalence of a specific psychiatric disorder in the general population (perhaps for planning or administrative purposes), a probability sample for the general population should be selected. This approach is similar to that used for the ECA study (Regier *et al.*, 1984). This design can be considered as "descriptive epidemiology," or a population survey.

If, however, the primary interest is in estimating the morbidity risk of a disorder among the relatives of probands with the same disorder, assuming no familiarity (as is the case in most family studies), "general population risk" would not be a good estimate of this "null expected risk," because if, in fact, familiarity exists, the general population risk would be a mixture of risks related and unrelated to familiarity; that is, the general population sample would include familial cases of the disorder under study. Consequently, the magnitude of the difference between the rate for family members of the index cases and the general population would be diminished. Therefore, when the intent is to compare rates of psychiatric illness among relatives of probands with those among relatives of controls, the controls should be normals who do not meet diagnostic criteria for the disorder under study. Obviously, by omitting the cases, the normals are not representative of the general population, but they can still be chosen to serve as the controls for the purpose of the family study. However, as stated by Baldessarini (1984), "normality" (no disorder) can also run in families, and this could lead to a lowered rate of disorder among the family members of "normal controls."

The tenability of Baldessarini's argument can be examined using extreme examples. Suppose that all cases of a psychiatric disorder were attributable to familiarity. The expected rate under no familiarity would be 0 and, therefore, the "general population rate" would not be a good estimate of this expected rate. This example is so extreme that even normal probands that have symptomatic family members would have to be excluded as controls. Now suppose that all cases of another psychiatric disorder were never attributable to familiarity. The expected rate under no familiarity would be the observed rate in the population. Since no familiarity exists, the rate among relatives of normal probands (or any other index subjects for that matter) would constitute the expected rate. In reality, the familiarity of psychiatric disorders falls between these two extremes, but how one should obtain "expected rate under no familiarity" deserves further thought and investigation.

There is yet another issue involved in the research of Weissman *et al.* (1982). As stated earlier in this chapter, epidemiological investigation seeks to explore the relationship between a risk determinant and an outcome. In the case under discussion, the risk determinant is the psychiatric status (depressed or normal) of the index subject, and the outcome of interest is the occurrence of a particular psychiatric disorder (i.e., affective disorder) among the first-degree relatives. The contrast is between index subjects with an illness, whose relatives are "at risk," and normal subjects without the illness, whose relatives are "not at risk."

It is therefore clear that the relatives are the study subjects and their outcome is the object of the study. Their enrollment in the study is based on their exposure status (having or not having a depressed index relative) and not on their outcome status (having or not having an affective illness) (see the section on cohort and case–control study). Consequently, "case–control study" is not a good description of this design (M. M. Weissman, personal communication, February 15, 1989). Depending on the time sequence between exposure and outcome, and the timing of data collection, this type of study should be categorized instead as a cross-sectional study, a prospective cohort study, or a retrospective cohort study. For example, if the study outcome is the lifetime cumulative incidence ("lifetime prevalence") of affective disorders among the relatives, the design then resembles that of a retrospective cohort study.

Some of the confusion in describing the various types of family studies has occurred as a result of the different ways in which design components are labeled. Based on the classification scheme described in this chapter, the use of the term *controls* should be avoided in this type of study and be replaced with terms like *proband of the comparison group, contrasting proband,* or *comparison proband*. For now, it is important to know in what sense and in which design the terms *cases* and *controls* are being used, since the concept and criteria of a control can be very different among different studies (e.g., Schwartz & Link, 1989; Tsuang, Fleming, Kendler, & Gruenberg, 1988).

Tsuang *et al.* (1988) proposed the use of several comparison proband groups in family studies of the major psychoses, including major depression. The selection of several types of comparison proband groups in a family study will allow the investigators to empirically examine the issues raised earlier (i.e., which is the correct comparison group to be used in testing the hypotheses of familiarity). For our current discussion, we will focus on two comparison groups: *screened* and *unscreened*. *Screened* means that the comparison group contains only subjects without major depression or any history of psychiatric symptoms, in effect, a "supernormal" proband group. *Unscreened* means that the comparison groups does not contain subjects with major depression but may contain individuals with a history of other psychiatric symptoms.

If one assumes that other validity issues (such as matching, blind interviewing, study execution in similar environments or under similar circumstances, controlling of covariables in the analysis) have been properly dealt with, then the major design issue becomes the correct formulation of the comparison groups to achieve comparability of effects and to afford proper inference. When selecting a contrast in a family study, it is always good to bear in mind that one is attempting to measure an "expected effect" of an exposure under the null hypothesis of "no familiarity." Obviously, in psychiatric family studies, this depends on what effect one is interested in studying or teasing out. Using major depression as an example, if one selects a screened comparison group where none of the subjects meet criteria for major depression or have other psychiatric symptoms, then the total effect (measured as "risk in the relatives") is attributable to major depression and other psychiatric symptoms in the proband. However, if the unscreened comparison group is chosen, the contrast is between the relatives of probands with major depression versus the relatives of subjects without major depression, who, however, may have other psychiatric symptoms which the probands with major depression also possess (i.e., the major effect is attributable to the depression). This latter approach would be appropriate if the effect of major depression is the main variable of interest rather than the joint effects of major depression and other psychiatric symptoms.

SUMMARY

In this chapter, we explored various aspects of group comparison approaches in psychiatric research. Comparative population research has become essential to the development and testing of psychiatric hypotheses, whether the topic is psychopharmacology, nosology, clinical interventions, or familiarity.

Given the nature and complexity of psychiatric disorders, the use of group comparison methodology in psychiatry presents some special challenges. In this chapter, we focused on how these challenges have been addressed by psychiatric researchers both in principle and in specific examples.

We began with an examination of measures of outcome and measures of strength of association or relation. This was followed by a discussion of types of comparison studies that explored experimental designs and such important nonexperimental designs as cross-sectional and longitudinal (including retrospective and prospective cohort and case–control) studies. Questions concerning validity in relation to nonexperimental designs were examined at some length. We concluded the chapter with a discussion of the formulation of comparison groups in family studies.

APPENDIX: ODDS RATIO AND ITS INTERPRETATION
IN CASE–CONTROL STUDIES

By definition, odds ratio is the ratio between two odds. An odds is, in turn, the ratio of the probability of an event to its complement (i.e., $1 -$ the probability). In studies of the relation between an exposure and a disease, there are two types of odds. The first is the disease odds, which is the ratio of probability of disease over the probability of no disease. The other is the exposure odds, which is the ratio of probability of exposure over the probability of no exposure.

In epidemiologic studies, odds ratio is commonly obtained from a case–control study. Procedure-wise, those with the disease are enrolled in the study as the cases and a sample of those without the disease are enrolled as the controls. These cases are then further categorized, for a dichotomous exposure variable, as the exposed or nonexposed; controls are similarly classified into the exposed and nonexposed groups. Odds ratio is obtained as the ratio of the exposure odds among the cases to that among the controls.

Most epidemiologists recognize that a case–control study is a method to sample the disease experience in a population. The interpretation of the exposure odds ratio obtained in a case–control study depends on the type of population experience and the method of sampling (Miettinen, 1976; Greenland and Thomas, 1982; Miettinen, 1985a). In the following we describe some of the possible ways of conducting a case–control study and the interpretation of the observed odds ratio derived from the study.

1. Case–control sampling from a fixed cohort with controls selected from the noncases

The classic rationale of a case–control study is based on a fixed cohort (a closed population). At the end of follow-up of a cohort, those who developed the disease are collected as the cases. The controls are then sampled from among those who did not develop the disease and, therefore, are noncases. This sampling method is illustrated as follows. In the table below, E_1 denotes that the subjects were exposed and E_0 not exposed.

	E_1	E_0	Total
Cases	a	b	M_1
Noncases	$N_1 - a$	$N_0 - b$	$T - M_1$
Total	N_1	N_0	T

With T subjects in the cohort at the beginning of the follow-up, N_1 were exposed and N_0 not exposed. At the end of follow-up, M_1 subjects developed the disease under study and these are enrolled as the cases. Among the M_1 subjects a were from the exposed group and b from the nonexposed group. The classical rationale samples the controls from among those who did not develop the disease at the end of follow-up. There are $T - M_1$ such subjects; $N_1 - a$ were from the exposed group and $N_0 - b$ from the nonexposed group. Suppose with a sampling fraction of k among $T - M_1$ subjects, M_0 subjects without the disease were obtained as the controls; among them c were from the exposed group and d from the nonexposed group. After the case–control sampling the resulted data are usually displayed as

	E_1	E_0	Total
Cases	a	b	M_1
Noncases	c	d	M_0
Total	$a + c$	$b + d$	$M_1 + M_0$

For this table, the observed odds ratio is obtained as the ratio of the exposure odds between cases and controls

$$OR = (a/b)/(c/d) \text{ or, more commonly}$$
$$= (ad)/(bd)$$

This odds ratio can be re-expressed as

$$OR = (a/c)/(b/d)$$

Applying the sampling function

$$c = k(N_1 - a), d = k(N_0 - b)$$

the odds ratio becomes $\{a/[k(N_1 - a)]\}/\{b/[k(N_0 - b)]\}$ which, after canceling k, is $[a/(N_1 - a)]/[b/(N_0 - b)]$.

This expression is exactly the disease odds ratio or risk odds ratio or cumulative incidence odds ratio for the original cohort at the end of follow-up. If a and b are relatively small compared to N_1 and N_0 ("rare disease" assumption),

$$OR = \{a/[N_1(1 - a/N_1)]\}/\{b/[N_0(1 - b/N_0)]\}$$

$$= (a/N_1)/(b/N_0)$$

= risk ratio, cumulative incidence ratio, or "Relative Risk" in the original cohort.

This represents the classic rationale of conducting a case–control study and remains to be the only understanding of this methodology by many to this date (see, for example, Sandercock, 1989). However, there are other ways of sampling this same cohort.

2. Case–control sampling in a fixed population with controls selected from the beginning population

Similar to the above situation, at the end of follow-up, cases are collected and subdivided into the exposed/nonexposed groups. As for the controls, the samples are obtained from among the *total* starting population (rather than from just the noncases). In the first table of this Appendix a sampling fraction of k is applied to the $T (= N_1 + N_0)$ subjects; M_0 subjects were obtained: among them c were from the exposed group and d from the nonexposed group. As before, after the case–control sampling the resulting data are displayed as

	E_1	E_0	Total
Cases	a	b	M_1
Noncases	c	d	M_0
Total	$a + c$	$b + d$	$M_1 + M_0$

For this table, the observed odds ratio is obtained as the ratio of the exposure odds between cases and controls

$$OR = (a/b)/(c/d) \text{ or } (ad)/(bc)$$

The odds ratio can be re-expressed as

$$OR = (a/c)/(b/d)$$

Applying the sampling fraction

$$c = k(N_1), \ d = k(N_0)$$

the odds ratio becomes $\{a/[k(N_1)]\}/\{b/[k(N_0)]\}$ which, after canceling k, is $(a/N_1)/(b/N_0)$. Therefore, the observed odds ratio is a direct estimate of risk ratio (cumulative incidence ratio, "relative risk"). Unlike the classical method described in the previous section, the "rare disease" assumption is not needed in this procedure.

Clearly, this sampling method is conceptually superior to the preceding case–noncase sampling rationale. It is noted that cases are among the beginning population and can be among the samples selected to be controls. This is not a misclassification of outcomes. Misclassification of outcome concerns the classification of cases in the total population. Since case–control method is but a way of sampling the disease experience of a population, the samples should merely reflect the classification status in the population.

3. Case–control sampling of a fixed cohort with controls selected within the risk set for each case.

There is yet another way of sampling a fixed cohort. Usually the follow-up of a fixed cohort enables one to estimate the person-time accumulated in the study. The incidence rate (density, hazard, "force of morbidity or mortality") can then be estimated as number of cases over the amount of person-time for each exposure group. The ratio of the two incidence rates is known as the rate ratio, incidence density ratio, or hazard ratio. "Relative risk" has also been used very often to describe the incidence rate ratio. This usage somewhat confuses many on the distinction between risk ratio and rate ratio. The previous two methods (case–noncase, case–beginning population) of sampling a fixed cohort cannot provide an estimate of incidence rate ratio which is estimable inherently in the fixed cohort. Also, the ability of these two methods to provide risk odds ratio and risk ratio estimates depends on whether the follow-up of every subject in the cohort is complete, i.e., without censoring.

Without conducting a case–control sampling, the full data obtained from a fixed cohort (e.g., subjects in a clinical trial) can be analyzed using the proportional hazards model (Cox, 1972; Woolson et al., 1980). The model assumes constant hazard ratio over the follow-up period and puts no restriction on the baseline hazard (i.e., the incidence rate in the nonexposed group) over time. The construction of this model is based on the likelihood of observing a case occurring at a particular follow-up time point among the cohort members who are eligible at that time. The eligible members would have a follow-up time at least as long as that of the case. These members form the risk set (candidate set) for that particular case. After fitting with the data with the likelihood that among these candidates the case has the observed exposure status, the model can provide an estimate of the incidence rate ratio under the proportional hazards assumption.

Instead of including every member of the risk set in the analysis, a case–control sampling can be applied. For each case occurred, a fraction of the members in the risk set will be sampled as the controls. In effect, the controls are matched to the cases on the time of follow-up. Analytic methods conditionally on the matched time will need to be performed. Conditional logistic regression, which shares a similar likelihood formulation as the proportional hazards model, is among them. With case–risk set sampling, under the proportional hazards (constant rate ratio) assumption, the observed odds ratio from a matched analysis is an estimate (has the interpretation) of the incidence rate ratio (density ratio, hazards ratio, "relative risk").

4. Case–control sampling from a dynamic population with the steady state assumption.

In a dynamic population, the subjects can enter the study at any time, and they may leave it (by dying or leaving town or through termination of the study) at any time. The exposure represents a status, of being exposed or nonexposed, which continues over time. In such a population, cases arise out of a pool of human experience whose size is measured in units of person-time. Since a subject may represent a quantity of observation that ranges anywhere from days to years, the calculation of cumulative incidence (e.g., cases per 100 subjects) is not meaningful. Calculation of incidence rate (e.g., cases per 100 subject-years), on the other hand, is possible; so is the incidence rate ratio comparing the incidence rates between the two groups. Suppose that in this dynamic population over a defined time-period a cases arise out of the P_1 exposed person-years and b cases arise out of the P_0 nonexposed person-years. In this pool of experience, the incidence rate ratio is, therefore, $(a/P_1)/(b/P_0)$. Diseases which do not occur frequently within a short time require large number of subjects over many years. The expense of maintaining information on a large enough number of in-transient persons at risk may be prohibitive. Epidemiologists deal with this common situation through a case–control sampling design, collecting data not on all persons in the dynamic population but only on samples (cases and controls). Most often this type of sampling is conducted where a complete registry of the cases (or a similar case-ascertainment mechanism) exists in the population studied.

The assumption of steady state means that the number of subjects who are entering and leaving this dynamic population has reached an equilibrium (i.e., if a subject dies or leaves, another subject with the same characteristics enters the population to replace him/her) so that the relative pool of experience contributed by the exposed to that by the nonexposed remains constant throughout the period of study. With a constant exposed/nonexposed ratio throughout the study period, subjects sampled at any point in time would reflect this exposed/nonexposed ratio. This forms the basis for conducting a case–control study. The odds ratio from this case–control study is an estimate of the incidence rate ratio. This sampling method is illustrated as follows. The table below represents the pool of population experience contributed by the exposed and the nonexposed subjects over time, and the number of cases occurred from each pool.

	E_1	E_0	Total
Cases	a	b	M_1
Person-time	P_1	P_0	$P_1 + P_0$

A case–control study would then (1) obtain all the cases (or a fraction of them) M_1 and subdivide them into a exposed and b nonexposed and (2) sample from the population at any time a total of M_0 subjects as the controls and subdivide them into c exposed and d nonexposed. With the steady state assumption described above, c/d is an estimate of P_1/P_0. Therefore, the exposure odds ratio between cases and controls is

$$OR = (a/b)/(c/d)$$
$$= (a/b)/(P_1/P_0)$$
$$= (a/P_1)/(b/P_0) = \text{incidence rate ratio}$$

5. Case–control (random time, random sample) sampling from a dynamic population by selecting randomly both the time points and the subjects

For some geographically defined dynamic populations, the sampling of controls can be entirely straightforward, without the steady state assumption. In many places, it is possible to obtain a complete list of residents. In this event the following procedure can be considered (Walker, 1991): (1) select a date at random from the case accrual period; (2) select a person at random from the population list and, if the subject selected was actually resident in the study area at the random date chosen, the subject is enrolled as a control for the case–control study as of the randomly sampled day; (3) classify the control selected as to the exposure status; (4) repeat the above three steps until the desired number of controls has been chosen. In the dynamic population person-time (P_1 and P_0), rather than persons, is meaningful and the incidence rate, as well as incidence rate ratio, can be calculated. The double-selection process (choosing a random time point from the case accrual period and a random subject from the population under study) samples person time rather than people. Again, c/d is an estimate of P_1/P_0, and the odds ratio obtained estimates the incidence rate ratio in the dynamic population during the study period.

6. Case–control sampling with cases accrual from an incomplete registry (e.g., a hospital).

Similar rationale can show that the observed odds ratio estimates the incidence rate ratio in a hospital-based case–control study. However, it is more difficult to conceptualize the appropriate population to be sampled as compared with the population experience which has a complete registry of cases as discussed in Sections 4 and 5 above (Miettinen, 1985b). The issue is that in some hospital-based case–control studies, cases are ascertained from one or a few institutions; they represent only a fraction of those which arose from the catchment area, and they could have some particular referral patterns. Thus, they may not be all the cases occurred in the catchment area. Therefore, the real source population needs additional definitions. It has been proposed that the source population in this case be defined as those who, had they had the same diagnosis as the cases, would have come to these particular institutions. Controls are selected based on this criteria. More detailed discussion of this issue can be found in the reference cited (Miettinen, 1985a, 1985b). Again, the odds ratio observed is an estimate of the incidence rate ratio in the real source population, however defined, during the study period.

Acknowledgments. The studies that were presented in this chapter were supported in part by grants MH-43518, MH-44277, MH-46318, and DA-04604 from the National Institute of Mental Health and the National Institute of Drug Abuse, and by a Veterans Administration Medical Research Merit Review Grant to Dr. Tsuang. The authors would like to thank Leslie Young for her assistance in the preparation of this chapter. This paper was partially completed while Dr. Ming Tsuang was the Fritz Redlich Fellow at the Center for Advanced Study in the Behavioral Sciences. Dr. Tsuang is grateful for financial support provided by the John D. and Catherine T. MacArthur Foundation and Foundation Fund for Research in Psychiatry Endowment.

REFERENCES

Anderson, S., Auquier, A., Hauck, W. W., Oakes, D., Vandaele, W., & Weisberg, H. I. (1980). *Statistical methods for comparative studies*. New York: Wiley.

Baldessarini, R. J. (1984). Risk rates for depression (letter). *Archives of General Psychiatry, 41,* 103–104.

Berkson, J. (1946). Limitation of the application of fourfold table analysis to hospital data. *Biometrics Bulletin, 2,* 47–53.

Campbell, D. T., & Stanley, J. C. (1963). *Experimental and quasi-experimental designs for research.* Chicago: Rand McNally.

Chiang, C. L. (1968). *Introduction to stochastic processes in biostatistics.* New York: Wiley.

Cox, D. R. (1972). Regression models and life tables (with discussion). *Journal of the Royal Statistical Society (B), 34,* 187–220.

Eaton, W. W., & Kessler, L. E. (1985). *The (NIMH) epidemiologic catchment area program.* New York: Academic Press.

Eaton, W. W., Holzer, C. E., Von Korff, M., Anthony J. C., Helzer, J. E., George, L., Burnam, M. A., Boyd, J. H., Kessler, L. G., & Locke, B. Z. (1984). The design of the epidemiologic catchment area surveys. *Archives of General Psychiatry, 41,* 942–948.

Elandt-Johnson, R. C. (1975). Definition of rates: Some remarks on their use and misuse. *American Journal of Epidemiology, 102,* 267–271.

Elwood, J. M. (1988). *Causal relationships in medicine: A practical system for critical appraisal.* New York: Oxford University Press.

Feighner, J. P., Robins, E., Guze, S. B., Woodruff, R. A., Winokur, G., & Munoz, R. (1972). Diagnostic criteria for use in psychiatric research. *Archives of General Psychiatry, 26,* 57–63.

Gershon, E. S. (1984). Risk rates for depression (letter). *Archives of General Psychiatry, 41,* 104–105.

Greenland, S., & Thomas, P. (1982). On the need for the rare disease assumption in case–control studies. *American Journal of Epidemiology, 116,* 547–53.

Hennekens, C. H., & Buring, J. E. (1987). *Epidemiology in medicine.* Boston: Little, Brown.

Kramer, M. (1957). A discussion of the concepts of incidence and prevalence as related to epidemiologic studies of mental disorders. *American Journal of Public Health, 47,* 826–840.

Lewis, G., & Pelosi, A. J. (1990). The case-control study in psychiatry. *British Journal of Psychiatry, 157,* 197–207.

Miettinen, O. S. (1976). Estimability and estimation in case-referent studies. *American Journal of Epidemiology, 103,* 226–35.

Miettinen, O. S. (1985a). *Theoretical epidemiology.* New York: Wiley.

Miettinen, O. S. (1985b). The "case-control" study: Valid selection of subjects. (with discussions). *Journal of Chronic Disease, 38,* 543–558.

Monson, R. R. (1990). *Occupational epidemiology* (2nd ed.). Boca Raton, FL: CRC Press.

Morrison, J., Clancy, J., Crowe, R., & Winokur, G. (1972). The Iowa 500: I. Diagnostic validity in mania, depression and schizophrenia. *Archives of General Psychiatry, 27,* 457–461.

Regier, D. A., Myers, J. K., Kramer, M., Robins, L. N., Blazer, D. G., Hough, R. L., Eaton, W. W., & Locke, B. Z. (1984). The NIMH epidemiologic catchment area (ECA) program: Historical context, major objectives, and study population characteristics. *Archives of General Psychiatry,* *41*, 934–941.

Sandercock, P. (1989). The odds ratio: A useful tool in neurosciences. *Journal of Neurology, Neurosurgery and Psychiatry, 52,* 817–20.

Schlesselman, J. J. (1982). *Case-control studies: Design, conduct, analysis.* New York: Oxford University Press.

Schwartz, S., & Link, B. G. (1989). The "well control" artefact in case/control studies of specific psychiatric disorders. *Psychological Medicine, 19,* 737–742.

Tsuang, M. T., & Dempsey, G. M. (1979). Long-term outcome of major psychoses: II. "Schizoaffective" disorder compared with schizophrenia, affective disorders, and a surgical control group. *Archives of General Psychiatry, 36,* 1302–1304.

Tsuang, M. T., Woolson, R. F., & Fleming, J. A. (1979). Long-term outcome of major psychoses: I. Schizophrenia and affective disorders compared with psychiatrically symptom-free surgical conditions. *Archives of General Psychiatry, 36,* 1295–1301.

Tsuang, M. T., Winokur, G., & Crowe, R. R. (1980). Morbidity risks of schizophrenia and affective disorders among first-degree relatives of patients with schizophrenia, mania, depression and surgical conditions. *British Journal of Psychiatry, 137,* 497–504.

Tsuang, M. T., Fleming, J. A., Kendler, K. S., & Gruenberg, A. S. (1988). Selection of controls for family studies: Biases and implications. *Archives of General Psychiatry, 45,* 1006–1008.

Walker, A. M. (1991). Observation and inference. An introduction to the methods of epidemiology. Chestnut Hill: Epidemiology Resources, Inc.

Weissman, M. M., Kidd, K. K., & Prusoff, B. A. (1982). Variability in rates of affective disorders in relatives of depressed and normal proband. *Archives of General Psychiatry, 39,* 1397–1403.

Weissman, M. M., Kidd, K. K., & Prusoff, B. A. (1984). Risk rates for depression [Letter to the editor]. *Archives of General Psychiatry, 41,* 105–106.

Woolson, R. T., Tsuang, M. T., & Fleming, J. A. (1980). Utility of the proportional-hazards model for survival analysis of psychiatric data. *Journal of Chronic Disease, 33,* 183–95.

CHAPTER 5

Correlational Approach

GERALD GOLDSTEIN

INTRODUCTION

Correlational methods are often described by contrast with group comparison approaches. In group comparison approaches, as described in Chapter 4, groups are constructed and controls are imposed. Generally, correlational methods are not thought of as being used in controlled studies, but rather in dealing with relationships among phenomena as they exist in natural situations. A correlation can be defined in numerous ways: as the strength of association between phenomena, as the degree to which one phenomenon can be predicted from another phenomenon, or as the degree to which phenomena covary. In a sense, it is a scientific version of the kinds of natural observation in which one relates one thing to another. Underlying these observations, we can usually find some theoretical inference concerning those relationships. For example, the clinician may observe that child abusers are often individuals who have suffered abuse themselves. A formal study of this observation would involve obtaining some response measure of child abuse and of experiencing abuse in the same set of individuals. The measure need only be the presence or absence of the experience. We can then tabulate these data in a contingency arrangement of the type shown in Figure 1. It can be seen there that the high numbers are in those cells that are completely positive or negative for the two phenomena (i.e., abusers with abusive parents and nonabusers with nonabusive parents). We can

Gerald Goldstein • Highland Drive, Veterans Administration Hospital, Pittsburgh, Pennsylvania 15206.

Research in Psychiatry: Issues, Strategies, and Methods, edited by L. K. George Hsu and Michel Hersen. Plenum Press, New York, 1992.

		COMMITTED CHILD ABUSE	
		Yes	No
ABUSING PARENT?	Yes	12	3
	No	2	14

Figure 1.

therefore say that there is a high correlation between having been abused and committing child abuse. However, in research applications, it is necessary to know how high. The value typically used to express how high the correlation is, or the strength of association, is called the *correlation coefficient*. A correlation coefficient is an index of the strength of association between two variables. It is a number that can range between −1 and +1. A value of 0 reflects complete absence of correlation; a −1 indicates a perfect negative correlation, whereas a +1 represents a perfect positive correlation. A positive correlation occurs when both values go up (e.g., height and weight in children), and a negative correlation occurs when one value goes up as the other goes down (e.g., days of drought and size of wheat crop). Correlations are rarely perfect, and most correlation coefficients are values such as .67 or −.35. The problem then becomes one of evaluating strength of association from these values. There are two considerations here: statistical significance and amount of explained variance. The statistical significance of a correlation coefficient involves the determination at a particular confidence level as to whether or not the coefficient is different from 0. Typically, statistical analysis in the behavioral sciences utilizes the .05 (occurrence by chance 5 times out of 100) or .01 (1 time out of 100) level. Thus, working at the .05 level, a given correlation coefficient would be appreciably significant if it could occur by chance less than 5 out of 100 times. Nonsignificant correlations are sometimes referred to as zero-order correlations. The statistical significance of a correlation coefficient is generally considered to be a relatively trivial matter in most research, but particularly when the purpose of the research is that of generating predictions from an unknown variable to a known variable. Highly significant correlation coefficients can have exceedingly low predictive value. Generally, a more important consideration is the percentage of explained variance: that percentage is the squared correlation coefficient. Thus, a correlation coefficient of .40 yields a 16% explained variance. That is, 16% of the variance in the unknown variable can be accounted for by variance in the known variable. The remaining variance in the unknown variable has to be accounted for by unknown factors.

Generally, correlation coefficients are derived from *regression analyses*. Regression provides estimates of unknown (y) values from known (x) values through the generation of equations. Thus, application of a regression equation can provide a predicted score for the unknown variable based upon the known variable score. The correlation coefficient is a measure of the gain in precision of predicting y from knowledge of x. Thus, a coefficient of 0 means absolutely no gain, whereas +1 or −1 means complete predictability. It is often useful for the investigator to examine regression equations diagrammatically so that the pairing of x and y variables can be seen in individual cases. This step may be accomplished by the plotting of a scatter diagram or scattergram. On a scattergram, the x scores are plotted along the X axis and the y scores along the Y axis. Individual score pairs are plotted as points at their meeting places. Thus, the point for a score of $x = 5$ and $y = 6$ would be plotted at 5 units along the X axis and 6 units up the Y axis. The scattergram is helpful in providing a picture of what the bivariate distribution looks like. That is, one can tell at a glance whether it is linear, curvilinear, or random.

There are many variants of regression analysis and many types of correlation coefficients. The major reason for choosing among the various types has to do with the mathematical assumptions upon which the statistic is based. Most notably, there is an assumption of linearity of the bivariate distribution for most correlation coefficients. However, many strong associations may not be linear. They may be U-shaped or may have some other configuration. Appropriate statistics have been devised for situations in which the assumption of linearity cannot be made. We will go no further into the mathematics of regression and correlation here, since these matters are covered in extensive detail in numerous statistics texts (e.g., Bruning & Kintz, 1987).

CORRELATION AND CAUSATION

Probably the most controversial issue involved in correlational data analysis has to do with the matter of *causality*. There is a commonly stated dogma that correlation is not causation. Because the correlation coefficient relating A to B is high, that does not mean that A causes B. The reasons for absence of causality may be simple co-occurrence of phenomena with no actual cause-and-effect relationship, or the presence of a third variable that is correlated with the two variables under study, but that is the real causal variable. For example, loss of teeth may be correlated with slowing of gait, but it might seem apparent that one does not cause the other. It seems more likely that the high correlation coefficient occurs because both variables are correlated with age. It may be recalled that this issue became particularly controversial during the time of the early cigarette smoking and cancer research. Despite the high correlations found, it was nevertheless argued by some that smoking was not the cause of cancer. The argument was based upon the considerations raised above. Either smoking and cancer frequently co-occurred in the same people, without evidence of a direct cause-and-effect relationship, or, alternatively, that both the inclination to smoke and cancer were actually caused by a third unknown variable. Thus, many scientists view correlation research as merely descriptive in nature, and definitive, causative findings must await specification of clearly defined independent and dependent variables followed by experimental interventions.

It is noted that independent and dependent variables are often not specified in correlational research. They may be either implied but not specified, or the investigator may simply be seeking relationships among phenomena without any need for specification. In this regard, a distinction may be made between what may be termed *transitive correlation* and *intransitive correlation*. In *transitive correlation*, the relationship between two variables is reciprocal. One cannot say that one is the independent and the other the dependent variable, nor can it be reasonably stated that one variable is the cause and the other the effect. The correlation between abilities would be an example of a transitive relationship. Because mathematical and reading abilities are highly correlated, it cannot be interpreted to mean that one ability caused the performance level of the other. They both, in fact, may have been caused by other considerations, such as quality of education or general intelligence. On the other hand, if one considers the correlation between size of wheat crop and amount of rainfall, no reasonable person would argue that wheat growing causes it to rain. Thus, the relation between correlation and causation would appear to resolve to logical analysis specifying independent and dependent variables, or the lack of pertinence of that distinction to the matter under study. For example, in an advanced form of correlational analysis called *factor analysis*, there is typically no interest at all in independent and dependent variables, since the purpose of the analysis is purely that of seeking relationships among variables. In summary, although one should not naively assume that correlation implies causation, neither should one naively assume that it does not. The mathematics of correlation is neutral to the matter of causality, and the issue can only be dealt with through logical analysis of the variables under consideration, particularly with regard to their transitive or nontransitive relationship. It may be noted that statisticians have attempted to deal directly with the matter of causal contribution through an advanced procedure called *path analysis* (Jöreskog, 1979).

CORRELATION IN BEHAVIORAL RESEARCH

In the remainder of this chapter, I will deal with what are probably the two most extensive areas of correlational research in the behavioral sciences: *psychometrics* and *epidemiology*. *Psychometrics* is the branch of behavioral science that has to do with the development and application of objective assessment and evaluation procedures. Psychiatric *epidemiology* technically deals with the incidence and prevalence of mental disorders, but is actually a broader field that does community and crosscultural longitudinal and cross-sectional studies of mental illness. Both of there fields make extensive use of correlational methods, but in different ways.

Psychometrics

There are three major applications of correlational statistics in psychometrics. They are determination of validity, reliability, and interrelationships among tests or test items. *Validity* is the appropriateness of a test for the purpose for which it is used. Tests may be used for classification, prediction of future performance, or, in clinical contexts, as an aid to diagnosis and prognosis. The extent to which they perform these functions well is referred to as their validity. Validity is generally established by correlating scores from the test under scrutiny with what is referred to as a *criterion*. A *criterion* is a quantified measure of the outcome that the test is purported to predict. Within the context of psychiatric research, the criterion used is frequently expert clinical judgment. Depending upon the level of sophistication of the psychometric research being accomplished, varying criteria may be established for the reliability of those judgments. For example, a stringent criterion might be complete agreement on the judgment among three board-certified psychiatrists. Many psychological tests, such as the Minnesota Multiphasic Personality Inventory-2 (MMPI-2) (Butcher, Graham, Dahlstrom, Tellegen, & Kaemmer, 1989) have been validated against clinical judgments of this type. In this case, what we obtain is called *concurrent validity*, or the ability of the test to predict to a contemporary criterion. Another type of criterion-related validity is called *predictive validity*. Tests are often used to predict future performance, such as level of functioning on a job or treatment outcome. In this case, there must be a waiting period between administration of the test and acquisition of the outcome information that is used as a criterion. In both concurrent and predictive validity establishment, a validity coefficient, which is in fact a correlation coefficient, is typically computed in order to determine the degree of association between the test scores and the criterion ratings. Low coefficients suggest that the test is not suitable for the purpose for which it is being used. There is no hard-and-fast rule for determining acceptability of a validity coefficient, but we are generally impressed when they get into the .8 to .9 range, and unimpressed when they are less than about .6.

Reliability has to do with the stability or consistency of an instrument. The concept of reliability cannot be intuited as readily as that of validity, probably because the stability of instruments we use clinically on a routine basis is assumed. However, imagine a thermometer that gave readings that were different over the course of a day even though evidence was available that the patient's temperature had not changed at all. What we would have is an unreliable thermometer, and we would probably discard it. In the case of psychometric procedures, the problem is that it is not scientifically justifiable to presume that a new psychological test is a stable measuring instrument that provides consistent data. Part of test development always includes a determination of degree of stability. That procedure is referred to as establishing the reliability of the test.

In psychometrics, there is a distinction between two types of reliability, both of which are assessed with the correlation coefficient. The first type is internal consistency and the other is repeatability. A test typically consists of numerous items that are thought to measure some trait or other dimension. If it does so reliably, then various alternate or parallel forms of the test should agree with each other. Within the framework of our present discussion, we mean that the scores should be highly correlated with each other. Thus, one method of determining reliability involves administering both alternate forms to the same group of individuals and computing the correlation coefficient between the two sets of scores. If alternate forms are not available, the single test itself can be split in half and the odd-numbered items can be correlated with the even-numbered items. Determining reliability in this manner provides information concerning the internal consistency of the test.

The matter of repeatability comes closer to the thermometer example. If the subject does not change, then we would want a measure to provide about the same scores over numerous testing occasions. This kind of evaluation is done with what is called the *test–retest reliability method*. It simply involves giving the same subjects the same test on at least two occasions, and computing correlations between the scores obtained the first time with those obtained the second time. This method, while commonly used, is somewhat hazardous. First of all, retesting often produces a "practice effect" such that the subject may improve on the second testing as a result of experience with the first testing. This problem is somewhat attenuated by the fact that the mathematics of correlation is based mainly on the relative rankings of scores, and as long as the rankings remain stable across testing occasions, the correlation should not be greatly affected. Thus, it is possible that the average score for the group may be substantially higher on the second testing occasion than it was on the first, but the correlation coefficient may nevertheless be quite high. In clinical situations, the test–retest method is often not applicable because of the high probability of there being rapid fluctuations in the conditions of patients. The test–retest method really depends upon sampling in a stable population.

The common wisdom is that there cannot be validity without reliability, since an unstable procedure cannot predict accurately to any criterion. Nevertheless, it is quite possible to have satisfactory reliability without validity. If one used the bull's-eye of a target as an analogy for the criterion, one could consistently hit some precise area time after time, but that area may be quite distant from the bull's-eye. As in the case of validity, there is no commonly accepted single value for determining whether a reliability coefficient is satisfactory or not. However, there is a helpful statistic in psychometrics called the *probable error of measurement*. Without going into detail, it is generally assumed that there is some error in testing so that a single test score is viewed as a point in a range of scores. That range is a function of the test's reliability. Thus, changes in test scores may reflect actual change in the subject or chance fluctuations within the probable error of measurement. Reliability is considered to be unsatisfactory to the extent that the probability of error of measurement of the score of a single subject ranges over an entire distribution of scores.

Reliability of Judgment

Here we will consider the situation in which decisions are reached not by administering quantitative tests but through the process of clinical judgments. From the point of view of quantification, clinical judgments are different from tests in that they constitute nominal rather than metric scales. That is, a phenomenon is said to be present or absent, and the clinician is, in essence, the test. The role of correlation in this context is frequently that of assessing the reliability of these judgments. Reliability of clinical judgment may be evaluated by having a clinician make nominal judgments concerning the same case over several occasions, by having a clinician make judgments and then contrasting them with nominal judgments made by a procedure different from clinical judgment, or by contrasting the clinical judgments made by more than one clinician concerning the same case, assuming that these judgments are made independently. In psychiatry, the third alternative is the one most commonly used. I will therefore take examples from those kinds of comparisons and try to show that the evaluation procedure used is quite comparable to procedures carried out in determining the reliability of quantitative tests.

Most of us are familiar with the problem of the reliability of psychiatric diagnosis, and with the major effort made by the science and profession of psychiatry to improve that reliability, which has led ultimately to the development of the objective diagnostic criteria codified in the *Diagnostic and Statistical Manual of Mental Disorders* (DSM-III) (American Psychiatric Association, 19890) and revised later in the DSM-III-R (American Psychiatric Association, 1987). Since there are few objective criteria for most of the mental disorders, in the sense of definitive laboratory or related biological indicators, the emphasis was placed on the application of structured clinical interviews, and the extent of agreement among clinicians on conclusions reached on the basis of these interviews. It is noted that the interviews were typically not used as psychological tests yielding quantitative scores, but rather as procedures used to aid clinical judgment. Thus, the representative research study was one in which two or more clinicians independently interviewed the same patients and made judgments concerning their diagnoses. As Cohen (1960) pointed out, it then becomes possible to view the clinicians as analogous to alternate forms, and the judgments as analogous to test scores. The statistical problem then becomes quite similar to what is involved in determining the reliability of psychological tests. The major difference is in the nature of the data, which are on a metric scale in the case of psychological tests and on a nominal scale in the case of clinical judgment.

Let us begin with the simplest possible case to develop an example: two clinicians making independent judgments concerning the presence or absence of a single diagnosis. How well do they agree with each other (i.e., what is their interjudge reliability?). Let us say that they both independently interviewed 30 patients and had to judge whether or not these patients were schizophrenic. Their data can be cast in a 2 × 2 contingency schema (Figure 2). Note that the agreements are on one diagonal and the disagreements are on the other. There is 80% agreement (24/30). Does that figure constitute satisfactory reliability? In order to answer that question, the first matter to consider is that some of the agreement could have occurred by chance. In this case, the judges would agree with each other half of the time by chance. Is 80% significantly better than 50%?

		JUDGE 1	
		SCHIZOPHRENIC	NONSCHIZOPHRENIC
JUDGE 2	SCHIZOPHRENIC	12	4
	NONSCHIZOPHRENIC	2	12

Figure 2.

As simple as the question may seem, no method was generally available to answer the question until the statistician Jacob Cohen (1960) published his research describing a statistic that he called *kappa* (κ). Those familiar with contingency tables might suggest that chi-square (χ^2) would be the appropriate statistic for determining significance, and that the chi-square-related correlation coefficients, the phi (ϕ) or contingency (C) coefficients, would be the appropriate reliability coefficients. However, Cohen pointed out that chi-square simply tests for association and not for agreement. Indeed, it would be possible to obtain a highly significant chi-square if there were complete disagreement between the judges. A statistic was needed that dealt with only the values along the agreement diagonal, thus testing the null hypothesis that the obtained proportions of agreement could have occurred by chance. Kappa is computed with the following equation:

$$\kappa = \frac{f_o - f_c}{1 - f_c}$$

That is, it is equal to the number of agreements obtained subtracted from the number of agreements that would be obtained by chance divided by 1 minus the number of agreements that would be obtained by chance. Kappa may range from 0 to 1, with 1 representing perfect agreement. The hypothesis that an obtained kappa is significantly different from 0 may be obtained by converting kappa to a z score and referring to a normal distribution table. Testing for the significance of a difference between two kappas can be accomplished in a similar manner. Of course, kappa can be generalized beyond the 2 × 2 table situation. Various elaborations of kappa, including a weighted kappa in which serious disagreement can be quantified, is presented in Fleiss (1981).

As in the case of the correlation coefficient, the finding that kappa is significantly different from 0 is often trivial, since such significance can occur in the presence of substantial disagreement. Citing a study by Landis and Koch (1977), Fleiss presents a rating scale for kappas in which values above .75 reflect excellent agreement, values below .40 represent poor agreement, and values in between represent fair-to-good agreement exceeding chance expectation.

Correlational methods are probably found in their most elegant form in research concerning relationships among abilities. Historically, this research began with the study of the structure of intelligence. At one time, there was a great debate over whether intelligence was a global ability or a series of separate functions. The scientific activity associated with this debate largely involved correlational methods, with the database consisting of subscales of intelligence and related mental ability tests. The names of Spearman, Burt, and Thurstone are most prominently associated with this movement.

Rather than pursuing the substantive matter of the nature of intelligence, I will supplement the remarks made about correlational statistics at the beginning of this chapter, since the research in intelligence is based primarily on these more advanced applications of correlation. First, it is frequently necessary to deal with more than one correlation at a time. That is, the investigator may be interested in interrelationships among more than one bivariate at a time; for example, the relationship among age, height, weight, and blood pressure. If we paired each of these variables, there would be 16 possible pairs, although 6 of them repeat themselves (e.g., height vs. weight and weight vs. height), and 4 cases would represent the correlation of the variable with itself. Therefore, there would be only six meaningful correlations. In general, the number of intercorrelations is equal to the square of the number of tests minus 1 divided by 2. Generally, the correlations are presented in tabular form called a *correlation matrix*. Table 1 provides an example of a correlation matrix. Note the triangular shape of the matrix reflecting the fact that redundant correlations are generally not entered, nor are the "1s" that reflect the correlation between the variable and itself. When working with multiple variables, it is often useful to construct a correlation matrix in order to look for patterns of relationships among variables (i.e., clusters of variables that are highly correlated among themselves, but not with other variables).

The situation often arises in which it is thought that a combination of many factors may be contributing to a single outcome or criterion. The procedure for performing this kind of evaluation is called *multiple regression and correlation*. Instead of an x variable and a y variable, there are at least two x variables and one y variable. It is possible to compute regression equations and correlation coefficients for these situations, but the mathematical computations required are far more complex than is the case for bivariate correlation. Using the example mentioned above, suppose we wanted to know the correlation between the combined effects of age, height and weight on blood pressure. Age, height, and weight are then characterized as *predictor* or independent variables and blood pressure is called the *criterion* or dependent variable. A multiple regression equation is written with the independent variables on the left-hand side and the

Table 1.   Interrelationships among Age, Height, Weight and Blood Pressure

	Age	Height	Weight	Blood pressure
Age		.85	.78	.63
Height			.91	.57
Weight				.62
Blood pressure				

dependent variable on the right-hand side. The correlation coefficient is called *multiple R* or simply *R*. *R* is not simply an additive function of the simple correlation coefficients but rather reflects the interaction of the weights they contribute to the multiple regression equations. These weights, sometimes called *beta weights* or *partial regression coefficients*, are used in calculating *R*. It is also possible to compute individual predicted *Y* scores from the regression equation. Some investigators use the so-called residual scores or the differences between actual and predicted scores in their analyses. The major reason for their use is that when estimating scores from a regression equation, the accuracy of the estimate may depend on the location of the score on the distribution. Typically, extreme scores are estimated with relatively less accuracy. Before leaving this topic, it should be emphasized that while these multivariate procedures are quite powerful, they often require large numbers of subjects. As a general rule of thumb, a ratio of 10 subjects to 1 variable is desirable.

As indicated above, two variables are sometimes correlated with each other within the context of both being correlated with a third variable. For example, two abilities may be correlated with each other because they are both correlated with general intelligence. The method used to evaluate this third variable effect is called *partial correlation*. Thus, one can compute the correlation between reading and mathematics ability to account for the variance associated with general intelligence. This third variable is called a *covariate* or a *control variable*. The coefficient derived from this process is called the *partial correlation coefficient*. It is an index of the strength of association between two variables following removal of the variance produced by a third variable. Partial correlation may be extended by utilizing several covariates. In the present example, one might want to use general intelligence and years of education as covariates. Partial correlation is particularly useful in behavioral research when one wants to account for variance contributed by some demographic variable. Thus, age, education, and socioeconomic status are often used as covariates.

The most elegant and complex form of correlational analysis is a procedure called *factor analysis*. Factor analysis is both an art and a science, and requires advanced training to master. It is rather commonly used now because of the general availability of statistical packages designed for use with high-speed computers, although interpretation of the output of these packages if often problematic for the individual who lacks appropriate training. As indicated, a correlation matrix can be inspected to see which correlation coefficients cluster together; that is, are correlated with each other but not with other clusters of correlations. For example, if we had a correlation matrix containing intelligence test subscales, one might note that the verbal tests are correlated with each other, but not with the performance tests, for which the reverse is true. Factor analysis is a formal method of doing this clustering.

The mathematical procedures employed to do a factor analysis may be divided into two components: one to derive the factor matrix and the other that rotates the matrix to an interpretable structure. This distinction is important because there are numerous paradigms for doing the initial factoring as well as numerous methods of rotation. With some restrictions, it is possible to interchange initial factoring methods and rotation methods. Thus, Factoring Method A may be used in combination with Rotation Methods A, B, or C. The investigator needs to choose one of each, and, ideally, to provide some rationale for that choice.

The bottom line of a factor analysis for most behavioral science investigators is called the *matrix of rotated factor loadings*. A factor is what the mathematics of the method used determines to be a cluster of correlations (as discussed above). A loading is the correlation between an individual variable and the factor. The matrix of rotated factor loadings tells us how many meaningful factors were extracted and what the loading pattern is. Ideally, the goal of rotation should be that of obtaining simple structure, or a matrix in which the individual variables load on unique factors. A factor analysis solution in which the same test loads substantially on several factors is often not helpful, particularly when one is seeking the underlying dimensions of the series of measures under investigation. A good general introduction to factor analysis can be found in Rummel (1970).

In contemporary behavioral investigation, factor analysis is viewed mainly as an exploratory procedure to be followed by more specific experimental investigations. It is commonly used as a data reduction method when the investigator has an excessively large number of variables and has to make sense out of how they relate to one another. A large correlation matrix can be bewildering, and factoring can provide a much more coherent picture of the structure of the data. It is also possible to reduce the number of variables used in subsequent studies through factor analysis. The two most commonly used ways of doing this are to use only the variables with the highest loadings on each factor or to use factor scores. Factor scores are the scores of each subject on each factor.

Epidemiology

As Bromet, Davies, and Schulz (1988) have illustrated, psychiatric epidemiology is not restricted to rate estimation. In addition to that area of investigation, which they term *descriptive epidemiology*, there is also an analytic and experimental epidemiology. *Analytic epidemiology*, with which we will be mainly concerned here, includes case–control, longitudinal, and prospective studies. It is largely concerned with causes of rate differences in different groups, and so looks at risk factors, the natural history of various disorders, the role of environmental factors, and the prediction of outcome. Implicitly or explicitly, much of this research is correlational in nature. A typical clinical research design in psychology or psychiatry may have a group comparison component, generally based on diagnosis, but once the groups are established, the remainder of the procedure is correlational in nature. In his Chapters 5 and 6, Fleiss (1981) provided information concerning specific statistical methods that are useful in naturalistic, prospective, and retrospective studies.

Let us use a risk study as a simple example. What is the risk of developing schizophrenia if one has a schizophrenic parent? As in examples used above, we can cast the data in a 2 × 2 contingency arrangement (Figure 3). It will be noted that 12 of the 26 schizophrenics had schizophrenic parents, while 8 of the 24 nonschizophrenics had schizophrenic parents and the remaining 16 did not. It would be appropriate to use the phi coefficient in this case as the measure of association. However, Fleiss (1981) described a statistic that is a measure of association but is more meaningful in risk research. It is called the *odds ratio*, and provides an estimate of the probability that *B* will occur when *A* is present and when it is absent. In this case, we would have the odds of there being a schizophrenic offspring when there was a schizophrenic parent. Information in this form may be more useful to the investigator than it would be in the form of a correlation coefficient.

Zigler and Glick (1986) utilized correlational evidence quite extensively in their work on the relationship between premorbid competence and psychiatric hospitalization. In one analysis they tested the hypothesis that more competent individuals, as measured by a scale they developed, would be hospitalized at a later age than would less competent individuals. They correlated age at first hospitalization with score on the competence test and obtained correlation coefficients that were somewhat consistent with the hypothesis. They also factor analyzed their premorbid competence scale, finding that it was multifactorial rather than based on a single dimension. Three factors were identified: one representing education and occupation, the second receiving high loadings only from age and marital status, and the third reflecting employment history.

Application of partial correlation is commonly seen in prospective or retrospective field studies when there is a need to adjust or correct the data for some demographic variable. For example, one may wish to attribute some characteristic to a particular diagnostic group, but may subsequently find that the characteristic is sensitive to age, educational, or gender differences. It then becomes appropriate to use these variables as covariates in partial correlation analyses. As a rather dramatic example of the effects of such an analysis, Goldstein, Zubin, and Pogue-Geile (1991) recently studied the degree of association between length of hospitalization and cognitive decline in schizophrenic inpatients. Initially, we computed simple correlation coefficients and found many robust correlations between performance on cognitive tests and years of hospitalization. However, when we repeated these analyses, using chronologi-

		SCHIZOPHRENIC PARENT	
		Yes	No
SCHIZOPHRENIC	Yes	12	14
	No	8	16

Figure 3.

cal age as a covariate, these robust relationships essentially disappeared, and we had to conclude that there was no significant association between years of hospitalization and cognitive decline. However, as people remain hospitalized they also get older, and it seems that advancing age was the key factor in producing the decline rather than the institutionalization. In this case, the application of partial correlation helped to detract from the correctness of a hypothesis that had some support in the literature.

A matter of particular interest in clinical research is prognosis or prediction of outcome. In prospective studies designed to evaluate accuracy of prediction, a mixed design is often devised in which both group comparison and correlational methods are used. The groups may be divided along numerous dimensions, but perhaps most often diagnostic or treatment variables are used. In the case of treatment research, the question may involve either comparisons of different treatments or simply an active treatment against a placebo control. The specific treatment effect may be directly evaluated with group comparison statistics, but components of the study that may be characterized as more "epidemiological" in nature would involve correlational statistics. For example, in many treatment studies, although the active treatment group may have improved relative to the control group, not all the patients in that group get better, or some patients do not improve as much as others. If pertinent demographic, diagnostic, and other clinical data are collected, then it is possible to correlate these data with outcome. Such questions as to whether age is associated with treatment response, or whether women improve more than men, or whether a particular laboratory finding is associated with outcome may be answered in this manner. These analyses aid in refining the findings and in identifying those individuals for whom the treatment is most promising.

Sometimes the investigator is simply interested in the prediction from baseline data to outcome. Such a question as "What patient characteristics are most predictive of outcome following treatment for depression?" are typical of those that are asked in this type of research. The most direct way of answering this question is by the method described above of obtaining the predictive validity of tests. Here the tests are replaced by the baseline measures, and the criteria are measures of outcome that are obtained some time after the baseline period. In many instances, univariate predictors are not adequate, but it is possible to use multiple predictors by applying multiple regression and correlation methods if enough subjects are available. Sometimes outcome is also complex and cannot be sufficiently captured by one variable. For example, relief from symptoms, return to work, and improved family relations may all be outcomes of some treatment. Although separate regression equations could be computed for each criterion, a more elegant way of analyzing the data would be to employ an advanced statistical procedure called *canonical correlation*. A *canonical correlation* permits more than one variable on both the left- and right-hand sides of the multiple regression equation, thereby allowing for associating multiple predictors with multiple criteria.

Outcome is sometimes conceptualized as change on the same measure.

Such a conceptualization is extremely common in treatment research. Treatment with a diuretic may change blood pressure; treatment with a neuroleptic may change the Brief Psychiatric Rating Scale (BPRS) score, etc. It may appear that change can be directly evaluated by taking the difference between a measure taken on the first occasion and measures taken on subsequent occasions. Even though that is sometimes true, it is unfortunately not always true. The basic reason why it is not always true is that not all phenomena lie on equal interval scales. Probably the best way to illustrate this point is with an athletic example. An accomplished runner may set a new world record on the basis of a fraction of a second, whereas an amateur runner may improve running time by several seconds over many occasions without the same significance. Running times are therefore not on an equal interval scale. At the extreme limit of human performance, changes of fractions of a second appear to require substantially more ability and effort than do changes at less extreme points in the range of performance. Making the same observation in the case of psychophysiological measurements, Lacey (1956) characterized this phenomenon in a general way as the "law of initial values." How then do we evaluate change if the significance of a particular magnitude of change varies with the point on the scale at which it lies? A commonly used procedure is sometimes called *correction for baseline* and involves the use of correlation. More specifically, it involves the regression equation relating initial values to values obtained on subsequent occasions. Taking a two-occasion example, we can solve a regression equation and compute a correlation coefficient relating the scores of a sample on the first occasion to their scores on the second occasion. The regression equation allows us to predict second occasion (y) scores from performance on the first occasion (x) scores, as we have discussed previously. We then compare this predicted score with the score actually obtained and take the difference between them. This difference is known as a *residual change score*. Large residual change scores mean that the subject has changed substantially beyond what would be predicted for an individual with his or her initial level. Small residual change scores mean the opposite, and any change obtained is not much different from what would be predicted from initial performance. Thus, we have factored initial performance out reasonably well and have obtained a purer measure of meaningful change through the use of correlation and regression.

SUMMARY

In this chapter, I have introduced some basic concepts of regression and correlation and have provided some illustrations of how these methods are typically applied in behavioral research. Illustrations were taken from psychometrics and from descriptive, epidemiological studies in the behavioral sciences; but essentially regression and correlation are used in all applications of statistical methods. It should be emphasized that though the term *correlational research* has some connotations of being merely descriptive, exploratory, and preliminary, probably more often than not correlational methods are used in combination with group comparison, experimental studies. Sometimes a stated preference for "experimental" rather than "correlational" studies may be based upon some degree of mathematical naïveté. For example, one may compare two groups on some measure and determine whether or not their means differ significantly from each other using Student's t test or some similar statistic. If they are not significantly different from each other, that probably means that the scores obtained by one group are reasonably highly correlated with the scores of the second group. A correlation coefficient can be computed from precisely the same data that were evaluated by the t test. The point is that the use of correlational statistics should not produce the assumption that the research being done is preliminary, exploratory, or purely descriptive.

As specialized fields in statistics develop, they tend to become increasingly mathematically complex. That appears to be the case in correlation and regression, but I should nevertheless point out that this area has not been completed, and research producing new methods is still being actively conducted. Furthermore, there are outstanding needs for new developments that are only in their early stages. For example, there is a great need for methods that can deal with multivariate analysis of nonlinear relationships.

Recent interest has focused on three significant areas. First, there is the problem of correlation and causality. Developments in a technique called *path analysis* have addressed this problem directly (Jöreskog, 1979), and the early concept that correlation does not imply causality appears to be changing. Our ideas about the exploratory nature of factor analysis are also changing. Methods have been developed for what is called *confirmatory factor analysis* that allow for testing of specific hypotheses through factor analysis. Investigators now often make the distinction between exploratory and confirmatory factor analysis in describing their work.

Our emphasis thus far has been on correlation of tests and other methods, but one can also correlate people. We do this naively when we make such a statement as John is like Harry because they are both tall and have red hair. When we do this more formally, it is called *classification*. John and Harry are both schizophrenics because they have delusions, hallucinations, bizarre language, and meet other criteria. Classification is based upon similarities and differences, but may be accomplished in a variety of ways (e.g., intuitively, using objective rules, or empirically). The two most widely used empirical methods are called *Q-type factor analysis* and *cluster analysis*. In either case, they can be thought of as factor analyses of people rather than tests. As in the case of factor analysis of tests, these methods are complex and require special training to use. However, cluster analysis in particular appears to be growing in popularity, apparently because of its growing availability in statistical computer packages.

In conclusion, correlation and regression are important statistical tools that are applicable in a variety of research settings. It is probably inappropriate to think of their use as restricted to a particular type of research, which is generally characterized by such terms as descriptive, naturalistic, hypothesis-seeking, or preliminary. The mathematics of correlation and regression are neutral to the kind of research in which the investigator is interested. Furthermore, new developments in these mathematics are changing our previously held views that correlational statistics cannot deal with causality or hypothesis testing.

REFERENCES

American Psychiatric Association. (1980). *Diagnostic and statistical manual of mental disorders* (3rd ed.). Washington, DC: Author.
American Psychiatric Association. (1987). *Diagnostic and statistical manual of mental disorders* (3rd ed., rev.). Washington, DC: Author.
Bromet, E. J., Davies, M., & Schulz, S. C. (1988). Basic principles of epidemiologic research in schizophrenia. In H. A. Nasrallah (Ed.), *Handbook of schizophrenia, Volume 3* (pp. 151–168). Amsterdam: Elsevier.
Bruning, J. L., & Kintz, B. L. (1987). *Computational handbook of statistics* (3rd ed.). Glenview, IL: Scott, Foresman.
Butcher, J. N., Graham, J. R., Dahlstrom, W. G., Tellegen, A. M., & Kaemmer, B. (1989). *MMPI-2 Manual for administration and scoring*. Minneapolis: University of Minnesota Press.
Cohen, J. (1960). A coefficient of agreement for nominal scales. *Educational and Psychological Measurement, 20,* 37–46.
Fleiss, J. L. (1981). *Statistical methods for rates and proportions* (2nd ed.). New York: Wiley.
Goldstein, G., Zubin, J., & Pogue-Geile, (1991). Hospitalization and the cognitive deficits of schizophrenia: The influences of age and education. *Journal of Nervous and Mental Disease, 179,* 202–206.
Jöreskog, K. G. (1979). *Advances in factor analysis and structural equation models*. Cambridge, MA: Abt Books.
Lacey, J. I. (1956). The evaluation of autonomic responses: Toward a general solution. *Annals of the New York Academy of Science, 67,* 123–164.
Landis, J. R., & Koch, G. G. (1977). The measurement of observer agreement for categorical data. *Biometrics, 33,* 671–679.
Rummel, R. J. (1970). *Applied factor analysis*. Evanston, IL: Northwestern University Press.
Zigler, E., & Glick, M. (1986). *A developmental approach to adult psychopathology*. New York: Wiley.

CHAPTER 6

Basic Statistical Principles

JOEL B. GREENHOUSE AND BRIAN W. JUNKER

INTRODUCTION

In a randomized controlled clinical trial for the prevention of the recurrence of depression, it is reported that imipramine is more effective than lithium or placebo in delaying the recurrence of a depressive episode. In another study, a randomized controlled clinical trial of the comparative efficacy of interpersonal therapy, cognitive behavioral therapy, imipramine, and placebo for the treatment of depression, it is found that the psychotherapies and the drug are almost equally effective. In a nonrandomized comparative study, it is reported that depressed patients have a decrease in rapid-eye movement latency relative to healthy subjects. As consumers of statistics there are many questions we should ask about these studies, including: How were these conclusions reached? What do these conclusions mean? and How should we evaluate the merits of these studies and their results?

The purpose of this chapter is to introduce statistical methods to describe and summarize the results of studies and to introduce statistical principles that will guide the psychiatric researcher in the evaluation and interpretation of clinical research. We share the view expressed by Arnold Relman (1986), former editor of the *New England Journal of Medicine*, that

> No one who reads the current medical literature, and certainly no one who performs clinical studies these days, can be unaware of the growing importance of

Joel B. Greenhouse and Brian W. Junker • Department of Statistics, Carnegie-Mellon University, Pittsburgh, Pennsylvania 15213.
Research in Psychiatry: Issues, Strategies, and Methods, edited by L. K. George Hsu and Michel Hersen. Plenum Press, New York, 1992.

statistics. Sound clinical research, as well as the ability to understand published
results of research, increasingly depends on a clear comprehension of the fundamental
concepts of statistical design and analysis. (p. xi)

Statistics is concerned not only with the collection and presentation of data in the
form of figures and tables but also with making inferences from data; that is,
assessing the evidence provided by the data for or against a research hypothesis.
In this chapter, we examine the underlying logic of the practice of statistics as
applied to clinical psychiatric research. Our emphasis will be on how to think
about and interpret data and to reason statistically rather than on mathematical
formulas and calculations.

In the first section of this chapter, we will discuss relatively easy-to-use and
informal methods for describing and comparing data. Our aim is to develop
methods for investigating relationships among variables in order to learn about
the effect of one variable upon another. Specifically, we want to characterize
changes in the features of the distribution of one of the variables as values of the
other variable change. We will introduce methods to describe features of the
distribution of quantitative variables; that is, variables that are measured, such
as the length of time to the recurrence of illness or blood plasma levels of
imipramine, as well as methods for categorical variables, which are variables
that indicate which category an individual falls into (e.g., gender, male or
female, recovered from illness, yes or no, or treatment group assignment,
psychotherapy, drug, or placebo).

For the purpose of describing relationships among variables, it is also
useful to distinguish between response variables and explanatory variables. A
response variable measures an outcome of a study and an *explanatory variable*
attempts to explain the observed outcome. For example, in a treatment study the
response variable might be recovery from illness and the explanatory variable
might be treatment group: either psychotherapy, drug, or placebo. Response
and explanatory variables can be either quantitative or categorical.

In the second section of this chapter we discuss and illustrate principles
related to the evaluation of the nature of the association among variables. Once
we have observed an apparent relationship between variables, an important
question to be addressed is whether or not the observed relationship is causal, in
the sense that changes in one variable elicit changes in another. We will also
introduce basic principles for the design of studies to investigate a primary
research question. These principles will be useful in designing studies that yield
unambiguous answers to well-posed research questions. Throughout this
chapter principles and methods will be illustrated using examples and case
studies based on data sets primarily from the psychiatric research literature.

DESCRIBING AND COMPARING DISTRIBUTIONS: QUANTITATIVE RESPONSE VARIABLE

Reports of research results are replete with statements about variables such
as "the mean Hamilton score at baseline" or "the median number of previous

episodes of depression" or "the proportion of patients responding to clozapine." Each of these statements is an attempt by the investigator to reduce a collection of measurements to a single numerical summary. We might ask why after going to all the trouble to obtain measurements on each subject would we reduce this information down to a single number? Consider the measurements of rapid eye movement (REM) latency obtained from a group of 19 depressed patients and 20 healthy subjects displayed in Table 1. *REM latency* is defined to be the time in minutes from sleep onset to the beginning of the first REM period. It is not easy from looking at these lists of numbers to discern any patterns or features of the data from which we can characterize the distribution of REM latency in each group. Therefore, if we want to compare the two groups to determine whether or not there was a difference in the distribution of REM latency between depressed patients and healthy controls, it would be difficult based only on a simple inspection of the two lists of numbers. One approach to this problem is to obtain a summary measure of each list, such as the mean REM latency for each group and to compare them. For example, the mean REM latency for the depressed patients is 37.7 min and for the healthy subjects is 71.5 min. The mean is a measure of central location, that is, a single number summarizing the most typical values of the data. Based on a comparison of the means in each group we might conclude that REM latency is reduced in depressed patients. However, in this discussion of basic statistical principles, our goal is to emphasize that there are other features of a distribution, such as spread, shape, and atypical or unusual values, that are often as important to describe and summarize as central location. In this section, we will discuss methods for summarizing and describing distributions, with the objective to learn as much as possible about any patterns or features of the data.

The approach described here, known as *exploratory data analysis* (EDA), is based on the premise that the more is known about the data, the more effectively data can be used to develop, test, and refine theory. Methods for exploratory data analysis should be relatively easy to do with or without a computer, quick to use so that a data set may be explored from different points of view, and robust in the sense that they are not adversely influenced by such misleading phenomena as extreme cases, measurement errors, or unique cases that need special attention. Two methods to be discussed here for quantitative response variables, the stem-and-leaf plot and the boxplot, are graphical methods that satisfy these requirements and are powerful tools for developing insights and hypotheses about a data set.

Table 1. *REM Latency Times for Depressed Patients and Healthy Subjects*

Group	Time (in minutes)
Depressed patients	87 2 39 5 81 81 47 6 10 25 65 48 15 21 52 17 48 19 48
Healthy subjects	47 90 95 51 87 60 69 51 19 54 66 138 64 66 60 84 137 60 69 63

Stem-and-Leaf Plot

In a stem-and-leaf plot, the data values are sorted into numerical order and brought together quickly and efficiently in the form of a graphic display. The stem-and-leaf plot uses all the data and illustrates nicely the shape of a distribution; that is, whether it is symmetric or skewed, single or multiple peaked, and whether it has outliers (atypical extreme values) or gaps within the distribution. Figure 1 shows the stem-and-leaf plot for the values of REM latency for the 20 healthy subjects. The first digit of each REM latency is designated the *stem* and the last digit the *leaf*. The possible stem values are listed vertically in increasing order from top to bottom and a vertical line is drawn to the right of the stems. The leaves are recorded directly from Table 1 onto the lines corresponding to their stem value to the right of the vertical line. Within each stem the leaves should be arranged in increasing order away from the stem.

From Figure 1 we can now begin to see important features of the distribution of REM latency for the healthy subjects:

1. *Typical values:* It is not difficult to locate by eye the typical values or central location of the distribution by finding the stem or stems where most of the observations fall. For the distribution in Figure 1, we see that the center seems to be in the 60s.

2. *Shape:* Does the distribution have one peak or several peaks? Is it approximately symmetric or is it skewed in one direction? A distribution is symmetric if the portions above and below the center are approximately mirror images of each other. It is skewed to the right (positive) if the right tail (higher values) is much longer than the left tail (lower values) or skewed to the left (negative) if the left tail is much longer than the right tail. We see that the distribution in Figure 1 has a single peak and is approximately symmetric.

3. *Gaps/atypical values:* The stem-and-leaf plot is useful for identifying

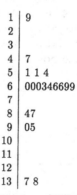

Figure 1. Stem-and-leaf plot of the distribution of REM latency (in min) for healthy subjects (Legend: 13|7 = 137 min).

atypical observations which are usually highlighted by gaps in the distribution. For example, the subject with a REM latency of 19 minutes and the two subjects with REM latencies of 137 and 138 minutes, respectively, are three unusual observations that may not have been noted very easily from just looking at the values in Table 1.

Sometimes a stem-and-leaf plot will be so concentrated that it is too difficult to discern the shape of the distribution. When this happens, it is possible to make a two-stem stem-and-leaf plot which uses each stem line twice with the first stem line containing values of leaves from 0 to 4 and the second stem line containing values of leaves from 5 to 9 (see Koopmans, 1987, pp. 19–22, for examples and further modifications).

It is useful to compare two related distributions by making a *back-to-back* stem-and-leaf plot. Figure 2 presents a back-to-back stem-and-leaf plot comparing the distribution of REM latency for the depressed patients and the healthy subjects. Such a display makes it relatively easy to compare the important features of the two distributions. For example, it is easy to see differences in central location between the groups, and that the distribution of REM latency for the healthy subjects has a single peak whereas the distribution for the depressed patients has several peaks. We will provide more details about the comparison of these two distributions below.

Boxplot

As noted earlier, major features of a distribution include the central location of the data, how spread out the data are, the shape of the distribution, and any unusual observations, called *outliers*. The boxplot is a visual display of numerical summaries, based in part on sample percentiles, that highlights the major features of a distribution. The boxplot summarizes the behavior of a data set by providing a clear picture of where the middle of the distribution lies, how spread

Depressed			Normal
652	0		
9750	1	9	
51	2		
9	3		
8887	4	7	
2	5	114	
5	6	000346699	
	7		
711	8	47	
	9	05	
	10		
	11		
	12		
	13	78	

Figure 2. Back-to-back stem-and-leaf plot for comparing the distribution of REM latency (in min) for depressed patients and healthy subjects (Legend: 13|7 = 137 min).

out the middle is, the shape of the distribution, and the identification of outliers in the distribution. A boxplot differs from a stem-and-leaf plot in several ways. The boxplot is based on numerical summaries of the distribution but not on every observation as is the stem-and-leaf plot. Furthermore, it provides a much clearer picture of the tails of the distribution and it is better at identifying outliers than the stem-and-leaf plot.

The boxplot is based on sample percentiles because percentiles, such as the median (50th percentile), are robust measures of location. For example, consider three numbers: 1, 2, 3. The mean of these numbers is 2 and the median (the middle value of the distribution) is also 2. But if we make a mistake in writing down the numbers and write 33 instead of 3, we find that the mean of 1, 2, and 33 is 12, whereas the median is still 2. We see that the mean is not a robust measure of central location because it is influenced by atypical observations. Formally, the p-th percentile of a distribution is the value such that $p\%$ of the observations fall at or below it. For example, the 25th percentile, also called the *first quartile*, is the value such that 25% of the observations fall at or below it and 75% fall above it.

Figure 3 presents a boxplot of the distribution of REM latency for the healthy subjects produced by the statistical software package MINITAB (Ryan, Joiner, & Ryan, 1985). We describe the features of this boxplot. The box itself is drawn from the first quartile ($Q_1 = 54$) to the third quartile ($Q_3 = 87$). The "plus" inside the box denotes the median ($m = 65$). The difference or distance between the third quartile and first quartile ($Q_3 - Q_1 = 87 - 54 = 33$) is called the *interquartile range* (IQR) and is a robust measure of variability. The IQR corresponds to the length of the box in Figure 3. Measures of variability, such as the IQR or the standard deviation, are measures of distance and indicate how spread out a distribution is. They are nonnegative, and smaller values indicate a more concentrated distribution than larger values. The dotted lines going in either direction from the ends of the box (i.e., away from Q_1 and Q_3, respectively) denote the tails of the distribution. The two asterisks in Figure 3 denote outliers or atypical values (137 and 138 min) and are so defined because they are located a distance more than 1.5 times the IQR from the nearest quartile. The dashed lines extend to an observed data point within 1.5 times the IQR from each respective quartile to establish regions far enough from the center of the distribution to highlight observations that may be atypical or outliers (see Koopmans, 1987, pp.

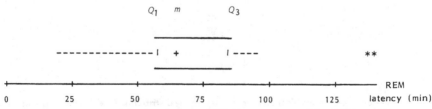

Figure 3. Boxplot of the distribution of REM latency (in min) for healthy subjects.

51–57). Note that the mean REM latency is 71.5 minutes and is larger than the median because of the influence of the two large atypical values among the healthy subjects.

A basic question in clinical research is whether or not two groups (say, one healthy and one diseased, or one treated and the other not treated) differ. In the language of statistics, we wish to know whether the features of the distribution of a response variable are different for the different categories of a categorical explanatory variable. When the response variable is quantitative, boxplots are particularly useful for comparing distributions because they graphically highlight important features of the data. For example, to investigate whether the distribution of REM latency is different for depressed patients compared to healthy subjects, we present in Figure 4 the boxplots for the distributions of REM latency for each group. Table 2 gives the relevant numerical summary measures for each group. A comparison of the two distributions reveals the following:

1. *Central Location.* The distribution of REM latency for the depressed patients is shifted to the left relative to the distribution for the healthy subjects, indicating reduced REM latency times. The boxes do not overlap, indicating that 75% of the depressed patients have REM latency times below $Q_1 = 54$ min for the healthy subjects. The median REM latency for the depressed patients is 39 min, which is much smaller than the median for the healthy subjects.

2. *Spread.* Judging by the IQRs for each distribution (i.e., the length of the boxes in Figure 4), the spread is about the same for the two distributions: 33 for the healthy subjects and 37 for the depressed patients. Note, however, that the ranges of the two distributions (the maximum value minus the minimum value) are very different: 85 for the depressed patients and 119 for the healthy subjects. The range is not a robust measure of spread because it is influenced by extreme values.

3. *Shape.* The shape of the middle 50% of the distribution of REM latency (i.e., the box, for the depressed patients) is skewed to the left. Note that the median is closer to Q_3 than to Q_1. Yet in the tails we see that the right tail is longer than the left. The shape of the middle 50% of the distribution of REM latency for the healthy subjects is skewed to the right; the

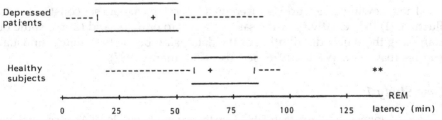

Figure 4. Comparative boxplots of the distribution of REM latency (in min) for depressed patients and healthy subjects.

Table 2.   Numerical Summary Measures for the Distribution
of REM Latency for Depressed Patients and Healthy Subjects

	Depressed patients	Healthy subjects
n	19	20
Median	39	65
Mean	37.7	71.5
Q_1	15	54
Q_3	52	87
IQR	37	33
Range	85	119

median is closer to Q_1 than to Q_3. Yet again we see a different shape
in the tails; the left tail is longer than the right tail.

4. *Outliers*. There are no outliers identified among the depressed patients,
   whereas as noted earlier there are two outliers among the healthy
   subjects (137 and 138 min). These two observations call for further
   investigation. Are they due to coding errors, that is, might they be 37 and
   38 minutes, respectively? Or perhaps the first REM period was not
   recorded or was just missed by the sleep technician, so that these values
   may actually represent the latency times for the second REM period.

Inspection of the stem-and-leaf plots and the boxplots together suggests
that the distributions of REM latency in the depressed patients and the healthy
subjects might really be mixtures of two or more subgroups. The stem-and-leaf
plot for the depressed patients has multiple peaks, and there are gaps in the
distributions for both the depressed patients and the healthy subjects. From the
boxplots we see that the distributions of REM latency have relatively long tails:
the right tail for the depressed patients and the left tail for the healthy subjects.
Also, the skewness in the box goes in a different direction from the skewness in
the tails. Taken together, these unusual features suggest that within each group
these subjects are not homogeneous. For example, there may be heterogeneity
because of differences among the depressed patients in terms of the severity of
illness, and there may be heterogeneity among the healthy subjects because of a
combination of the natural variability of REM latency in the general population
plus the effect of some other uncontrolled source of variability, such as a bias that
is due to self-selection since these subjects were all volunteers.

The following case study is based on a hypothetical data set constructed to
illustrate (1) the sensitivity of the sample mean to outliers, and (2) the value of
examining the whole distribution of the data using boxplots to detect unusual
features (based on Wainer, 1976; see also Koopmans, 1987).

Case Study 1

Suppose that the data in Table 3 are the scores on the Global Assessment Scale
(GAS) (Endicott, Spitzer, Fleiss, & Cohen, 1976) obtained as patients are admitted

Table 3.   Hypothetical Global Assessment Scale Scores by Clinic

Group	Scores
Clinic 1:	88 49 31 86 41 26 52 39 46 40 37 58 97 43 90 34 54 28 48 40 89 22 32 35 45
Clinic 2:	54 48 36 53 45 31 49 42 46 44 41 51 63 45 59 39 50 33 47 43 57 27 37 40 46
Clinic 3:	59 51 0 58 45 0 53 41 50 44 38 56 68 47 64 32 55 0 50 42 62 0 0 36 49

into a study being conducted in three different clinics using a common protocol. The GAS is scored from 0 to 100, with high scores reflecting good functioning. The sample means for each clinic are 50, 45.04, and 40, respectively. Based on the sample means alone, it might be concluded that the patients in Clinic 2 and 3 are more severely ill than the patients in Clinic 1, and that the patients in Clinic 3 are more severely ill than the patients in Clinic 2. As a result of this examination of sample means, the principal investigator of this study may be concerned that, because the patients in the three clinics appear to be different with respect to functioning, it will not be possible to draw general conclusions from the study because the investigator will not be able to combine data from the three clinics.

Figure 5 presents a comparative boxplot for the three clinics. It is clear from the boxplots that the observed differences in the mean GAS scores in the three clinics are due to the outliers in Clinics 1 and 3. The large outliers in Clinic 1 pull the mean of those patients up, and the small outliers in Clinic 3 pull the mean of those patients down. Examining the median GAS scores (43, 45, and 47, respectively) and observing the overlap in the boxes, we see that the middle 50% of the distributions of GAS scores in the three clinics are really quite similar. The boxplots allow the principal investigator to quickly inspect the data and to screen the data for unusual features. In this example, the unusual features are the four large outliers in Clinic 1, which may indicate that this clinic is not being careful about who is admitted into the study with respect to severity of illness criteria, and the five small outliers equal to zero in Clinic 3, which may be the result of a coding or

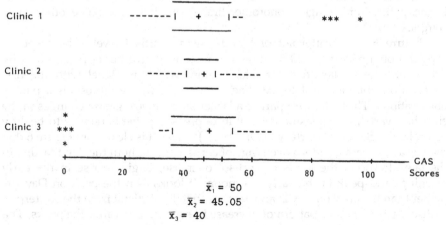

Figure 5. Comparative boxplots of the distribution of hypothetical GAS scores by clinic.

transcription error. In any case, the principal investigator has been alerted to possible problems in the clinics with respect to the collection of the GAS scores.

Exploratory Regression Analysis

As we have seen, stem-and-leaf plots and boxplots are useful methods for exploring the relationship or association between a quantitative response variable and a categorical explanatory variable (e..g, group membership). We next consider a collection of methods, which we will refer to as *exploratory regression analysis*, for the case when both the response variable and the explanatory variable are quantitative. An observation for each subject consists of a pair of measurements (an explanatory variable and a response variable) such as *blood plasma levels* of imipramine and *weight change, age* and *number of days* since the previous episode of depression, or *time* of day and *plasma cortisol level*. Our objective is to characterize, either for descriptive purposes or for the purpose of making predictions, how changes in the response variable depend on changes in the explanatory variable. A question of interest, for example, might be to describe changes in plasma cortisol levels with changes in the time of day; that is, to describe the circadian variation of cortisol. Or interest might be in predicting weight changes in patients based on blood plasma levels of imipramine.

A simple graphic display, called a *scatterplot*, presents a plot of the values of the response variable and the explanatory variable for each subject. The response variable appears on the vertical axis with increasing values going up, and the explanatory variable on the horizontal axis with increasing values going to the right. We use scatterplots to investigate the nature of the relationship between the two variables. For example, does the response variable increase with increasing values of the explanatory variable, indicating a positive relationship between the variables, or does it decrease indicating a negative relationship? Or perhaps the response variable does not change at all with changes in the explanatory variable, indicating no relationship between the two variables. Is the pattern of change monotonic, linear, quadratic, or some other more complex form?

Figure 6 is a scatterplot of blood plasma cortisol levels (the response variable) obtained every 20 minutes for 54 consecutive hours from a healthy volunteer. The explanatory variable is time, which we label with the first observation obtained at 4:40 P.M. Each star in the figure represents a pair of observations. These data are part of a larger study investigating changes in the circadian variation of plasma cortisol in depressed patients relative to healthy control subjects (data courtesy of Dr. David Jarrett). It is clear from Figure 6 that there is a systematic pattern of change of cortisol throughout the day. Starting in the late afternoon the levels of cortisol decrease, begin to rise in the early morning, and peak in the early afternoon. It looks as if the peak on Day 1 is higher than the peak on Day 2, and we note that it is difficult from the scatterplot to discern a systematic pattern of decrease in cortisol levels after the peaks. The

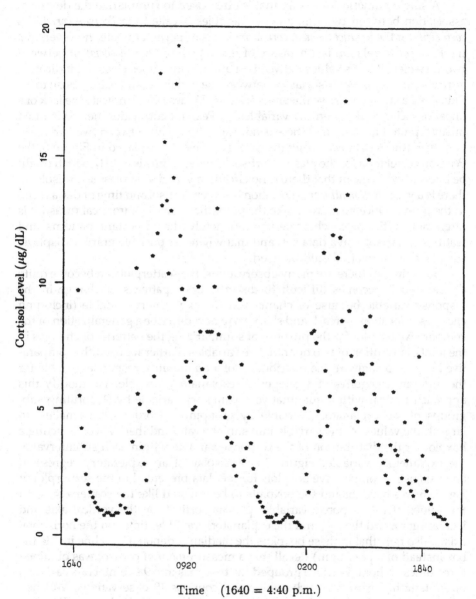

Figure 6. Scatterplot of cortisol level versus time of day.

scatterplot is a particularly rich display often revealing many interesting features of the joint distribution of two quantitative variables.

A single numerical measure that is often used to summarize the degree of association between two quantitative variables is called the *Pearson correlation coefficient* (or the *product moment correlation*). It is important to note, however, that the Pearson correlation is a measure of the degree of *linear association* between two variables. It takes values between −1 and 1, with values close to 1 indicating a strong positive linear association between the variables, and values close to −1 indicating a strong negative linear association. Values near 0 indicate the lack of a linear association between the variables. A Pearson correlation near 0 is often misinterpreted to mean that there is no association at all between two variables. However, this is not necessarily the case. For the data displayed in Figure 6, the Pearson correlation for the plasma cortisol levels and time is −0.117 which might be interpreted to mean that there is no circadian variation in plasma cortisol. Yet there is a very clear *nonlinear* association between cortisol and time of day as seen in the figure. Once again we make the point that a single numerical measure is often not sufficient to characterize completely the important patterns and features of variables in a data set, and that whenever possible graphic displays, such as a scatterplot, should be used.

Sometimes if there are many observations, the scatterplot can become quite dense, and it becomes difficult to discern subtle patterns of change in the response variable because of changes in the explanatory variable (including changes in location, spread, and shape). We next describe a generalization of the comparative boxplot for the purpose of summarizing the patterns of changes in the joint distribution of two quantitative variables. Earlier we used the comparative boxplot to compare the distribution of a quantitative response variable for the different categories of a categorical explanatory variable. We modify this approach to deal with a quantitative explanatory variable by (1) forming subgroups of the explanatory variable by grouping, in order from smallest to largest, the values of this variable into subintervals, and then (2) constructing a boxplot for the distribution of the response variable within each subinterval of the explanatory variable. Figure 7 is a display of an exploratory regression analysis using comparative boxplots for the data presented in the scatterplot in Figure 6. We have rotated the boxplots to be oriented like the scatterplot, with the values of the response variable, plasma cortisol, on the vertical axis and increasing toward the top, and the explanatory variable, time, on the horizontal axis. (Also note that in these boxplots the median is denoted by a line inside the box instead of a plus sign.) Recall that a measurement of cortisol was obtained three times an hour. We have grouped the time axis into 9 subintervals each of 6 hours length. Therefore, each subinterval contains 18 observations. We then construct a boxplot for each subinterval using the methods described earlier. Each boxplot provides a display of the distribution of cortisol given a particular 6-hour period centered at the midpoint of the interval. Such a distribution for a particular value or subinterval of the explanatory variable is known as the *conditional distribution* of the response variable, given the specified values of the

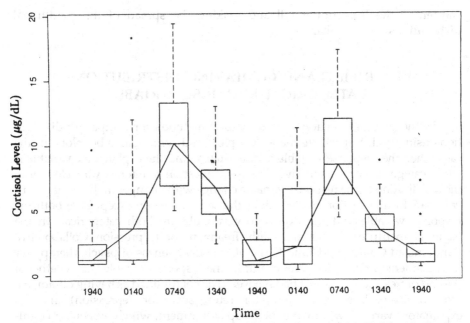

Figure 7. Exploratory regression analysis of cortisol level versus time of day. Each boxplot displays the conditional distribution of plasma cortisol centered at the midpoint of a 6-hour period during the day.

explanatory variable. For example, the first boxplot in Figure 7 describes the conditional distribution of plasma cortisol level conditional on measurements being obtained in the time interval between 4:40 P.M. and 10:40 P.M. on Day 1, centered at 7:40 P.M.

Figure 7 makes it clear that there is a systematic and repeatable pattern of change in the conditional distribution of cortisol with time of day. The continuous line connecting the medians in each of the conditional distributions is called an *exploratory regression curve* and traces out a pattern of change in central location that appears here much like a sinusoidal function of time. Note that each conditional distribution is positively skewed with a long upper tail toward larger values. There are several observations that are identified as outliers. We also see that the spread or variability in each of the conditional distributions is not constant, as measured by the length of the box (i.e,. the IQR), and, in fact, appears to change in a systematic fashion. Specifically, the spread appears to increase as the median level of cortisol increases. Whenever the variability of a measure seems to depend on the level or central location of that measure, it is usually a good idea to consider a transformation of the values of that measure, using either a logarithmic, or a square root, or other power transformation (see Koopmans, 1987, p. 392). Taking the logarithm of each cortisol value would have several effects here, including making the distributions more symmetric by shortening the long upper tail and making the spread of the conditional distributions more similar.

DESCRIBING AND COMPARING DISTRIBUTIONS: CATEGORICAL RESPONSE VARIABLE

In the previous sections, we described methods for comparing distributions using back-to-back stem-and-leaf plots and comparative boxplots for the case when the response variable is quantitative and the explanatory variable is either categorical or quantitative. The basic question of interest was: How does the distribution of the response variable change with changes in the explanatory variable? In this section, we consider the same question except here both the response variable and the explanatory variable are both categorical. In the National Institute of Mental Health Treatment of Depression Collaborative Randomized Controlled Clinical Trial of the effectiveness of psychotherapy for the treatment of depression, for example, the response variable was whether at the end of treatment a patient had recovered or not (defined as having obtained a score of six or less on the Hamilton rating scale for depression), and the explanatory variable was treatment group assignment, which was either cognitive behavior therapy (CBT), interpersonal therapy (IPT), imipramine (IMI), or placebo (PLA) (Elkin *et al.*, 1989). Elkin *et al.* (1989, Table 2) reported the patients who completed between 12 and 15 weeks of treatment and the frequency counts of the number of patients who recovered in each treatment group. These data are presented in Table 4 in the form of a *two-way classification table*, also known as an R × C (read "R by C") table, where R equals the number of rows, in this case 4, and C equals the number of columns, in this case 2.

The exploratory approach to analyzing the data in Table 4 is to calculate appropriate percentages from the frequency counts given. In this particular example, the appropriate percentages are found from the proportion of patients who recover among those in a particular treatment group. So the proportion of patients who recovered among the 37 who received CBT is 19 out of 37 = 0.51. Note that in the CBT group the proportion who recover and the proportion who

Table 4. *Percentage of Patients Who Recovered among Treatment Completers in the NIMH Treatment of Depression Study by Treatment Group*

	Patient Status recovered		
Treatment group	Yes	No	Total
Cognitive behavior theory (CBT)	19 (51%)	18 (49%)	37 (100%)
Interpersonal therapy (IPT)	26 (55%)	21 (46%)	47 (100%)
Imipramine (IMI)	21 (57%)	16 (43%)	37 (100%)
Placebo (PLA)	10 (29%)	24 (71%)	34 (100%)
Total	76 (49%)	79 (51%)	155 (100%)

do not recover add to 100%. (This is true for each of the treatment groups.) The two proportions together make up the *conditional distribution* of recovery, given that a patient is in the CBT group. To determine whether treatment has an effect on the likelihood of recovery, we compare the conditional probability of recovery (given in the first column of Table 4) to each other and to the total or marginal proportion recovered at the bottom of the table (i.e., 49%). It is clear that the proportion who recover is not very different in the CBT, IPT, and IMI treatment groups, but the proportion who recover in these three groups is greater than the proportion who recover on placebo (29%). Formal statistical procedures for determining whether or not these differences in proportions are statistically significant (i.e., not explainable by chance variation alone) can be found in Fleiss (1981).

Case Study 2

In a reanalysis of the results of the NIMH Collaborative Study of Maintenance Treatment of Recurrent Affective Disorders (Prien, Kupfer, Mansky, Small, Tuason, Voss, & Johnson, 1984), Greenhouse, Stangl, Kupfer, and Prien (1991) investigated the effects of abrupt discontinuation of imipramine on the probability of an early recurrence of depression among unipolar patients who have been stabilized on imipramine for at least 8 weeks. The response variable, an early recurrence of illness, is defined by having (1) a definite major depressive disorder based on Research Diagnostic Criteria, (2) a score of 60 or below on the GAS, and (3) the recurrence occurs within 8 weeks of being discontinued from imipramine. In this study 71 patients out of the 150 who stabilized were selected at random to be discontinued from imipramine and the remaining 79 remained on imipramine. Being discontinued or not from imipramine is the explanatory variable. The results are given in Table 5 in the form of a 2 × 2 table.

We see that 26 out of 71 or 37% of the patients who were discontinued from imipramine had an early recurrence, whereas only 7 out of 79 or 9% of the patients who were not discontinued had an early recurrence. This appears to be a large difference, suggesting that there is an association between abrupt discontinuation of imipramine and the likelihood of a recurrence. Greenhouse *et al.* (1991) confirmed this result using more formal statistical procedures.

There are many single numerical measures available to summarize the degree of association between the response and the explanatory variable for the special case of a 2 × 2 classification table (see Fleiss, 1981). Here we introduce one

Table 5. Summary of Recurrence Status of Illness by Discontinuation Status of Medication

	Early recurrence of depression (0–8 weeks)	No early recurrence of depression	Total
Discontinued from imipramine	26 (37%)	45 (63%)	71 (100%)
Not discontinued from imipramine	7 (9%)	72 (91%)	79 (100%)
Total	33 (22%)	117 (87%)	150 (100%)

such measure called the *odds ratio*, which turns out to be useful not only as a summary measure but also in the interpretation of more complex statistical models of association such as the logistic regression model (Greenhouse, 1991). We refer to Case Study 2 in which we considered the relationship between discontinuation status and recurrence status in a randomized clinical trial for the prevention of the recurrence of depression. Let P_D denote the conditional probability of an early recurrence, given that a patient was discontinued from imipramine; and let P_{ND} denote the conditional probability of an early recurrence, given that a patient was not discontinued. From Table 5, estimates of these values are 37% and 9%, respectively. The definition of the odds, for example, the odds of an early recurrence given discontinuation is $P_D/(1 - P_D)$. Specifically, this is the ratio of the probability of a response, that is, an early recurrence, to the probability of not having an early recurrence for patients who were discontinued. Similarly, the odds of an early recurrence for patients who were not discontinued is $P_{ND}/(1 - P_{ND})$. The odds ratio, then, is the ratio of the odds of responding given a patient was discontinued to the odds of responding given a patient was not discontinued and is written as

$$\psi = \frac{P_D/(1 - P_D)}{P_{ND}/(1 - P_{ND})}$$

Substituting the conditional probabilities from Table 5 into the above equation, an estimate of ψ is

$$\psi = \frac{.37/.63}{.09/.91} = 5.8$$

The interpretation of ψ is that patients who are discontinued from imipramine are estimated to be almost six times as likely to have an early recurrence as patients who remain on imipramine , a fairly substantial increase in risk. If there were no increase in the risk of an early recurrence for patients who were discontinued, then the odds ratio would be equal to one, indicating that the odds of a response in each group are the same. The larger the odds ratio the greater the risk of a response for patients in one category of the explanatory variable relative to the other category. The odds ratio is also called the *cross product ratio* because we can write ψ as the cross product of the cell frequencies from the 2 × 2 table, for example,

$$\psi = \frac{26 \cdot 72}{7 \cdot 45} = 5.8$$

ASSESSING THE NATURE
OF ASSOCIATIONS AMONG VARIABLES

We have developed methods that can be used to investigate how features of the distribution of the response variable change with systematic changes in the explanatory variable. Once we have observed an apparent association among variables, an important question to be addressed is whether or not this observed relationship is causal; that is, do changes in the explanatory variable cause changes in the response variable? In this section, we discuss and illustrate some of the issues related to evaluating the nature of associations among variables.

In a discussion of statistical relationships and proof in medicine, Cornfield (1959) observed that in investigations of causal relationships, if important alternative hypotheses are compatible with available evidence, then the primary research question is unsettled. In other words, in evaluating whether or not an association is causal, it is necessary to consider additional explanations for the observed association and to evaluate the alternative explanations in light of the evidence provided by the data. For example, in the NIMH Collaborative Study of Maintenance Treatment of Recurrent Affective Disorders, it was concluded that for patients who stabilize on imipramine after an acute episode of depression, maintenance levels of imipramine are effective in preventing or delaying the recurrence of depression (Prien et al., 1984). However, as we observed in Case Study 2, an alternative explanation for the difference in the recurrence rates between patients who are maintained on imipramine and those who are not is the effect of the abrupt discontinuation of imipramine at the beginning of maintenance. Thus, it may not be that imipramine prevents the recurrence of depression, but, rather, the patients who are abruptly withdrawn from imipramine may experience a drug withdrawal reaction that precipitates an episode of depression or these patients may develop symptomatology that mimics a depressive episode. A variable, such as discontinuation status, that is associated with the response variable and interferes with our ability to determine the nature of the relationship between the response variable and the explanatory variable, is called a *confounding* variable.

In the evaluation of statistical relationships between variables, Lilienfeld and Lilienfeld (1980) suggested a useful classification of associations into three categories: (1) spurious; (2) indirect, and (3) causal. We consider each of these three categories separately.

Spurious Association

When an observed association occurs as a result of the presence of a confounding variable, such as a flaw in the design of the study, or as a result of biased methods of selecting study subjects, or as a result of biased methods of obtaining information from patients, then the association is said to be *spurious*. Consider a randomized study to compare two treatments for depression. Let us assume that the psychiatrist who evaluates each patient's response to treatment also knows which treatment the patient is receiving. If either consciously or unconsciously the psychiatrist believes in the effectiveness of one of the therapies over the other, his or her evaluation of the patient's response to treatment might be so influenced, resulting in an apparent association between treatment and response which might not be causal. Or, in epidemiologic studies of occupation and health, it is often found that workers experience less morbidity and mortality than the general population. An explanation for this association is that generally less healthy workers do not remain in the workforce, thus the workers who remain are relatively healthier than the general population. This selection bias is known as the healthy worker effect and suggests that the general population is not an appropriate comparison group for these types of studies. An example of a spurious association that is due to selection bias in a randomized controlled clinical trial is illustrated in the next case study.

Case Study 3

Greenhouse *et al.* (1991) discussed another explanation for the observed association between maintenance treatment and the likelihood of the recurrence of a depressive episode in the NIMH Collaborative Study of Maintenance Treatment of Recurrent Affective Disorders. The design for this study called for patients in an acute episode of depression to be entered into a preliminary phase during which the index episode is controlled and the patient's clinical condition is "stabilized." After completing an 8-week stabilization period, patients are then randomized to a maintenance therapy, the primary experimental phase of the study discussed earlier. Approximately 90% of the patients were treated for the index episode and stabilized on imipramine during the preliminary phase. There were 343 patients who entered the preliminary phase, and only 150 of these patients completed the preliminary phase and hence were randomized to a maintenance therapy.

In this trial, imipramine was found to be an effective maintenance therapy for the prevention or delay of the recurrence of depression. However, this result could have been obtained either because imipramine is, in fact, more effective than the other maintenance treatments considered, or because by virtue of the design of the study only patients who are imipramine responders are selected into the maintenance phase. That is, even if imipramine is not any more effective than the other maintenance therapies in the *general* population of patients with recurrent disorder, because of the effect of selection, it would appear to be so. Instead of having an unambiguous answer at the conclusion of this trial as to whether imipramine is more effective than the other maintenance therapies for the *population* of patients with recurrent disorder, we are in the situation where the results of the trial are compatible with at least one alternative explanation (i.e., selection bias) leaving the primary question unanswered. Clearly, part of the problem here is that a large fraction of the patients who enter the preliminary phase never were in the maintenance phase because they were unable to stabilize successfully on imipramine. Thus, the observed association found in the maintenance phase may well be spurious.

Indirect Association

An *indirect association* occurs when two or more variables are associated because each is influenced by a third variable. In the 1950s, an alternative explanation for the observed association between smoking and lung cancer was put forward based on the possible existence of a third factor, such as a genetic disposition, that was associated with both smoking and lung cancer. It was argued that this genetic factor caused cancer and also caused people to smoke.

Thus, quitting smoking would not change the genetic factor and would not change the likelihood of getting cancer. (It should be noted that no evidence of sufficient strength has been found in any study to support the hypothesis of a third variable, such as a genetic factor, to explain the strong relationship between smoking and lung cancer that has been consistently observed.) For a very nice discussion of the issues involved in establishing a causal association between smoking and lung cancer see Brown (1978).

Causal Association

As noted earlier, an association is said to be *causal* when a change in the explanatory variable directly causes changes in the response variable. The establishment of causality is not easy. Randomized controlled double-blind clinical trials in which the putative causal agent is randomly assigned to a portion of a sample of the relevant population remain the "gold standard" to establish causality. There are, however, many circumstances, for example, because of ethical reasons, in which it is impossible to randomly assign a putative causal agent. If an experiment cannot be designed to study directly the question of causation, then the establishment of causality usually proceeds by demonstrating that the observed association is not spurious or indirect. This requires a combination of approaches, including: (1) establishing the association in different studies among different subgroups of subjects, i.e., the establishment of the consistency of the association; (2) demonstrating the strength of the association, for example, the larger the odds ratio the stronger the evidence for association; (3) demonstrating a temporal association between the variables, that is, the explanatory variable (cause) must precede the response (effect); and (4) establishing a plausible biological explanation for the observed association. Typically, many such studies are needed to establish a presumption of causality. For a more detailed discussion of approaches to assess the causal nature of an observed association from an epidemiologic and chronic disease perspective, see Lilienfeld and Lilienfeld (1980).

Case Study 4

Since a large proportion of patients with depression resist suppression of blood cortisol levels following a dose of dexamethasone given the night before (Carroll, 1980), the dexamethasone suppression test (DST) has become widely used in psychiatry as a diagnostic tool for depression. Thus, it appears that there is a relationship between the lack of suppression of blood cortisol levels following a dose of dexamethasone (the response variable) and depression (the explanatory variable). To argue that the relationship is causal, we must rule out the possibility of an indirect association which would occur if depression and DST were related only because some third variable causes both and the possibility of a spurious association, which would occur if the relationship between depression and DST were somehow confounded by the action of a third variable. For example, it has been argued that weight loss can increase the escape from dexamethasone suppression. It has also been observed that depressed patients often experience loss of weight. If weight loss caused both depression and a positive DST response, then the association between depression and DST would be indirect. If depression and weight loss were merely associated (or if depression caused weight loss), and if loss of weight alone could also increase the escape from dexamethasone suppression, then the association between depression and DST might be spurious; in other words, the apparent association between depression and DST could equally well have been due to the confounding variable, weight loss.

To investigate the question of "spurious association," Mullen et al. (1986) designed a study in which normal healthy volunteers were placed on a restricted caloric intake of a period of 18 days. The DST was administered at baseline (before beginning the diet) and again after the 18 days. The subjects experienced an average weight loss of 4.3 kg. The authors reported that by restricting caloric intake in normal subjects they were able to reproduce "the pattern of response to dexamethasone said to characterize depressive illness" and that this response "cannot be explained by the induction of a mood disorder since no subject became depressed" (p. 1054). This study nicely illustrates the investigation of an alternative explanation for an association by directly studying the effect of the confounding variable.

Because the Mullen et al. study indicates that weight loss does not cause depression (or more precisely, does not have an effect on diagnostic measures of depression that would indicate pathology), this tends to rule out the possibility that the association between depression and DST is indirect: at least, this association is not caused by the putative common influence of weight loss. At the same time, Mullen et al. show that weight loss can increase the escape from dexamethasone suppression (among "normal" patients, anyway), which suggests a spurious association: weight loss is associated with depression in some way, and weight loss can cause a positive DST response. To evaluate the confounding effects of weight loss on the DST more carefully, we would need to know whether depressed patients who have lost weight escape from dexamethasone suppression to the same degree as depressed patients who have not lost weight. If depressed patients who have lost weight respond to the DST and those who have not lost weight do not, then perhaps the DST is specifically detecting patients with weight loss, and only incidentally detecting some depressed patients because of the association between depression and weight loss. On the other hand, if depressed patients who have not lost weight respond to the same degree to the DST as those who have, then the DST may be detecting two separate but overlapping groups: depressed patients and those who have recently lost weight. Clearly, very carefully designed and controlled studies are needed to resolve these questions.

As suggested in Case Study 4, the most direct approach to establish a causal relationship between variables is to perform a designed experiment. In a designed experiment, the investigator takes active steps to control for different sources of bias that are due perhaps to spurious or indirect associations, by the manipulation of variables, and by experimental conditions. In the various examples and case studies discussed in this chapter, we have mentioned or alluded to some of the principles of designed clinical experiments that help to avoid conclusions based on spurious or indirect associations. These principles include the use of a control/comparison group, randomization, blinding, and the control of variation.

If we are trying to demonstrate that a particular explanatory variable, say an intervention or a treatment, is causally related to a response variable, then subjects who receive the intervention or treatment (the *treatment* group) should be compared to a group of subjects who do not receive the intervention or treatment (the *control* group). The control group should be as similar to the treatment group as possible, except for the fact that these subjects do not receive the intervention. Usually, it is hard to judge the effect of a treatment or intervention properly without comparing it to something else. In particular, subjects who do not receive a treatment or intervention often show a positive response just by the fact that they are participating in a study—a phenomenon known as the *placebo effect* (Beecher, 1955). For example, in the NIMH Treatment of Depression Study (Elkin *et al.*, 1989) nearly 30% of the patients in the placebo group recovered (see Table 4). If the treatment group is just like the control group, apart from the intervention, then an observed difference in the responses of the two groups is likely to be due to the effect of the intervention and not to a confounding variable.

The best way to ensure that the treatment group is like the control group is to assign subjects to each group at random. *Randomization* is a mechanical procedure using chance to assign subjects to one group or the other. Flipping a coin, for example, is a simple mechanical procedure based on chance to assign subjects to one of two groups: If the coin comes up heads, the subject is assigned to the intervention group, and if it comes up tails, the subject is assigned to the comparison group. The effect of using randomization to assign subjects to a group should be to balance equally the distribution of known and unknown confounding variables between the treatment group and the comparison group.

Whenever possible a study should be *double-blinded*, which means that both the subjects and the investigators who evaluate the subjects' response do not know to which group (treatment or control) the subject has been assigned. Use of blinding in a study should help guard against spurious associations. To assure double blindness in the NIMH Treatment of Depression Study (Elkin *et al.*, 1989), the clinicians responsible for the evaluation of outcomes were not the same therapists who treated the patients. Blindness, either double or single (i.e., either the clinician or the patient is blind but not both), is an ideal to strive for, but obviously there are interventions for which it is possible to maintain blindness, such as a study of electroconvulsive therapy (ECT) or of a new surgical procedure.

There is another notion of control in statistics other than a control group which has to do with the *control of variation*. We have seen in Figure 7 how plasma levels of cortisol change with the time of day. Therefore, in a study of the DST, such as described in Case Study 4, we would want to assess subjects at the same time in their circadian cycle of cortisol in order to control for differences in levels of cortisol that are due solely to circadian variation. The time of measurement of cortisol, if not controlled for, could be a confounding variable in studies of the DST. The area of statistics known as the *design of experiments* is concerned with statistical methods for the control of variation (see for example, Cox, 1959; Fleiss, 1986; Neter, Wasserman, & Kutner, 1990).

We recognize that in the practice of clinical research it may be difficult to implement each of these principles in the design of every study. However, the good practice of statistics requires that in the planning stages of a study each of these principles should be considered as an ideal to strive for and the implications of the failure to use any one of these principles in the interpretation of the results of the study should be carefully and thoroughly evaluated.

SUMMARY

The practice of statistics requires an understanding of the research questions being asked, where the data come from, how the study that produced the data was designed, what features best describe the data, how the conclusions from the study are influenced by unusual features in the data, and what alternative hypotheses might explain the results. In this chapter, our approach has been to focus on statistical concepts and methods for learning from data, rather than on mathematical formulas and calculations.

We have chosen to emphasize exploratory data analysis (EDA) methods. These methods are effective and powerful tools for learning about data, and, as we have tried to illustrate, they are relatively easy to use and are quick and robust (Koopmans, 1987; Velleman & Hoaglin, 1981). In particular, stem-and-leaf plots and boxplots are two very useful graphical displays that highlight important features of a distribution, such as central location, spread, shape, and outliers. Our aim throughout the chapter has been to use these methods to investigate relationships among variables. Specifically, we have introduced the back-to-back stem-and-leaf plot, the comparative boxplots, and two-way classification tables to display changes in the conditional distribution of a response variable that coincide with changes in an explanatory variable. The notion of a conditional distribution has played a central role in this discussion. It should be noted that in addition to EDA there are more formal statistical procedures for investigating relationships and drawing conclusions from data. For a discussion of these methods, we recommend several excellent introductory textbooks, such as Ingelfinger, Mosteller, Thibodeau, and Ware (1983), Moore and McCabe (1989), and Snedecor and Cochran (1980).

Once an association among variables is observed, an important question to be addressed is whether or not this observed relationship is causal. We have discussed and illustrated some of the issues related to evaluating the nature of associations among variables and have described some basic principles of experimental design for establishing causality. The most direct approach for investigating causal relationships is by performing a designed experiment. It is now well accepted that the randomized controlled clinical trial is the most definitive clinical research tool for evaluating the efficacy of a new therapy in human subjects. For a more detailed discussion of the principles, methods, and practice of conducting clinical trials, we recommend Friedman, Furberg, and DeMets (1984), and Meinert (1986). Even though the randomized controlled trial is considered the gold standard of study designs, there are, of course, other important approaches that are fundamental to the practice and to the advancement of biomedical research, including observational and epidemiological studies. For further discussions of these approaches, see Lilienfeld and Lilienfeld (1980) and Schlesselman (1982).

Our objective has been to introduce statistical methods that highlight important features and relationships in data. We would be remiss, however, if we did not stress again the central role of subject matter knowledge in the consideration of alternative explanations for observed associations and for the evaluation of causal relationships. This point is made by Moses (1986) in his parable about an experiment in which subjects were randomly given either large drinks of whiskey and water, run and water, or brandy and water, and all showed signs of intoxication. Moses noted that "It is 'outside knowledge' that supports the conclusion that the effect was due to the alcohol, not the water" (p. 9). Even though statistics and statistician play an increasingly important role in clinical research, ultimately it is the clinical investigator who must make decisions about the interpretation of data and the results of studies. As Cornfield (1959) wisely observed,

> Enthusiasm for statistical tools, while deserved, should be tempered with recognition of the importance of insight, imagination, and intimate knowledge of one's field. The statistician functions as a devil's advocate against the admission of new evidence, and in this capacity has an important influence on the quality and cogency of the evidence submitted. The investigator must pay close attention to this advocate, but it is his and not the advocate's responsibility to decide when he must stop listening. (p. 251)

Acknowledgment. This work was supported in part by the National Institute of Mental Health, MHCRC Grant MH-30915, a National Research Service Award MH-15758, and a grant from the John D. and Catherine T. MacArthur Research Network on the Psychobiology of Depression.

REFERENCES

Beecher, H. K. (1955). The powerful placebo. *Journal of the American Medical Association, 159,* 1602–1606.

Brown, B. W. (1978). Statistics, scientific method, and smoking. In J. Tanur, F. Mosteller, W. Kruskal, R. Link, R. Pieters,, G. Rising & E. Lehmann (Eds.): *Statistics: A Guide to the Unknown* (pp. 59–70). Oakland, CA: Holden-Day.

Carroll, B. J. (1980). Dexamethasone suppression test in depression. *Lancet,* 1249.

Cornfield, J. (1959). Principles of research. *American Journal of Mental Deficiency, 64,* 240–252.

Cox, D. R. (1958). *Planning of experiments.* New York: Wiley.

Elkin, I., Shea, M. T. Watkins, J. T., Imber, S. D., Sotsky, S. M., Collins, J. F., Glass, D. R., Pilkonis, P. A., Leber, W. R., Docherty, J. P., Fiester, S. J., & Parloff, M. B. (1989). National Institute of Mental Health treatment of depression collaborative research program: General effectiveness of treatments. *Archives of General Psychiatry, 46,* 971–982.

Endicott, J., Spitzer, R. L., Fleiss, J. L., & Cohen, J. (1976). The Global Assessment Scale. A procedure for measuring the overall severity of psychiatric disturbance. *Archives of General Psychiatry, 33,* 766–771.

Fleiss, J. L. (1981). *Statistical methods for rates and proportions* (2nd ed.). New York: Wiley.

Fleiss, J. L. (1986). *The design and analysis of clinical experiments.* New York: Wiley.

Friedman, L.M., Furberg, C. D., & DeMets, D. L. (1984). *Fundamentals of clinical trials.* Boston: John Wright.

Greenhouse, J. B. (1991). *Logistic regression: An introduction to statistical modeling.* Department of Statistics Technical Report #495. Pittsburgh: Carnegie Mellon University.

Greenhouse, J. B., Stangl, D., Kupfer, D. J., & Prien, R. (1991). Methodological issues in maintenance therapy clinical trials. *Archives of General Psychiatry, 48,* 313–318.

Ingelfinger, J. A., Mosteller, F., Thibodeau, L. A., & Ware, J. H. (1983). *Biostatistics in clinical medicine.* New York: Macmillan.

Koopmans, L. H. (1987). *Introduction of contemporary statistics methods.* Boston: Duxbury Press.

Lilienfeld, A. M., & Lilienfeld, D. E. (1980). *Foundations of epidemiology.* Oxford: Oxford University Press.

Meinert, C. L. (1986). *Clinical trials: Design, conduct and analysis.* New York: Oxford University Press.

Moore, D. S., & McCabe, G. P. (1989). *Introduction to the practice of statistics.* New York: W. H. Freeman.

Moses, L. E. (1986). Statistical concepts fundamental to investigations. In J. C. Bailar, III, & F. Mosteller (Eds.), *Medical uses of statistics* (pp. 3–27). Waltham, MA: NEJM Books.

Mullen, P. E., Linsell, C. R., & Parker, D. (1986). Influence of sleep disruption and calorie restriction on biological markers for depression. *Lancet,* 1051–1054.

Neter, J., Wasserman, W., & Kutner, M. H. (1990). *Applied linear statistical models* (3rd ed.). Homewood, IL: Irwin.

Prien, R. F., Kupfer, D. J., Mansky, P. A., Small, J. G., Tuason, V. B., Voss, C. B., & Johnson, W. E. (1984). Drug therapy in the prevention of recurrences in unipolar and bipolar affective disorders. *Archives of General Psychiatry, 41,* 1096–1104.

Relman, A. (1986). Preface. In J. C. Bailar, III, & F. Mosteller (Eds.), *Medical uses of statistics* (pp. xi–xiii). Waltham, MA: NEJM Books.

Ryan, B. F., Joiner, B. L., & Ryan, T. A., Jr. (1985). *Minitab handbook.* Boston: Duxbury Press.

Schlesselman, J. J. (1982). *Case-control studies: Design, conduct, analysis.* New York: Oxford University Press.

Snedecor, G. W., & Cochran, W. G. (1980). *Statistical methods* (7th ed.). Ames: Iowa State University Press.

Velleman, P. F., & Hoaglin, D. C. (1981). *Applications, basics, and computing of exploratory data analysis.* Boston: Duxbury Press.

Wainer, H. (1976). Robust statistics: A survey and some prescriptions. *Journal of Educational Statistics.* 1, 285–312.

PART III

ASSESSMENT ISSUES

CHAPTER 7

Structured and Semistructured Inventories

WENDY REICH

INTRODUCTION

Structured and semistructured interviews are methods of collecting data on psychiatric disorders according to specific diagnostic criteria. They are used primarily for research, but clinicians also find them helpful in clarifying psychiatric diagnoses. The interviews are particularly important because they are the means by which the data are systematically collected for much of modern psychiatric research. Moreover, the validity of research results in many instances depends on the effectiveness of these instruments.

Prior to the 1960s, little effort was put into the formal classification of psychiatric disorders because researchers tended to be concerned with etiology rather than with description and classification. This meant that since clinicians and researchers were often using different criteria to diagnose individual patients, it was not possible to reliably compare patients when they were diagnosed by different physicians (Spitzer, Endicott, & Robins, 1978). Thus, research results could not be compared, and advances in the field were often thwarted.

One of the earliest classifications systems was known as the "Feighner Criteria," which was developed at Washington University in St. Louis (Feighner,

Wendy Reich • Department of Psychiatry, Division of Child Psychiatry, Washington University School of Medicine, St. Louis, Missouri 63110.
Research in Psychiatry: Issues, Strategies, and Methods, edited by L. K. George Hsu and Michel Hersen. Plenum Press, New York, 1992.

Robins, Guze, Woodruff, Winokur, & Munoz, 1972). This classification system delineated criteria for 15 psychiatric disorders which the authors felt could be described in clear clinical terms, and which showed consistency over time. A subsequent classification system that was built on the Feighner Criteria was known as the Research Diagnostic Criteria (RDC) (Spitzer *et al.*, 1978). The RDC was developed specifically as part of the Collaborative Project on the Psychobiology of the Depressive Disorders which was sponsored by the Clinical Research Branch of the National Institute of Mental Health (NIMH). In the development of the RDC, a number of additional diagnoses were included, such as schizoaffective disorder as well as other diagnoses relevant to affective disorders and schizophrenia. The RDC offered 25 major diagnostic categories with some of these further subdivided.

THE SCHEDULE FOR AFFECTIVE DISORDERS AND SCHIZOPHRENIA—A SEMISTRUCTURED INTERVIEW

The Schedule for Affective Disorders and Schizophrenia (SADS) is a semistructured interview originally designed to operationalize the RDC criteria for the collaborative study on depression (Endicott & Spitzer, 1978). In a semistructured format, questions for each symptom of a diagnosis are written out and probes are suggested in the interview. However, interviewers are expected to make their own decisions as to whether or not a symptom is positive and how severe it is. The SADS is intended to be given by trained clinicians who use their knowledge of psychiatric disorders in making these decisions. Currently, there are a number of different versions of the SADS, including the SADS-L, a version that yields lifetime diagnoses. Other recent versions include the SADS-LA for use with anxiety disorders and the SADS-LB for studies of bipolar illness. There is also a version of the SADS-L that was modified by Elliot Gershon to make the diagnosis of unipolar depression more stringent.

The idea behind the development of the SADS was that interviewers in a research study would be able to use the RDC as a basis for their clinical judgment. The SADS interview would list the symptoms for each diagnosis, with suggested phrasing for questions and probes, as well as find out about such characteristics of a psychiatric diagnosis as duration, age of onset, and severity. Researchers who were studying a particular population would be assessing subjects according to similar criteria of known and acceptable reliability.

Two major sources of disagreement among clinicians with regard to psychiatric diagnoses are criterion variance and information variance. *Criterion variance* refers to the specific criteria the clinicians use in order to make psychiatric diagnoses. The RDC criteria used in the SADS interview would reduce the criterion variance since everyone who interviewed a patient would do so with the same diagnostic criteria.

Information variance occurs when clinicians have different amounts and kinds of information about patients. The use of the SADS interview would minimize the information variance because the organization of the interview (i.e., the kind of information elicited about the symptoms, as well as other information necessary for making a diagnosis) would ensure that clinicians had the same information about each patient. Thus, other investigators reviewing the data could be assured that a particular diagnosis was made using established criteria and the results of a uniform set of questions. Findings from different studies could then be confidently compared.

The first two editions of the American Psychiatric Association's *Diagnostic and Statistical Manual of Mental Disorders* (DSM) did not have explicit criteria for psychiatric diagnoses. Rather, they contained descriptions of psychiatric disorders, and researchers had to select diagnostic categories that most closely resembled the symptoms in the patients they were interviewing. In effect, other researchers could not really ascertain how subjects in a particular study had been diagnosed. However, more modern nosological schemes contained in the DSM-III and the DSM-III-R are based on explicit criteria, such as the Feighner and the RDC systems. The DSM-IV will also follow this style. Thus, the future direction of American psychiatric diagnosis will reflect a more explicit tradition.

THE DIAGNOSTIC INTERVIEW SCHEDULE (DIS)— A STRUCTURED INTERVIEW

The interest in psychiatric classification and the development of systems, such as the RDC and, later, the DSM-III and the DSM-III-R, led to the feasibility of the National Institute of Mental Health (NIMH) Epidemiologic Catchment Area (ECA) Program. The object of this ambitious yet highly successful study was to assess rates of prevalence and incidence of specific mental disorders, to study factors influencing the development and continuance of disorders, to estimate rates of health and mental health services use, and to study factors influencing use of services. The plan was to sample approximately 20,000 people in 5 sites: St. Louis, New Haven, Baltimore, Durham, North Carolina, and Los Angeles.

For the purposes of the study, it was important that the diagnoses be made according to the same criteria, and that all interviewers make the diagnoses in the same way. Because of the enormous size of the population to be surveyed, it would have been too costly to use clinicians as interviewers even when they were carrying out a prewritten interview, such as the SADS. The decision was made to devise an interview that could be given by lay interviewers. The result was the Diagnostic Interview Schedule (DIS) which was developed in St. Louis by Lee Robins and her colleagues. The DIS was based on the Renard Diagnostic Interview (RDI), an instrument developed by the St. Louis group which operationalized the Feighner Criteria (Helzer, Robins, Croughan, & Welner, 1981).

The DIS is a highly structured interview, which means that all the questions are written out, and the interviewers are expected to read them exactly as written. In addition, the interview contains a probing pattern that must be learned and skip instructions that must be followed precisely.

For the ECA study, between 50 and 100 interviewers were trained for each site. Many of them were professional interviewers working for research survey firms and were accustomed to doing surveys in which questions were posed precisely as written. Other interviewers had no experience at all and included teachers on vacation during the summer, graduate students taking a term off, and housewives looking for an opportunity to return to work. Few of the interviewers had much knowledge of psychiatric diagnoses.

The training period for these interviewers lasted approximately 1 week to 10 days, although the interviewers were expected to practice until they felt confident about their ability to administer the interview.

Designing an interview which could be used by lay interviewers who had approximately 1 week of training to make complex psychiatric diagnoses, including past diagnoses, was an extremely difficult and time-consuming task. Each question had to be phrased in lay language which could be understood by individuals of all educational levels, but which would not sound patronizing to more educated groups. The questions also had to be constructed so that they would convey all the subtleties of the symptom as well as explain certain conditions necessary for the symptom to be counted as positive. Some examples of these are as follows:

In the DSM-III-R criteria for Manic Episode, the first symptom reads: "A distinct period of abnormally and persistently elevated, expansive or irritable mood" (American Psychiatric Association, 1987, p. 217).

In addition to translating this criterion into a question that can be understood and answered by someone with only a sixth grade education, the researcher must be sure that the question complies with another DSM-III-R criterion which specifies that the mood disturbance be "sufficiently severe to cause marked impairment in occupational functioning or in usual social activities or relationships with others, or to necessitate hospitalization to prevent harm to self" (American Psychiatric Association, 1987, p. 217). By DSM-III-R criteria, the duration of the manic episode should be at least a couple of days.

After taking these criteria into consideration, the researchers then wrote this question for the latest version of the DIS:

> Has there ever been a period of days when you were so *happy or excited or high* that you got into trouble, or your family or friends worried about it, or a doctor said you were manic?

Note that the key words *"happy or excited or high"* are italicized and thus are meant to be emphasized by the interviewer. The term included in the DSM-III-R criteria that the mood disturbance be sufficiently severe to cause marked impairment is covered by adding the phrases "that you got into trouble, or your family or friends worried about it, or a doctor said you were manic."

Notice that according to the DSM-III-R criteria, the mood can also be irritable. However, asking about an irritable mood in the same question as one that describes a "happy, excited, or high mood" would be confusing. For this reason, the question about irritable mood is assessed after all the other symptoms of mania have been asked. After asking about all the symptoms of mania and establishing that some of them are positive, including the first question about the *happy* or *excited* or *high* mood, the following question is asked:

> You said you've had a period of feeling (high/own equivalent) and also said that you've had some feelings or experiences like (name symptoms that respondent has listed as positive). Has there ever been a period when the feelings of being excited or manic *and* some of these other feelings or experiences occurred together?

If the *happy* or *excited* or *high* mood has not been reported as positive, but other symptoms of mania have been, the interviewer then skips to another question which reads:

> You said you've had times when (list the positive moods given in the mania section). Was there ever a period when some of these feelings or experiences occurred together?

If the answer is no, then it is not possible for a manic episode to have occurred, and so the interviewer skips to the next section.

If the answer is yes, then it is possible for a manic episode to have occurred, if there has been a mood disturbance of some kind. However, it has been established that the mood was not *happy* or *excited* or *high*, because the respondent gave a negative response to this question. Remember, however, that the mood can also be irritable, so if it is established that there is a clustering of manic symptoms, the question about a possible irritable mood is asked. If the answer to the irritable mood question is yes, then the criteria for a manic episode have been met. Thus, the mood question, which includes elevated or irritable mood, has been broken into two questions, making it easier to ask about different kinds of moods.

Another criterion for mania is "excessive involvement in pleasurable activities which have a high potential for painful consequences, e.g., the person engages in unrestrained buying sprees, sexual indiscretions, or foolish business investments" (American Psychiatric Association, 1987, p. 217).

The examples in this mania question have been broken up into two questions. The first is:

> Has there ever been a period when you went on *spending sprees* spending so much money that it caused you or your family some financial troubles, or a period when you made foolish decisions about money?

The second question reads:

> Have you ever had a period when your *interest in sex was so much stronger than is typical for you that you* wanted to have sex a lot more frequently than is normal for you or with people you normally wouldn't be interested in?

A positive answer to either one of these questions would mean that the respondent would be scored as having the manic symptom. With respect to the second question, it is interesting to note that few people seem to mind questions about sex. The questions that people do not like to answer are those about how much money they make.

The questions in the DIS have been carefully thought out and thoroughly tested, and interviewers are expected to read them exactly as written. If the respondent does not understand the question, the interviewer is expected to reread the question, emphasizing those parts which the respondent does not seem to understand. Interviewers are advised against rephrasing the questions in case the new phrasing might inadvertently change the meaning of the question. The DIS is respondent based, meaning that the ultimate responsibility for the answer lies with the respondent. The interviewer does not make a judgment.

For example, one of the questions in the depression section is: "Did you ever attempt suicide?" Instead of answering the question directly, some respondents will describe their behavior:

> *Interviewer:* Did you ever attempt suicide?
> *Respondent:* Well, I took a bunch of Valium out of the bottle and held them in
> my hand.

It is very important to note that the interviewer is not expected a make a decision as to whether or not the patient has made a suicide attempt. The interviewer is expected to repeat the question.

> *Interviewer:* Let me repeat the question. Did you ever attempt suicide?
> *Respondent:* Well, I thought about it but I guess I didn't really make an attempt.

The interviewers then codes the question as no. Note that the decision as to whether or not a suicide attempt was made is at the discretion of the respondent.

Individual investigators do disagree over the relative merits of a structured versus a semistructured instrument. Advocates of the semistructured approach feel that no interview, no matter how well written, can be given by someone without clinical experience, especially when additional questions may be asked. The opposing view suggests that clinicians will bring their own subjective biases to the interview, and that the criteria will not be strictly followed. In actual practice, both types of interviews appear to show good results. Hesselbrock, Stabenau, Hesselbrock, Mirkin, and Meyer (1982) conducted a study that compared the DIS and the SADS. They showed that there was good agreement between instruments when both were used to diagnose the same individual. This finding suggests that the problem facing the researcher is not so much which instrument is better but which is most suitable for a particular study design. For example, in a study that included as large a number of people as did the ECA study, the cost of using clinicians for every interview would have been prohibitive. On the other hand, the SADS might be more appropriate for a study of affective disorders, since it was originally designed to assess psychopathology of that nature and covers an extensive range of affective symptoms.

HOW DO WE KNOW THAT THE INTERVIEWS WORK?

If any research project using structured interviews is to be successful, the instruments must be able to diagnose the subjects accurately. The difficulty is that there is no satisfactory way of judging in an absolute fashion whether or not the respondent, who is diagnosed by a particular interview, really suffers from that disorder. A logical method of determining the validity of an interview would be to compare the results of the interview to the diagnosis of that individual by a clinician. However, even since the advent of the diagnostic criteria, clinicians still show poor agreement with each other. Therefore, the validity of the instrument would depend on which clinician's diagnosis the interview was compared. The truth is that there is no "gold standard" with which to compare the interview, no absolute way of knowing whether or not a person who seems depressed, for example, as measured by a particular interview, really is depressed (Robins, 1985).

There are, however, a number of ways of testing the instruments to obtain a rough idea of how closely the interviews come to assessing "the truth."

Test–Retest Design

The test-retest design assesses the reliability of a particular instrument. That is, it measures whether or not the instrument will obtain the same results when it is administered to the same person on two different occasions by different interviewers. The test–rest design is conducted as follows: the respondent is interviewed by the first interviewer using a particular interview schedule. This is designated as Time I. A few days to a week later (Time II), the same respondent is interviewed by a second interviewer using the same interview schedule. If the results of the tests show high similarity between Time I and Time II, then the interview can be expected to elicit similar information from respondents even when given by different interviewers. Assuming that the respondent has been truthful and that the interviewers have been well trained, good reliability indicates that the interview is able to elicit the same information from a group of respondents.

Unfortunately, just because a particular interview is reliable does not automatically mean it is valid. The two interviews could be obtaining the same results, but both results could be wrong. The respondent could be depressed, but both interviews might not diagnose the depression. Therefore, both interviews could show identical results (e.g., anxiety) but these results would not be valid.

However, since an instrument cannot be valid unless it is reliable, the first step in evaluating these interview schedules is to test for reliability. Test–retest reliability studies on both the DIS and the SADS show good reliability (Endicott & Spitzer, 1978; Robins, Helzer, Croughan, & Ratcliff, 1981). As mentioned, the Hesselbrock et al. (1982) study proved that there was good agreement between the DIS and the SADS, which is another indication that both interviews are reliable.

Even though it is well known that agreement among clinicians is poor and does not constitute a reliable standard, the clinician's knowledge and experience are clearly important with respect to diagnosing psychiatric disorders.

Reliability and validity tests on the DIS have made use of the clinician's judgment in assessing the instrument. In a study by Robins, Helzer, Ratcliff, and Seyfried (1982), tests are conducted which attempted to use clinical expertise to assess the validity of the DIS. In one part of the study, 216 subjects were interviewed. Each was interviewed twice, once by a lay interviewer and once by a psychiatrist, both using the DIS. None of the lay interviewers had previous experience in interviewing and none had any clinical training. All were college graduates.

The psychiatrists were trained in the use of the DIS and administered it in the same manner as the lay interviewers. This ensured that all the psychiatrists would use the same criteria and cover the same material. This procedure would reduce poor agreement among clinicians, and between clinicians and lay interviewers. After completing the DIS, the psychiatrists scored their clinical impressions with respect to each diagnosis that was covered. They then had a free question period during which they could ask any further questions they wished, either to elicit new information or to clarify answers obtained during the interview. After the free answer period, they again scored their clinical impressions. The interviews given by the lay interviewers were scored by a computer.

The order in which the two interviews were given was randomized. Out of the 216 total subjects, 97 were given the first interview by the lay interviewer and 199 were given the first interview by the psychiatrists. The diagnoses were made on the basis of three criteria: Feighner, RDC, and the DSM-III. Diagnoses from the psychiatrists and the lay interviewers were compared using the kappa statistic, which corrects for agreement that is due to chance. The agreement for most diagnoses was considered quite satisfactory which indicates that when clinicians use the same methods as lay interviewers their results can be comparable. What is particularly important is that the free question period provided for the psychiatrists did not generally yield information that would change the diagnosis made using the DIS.

A study by Helzer, Clayton, Pambakian, and Woodruff (1978) at Washington University compared results of a structured interview with hospital charts. Interestingly, for many diagnoses, concordance was found to be high. In this study, however, the investigators were interested in seeing what information they could find out when there were discrepancies between the interview and the chart. The authors concluded that many of the discrepancies in the chart were due to information not asked by the physician. The inclusive nature of the structured interview means that it systematically elicits more information than is usually obtained in a clinical interview. On the other hand, diagnoses missed by the structured interviews seemed to be due to lack of a longitudinal clinical observation that could only have been made by a physician observing a patient through the course of a hospital stay, or possibly through repeated admissions.

Nevertheless, there were more diagnoses missed in the hospital charts than in the structured interviews. Consequently, the authors suggested that structured interviews are useful in routine initial evaluations of psychiatric patients.

Summary Diagnoses

Since there is no absolute standard by which to measure the interview, researchers and clinicians interested in finding out the "real" diagnosis if a particular respondent often use multiple sources of information. These include the interview itself and such other measures of psychiatric disorders as checklists, information from a clinician, the results of psychological testing, hospital records, and information from family members. The resulting diagnoses are based on all the information available and are usually referred to as *summary diagnoses* or *best estimate diagnoses*.

Interrater Reliability

Interrater reliability can be used to measure two procedures. First, it is a method of testing whether or not a given interviewer can elicit clear answers that other interviewers will interpret in the same way. Second, it is a method of testing how well the interviewers have been trained and how faithfully they carry out their interviewing techniques.

Interrater reliability can be tested by having one person administer the interview and then by having several other interviewers score the respondent's replies independently. This method tests the interview in the sense that the replies to the questions should be sufficiently clear so that each rater (interviewer) will code the same answer. On the other hand, it is a test, particularly in a semistructured interview, of the main interviewer's ability to probe correctly, as well as the experience of the other raters in being able to interpret the answers to both the questions and the probes.

In a discussion of a reliability study of the Present State Examination (PSE), a British semistructured interview developed by John Wing and his colleagues, Sanson-Fisher and Martin (1981) pointed out that one study showing good reliability of an instrument means only that the instrument has been used reliably at one particular time with a specific group of interviewers. It does not mean that it will be reliable in another study with a different group of interviewers. In fact, the authors found to their disappointment in their review of studies using the PSE, that only 77% of the interviewers had performed their own reliability testing.

According to Sanson-Fisher and Martin, it is not enough to conduct reliability testing at the beginning of data collection, but that rather reliability checks should be made throughout the study. One method of doing this is either to audiotape or videotape the interviews and then have another interviewer play the tape, score the interview, and compare the results with those of the first interviewer.

Sanson-Fisher and Martin also drew attention to the possibility that the group of raters as a whole might drift away from the original instructions by developing their own idiosyncratic style and moving off in their own direction. Interestingly enough, under these circumstances, raters could show a high degree of agreement but only because they are all making the same mistakes. In this case, all the interviewers must be brought back to the guidelines originally established at the beginning of the study.

OTHER STRUCTURED INTERVIEWS

The Structured Clinical Interview for the DSM-III-R

The Structured Clinical Interview for the DSM-III-R (SCID) yields DSM-III-R diagnoses and will undoubtedly be updated for the DSM-IV (Spitzer, Williams, Gibbon, & First, 1990). Of all the adult interviews available, the SCID is the least structured and therefore requires a good deal of clinical knowledge in order to administer it. The SCID was designed for three purposes: clinical diagnosis, research, and training.

There are two ways in which the SCID can be used by clinicians. In the first, the clinicians administer their usual interview and then follow it up with appropriate portions of the SCID to confirm a possible diagnosis. The advantage of using the SCID in this fashion is that the clinicians can check their diagnoses against DSM-III-R criteria, and make use of the SCID questions which have been shown to be efficient ways of obtaining diagnostic information. The second way the SCID can be useful to clinicians is to have the entire SCID administered as an intake procedure. This ensures that all the major DSM-III-R diagnoses are systematically evaluated.

With respect to research, the SCID is most often used to select a study population and to ensure that all the patients have a disorder that meets DSM-III-R criteria. The SCID is also used to exclude subjects with certain disorders. For example, researchers may wish to use the SCID to exclude all patients with a history of Psychoactive Substance Use Disorder. Finally, the SCID is often used to characterize a study population in terms of current and past psychiatric diagnoses.

The SCID is also a useful instrument for training students in the mental health professions because it teaches them how to use the DSM-III-R criteria, as well as allows them to become familiar with carefully thought out questions that help to elicit specific diagnostic information.

Specific Features of the SCID

When testing with the SCID begins, the interviewer obtains an overview of the patient's present illness and inquires about any past episodes of psycho-pathology. At the end of this overview, the interviewer should have enough information to formulate tentative diagnoses. In the SCID are many open-ended questions that encourage respondents to explain a problem as they understand it, rather than simply answer yes or no to a question as posed by the interviewer.

Unlike the DIS, the ratings of the diagnostic criteria in the SCID are not necessarily the respondent's answer to the question. Thus, in the suicide example that was chosen from the DIS, the interviewer would not take the respondent's word for whether or not having "a bunch of Valium" in hand would constitute a suicide attempt but rather would make a clinical judgment. In the introduction to the SCID, interviewers are instructed that if they are convinced that a particular symptom is present, they should challenge respondents with respect to their denial of the subject. The instructions are that if the respondent appears depressed during the interview but denies depressed mood, the interviewer should comment on the respondent's mood and probe further.

An addition to the SCID, the SCID-II is another interview schedule for evaluating personality disorders as defined by the DSM-III-R. It is not a part of any other of the widely used interview schedules. This feature of the SCID-II is particularly important because so much less work has been done on the personality disorders than on the Axis I disorders. Thus, the SCID-II provides an opportunity for diagnostic hypothesis testing of the personality disorders (Skodol, Rosnick, Kellman, Oldham, & Hyler, 1988).

A test–retest study of an earlier version of the Axis I SCID consisted of data on 506 pairs of interviews collected at 6 sites. The kappas for the test–retest studies were comparable to the DIS and the SADS. The kappas for the SCID-II on 226 subjects were similar to test–retest kappas reported for other personality assessment instruments (Spitzer, 1990).

The Composite International Diagnostic Interview

The Composite International Diagnostic Interview (CIDI), which is a combination of the Diagnostic Interview Schedule (DIS) and the Present State Examination (PSE), was developed by John Wing and his colleagues. The CIDI was commissioned by the World Health Organization with the goal of increasing the comparability between DIS and PSE based studies. As developed by Robins, Wing, and Helzer, the new CIDI has been structured to incorporate the latest version of the International Classification of Diseases (ICD-10), which is the diagnostic classification manual most commonly used in Europe, and, in addition, the Feighner, RDC, DSM-III, and DSM-III-R criteria that are used in the United States. Wing, who was first author of the PSE, reviewed the DIS to see which questions were close enough to the intention of the PSE items to be left unchanged. Then he and Robins and Helzer wrote new questions to fill the remaining gaps. Questions have been added about a general sense of well-being, chronic physical illness, and worry about physical illness. At the end of the interview, observations about slowness of speech and movement have been added. Draft versions of the interview have been tested in St. Louis, London, and several sites in Germany, most notably Munich, where WHO sponsored a CIDI/PSE comparison trial conducted by Uli Wittchen and his colleagues. Further tests of the CIDI are planned. For these tests the interview will be translated into several languages so that possible cross-cultural differences can be observed.

The CIDI-Substance Abuse Module

The CIDI-Substance Abuse Module (CIDI-SAM) includes the regular CIDI with an additional module which asks questions about substance use, abuse, and dependence. The CIDI-SAM yields diagnoses according to DSM-III, DSM-III-R, ICD-9, RDC, and Feighner criteria. The CIDI-SAM was first pretested in St. Louis. A unique feature of this test–retest assessment was that at the end of the second interview, the examiner produced a copy of the first interview and discussed the discrepancies with the respondent. The results showed that the most common reason for discrepant answers was that information had been forgotten at the time of one of the interviews or that the respondent did not understand the question during one of the interviews.

INTERVIEWING CHILDREN WITH STRUCTURED AND SEMISTRUCTURED INTERVIEWS

Constructing an interview schedule for adults that is reliable and that can be shown to approach validity is difficult, demanding, painstaking, and time consuming. Developing such instruments for children is even more so. Despite the difficulties, there are a number of interviews for children that are currently in use.

Until about 20 years ago, psychiatrists did not question children directly about their problems, but rather inferred these problems (or the etiology of the observed behavior) by observing children play, by engaging them in play, by using dolls or puppets, by analyzing drawings, or by other indirect methods. Of course, many of these methods are still in use and are particularly helpful with younger children. However, the changes in psychiatric methodology which focused on descriptive diagnostic categories have led to the view that childhood psychopathology typically consists of specific symptoms which run a predictable course and that even very young children could be asked to describe their symptoms. The pioneering work in the direct interviewing of children was carried out by Michael Rutter and his colleagues at the Maudsley hospital in London. They developed a semistructured interview in which the questions were posed directly to children. The group at the Maudsley also developed a parallel interview that asks the same questions of one of the child's parents, usually the mother. Like the adult semistructured interviews, Rutter's interview requires clinicians as interviewers.

The Diagnostic Interview for Children and Adolescents (DICA)

In the United States, one of the earliest interviews for children was the Diagnostic Interview for Children and Adolescents (DICA), which was developed by Barbara Herjanic at Washington University in St. Louis. The DICA was designed as a fully structured interview and was based on the Renard Diagnostic Interview (RDI), the forerunner of the DIS. Like the adult fully structured interviews, the DICA was designed to be used with lay interviewers. As with the adult interviews, the lay interviewers were considered ready to administer the instrument after a week's training with some practicing on their own. Like those in the RDI and in the DIS, the questions on the DICA were meant to be asked verbatim and the child's answer to be recorded. Because the interview was designed to be given to children between the ages of 6 to 17, the questions were phrased in such a way that children would be more likely to understand them. Many of the questions were asked in several different ways, so that the children would be able to understand them more easily.

Parent–Child Comparisons

When children have emotional or behavioral problems, they usually do not seek help on their own, but are brought to mental health professionals by adults, usually their parents, who report on the child's problems. For this reason, most of the standard interviews for children have both parent and child versions which ask the same questions.

When the systematic interviewing of children first started, it was assumed (although nowhere is this stated explicitly) that the parent was the gold standard (i.e, that the parent's report about the child was correct and that the way of determining the accuracy of the child's interview was to see how it compared to the parent's).

A study by Reich, Herjanic, Welner, and Grandhy (1982) compared 307 mother–child interview pairs who had been diagnosed by computer. Diagnoses on the mother–child interviews were compared using the kappa statistic. The kappas were not as high as the test–retest kappas from the adult reliability studies; however, there are two reasons that explain this. First of all, the two tests are not the same. In the test–retest format, the same respondent is interviewed on two separate occasions by different interviewers. In the parent–child design, however, two respondents (the parent and the child) are assessed by two different interviewers. Introduction of another person (the mother) into the parent–child format has the potential of introducing another source of error, assuming that the parent and child interviews are not identical. In the standard test–retest design, only one person (either the child or the parent) would be interviewed. The additional source of error in the parent and child test–retest ensures that the kappas would be lower than if one person were being tested.

Further analysis provided more interesting results; namely, that mothers and children reported significantly different information about the children's emotional and behavioral problems. Herjanic and Reich (1982) showed that mothers tended to report significantly more behavioral symptoms (e.g., symptoms of Attention Deficit Disorder and Oppositional Disorder), whereas children, even those in the 6 to 9 age group, reported significantly more subjective symptoms (e.g., depression and anxiety). Adolescents reported more symptoms of Conduct Disorder as well as tobacco use and drug and alcohol problems of which their parents appeared to be unaware.

Specifically, the reports of the parents were not an adequate measure about their child's behavior. Rather, they were just an additional, albeit important, source of information about the child. The lack of an absolute standard for children's diagnoses places child researchers in much the same position as those researchers who are looking for ultimate validity with respect to diagnoses obtained from the adult interviews. In fact, because there is less certainty as to the properties of diagnoses in children, the attempt to look for validity is much more difficult. As with the adult interviews, many current studies of children use several sources of information, including both parent and child interviews, teacher reports, and clinical evaluations when available, in order to make a summary diagnosis of the child.

Other Interviews for Children

The Kiddie-SADS (K-SADS), a version of the SADS to be given to children and their parents, was developed by Joaquim Puig-Antich and his colleagues. Like the SADS, it is semistructured and is designed to be administered by clinicians. Unlike the DICA, both mother and child are interviewed by the same person. The mother is interviewed first and then the child. The clinician makes a diagnosis based on the two interviews. If there is a discrepancy between parent and child reports, the interviewer is at liberty to bring the parent and child together and discuss the differences in the reports.

Test–retest agreement on both parent and child interviews of the K-SADS showed agreement comparable to that of the adult instruments (Chambers, Puig-Antich, Hirsch, Paez, Ambrosini, Tabrizi, & Davis, 1985). Originally the K-SADS yielded current diagnoses only. Later, however, new versions were developed which yielded lifetime diagnoses, as well as a version that contained enough diagnostic categories so that it could be used in epidemiological studies. As with the adult studies in which the interview is given by clinicians, very large studies mean a great deal of expense, as well as difficulty in finding enough clinicians who are willing do to the interviewing themselves.

Like the adult semistructured interviews, the questions in the K-SADS are written out, but the clinician is free to probe further if he or she feels it is necessary. The wording of the questions in all the versions of the K-SADS is satisfactory. Like the DICA, the same question is often asked in several different ways to facilitate the child's understanding and verify his or her comprehension of the question. The questions are written in a simple, concrete, and colloquial manner which is easy for children to understand. The K-SADS is designed to be given to young children, beginning at about age 6.

Since all the semistructured instruments require a long training period, to a very large extent the success in their administration depends on well-trained interviewers.

Other semistructured interviews for children include the Interview Schedule for Children (ISC) developed by Maria Kovacs and her colleagues at the University of Pittsburgh as part of a longitudinal study of the natural history of depressive disorders and focuses on the affective disorders. The ISC was modeled after the K-SADS, and the two instruments are quite similar. The ISC is noted for the excellent manner in which the questions are worded.

Another effective semistructured instrument for children is the Child Assessment Schedule (CAS) developed by Kay Hodges and her colleagues at the University of Missouri in 1978. This interview was also designed for clinical research, and is to be used by experienced researchers.

The Diagnostic Interview Schedule for Children (DISC)

Because of the success of the DIS and of the ECA program with adults, the NIMH decided to duplicate the ECA program for children and to design a highly structured interview for them that would be similar to the DIS. Initially, the committee designated to write this instrument consisted of Barbara Herjanic, Joaquim Puig-Antich, and Keith Conners. The first instrument that was produced—the Diagnostic Interview Schedule for Children (DISC)—resembled the DICA, because the DICA was closest to the DIS in design. Subsequent versions of the DISC were developed by A. J. Costello and colleagues at the University of Pittsburgh. The latest version of the DISC, which is currently being used in a child ECA study, was developed by David Shaffer, Prudence Fisher, and their colleagues at Columbia University. At this time, no data on the latest version have been published.

The current version of the DISC is designed for children aged 11 to 17. The highly structured nature of the instrument and the working of the questions that are carefully keyed with DSM-III-R criteria make it difficult to administer the DISC to children who are younger than 11. This version of the DISC also asks questions only about the past 6 months. This feature has advantages for the large-scale epidemiological study in which the data will represent rates of current psychiatric disorder among 11- to 17-year-olds. As currently designed, the interview does not lead to lifetime diagnoses.

As in the highly structured DIS, the questions and probes on the DISC are read verbatim, and the interviewers record the respondent's answers without exercising clinical judgment. In some instances, however, interviewers are asked to record the respondent's answer so that a clinician can be consulted if necessary.

The Diagnostic Interview for Children
and Adolescents—Revised (DICA-R)

In the past few years, the Diagnostic Interview for Children and Adolescents (DICA) has been extensively revised (Reich, Shayka, & Taibleson, 1991) to the point that it is now referred to as the DICA-R. Influenced by semistructured interviews, the authors revised the wording of the questions to make them more colloquial and easier for children to understand. The child interview was divided into two versions: the first for 6- to 12-year-olds, and the second for adolescents 13 to 17. This feature allows for age-appropriate wording of individual questions. For most questions, examples are given that describe the kind of behavior or emotion which the question is trying to elicit. Interviewers give the examples unless they feel the child clearly understands the question. For appropriate questions, such probes as "Is this a lot different from the way you usually feel?" are provided. The DICA-R is not as highly structured as the DISC and is intended to be used by lay interviewers, who may require a longer training period and should have a good understanding of the DSM-III-R requirements for each diagnostic category. All DICA-R interviews are reviewed by an editor with clinical experience or who has access to a clinician. The parent version of the interview is formatted so that up to three children can be asked about it during a single session.

To sum up, all of the interviews for children show good results, but more work needs to be done comparing interviews to determine which of the specific features of each works well with children and adolescents. There is also a need for other types of rigorous testing, such as those that have been conducted on the adult interviews.

SPECIAL PROBLEMS IN INTERVIEWING CHILDREN

Interviewing children is much more difficult than interviewing adults. Interviewers must be warm and friendly with children without being overwhelming. They must be careful not to lead the children. For example, if a child is not reporting bad behavior, the interviewer should not indicate approval. Nor should the interviewer indicate disapproval if a child is reporting Oppositional or Conduct Disorder symptoms. With younger children, interviewers must be able to determine when they are bored, when they are not paying attention, or when they do not understand a question. Obviously, it is useful to take a break under these circumstances.

Wording of the Questions

Probably the most difficult task in the development of interviews for children is to write the questions. The questions have to be clear, concrete, and written in language that the child can understand. For the younger children, this is most difficult because it is often necessary to explain quite complex ideas in very simple terms. It is also important that the questions be keyed to the criteria being used, which for most of these interviews is the DSM-III-R. This means that the authors must be careful to write the question so that it contains the exact meaning that the DSM-III-R wants to convey and not an approximation to it. Given the ambiguity of some of the DSM-III-R criteria, this elevates question writing to a high art form. It is probably impossible to overemphasize the importance of thoughtfully written questions in interviews that are designed for children. If the children do not understand the question, they cannot give accurate information. Without accurate information, data from the study are of little value.

This point is equally true with respect to interviewer training. A poorly trained interviewer, who forgets to ask a question, does not probe properly, or is not attuned to the way the child is reacting to the interview, will also produce data that should be directed to the paper shredder.

Interviewing Young Children

There is no consensus among researchers as to whether or not young children (ages 6 to 10) can be successfully interviewed. Unfortunately, insufficient numbers of formal studies have been carried out with respect to interviewing this age group. Thus, the different views on this subject tend to be based only on the clinical experiences of interviewing these young children.

Edelbrock, Costello, Dulcan, Karlas, and Conover (1986), and Verhulst, Althaus, and Berden (1987) suggested that the youngest children do not provide much information that is different from their parents. Herjanic and Reich (1982), however, found that even very young children were able to describe symptoms not reported by their parents. Moretti, Fine, Hale, and Marriage (1988) provided evidence to suggest that even young children can give valid self-reports of depressed symptoms. Clearly, further work needs to be accomplished on the assessment of very young children which will take their developmental level into consideration.

The Dominique

The Dominique Interview was developed by Jean-Pierre Valla and his colleagues at Laval University in Quebec, Canada. The interview consists of a series of cartoons, showing a little boy, named Dominique, engaged in activities that match the criteria in the DSM-III-R. For example, Dominique is shown stealing money from his mother's purse, setting a fire in a school locker, and being cruel to a cat by tying it by its tail to a clothesline. There are also some pictures in which Dominique is shown engaged in socially acceptable behavior, such as sharing toys with his friends. Children are shown the cartoons and are then asked "Are you like Dominique?" Preliminary tests of this delightful interview show good reliability and validity results.

Computerized Interviewing

Computer-administered interviews for both adults and children are currently being developed. To date, there is a computerized DIS and a computerized DICA-R. The DIS has both computer-assisted and computer-administered versions. With the computer-assisted DIS, the interviewer sits at the terminal which presents the DIS questions and probes in the appropriate sequence. The interviewer reads the questions to the respondent, evaluates the responses in the same manner as with the paper-and-pencil version, and inputs the final code using the keyboard number pad. This procedure has an advantage in that the information goes directly into the computer, thus reducing the inevitable errors that occur when the information has to be transferred from the interview to the computer. The computerized interview also greatly reduces the amount of training necessary, since it handles all the format conventions and the skip instructions. Postcollection "cleaning" of interview data is virtually eliminated, since the computer can be programmed not to accept logical inconsistencies and out-of-range codes.

Another method of administering the DIS by computer is simply to have the respondent sit in front of the screen and punch in the answers. A trained interviewer is always available to provide help when needed.

A computerized version of the DICA-R has been developed by Reich, Welner, and Herjanic at Washington University and by Multi Health Systems, a Toronto based firm. Like the paper-and-pencil DICA-R, the computerized interview includes a child, an adolescent, and a parent version. Preliminary studies of the interview show good test–retest reliability, as well as good child/ adolescent versus hospital chart agreement. Children of all ages appear to enjoy the computerized interview. Indeed, it may well prove to be an effective method of assessing psychopathology in this age group. Also, the method may be useful to engage the attention of younger children. Further studies will be conducted when the final versions of the interview are completed.

SUMMARY

Structured and semistructured inventories for children, adolescents, and adults are used in both clinical and research settings. They can be useful for clinicians in systematically screening patients and also for training purposes. In research, they are particularly important, as such data are often the chief source of information about subjects. In addition, structured and semistructured interviews enable data to be compared from many different studies so that hypotheses can be tested and confirmed and the results of different studies can be combined. For these reasons, it is vital to the accuracy of a study that the interviews be reliable and valid and that the interviewers be well trained and follow instructions faithfully.

A number of interview schedules have been developed for use with adults as well as with children. The interviews for adults have been well tested and appear to be reliable and valid, although each one has its particular strengths and weaknesses. The question, however, is not so much which interview is best but rather which one is most suitable for a particular research project. Nevertheless, further work on the adult instruments should be conducted.

The interviews for children and adolescents are more problematic because of the inherent difficulties in assessing individuals of this age group, particularly the younger ones. More studies need to be conducted on the child and adolescent interviews with respect to reliability and validity. Particular attention should be paid to the problems of using a number of different sources of information about the child in order to arrive at summary diagnoses. Additional methods of assessing children, for example, by means of cartoon and computer interviews, should also be explored further.

REFERENCES

American Psychiatric Association. (1987). *Diagnostic and statistical manual of mental disorders* (3rd ed., rev.). Wahington, DC: Author.

Chambers, W. J., Puig-Antich, J., Hirsch, M., Paez, P., Ambrosini, P. J., Tabrizi, M. A., & Davis, M. (1985). The assessment of affective disorders in children and adolescents by semi-structured interview. Test–retest reliability of the K-SADS-P. *Archives of General Psychiatry, 42,* 696–702.

Edelbrock, C., Costello, A. J., Dulcan, M. K., Conover, N. C., & Kala, R. (1986) Parent-child agreement on child psychiatric symptoms assessed via structured interview. *Journal of Child Psychology and Psychiatry, 27,* 181–190.

Endicott, J., & Spitzer, R. L. (1978). A diagnostic interview. The Schedule for Affective Disorders and Schizophrenia. *Archives of General Psychiatry, 35,* 837–844.

Feighner, J. P., Robins, E., Guze, S. B., Woodruff, R. A., Winokur, G., & Munoz, R. (1972). Diagnostic criteria for use in psychiatric research. *Archives of General Psychiatry, 26,* 57–63.

Helzer, J. E., Clayton, P. J., Pambakian, R., & Woodruff, R. (1978). Concurrent diagnostic validity of a structured psychiatric interview. *Archives of General Psychiatry, 35,* 849–853.

Helzer, J. E., Robins, L. N., Croughan, J. L., & Welner, A. (1981). Reliability and procedural validity of the Renard Diagnostic Interview as used by physicians and lay interviewers. *Archives of General Psychiatry, 38,* 393–398.

Herjanic, B., & Reich, W. (1982). Development of a structured psychiatric interview for children: Agreement between child and parent on individual symptoms. *Journal of Abnormal Child Psychology, 10,* 307–324.

Hesselbrock, V., Stabenau, J., Hesselbrock, M., Mirkin, P., & Meyer, R. (1982). A comparison of two interview schedules. The Schedule for Affective Disorders and Schizophrenia-Lifetime and the National Institute for Mental Health Diagnostic Interview Schedule. *Archives of General Psychiatry, 39,* 674–677.

Moretti, M. M., Fine, S., Hale, G., & Marriage, M. B. (1988). Childhood and adolescent depression: Child-report versus parent-report information. *American Academy of Child Psychiatry, 24,* 298–302.

Reich, W., Herjanic, B., Welner, Z., & Gandhy, P. R. (1982). Development of a structured psychiatric interview for children: Agreement on diagnosis comparing child and parent interviews. *Journal of Abnormal Child Psychology, 10,* 328–336.

Reich, W., Shayka, T., & Taibleson, C. (1991). *The Diagnostic Interview for Children and Adolescents–Revised.* Washington University.

Robins, L. N. (1985). Epidemiology: Reflections on testing the validity of psychiatric interviews. *Archives of General Psychiatry, 42,* 918–924.

Robins, L. N., Helzer, J. E., Croughan, J., & Ratcliff, K. S. (1981). The NIMH Diagnostic Interview Schedule: Its history, characteristics and validity. *Archives of General Psychiatry, 38,* 381–389.

Robins, L. N., Helzer, J. E., Ratcliff, K. S., & Seyfried, W. (1982). Validity of the Diagnostic Interview Schedule, Version II: DSM-III diagnoses. *Psychological Medicine, 12,* 855–870.

Sanson-Fisher, R. W., & Martin, C. J. (1981). Standardized interviews in psychiatry: Issues of reliability. *British Journal of Psychiatry, 139,* 138–143.

Skodol, A. E., Rosnick,L., Kellman, D., Oldham, J. M., & Hyler, S. E. (1988). Validating structured DSM-III-R personality disorder assessments with longitudinal data. *American Journal of Psychiatry, 145,* 1297–1299.

Spitzer, R. L. (1990). *Structured clinical interview for DSM-III-R multi-site test retest.* Unpublished Manuscript.

Spitzer, R. L., Endicott, J., & Robins, E. (1978). Research diagnostic criteria. *Archives of General Psychiatry, 35,* 773–782.

Spitzer, R. L., Williams, J. B. W., Gibbon, M., & First, M. (1990). *Users Guide for the Structural Clinical Interview for DSM-III-R.* Department of Psychiatry, Columbia University, Biometrics Research, New York State Psychiatric Institute.

Verhulst, F. C., Althaus, M., & Berden, G. F. M. G. (1987). The child assessment schedule: Parent–child agreement and validity measures. *Journal of Child Psychology and Psychiatry, Vol. 28, 3,* 455–466.

CHAPTER 8

Physiological and Behavioral Assessment

ROLF G. JACOB, CAROLYN BRODBECK, AND DUNCAN B. CLARK

INTRODUCTION

When addressing a research question in psychiatry and in the behavioral sciences, it is important to consider physiological and behavioral assessments in addition to self-report measures for two reasons. First, employing these methods allows the researcher to address questions that are only accessible in this manner; "physiological" questions often require physiological methods. Second, physiological measures and behavioral observations bypass certain problems involved in self-reporting, such as selective reporting, biases, forgetting, and the wish to please the experimenter.

We will begin this chapter by considering physiological measures, both in the laboratory setting and in ambulatory individuals. We will then consider behavioral measures. Among the behavioral measures, we will first consider certain behavioral indices of cognitive function that have recently been applied in clinical research. In the final section, we will discuss traditional methods of behavioral observation, including observations occurring in the natural environment and behavioral performance tasks. Thus, the first half of the chapter will concern objective measurements of variables within the individual, and the second half, of the individual acting on the environment.

Rolf G. Jacob and Duncan B. Clark • Department of Psychiatry, Western Psychiatric Institute and Clinic, University of Pittsburgh School of Medicine, Pittsburgh, Pennsylvania 15213.   Carolyn Brodbeck • Division of Psychology, Hahnemann University, Philadelphia, Pennsylvania 19102.
Research in Psychiatry: Issues, Strategies, and Methods, edited by L. K. George Hsu and Michel Hersen. Plenum Press, New York, 1992.

PSYCHOPHYSIOLOGICAL ASSESSMENT

Physiological assessments use measurements of biological parameters, such as the electroencephalogram, heart rate, and blood pressure as markers of psychological or psychopathological states. A considerable body of information is available for such assessments; this information forms the basis for the science of *psychophysiology*. Defined as "the study of the relation between psychological manipulations and resulting physiological responses, measured in the living organisms, to promote understanding of the relation between mental and bodily processes" (Andreassi, 1989, p. 2), the study of psychophysiology provides data that are central to applied sciences, such as psychosomatic medicine and behavioral medicine. Psychophysiology has also contributed to our understanding of psychopathological processes.

We will limit our discussion to measures used frequently in psychiatric or behavioral research. Further information can be obtained in textbooks or handbooks of psychophysiology, such as Andreassi (1989), Coles, Donchin, and Porges (1986), and Martin and Venables (1980). Many psychophysiological measures are technically complex to obtain, difficult to interpret, and require investment in hardware. The novice scientist should seek advice from an expert in psychophysiology before undertaking a study using complex psychophysiological measures. In fact, unfamiliarity with technical aspects of method can lead to serious mistakes in interpreting the significance of the results (Cacioppo & Tassinary, 1990).

Psychophysiological measures can be subdivided heuristically into those directly reflecting brain function and those reflecting the function of the peripheral nervous system or its effector organs. Frequently used measures of brain function include the electroencephalogram (EEG) and event-related potentials (ERPs). Other measures include the electromagnetogram and measures of cerebral blood flow, but these measures will not be discussed in this chapter. We also will discuss the measurement of eye movements as an index of central nervous system processes. Peripheral measures to be discussed include the electromyogram, respiration, cardiovascular measures (heart rate, blood pressure, blood volume), and electrodermal measures (skin conductance and skin potential). Psychophysiologists are interested not only in variations in individual measures but also in the covariation among multiple measures and between patterns of responses and psychological states. We will discuss a few of these patterns after the individual measures have been presented.

Central Nervous System Measures

Central nervous system (CNS) measures are most commonly employed to study the neurological basis for various psychological processes; they also can be used as markers for different psychological states, such as sleep, dreams, and meditative states.

Electroencephalogram

Discovered by Richard Caton in 1875 and developed for humans by Hans Berger in 1929, the electroencephalogram (EEG) has a long tradition. As a research tool, it can be used to study a variety of psychological states. Degree of alertness, for example, can be determined by measuring the degree of EEG "activation," or "desynchronization," which involves a change from slower (alpha) waves to faster (beta) waves. Similarly, the various stages of sleep are characterized, and now defined, by certain patterns in the EEG and eye-movement recordings (e.g., Andreassi, 1989). Besides sleep and alertness, EEG measures have been used to characterize other states of consciousness. For example, extensive debate has developed concerning the attributes of "altered states of consciousness" (Tart, 1969) induced by various meditative techniques. Some meditative states are associated with a predominance of alpha waves (see Shapiro & Walsh, 1984) or theta waves (Corby, Roth, Zarcone, & Kopell, 1977), but some "meditating" subjects actually may be sleeping (Pagano, Rose, Stivers, & Warrenburg, 1976).

Besides its use in examining various psychological states, the EEG also can be employed to study brain function. Thus, EEG asymmetries may reflect differences between the two hemispheres in the processing of a particular task. Such findings have contributed to the development of the popular notions of "right brain" and "left brain" activities (Miran & Miran, 1984). For example, nonmusically trained subjects whistling a tune showed greater activation of the right hemisphere (Davidson & Schwartz, 1977, cited by Andreassi, 1989) suggesting that the production of music represents a right hemispheric activity in these subjects. Davidson, Ekman, Saron, Senulis, and Friesen (1990) and Ekman, Davidson, and Friesen (1990) have examined the question of EEG correlates with emotions. These investigators have found evidence supporting their hypothesis that emotions involving "withdrawal" involve right frontal and right anterior temporal activation, whereas emotions involving "approach" involve left-sided activation.

The above studies used relative degrees of activation over different areas as a means to map brain topological function. More detailed inferences concerning the functional relationships between different structures of the brain can be made with *coherence analysis*. This form of computer-based statistical analysis examines the degree of covariation of the momentary EEG signals in different locations. Structures showing a high degree of coherence are thought to be structurally related (Andreassi, 1989, p. 41).

Event-Related Potentials

Event-related potentials (ERPs) are methods that record EEG responses to visual, auditory, or somatic stimuli. With these methods, psychological phenomena, such as perception, attention, and information processing, can be studied. Specifically, ERPs are EEG signals that occur at specified times after a given stimulus. The ERPs are superimposed on the background "noise" of unrelated EEG activity. Because the signal-to-noise ratio of one ERP recording is very small, the stimulus must be administered repeatedly for the ERP signal to be discerned. Averaging techniques allow the ERP apparatus to isolate EEG response specific to the stimulus, while simultaneously canceling out the background noise. Most modalities can be used as stimuli for ERP recordings. The most common measures are the auditory and the visual ERP.

The ERP tracing has a characteristic pattern of positive peaks and negative valleys. The early components of the ERP reflect activities in the initial relay stations, such as the brainstem, while the later ones reflect higher cortical activities. For example, the auditory ERP has an initial set of waves (termed wave I-VI) that reflect eighth nerve and brainstem function. The later components of the ERP, usually starting at 100 ms after the stimulus, reflect higher nervous system activities. These later components are labeled by using the letters P or N (for positive or negative deflections) combined with a number that indicates how many milliseconds after the stimulus (latency) the wave occurred. Thus, N100 refers to a negative deflection about 100 ms after the stimulus, and P300 designates a positive peak occurring at 300 ms. In more recent terminology, N100 is called "N1" and P300, "P3."

N1 is affected by the physical and temporal aspects of a stimulus as well as the level of wakefulness or motivation (Naatanen & Picton, 1987). Importantly, N1 has a wider and less peaked shape when the subject is attending to a stimulus compared to when he or she is not attending. The difference in N1 to an attended versus a non-attended stimulus is called the N_d component or *processing negativity*. Thus, the N_d component can be used to study attention. A recent study by Michie, Fox, Ward, Catts, and McConaghy (1990) found differences between schizophrenics and normal subjects in the N1 and N_d components; this finding suggests that schizophrenics have a deficiency in their ability to discard irrelevant stimuli that is present at the very earliest stages of perception.

The P3 is observed when the subject attends to stimuli that are unexpected (surprising) but relevant for the task at hand (Donchin, Karis, Bashore, Coles, & Gratton, 1986). P3 is larger or more delayed when the probability of the stimulus is low, when the stimuli and the tasks are complex, and when the stimulus is relevant for the task (Johnston & Dark, 1986). Impaired P3 responses occur in disorders of attention, such as psychosis. Kutcher, Blackwood, St. Clair, Gaskell, and Muir (1987) studied P3 in schizophrenics, patients with borderline personality disorder, patients with depression, patients with nonborderline personality disorders, and in normal controls. The method in which the P3 was elicited involved subjects listening to two types of tones delivered via earphones: frequent, low-pitched tones and infrequent high-pitched tones. The infrequent high-pitched tones (the target tones) were presented in random fashion. Subjects were instructed to count these tones silently. A P3 can be expected to develop specifically to the infrequent randomly occurring high-pitched tones (i.e., those that the subjects were supposed to count). The results indicated that borderlines did not differ from schizophrenics but did differ from the other diagnostic groups. Specifically, borderlines and schizophrenics had longer P3 latencies and lower P3 amplitudes. The authors concluded that because borderlines had an abnormality typical for schizophrenia, while differing from depressives, a hypothesized link between borderline personality disorder and depression was not supported. In contrast to borderlines and schizophrenics who have decreases in P3 responses, sociopaths appear to have enhanced P3 responses. Raine and Venables (1987, 1988) found an increased P3 amplitude and delayed P3 recovery to target stimuli in sociopaths, suggesting that these individuals have an enhanced ability to attend to events of immediate relevance.

ERPs occur *after* a specific stimulus. Other EEG events can be elicited *before* an expected stimulus or response. These measures can reflect anticipation of future events or intentions of engaging in a behavior. One such measure is the *contingent negative variation* (CNV), which refers to the negative potential's developing when the subject imminently expects a stimulus that requires a response (Andreassi, 1989, p 144). Reduced CNV might mean that the subject was distracted or unable to anticipate the event. For example, schizophrenics have reduced CNV (Pritchard, 1986).

Eye Movements

Because the eye is an electric dipole, its movements can be recorded from electrodes placed around it. The resulting tracing is called the *electro-oculogram* (EOG). More sophisticated techniques, such as the infrared oculogram, have recently become available. Eye movements are under intricate CNS reflex control. Therefore, although technically a "peripheral" measurement, the movements are often used as an indicator of brain function. There are six common forms of eye movements (Andreassi, 1989, p. 242; Ogilvie, McDonagh, Stone, & Wilkinson, 1988). These include: (1) saccades; (2) smooth pursuit; (3) nystagmus; (4) rapid eye movements; (5) low rolling eye movements associated with drowsiness and sleep onset; and (6) eye blinks.

Saccades are the quick movements that occur between successive eye fixations, usually lasting only .02 to .1 seconds. The speed of the saccades is reduced by certain drugs, such as diazepam, almost in a linear dose–response relationship. In a recent study, Roy-Byrne, Cowley, Greenblatt, Shader, and Hommer (1990) found that the saccades of patients with panic disorder were not affected by diazepam to the same degree as those of normals. This finding suggested that patients with panic disorder may have reduced benzodiazepine sensitivity.

Emotional and cognitive activity is often accompanied by characteristic eye movements. For example, Schwartz, Davidson, and Maer (cited by G. E. Schwartz, 1986) observed that emotional processing was associated with eye movements to the left, whereas verbal activity was associated with eye movements to the right. The investigators attributed these differences to a predominance of right hemispheric activity during emotional processing and left hemispheric activity during verbal processing.

Smooth pursuit movements are the slow movements that occur when the eye is pursuing a moving target. Impairment in these movements is considered a marker for schizophrenia (Holzman, Levy, & Proctor, 1976). Such movements are also impaired in patients with schizotypal personality disorder (Siever, Keefe, Bernstein, Coccaro, Klar, Zemishlany, Peterson, Davidson, Mahon, Torvath, & Mohs, 1990). For a comprehensive review, see Clementz and Sweeney (1990). *Nystagmus* consists of two alternating eye movements: a slow phase that enables individuals to focus on a target while quickly moving their heads, and a quick phase that resets the eye to its initial position. Nystagmic eye movements are controlled by the vestibular-ocular reflex. Patients with panic disorder and agoraphobia tend to have abnormalities in this reflex (Jacob, 1988; Jacob, Moller, Turner, & Wall, 1985; Jacob, Lilienfeld, Furman, & Turner, 1989).

Rapid eye movements are a marker for the stage of sleep called REM (rapid eye movement) sleep, which is commonly associated with dreaming. It should be noted that even this well-accepted association has been the subject of some controversy. Using improved EOG recording methods, Jacobs, Feldman, and Bender (1972, cited by Boukadoum & Kontas, 1986) reported that the association between REM sleep and dreams was not as close as previously thought. Although it had long been assumed that REMs are the equivalent of saccades occurring during sleep, more detailed recordings show that the saccades are generally faster, with a peak velocity of 200 to 325 degrees per second, compared to 150 to 180 degrees per second for REMs (Asperinsky, Lynch, Mack, Tzankoff, & Hum, 1985). Furthermore, the duration of REMs is longer than the duration of saccades.

Eye blinks are an expression of the blink reflex, which often is used as a marker for the startle reflex (Blumenthal & Levey, 1989; Ornitz & Guthrie, 1989). The startle reflex will be discussed in a later section. Besides the EOG, the electromyogram (see below) of the orbicularis oculi muscle can be used as an indicator of eye blinks (Lang, Bradley, & Cuthbert, 1990).

Peripheral Psychophysiological Measures

Peripheral psychophysiological measures include the electromyogram, measures of respiration, and measures reflecting autonomic nervous system activity, such as cardiovascular and electrodermal measures.

Electromyogram

The electromyogram (EMG) measures muscle potentials with underlying surface or needle electrodes. EMG measures are widely used in neurology for assessment of neuromuscular disorders. In the behavioral sciences, the EMG is perhaps best known for its use in biofeedback treatments, where it is often employed to induce a state of relaxation (e.g., Jacob, Chesney, Williams, Ding, & Shapiro, 1991). EMG feedback is also used to treat specific disorders characterized by abnormal skeletal movements.

Consistent with the facial movements that are characteristic of different emotions, EMG measures can be used to differentiate among emotional states. Happiness tends to be associated with an increase in zygomatic muscle activity, whereas sadness is associated with an increase in corrugator activity (for reviews, see G. E. Schwartz, 1986; Dimberg, 1990). Similarly, anger and anxiety can be distinguished by different temporal patterns of the frontalis, corrugator, orbicularis oculi, and orbicularis oris muscles. These measures can also be used in children; EMG recording of the corrugator muscle in children may be an indicator of distress or anxiety (Turner, Beidel, & Epstein, 1991). Finally, EMG measures are also routinely included in sleep recording. For example, REM sleep is characterized not only by rapid eye movements and certain EEG patterns but also by a drastic reduction in chin EMG.

For an extensive discussion of the technical aspects of electromyography, see Basmajian (1978) and Fridlund and Cacioppo (1986). For optimal electrode placement for facial muscle EMG recordings, see Tassinary, Cacioppo, and Green (1989).

Respiration

Measures of respiration may become important in the study of anxiety disorders, particularly panic disorder. Hyperventilation occurs frequently during panic attacks (Gorman, Fyer, Goetz, Askanazi, Liebowitz, Fyer, Kinney, & Klein, 1988). In fact, one theory of panic disorder proposes that panic attacks are a consequence of hyperventilation (Ley, 1985; see also Jacob & Rapport, 1984). Given such discussion, it is surprising that measures of respiration have not been used more often in the study of anxiety disorders.

Three strategies exist for measuring respiration. The first involves the attachment around the chest and abdomen of one or two bands that are sensitive to distention. Respiratory movements are then transformed into a tracing from which respiration frequency and amplitude can be determined; pulmonary ventilation also can be determined from these measures. The second strategy is to measure the air temperature via a sensor placed under the subject's nostril; the temperature will increase during each exhalation. The latter method yields only a frequency measure of respiration. The final strategy is to measure arterial or venous blood gases; a noninvasive method is to measure carbon dioxide tension transcutaneously (see the section on Physiological Ambulatory Monitoring below).

Electrodermal Activity

Electrodermal activity (EDA) measures, including skin conductance and skin potential, reflect the degree of hydration of the skin, including sweat gland activity. Skin potential measures are innervated by the sympathetic nervous system. Electrodermal measures, therefore, are commonly used as indices of generalized sympathetic activity or *arousal* (Fowles, 1986). With increased arousal, secretion of sweat increases.

The main electrodermal measures are skin conductance (SC) and skin resistance (SR). These two measures are obtained by applying a minute electrical current between two electrodes on the skin. With fixed voltage, the amount of current going between electrodes is directly proportional to SC and inversely proportional to SR. Skin conductance or skin resistance measures tend to be quite variable, depending on environmental factors and behavior. Changes will occur in response to a diverse array of stimuli, including sudden loud noise or the subject's taking a deep breath. Short-term changes are labeled *responses* (e.g., skin conductance response [SCR]). SCRs also occur even when an eliciting stimulus is not apparent; such responses are called *spontaneous* SCRs. The average level on which the SCRs are superimposed is called the *skin conductance level* (SCL). Because electrodermal activity can be affected by many variables, the assessment needs to be standardized. The student contemplating using electrodermal measures should start by consulting Fowles, Christie, Edelberg, Grings, Lykken, and Venables (1981); Barry (1990); and Mahon and Iacono (1987).

Electrodermal measures have been helpful in clarifying the concept of sociopathy. Compared to normal subjects, sociopaths tend to show decreased electrodermal activity in anticipation of avoidable aversive events (see review by Zahn, 1986). These findings are consistent with the notion that sociopaths have a diminished anticipatory fear response or impaired avoidance learning. Electrodermal measures have also been used extensively in the study of anxiety disorders. Among various physiological measures, skin conductance measures tend to have high correlations with self-report measures of anxiety (see review by Zahn, 1986). Children with anxiety disorders, compared to normal children, had more spontaneous skin conductance responses during baseline and while being exposed to loud tones or viewing pictures of snakes (Turner *et al.*, 1991). Electrodermal measures can also differentiate between retarded and agitated depressions, the former having decreased SCL. The skin conductance orienting response (SCOR, i.e., SCR to new stimuli) tends to be decreased in retarded depression. A considerable amount of research has been focused on electrodermal responding in schizophrenia. A relatively consistent finding is that many schizophrenics have fewer SCORs (Zahn, 1986), suggesting a disorder of attention.

Cardiovascular Measures

Cardiovascular measures include heart rate, blood pressure, and various measures of blood flow.

Heart Rate. Heart rate is fairly easily measured and has therefore been used extensively in behavioral research. Of interest are both *tonic* heart rate levels (i.e., changes in average heart rate extending over several minutes) and *phasic* heart rate changes (i.e., responses over a time frame of 15 sec or less). Phasic heart rate changes are often the result of complex interplays between sympathetic and parasympathetic activity and can reflect a multitude of subtle physiological and cognitive processes, as well as physiological homeostatic mechanisms.

The primary determinant of heart rate is general somatic activity (Obrist, 1982). In the exercise test, heart rate responses to specific work loads form the basis for determining a person's physical fitness (Astrand & Rodahl, 1986). In behavioral research, heart rate is often used as a measure of anxiety or "stress." For example, Foster, Evans, and Hardcastle (1978), measuring ambulatory heart rates in surgeons, found heart rates averaging 121 beats per min during operations. The heart rate induced by stress is superimposed on that required by metabolic demands (e.g., Carrol, Turner, & Hellawell, 1986).

Heart rate is commonly used as a measure of anxiety. During exposure to feared stimuli, agoraphobics have been reported to have extremely high heart rates (Mavissakalian & Michelson, 1982; Michelson, Mavissakalian, & Marchione, 1985; Michelson, Mavissakalian, Marchione, Ulrich, Marchione, & Testa, 1990). Similarly, social phobics have substantial increases in heart rate when exposed to performance situations (Beidel, Turner, Jacob, & Cooley, 1989; D. C. Clark & Agras, 1991). Even imagining feared stimuli can result in increases in heart rate (e.g., Lang, Levin, Miller, & Kozak, 1983; Vrana, Cuthbert, & Lang, 1986, 1989). The relationship between heart rate and anxiety, however, is complex. For example, the correlation between self-report of anxiety and heart rate change is far from perfect (Lang, 1968). Furthermore, in conditioning experiments in which animals are exposed to stimuli signaling the possibility of unavoidable shock, heart rate deceleration is sometimes observed (see review by Fowles, 1982). Similarly, measures of heart rate in blood phobics during exposure to feared stimuli can decrease dramatically (Ost, Sterner, & Lindahl, 1984), suggesting that the blood phobic response (which includes fainting) might be physiologically different from other fear responses.

More subtle changes in heart rate than those occurring with anxiety and stress are also of interest. For example, when a person attends to a novel stimulus, small decreases in heart rate and respiration rate tend to occur (Jennings, 1986). Rhythmic changes in heart rate occur in synchrony with respiration; the magnitude of this "respiratory sinus arrythmia" is an indicator of parasympathetic activity or "vagal tone" (e.g., Allen & Crowell, 1989; Porges, McCabe, & Youngue, 1982). In normal subjects, both lactate infusion and hyperventilation were associated with an increase in heart rate and a decrease in vagal tone (George, Nutt, Walker, Porges, Adinoff, & Linnoila, 1989). Because lactate infusion and hyperventilation can induce panic attacks in patients with panic disorder, this finding suggests that the heart rate increases seen in panic attacks may be vagally mediated.

Technically, heart rate measures are derived either from the electrocardiogram (EKG) or from some measure of blood flow, such as blood flow to the finger. When momentary heart rate and its variability are of primary interest, the EKG is preferable because the onset of systole (i.e., the R wave) can be determined more precisely. Some heart rate recorders measure heart rate directly by counting the number of beats within a certain interval; other recorders measure the time between successive heart beats, or *interbeat interval* (IBI). The interbeat intervals can then be transformed to heart rate. This is done on a beat-by-beat basis by calculating the inverse of the IBI, or by deriving a "local" heart rate as a function of time (e.g., Berger, Akselrod, Gordon, & Cohen, 1986).

Blood Pressure. Like heart rate, *systolic* and *diastolic blood pressure* tend to increase when a person is anxious. Therefore blood pressure rates can be used as a correlate of anxiety (Beidel *et al.*, 1989). The possibility that measures of diastolic pressure could differentiate anger from anxiety has generated considerable interest (e.g., Ax, 1953; see also review by G. E. Schwartz, 1986), but the issue of whether emotions can be differentiated based on autonomic measures alone remains unresolved (Stemmler, 1989). A disadvantage of most available noninvasive devices for blood pressure measurement is that measures are obtained only intermittently. This means that the device may miss the effect of important stimuli because they occurred at times when blood pressure was not being measured. Recently available, however, are noninvasive techniques with the ability to track blood pressure continuously through blood pressure cuffs, which rapidly adjust pressure so that the pressure gradient across the arterial wall remains constant at all times during each individual pulse wave (Larsen, Schneiderman, & DeCarlo-Pasin, 1986).

Another method that has been used to circumvent the problem with intermittent blood pressure measurements is to measure *pulse transit time* (PTT). For example, R-wave to finger pulse transit time measures the time between the R-wave on the EKG and the arrival of the pulse wave to the finger. Commonly used PTT measures are R-wave to finger, R-wave to earlobe, R-wave to radial pulse, and the time between two peripheral artery sites (e.g., between brachial and radial arteries). PTT tends to be inversely related to blood pressure (i.e., an increase in blood pressure is associated with a decrease in PTT). However, Lane, Greenstadt, Shapiro, and Rubinstein (1983), comparing intra-arterial blood pressure to various PTT measures, found only modest correlations between these variables. PTT may track myocardial contractility and sympathetic tone rather than blood pressure *per se* and is also affected by local factors in the arterial wall (Larsen *et al.*, 1986). Thus, considerable caution is in order when interpreting the results of studies using PTT. T. Weiss, del Bo, Reichek, and Engelman (1980) have found that the relationship between changes in PTT and changes in mean arterial blood pressure (a weighted mean of systolic and diastolic pressure) depends on what underlying autonomic mechanism produced the change. For example, decrease in PTT was accompanied by an *increase* in mean arterial blood pressure if the changes were induced by vagal blockade or alpha-adrenergic stimulation, but by a *decrease* in blood pressure if the underlying mechanism was that of beta-adrenergic stimulation.

Blood Flow. Blood flow measures record some variable that is proportional to blood perfusion which, in turn, is affected by the degree of vasodilation or vasoconstriction. Temperature and color can be used as indices of cutaneous blood flow. For example, blushing represents an increase in blood flow to the skin of the face (Hassett & Danforth, 1982). Skin temperature can be measured with a thermistor attached to the skin. Anxiety tends to be associated with decreased finger temperature, whereas anger increases temperature (Ekman, Levenson, & Friesen, 1983; Levenson, Ekman, & Friesen, 1990); however, panic attacks may be associated with an increase in finger temperature (Cohen, Barlow, & Blanchard, 1985). Schizophrenics also tend to have digital vaso-constriction, as indicated by the color of their nail beds (Maricq, 1963, cited by Zahn, 1986).

Besides temperature measurement, blood flow can be determined by devices generically called *plethysmographs*. These devices include (1) hydraulic or pneumatic systems that respond to volume changes; (2) devices measuring the resistance (impedance) to high-frequency alternating currents; and (3) photo-electric transducers that measure changes in transmitted or reflected light from a light source (*photometers* or *photoplethysmographs*, cf. Jennings, Tahmoush, & Redmond, 1980). The simple devices that measure heart rate in exercise facilities tend to be based on photometric blood flow measures to the finger. Forearm blood flow is often measured with the venous occlusion plethysmograph. In contrast to blood flow to the finger, forearm blood flow largely reflects the blood flow to the skeletal musculature (R. B. Williams, 1984). Cardiac blood flow can be measured using impedance cardiography, a technically complex procedure (see Sherwood, Allen, Fahrenberg, Kelsey, Lovallo, & van Doornen, 1990; Larsen *et al.*, 1986; Tursky & Jamner, 1982).

Forearm blood flow (FBF) is an important measure in cardiovascular psy-chophysiological research in that it can discriminate between alpha-adrenergic and beta-adrenergic activity. Sympathetic nerve stimulation of alpha-adrenergic receptors results in vasoconstriction and decrease in FBF, whereas beta-adrenergic stimulation results in vasodilation due to stimulation by epinephrine (R. B. Williams, 1984). R. B. Williams, Bittker, Buchsbaum, and Wynne (1975) showed that certain types of cognitive tasks were associated with increases in FBF, whereas others were associated with little change in FBF. Specifically, mental arithmetic, a task characterized by high mental activity and relative disregard for external stimulation, was associated with a marked increase in FBF. On the other hand, a word identification task (requiring a high degree of attention to external stimuli) resulted in a slight decrease in FBF. This experi-ment confirmed the hypothesized differences in autonomic responding to tasks involving two basic cognitive processes, *sensory intake* versus *sensory rejection*, the latter being associated with increase in FBF.

Blood Flow Measures of Sexual Arousal. One application of blood flow meas-ures lies in the assessment of sexual arousal. Most measures of sexual arousal involve devices that reflect blood flow to the genital organs. In men, sexual arousal can be measured using a strain gauge device that senses the circum-ference or volume of the penis (Geer, O'Donohue, & Schorman, 1986). For women, a vaginal photometer that measures vaginal blood flow and blood pooling has been developed (Geer *et al.*, 1986). This measure has shown good correlations with subjective measures of sexual arousal (Korff & Geer, 1983). A study by Abel, Blanchard, Barlow, and Mavissakalian (1975) provided an example of the skillful use of the penile strain gauge to measure sexual arousal patterns, including those considered "deviant." Sexual fantasies were presented to the patient on audiotapes, starting with the patient's own self-reported fantasies. The investigators examined the penile volume pattern while specific aspects of the fantasy were presented. Observing penile responses to certain fantasies but not to others, the investigators could identify those sexual cues that were genuinely arousing. Interestingly, it appeared that the subjects themselves were not always correct in identifying the specific stimuli that tended to arouse them.

Combinations of Physiological Measures

Although investigators sometimes are interested in a particularly physiological measure for its own sake, they frequently use the measure as an index of underlying hypothetical constructs. They employ multiple measures that converge on the phenomenon to be examined. We are unable, within the allotted space, to cover such issues in depth. Nevertheless, some concepts occur so frequently in the psychosomatic and physiological literature that we will mention them here briefly: arousal level, the orienting response, the defense response, and the startle reflex.

Arousal, also called *activation*, refers to parallel increases in heart rate, skin conductance, blood pressure, and EMG paired with EEG desynchronization (Andreassi, 1989). On many tasks, performance tends to be associated with arousal along an inverted U-shaped relationship. Specifically, performance tends to be low at both low levels of arousal and at high levels of arousal while the optimal performance occurs at moderate levels of arousal. Because covariation between the different physiologic measures of arousal is not perfect, concerns have been raised that the concept of arousal has been used inappropriately (Anderson, 1990; Neiss, 1988, 1990).

The *orienting response* refers to changes that occur in response to a novel stimulus. The changes are similar to those listed above for general arousal, except that heart rate and respiration *decrease* rather than increase. The orienting response is considered a sign of increased attention or information-processing (Jennings, 1986). Repeated presentation of the same stimulus quickly leads to *habituation*; that is, the orienting response diminishes until it no longer occurs. The orienting response is sometimes contrasted with the *defensive response*, which occurs with stressful stimuli. The defensive response includes an *increase* in heart rate. This increase has a long latency (more than 2 sec), and habituation occurs less easily (Turpin, 1986).

The *startle reflex* is elicited by sudden new stimuli. It differs from the defensive response in that the latency is shorter (less than 2 sec) and the reflex habituates more quickly. The startle reflex is of interest in the study of emotional states, particularly anxiety. For example, Lang *et al.* (1990) and Bradley, Cuthbert, and Lang (1990) have shown that people startle more easily when they are viewing slides of mutilations, spiders, or snakes than when they are viewing pleasant slides. Interestingly, an increased startle response is a phenomenon that has been included in the DSM-III-R diagnostic criteria of Generalized Anxiety Disorder and Post-traumatic Stress Disorder (American Psychiatric Association, 1987).

Physiological Ambulatory Monitoring

Measurement of physiological variables in the patient's natural environment can be obtained through the use of miniature monitoring devices. The technology for this assessment method, often referred to as *ambulatory monitoring*, has rapidly improved in recent years. Ambulatory monitors are available for measurement of heart rate, blood pressure, carbon dioxide pressure (pCO_2) and respiratory rate, temperature, skin conductance, and the electroencephalogram. Most of these devices can collect and store data over many hours or even days. Ambulatory monitoring has been extensively used in the study of panic disorder (see Clark, Taylor, & Hayward, 1990, for review). The advantages of using ambulatory monitoring compared with laboratory assessment include improved ability to capture infrequent physiological events, improved external validity of measurements made in the subject's natural environment, and the possibility of assessing subjects during unrestricted activities.

Objective physiological measurements are often carried out in the laboratory, but many important clinical phenomena are difficult to reproduce there. For example, spontaneous panic attacks are generally infrequent and therefore unlikely to occur during the limited time of a laboratory assessment session. In addition, observations of normal activity may be curtailed by differences in patient behavior between the natural environment and the laboratory or inpatient hospitalization. For example, the study of diurnal variations in physiological variables requires continuous measurement for days or even weeks, requiring either that the subject stay in the laboratory for prolonged periods of ambulatory monitoring. Since the activities of the subject are curtailed in the laboratory, measurement of diurnal variation in physiological variables may have compromised validity.

Although many clinical phenomena can be simulated in the laboratory, the validity of certain of these simulations has been questioned. For example, investigators have developed methods to induce panic attacks in the laboratory with lactate infusion, hyperventilation, carbon dioxide or sympathomimetic drugs (see Shear and Fyer, 1988, for review). These methods are more successful in inducing panic attacks in patients with panic disorder than in normal controls. Some investigators argue, however, that such differences between panic patients and controls are the result of differences in baseline anxiety levels that are due to anxiety induced by the laboratory setting (Margraf, Ehlers, & Roth, 1986). Thus, even though investigators generally assume that the laboratory is a neutral setting, allowing the collection of baseline data, there is increasing evidence that, for some subjects, the laboratory setting itself may provoke anxiety. For example, laboratory studies of panic disorder patients have consistently shown them to have higher resting heart rate than controls (e.g., Charney & Heninger, 1986; Dunner, 1985; Nesse, Cameron, Curtis, McCann, & Huber-Smith, 1984; Shear, Harshfield, Polan, Mann, & Frances, 1983). However, D. B. Clark, Taylor, Hayward, King, Margraf, Ehlers, Roth, and Agras (1990) have demonstrated—using ambulatory monitoring and controlling for activity level, medication use, and fitness—that panic disordered patients studied outside the laboratory do not evidence elevated mean waking or sleeping heart rates. This finding suggests that anxiety induced by phobic elements of the laboratory are responsible for the increases in "resting" heart seen in laboratory studies of panic patients.

Several investigators have used ambulatory monitoring to study heart rate during naturally occurring panic episodes (e.g., Freedman, Ianni, Ettedgui, & Puthezhath, 1985; Gaffney, Fenton, Lane, & Lake, 1988; Taylor, Telch, & Havvik, 1983; Taylor, Sheikh, Agras, Roth, Margraf, Ehlers, Maddock, & Gossard, 1986). These studies indicate that, consistent with patients' reports of symptoms, most panic episodes are accompanied by heart rate increases. Ambulatory blood pressure shows similar increases during panic episodes (White & Baker, 1986, 1987). A device for the continuous, ambulatory monitoring of transcutaneous pCO_2 has been used to study panic attacks (Hibbert & Pilsbury, 1988; Pilsbury & Hibbert, 1987). Because expected changes in pCO_2 did not occur in all panic episodes, these results demonstrated that hypocapnia is not necessary for panic symptoms to occur. An ambulatory monitoring device for the measurement of respiratory rate is also available and has been used in studying panic patients in the laboratory (Gorman et al., 1988), but not yet in the natural environment. Finger-ambient temperature differences can be recorded by a monitoring device and, consistent with patient subjective report, substantial temperature fluctuations have been observed in panic episodes (Freedman et al., 1985).

The use of ambulatory monitoring is, of course, not limited to the study of panic disorder. Ambulatory blood pressure devices have been used in the study of treatment effects for hypertension, including behavioral treatments. Thus, Jacob, Shapiro, Reeves, Johnsen, McDonald, and Coburn (1986) and Jacob, Shapiro, O'Hara, Portser, Kruger, Gatsonis, and Ding (1992) found that relaxation exercises did not result in generalized decreases in blood pressure, although drug treatment with atenolol or chlorthalidone did.

Less frequently used devices for ambulatory monitoring include those monitoring the electroencephalogram (EEG) or skin conductance. An electro-encephalograph monitor has been developed and is commercially available. Brain electrical activity can be monitored for up to 24 hours, and four channels of EEG data can be derived (Leroy & Ebersole, 1983). For example, Torsvall, Akerstedt, Gillander, and Knutsson (1989), in a study of night shift workers, showed that 20% of the subjects had sleep episodes during the night shift hours. The feasibility of using this device in psychiatric studies has also been demonstrated. Stevens, Bigelow, Denny, Lipkin, Livermore, Rauscher, and Wyatt (1979) demonstrated EEG abnormalities consisting of focal slow or spike activity over temporal regions in 39% of schizophrenic subjects using ambulatory monitoring. In this study, however, there was no temporal correlation between clinically abnormal events and EEG activity. Skin conductance can also be measured with ambulatory monitoring (Turpin, Shine, & Lader, 1983; Simpson & Turpin, 1983). Because ambulatory skin conductance levels are affected by ambient temperature, ambient temperature must be measured concomitantly (Turpin *et al.*, 1983).

Multichannel ambulatory monitors are now available that can concomitantly measure several physiological variables. For example, the monitor described by Thakor, Yang, Amaresan, Reiter, Hoen-Saric, and McLeod (in press) records skin conductance, ambient temperature, heart rate, respiration, and physical activity. In a current study in our laboratory, subjects wear two monitors: one for blood pressure and one for heart rate and activity. Because the size of the ambulatory monitors has decreased dramatically in recent years, it is possible to do such monitoring without undue interference with the subject's regular activities.

Behavioral Diaries during Ambulatory Monitoring

When undertaking a study involving ambulatory monitoring, patients typically monitor simultaneously their physical environment and behavior. The information elicited in the diary serves two purposes: (1) to provide information on specific behavioral stimuli relevant for the research question under study; and (2) to provide information on concomitant behavior with known effects on the physiological variable in question in order for the researcher to be able to control for these effects. A statistical technique to analyze ambulatory blood pressure recordings that takes diary information into account has been described by Marler, Jacob, Lehoczky, and Shapiro (1988). Figure 1 depicts the "behavioral diary" currently in use for ambulatory blood pressure monitoring in our laboratory. As shown, after each blood pressure measurement, subjects complete a brief questionnaire with questions about setting, social context, type of interaction, body position, mental activity, physical activity, and intake of food, caffeine, or alcohol. They also provide a brief verbal description of their activity. Finally, subjects report their predominant mood, using the Circular Mood scale (Jacob, Simons, Rohay, Manuck, & Waldstein, 1989). To test the validity of the mood rating, subjects also fill out a more extensive mood checklist on an infrequent basis, the Positive Affect-Negative Affect scale (Watson, Clark, & Tellegen, 1988). (This latter scale is not included in Figure 1).

When studying an episodic condition such as panic attacks with ambulatory monitoring, it is important to find ways to mark the event's occurrence exactly in time so that the physiological record and the information on symptoms can be juxtaposed. One such method is to have patients press an event marker on the ambulatory monitoring device each time the event of interest occurs. A disadvantage with event markers is that they only provide binary measures (i.e., present vs. absent). Audiotape recordings have been used as a form of spoken diary (e.g., Kenardy, Evans, & Oei, 1988), but this method best applies to recording over brief time periods.

A method for ambulatory monitoring of psychological symptoms using a

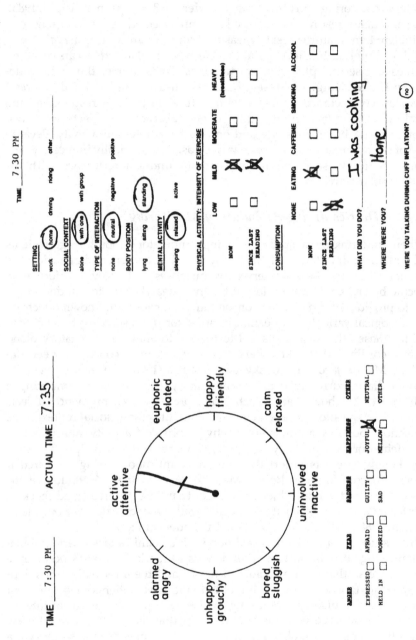

Figure 1. Front and back of a page in the behavioral diary used during ambulatory blood pressure monitoring. Each time blood pressure is recorded, subjects fill out one page.

pocket computer has recently been developed. This system, which eliminates many problems of written diaries or continuous audiotaped recordings, was pioneered by Taylor, Fried, and Klein (1990). Patients carry a small handheld, programmable computer (1" × 7" × 4") with a liquid crystal touch screen. Successive questionnaire items appear on this screen (e.g., specific panic symptoms), and the patients answer these questions by touching a designated area. The questions can be administered at predetermined intervals or initiated by the patient. The answers and the specific time of the entries are recorded in the computer memory. Using the built-in interface and an external disk drive, data can be downloaded from the handheld computer to a larger computer for permanent storage and data analysis.

Fried, Kenardy, Ironson, and Taylor (1989) used this method in a study of 20 women who had frequent panic attacks. Each subject recorded symptoms hourly from 7:00 A.M. to 11:00 P.M. for 7 days, yielding over 2,300 recordings with a compliance rate of 88%. Kenardy, Taylor and Fried (1989) used these data to examine diurnal variation in panic attacks and anxiety. Results showed substantial rises in anxiety during the late morning and early evening hours that coincide with diurnal variations in plasma norepinephrine.

Psychomotor Activity

Another method of measuring behavior concomitantly with physiological monitoring is to electronically assess activity levels. Recording of motor activity is also of interest for its own sake. Research has shown predictable relationships between psychomotor activity and psychiatric disorders, including depression (D. B. Clark, Taylor, Hayward, King et al., 1990; Kupfer, Weiss, Foster, Detre, Delgado, & McPartland, 1974), mania (B. L. Weiss, Foster, Reynolds, & Kupfer, 1974), anorexia nervosa (Falk, Halmi, & Tryon, 1985), agoraphobia (D. B. Clark, Taylor, Hayward, King et al., 1990), obesity (Chirico & Stunkard, 1960), and hyperactivity (Porcino, Rapoport, Behar, Sceery, Ismond, & Bunney, 1983).

The ambulatory measurement of activity typically uses a sensor, consisting of either mercury switches or an accelerometer, attached to the thigh or wrist. Devices with mercury switches have been extensively used in studying motor activity in psychiatric patients, but those using an accelerometer sensor are more accurate (Servais, Webster, & Montoye, 1984) and therefore likely to be more widely used in the future. An additional alternative is to measure electromyographic activity from muscles involved in locomotion. For example, Anastasiades and Johnston (1990) used a multichannel ambulatory monitor to record both heart rate and activities. The activity measure involved EMG recordings from the subject's thigh. This measure could discriminate among the activities of running, walking, and nonmovement. Furthermore, it provided significant correlations with heart rate.

Activity data collected with ambulatory monitoring devices show a relationship between affective state and activity. For example, D. B. Clark, Taylor, Hayward, King et al. (1990) suggested that patients with panic disorder without depression may be characterized by psychomotor agitation, and patients with simultaneous agoraphobia and depression, by psychomotor retardation. Personality characteristics have also been shown to be correlated with activity, including trait anxiety (Clark, Taylor, Hayward, King *et al.*, 1990), histrionic personality traits (King, Bayon, Clark, & Taylor, 1988), and interpersonal inhibition (Buss, Block, & Block, 1980; Korner, Zeenah, Linden, Berkowitz, Kraemer, & Agras, 1985). Moreover, mean daily motor activity may be a stable characteristic. In a study of children from 3 days old to early childhood, Korner and colleagues (1985) found that, despite differences in measuring devices and assessment situations, relative activity level was stable across this period. Animal studies have suggested that there may be an inheritable component to this characteristic, as it is possible to breed dogs for activity characteristics that covary with cardiovascular reactivity (Newton, Paige, Angel, & Reese, 1988).

BEHAVIORAL INDICES OF COGNITIVE PROCESSES

In the preceding section we considered the assessment of variables in the physiological domain. We will now begin to describe measures in the behavioral domain. The behavioral assessments of this section, like the physiological assessments of the previous section, can be employed as indices for hypothesized cognitive processes. Self-report measures can also be used to assess cognitive processes, but these will not be discussed.

The type of cognitive assessments to be described here all involve measurement of behavioral responses while subjects are presented with multiple classes of stimuli simultaneously that compete for attention. These methods offer promise in quantifying "unconscious" psychological phenomena. The prototype for this type of assessment is the Stroop Color and Word Test (Golden, 1978). In the test's original form, words designating different colors are printed on a series of test cards. The meaning of the word conflicts with the color of its ink (e.g., the word *RED* printed in blue). The subject is instructed to name the *ink* color for each stimulus word as quickly and accurately as possible. The Stroop interference mechanism involves the parallel processing of the color and the meaning of the word (Keele, 1986). Two measures of the degree to which the meaning of the word interferes with this task are the *error rate* and *response latency* for color naming. For example, the word *red* written in red ink would be expected to have a shorter latency than the word *red* written in green ink, and the time difference reflects the degree of interference.

Another way of creating interference in the Stroop task is to replace the words designating colors with words having affective significance. Suppose one card has the word *book* written on it in blue ink, and another, the word *murder* in blue ink. The subject is supposed to name the color of the print as opposed to the word itself. Because, to most people, the word *murder* has higher affective value than the word *book*, the latency to the word *murder* should exceed that of the word *book*. Psychiatric disorders may differ with respect to the specific themes that enhance interference. For example, depressed patients showed significantly elevated response latencies and error rates for stimuli associated with suicidal risk themes in comparison to negative and neutral affect lists (J. M. Williams & Broadbent, 1986). Interestingly, these interference effects attenuated as the depression remitted (Gotlib & McCann, 1984). Similarly, patients with generalized anxiety disorder who had primary somatic fears evidenced increased color-naming times for lists reflecting health-oriented threat cues (Mathews & MacLeod, 1985; Mogg, Mathews, & Weinman, 1987). Even after completed treatment for anxiety, interference effects specific for anxiety remained, suggesting a generalized vulnerability factor underlying the perceptual schemata in generalized anxiety disorder (Mathews, May, Mogg, & Eysenck, 1990).

In addition to these *specific* interference effects, the Stroop task can be scored to measure *global* interference effects. *Global interference* means that regardless of the thematic content, interference is increased. Schizophrenic inpatients, in comparison to psychiatric control subjects, show high global Stroop interference effects as well as other impairments for attention control mechanisms (Abramczyk, Jordan, & Hegel, 1983).

The Stroop type tasks represent a visual mode of presentation. An adaptation of the Stroop task to auditory mode involves presenting auditory stimuli concurrently with a visual task. Specific interference is reflected in the degree to which the thematic content of the auditory stimuli detracts from the performance of the primary visual task. A further adaptation of the auditory task involves presenting only stimuli in the auditory mode, but different stimuli to each ear (i.e., a *dichotic listening task*). In the dichotic listening task, separate auditory stimuli (e.g., clicks, tones, letters, digits, words, thematically related passages) are presented to the two ears by use of headphones. For example, subjects may be instructed to repeat ("shadow") or remember a passage from the right ear, while being exposed to distracting material in the left ear.

The dichotic listening task may be used to assess two types of attention: focused and divided. *Focused attention* refers to the subject's ability to discriminate between foreground stimuli and background "noise." It is evaluated by instructing the subject to listen to an *attended*, or primary, channel, and ignore stimuli presented to an *unattended*, or secondary, channel. *Divided attention* refers to the subject's ability to concurrently process and hold in memory information from multiple sources. Divided attention is evaluated by having the participant apply equal emphasis to stimuli presented to both ears. The divided attention tasks tend to be quite difficult. For example, the subject may be required to shadow material from one ear while concurrently searching for a "target" stimulus presented periodically to the other ear.

Dichotic listening procedures have been applied clinically to evaluate the specific interference effects of cues with specific affective value for patients with a particular disorder. For example, in the focused attention task, patients with generalized anxiety disorder showed interference when emotionally relevant information was presented to an unattended channel (Mathews & MacLeod, 1986). With these tasks, it has been shown that the effect of combat stress may have long-standing effects, regardless of whether the veteran develops "post-traumatic stress disorder." Trandel and McNally (1987) found that Vietnam-era veterans evidenced increased shadowing errors and elevated skin conductance reactivity when combat-related stimuli were presented to the unattended channel. For further in-depth review of this interesting type of research in depression or anxiety disorders see the recent study by Dalgleish and Watts (1990). Besides assessing specific interference effects, the dichotic listening task has also been employed to study global interference in patients with Alzheimer's disease and schizophrenia (Grady, Grimes, Patronas, Sunderland, Foster, & Rapoport, 1989; Wielgus & Harvey, 1988).

Recent progress in computer applications has further stimulated interest in cognitive assessment. The interested reader is referred to Graves and Bradley (1987), Maarse, Mulder, Sjouw, and Akkerman (1988), and Westall, Perksey, and Chute (1986). The IBM-compatible Micro Experimental Laboratory (MEL) software package may be of considerable practical value in setting up cognitive tasks and collecting data (Schneider, 1988). Methodological considerations for these tasks are reviewed by Berlin and McNeil (1976), Bradshaw and Burden (1986), Dyer (1973), and Bruder (1983).

BEHAVIORAL OBSERVATIONS

The measures discussed in the previous sections all concerned processes occurring *within* the individual. We now turn to measures of *individuals acting on their environment*. Two aspects of such actions lend themselves to objective quantitative measurement: performance and product. Behavioral *performance* refers to a person's movements. Examples of observations of behavioral performance include recording a hyperactive child getting in or out of his or her chair, an autistic child engaging in self-stimulatory behavior, a schizophrenic patient talking to himself, or a mother feeding her child.

Behavioral *product* refers to the enduring traces of behavior. Footprints in the snow, scores on a test, levels of income, and weights of psychiatric charts all can be viewed as product measures.

Observations of Behavioral Performance

Observations of behavioral performance are often done in the field in relatively defined or structured settings in which limits are placed on the range of behaviors to be observed. Thus, performance observations are widely used in classroom, clinical, and inpatient hospital settings. Typically, behavioral observers are placed unobtrusively in the location of interest. These observers record the presence or absence of a previously defined behavior at predetermined intervals. If two observers record the same individual, the extent to which the two observers agree (i.e., interrater reliability) can be determined. In other instances, videotaped recordings are made of the behavior. Behavioral observers then score the actions on the videotape. During observations, the target behaviors can be coded in different ways. For example, the behavior may be considered either *present* or *absent*. Other systems may record mutually exclusive alternative behaviors. The *intensity* of the behavior in question can also be recorded.

The recording procedure can vary. *Real time recording* involves noting the times of onset and offset for the behavior being observed. If several behaviors are observed simultaneously, the task quickly exceeds the attentional capacity of the observer. As an aid, *event recorders* have been constructed, allowing the observer to press a predefined button whenever the behavior occurs. *Frequency recording*, which involves making a recording at the onset of each instance of behavior, is particularly useful for behaviors that have short duration. Simple counting devices, like golf counters, can sometimes be used to simplify frequency recordings.

Interval recording involves recording the presence or absence of a behavior within a certain interval, say, 15 sec. One difficulty with interval sampling is that different results are obtained depending on the definition of a behavior as being "present." In *partial* interval recording, a behavior is considered "present" if it occurs in all or part of the interval. In *whole* interval recording, the behavior is considered present if it fills the entire amount of time. In *instantaneous* recording, also called discrete or momentary sampling (Suen & Ary, 1989), the behavior is considered present if it occurs at a discrete point in time. Interval recording is a commonly used technique of formal behavioral observations. However, unless the recording interval is very short compared to the typical duration of the behavior, these methods can provide misleading or biased estimates of the behavior's prevalence and incidence (Suen & Ary, 1989). Real time recording is the only technique through which each instance of the behavior is reconstructed with a high degree of fidelity.

Behavioral observations can be targeted toward one or multiple subjects. For example, Atkins, Pelham, and Licht (1988) observed each of 80 children for 2 sec 30 times per day at randomly selected times. This schedule resulted in a total of 7 min during 1 week for each child. Observations in which subjects are observed intermittently in this fashion are sometimes called *time sampling*. In the study by Atkins *et al.* (1988), observations focused on one subject at a time, but observational systems can also be designed in which specific interactional sequences between two or more persons are observed. Recordings of interactions are particularly useful for marital assessments: for example, the Martial Interaction Coding System-III (MICS-III) (R. L. Weiss & Summers, 1983) and the system used by Gottman and co-workers (Bakeman & Gottman, 1986). Similarly, for the inpatient setting, specific behavioral codes have been developed to observe interactional sequences between patients and staff (Paul, 1987; Paul & Lentz, 1977).

Behavioral observations of facial expressions can be used to measure emotional states. A comprehensive system to measure facial expression developed by Ekman and Friesen (1978) is the Facial Action Coding System (FACS).

This system was used in a study on the Type A Behavior Pattern by Chesney, Ekman, Friesen, Black, and Hecker (1990). The authors found that Type A's differed from Type B's with respect to two facial patterns: glare and disgust. *Glare* was defined as "the brows are lowered, the upper eyelid is raised, or the lower eyes are tensed, and the gaze is directed at the other person." The authors speculated that glare might be related to inhibited anger expression, to low levels of anger, or to the trait of hostility. In a different study, Ekman *et al.* (1990) investigate the emotion of happiness or joy. The authors coded the occurrence of the "Duchenne smile" in subjects watching a movie. The *Duchenne smile* was defined as involving both the orbicularis oculi and zygomaticus muscles and was thought to reflect genuine happiness (as opposed to "other" smiles). As expected, the Duchenne smile was associated with self-reports of enjoyment. It was also associated with increased asymmetry of the EEG over the two hemispheres. Besides facial expression, voice and speech patterns can be used as indices of emotions. For a review of this possibility, see Scherer (1987) and Bouhuys, Schutte, Beersma, and Nieboer (1990).

Behavioral observation systems have frequently been applied in the measurement of child behaviors. Almost any structured setting can be used for behavioral observations. For example, an observational system for hyperactive behavior during baseball games has been reported by Pelham, McBurnett, Harper, Milich, Murphy, Clinton, & Thiele (1990) and found to be sensitive to the effect of Ritalin. For the classroom setting, behavioral codes have been developed to observe children with attention deficit disorder and conduct disorder. The Hyperactive Behavior Checklist (Jacob, O'Leary, & Rosenblad, 1978) has six categories of behavior: solicitation of teacher attention, aggression, refusal to obey teacher commands, change of position (body position or locomotion), and "weird sounds" (e.g., making "Tarzan noises"). These behaviors are observed on a 10-sec observe, 5-sec record basis. In a formal classroom setting, the correlation between the hyperactive behavior score with the Conners Teacher Rating scale for hyperactive behavior was .78. Recently, Atkins *et al.* (1988) developed a comprehensive behavioral code for attention deficit and conduct disorders: the Classroom Observations of Conduct and Attention Deficit Disorder (COCADD). This behavioral code is based on DSM-III and DSM-III-R diagnostic criteria. The observational code is suitable for evaluation of behavioral performance in both classroom and playground settings. The observational system includes 32 specific codes, grouped under the 5 general headings of position, physical and social orientation, vocal activities, nonvocal activities, and play activities. Examples of individual categories are attending, listening, rule-breaking, proximity to adults, stealing/cheating, talking to others when not attending, verbal intrusion, and the like. The observers need specific training in which they are asked to memorize the item definitions, practice rating videotape recordings, and practice in the actual classroom or playground setting. Monitoring for reliability of behavioral observations can be performed through simultaneous observations by two different observers. Measures to calculate reliability can be found in Suen and Ary (1989) and House, House, and Campbell (1981).

Observational systems have also been developed for adult inpatient populations. The "Cadillac" of such observational systems is the one employed by Paul and Lentz (1977) in their assessment of the effect of milieu therapy versus token economy programs on chronic schizophrenics. The observational system used in this study provided the initial inspiration for the COCADD described above (Pelham, personal communication, December 7, 1990). Specific details of this observational system have been published by Paul (1986, 1987a,b).

Measures of Behavioral Product

As mentioned earlier, measures of behavioral product concern the lasting traces of behavior. Webb, Campbell, Schwartz, Sechrest, and Grove (1981) provided a comprehensive review of such measures. One problem with the observer-based measures described in the previous section is that of reactive measurement effects that are due to the presence of observers (Kazdin, 1979; Paul, Mariotto, & Redfield, 1986). For example, the observer's presence may inhibit occurrence of behaviors considered culturally undignified or sanctioned. Product measures are particularly likely to avoid observer effects if the actor is unaware that his behavior will be monitored. Besides being unobtrusive, behavioral product measures are highly cost-effective and can be extended over long time periods. For example, in a study by Miller (1987) to be described below, 75 patients could be observed over a time period of 278 days. In hyperactive children undergoing medication trials with stimulant medication, report cards were sensitive indicators of medication effects (Pelham & Milich, 1991).

One category of product measures involves *physical traces of behavior*. For example, the wear and tear of floor tiles in front of an exhibit can be used as an index of the exhibit's popularity. The number of empty beer cans or bottles of alcoholic beverages found in refuse containers can be used as an index of alcohol consumption in a household. In a study in which behavioral observations were developed to quantify hyperactive behavior in children, Atkins *et al.* (1988) used observations of behavioral products to quantify hyperactive behavior. One such measure simply involved academic achievement, such as grades. Another measure, developed to assess the DSM-III symptom "difficulty organizing work," was called "desk observations." Based on interviews with all the teachers in a school, the set of measures involved systematic quantification of the organizational status of the child's school desk. When the children were away from their classroom, observers would rate the child's desk for "neatness" and "preparedness," the latter referring to the presence or absence of required books and supplies.

An area in which product measures are frequently used is in the study of *patient compliance with prescribed medication regimens* (Dunbar, Dunning, & Dwyer,

1989). Frequency of *pharmacy refills* can be used as an unobtrusive measure of medication adherence over an extended time period. This measure, however, requires the patient to use only one specified pharmacy. *Pill counts* represent an alternative and potentially more exact measure of medication intake. To obtain pill counts, the investigator or pharmacist specifies the number of pills in the patient's bottle when dispensed and counts the number of remaining pills when the bottle is returned at the next appointment. The difference in dispensed and returned amounts represents the number of pills presumably taken by the patient. Of course, this measure assumes that the patient actually ingests the medication; if the patients are aware of being monitored, however, they might not return all of the unused medication. Pill counts provide average measures of compliance over an extended time period, but they cannot be used to study the *timing* of medication taking. Recently, *electronic monitors* have become available. The investigators dispense the medication in bottles equipped with a lid with a built-in computer chip and electronic circuitry designed to record the time points in which the lid has been opened or closed. A similar technique has also been described for eye-drop dispensers (Kass, Meltzer, & Gordon, 1984). Cramer, Mattson, Prevey, Scheier, and Ouellette (1989) used a monitor to determine compliance with prescribed medication in a small sample of patients with epilepsy. They found an overall adherence rate of 76%; adherence decreased as the dosage increased from one pill per day to four pills per day. They also showed that, compared to the monitor, pill counts overestimated adherence in patients whose compliance was low. Even this sophisticated method may be reactive to the patient's knowledge that compliance is being monitored. For example, Kruse and Weber (1990) reported a compliance rate in informed patients of 95%, whereas the compliance rate in patients who were unaware of being monitored was 77%.

Adherence measures have also been developed for behavioral interventions. To study adherence for home practice of relaxation exercises, Taylor, Agras, Schneider, and Allen (1983) equipped a tape recorder with an electronic device that would record every time a particular tape was played. A less "high-tech" variant of this method was used by Jacob, Beidel, and Shapiro (1984) to measure adherence to relaxation practice. Subjects were given several different relaxation tapes with identical content except for a final "relaxation word of the day" (e.g., "quiet," "serene," "calm"). The subjects were required to record the relaxation word on a self-monitoring sheet. Adherence could be determined based on the number of times the relaxation word was identified correctly.

Unobtrusive measures using computer technology can be employed in a study of behaviors more complex than compliance with treatment regimens. Miller (1987) developed a measure of "anhedonia" by recording patients' spontaneous sessions playing with computer games. The computer was placed in the inpatient unit. Patients participating in the study provided informed consent and were given a code name. At the beginning of a computer session, the computer prompted the subjects to enter their personal code names, their mood states (sad vs. happy), and their expectancies for success (poor vs. good). They could then use one of six games and select from several levels of difficulty. A total of 75 patients played a total of 7,744 games over the 278 days of the study. As expected, the rate of game playing was the greatest in the patients who did not have depression or schizophrenia. However, delusional depressives and secondary depressives also were active players. Schizophrenics and unipolar depressives were the least active. Delusional and secondary depressives tended to choose lower levels of difficulty than did bipolars, schizophrenics, or non-depressives. Thus, this preliminary study already provided rich and thought-provoking data. There was one problem with this assessment technique. Patients tended to play less as the number of hospital days increased. Thus, further development, perhaps by rotating the availability of specific games, would be needed before this procedure could be used as an outcome measure that is independent of length of stay.

The recording of *archival data* is another behavioral product measure. For example, frequency of physician visits, determined from clinic records, can be a measure of illness behavior (Mechanic & Volkart, 1960, 1961, cited in Jacob & Turner, 1984). Another measure of illness behavior of this kind is reflected by the amount of dollars spent on health care for specific individuals. This measure was used to assess the effect of a management approach for somatization disorder (Smith, Monson, & Ray, 1986). Even high school yearbooks can be used as archival measures. In one study, the premorbid personality of schizophrenics was assessed with high school yearbooks. It was found that future schizophrenics had significantly fewer voluntary social activities (Barthell & Holmes, 1968).

A study on the California drought by W. S. Agras, Jacob, and Ledebeck (1980) will serve as an example of research relying exclusively on archival data. The purpose of the study was to investigate the degree to which *stimulus control* (media coverage and appeals) and *outcome control* (fines for excessive water use) helped water conservation during the period of the drought. The outcome measure, water consumption, was obtained from the records of local water companies. Similarly, data on fines for excessive use were obtained from the water companies. Media coverage was measured by the number of issues per month of the *Palo Alto Times* with at least one reference to the drought. This measure had a high correlation with another measure: length in column inches of articles mentioning the drought. Articles specifically appealing for conservation and articles indicating that the "drought is over" were recorded separately. Records of rainfall (documenting the presence of a drought) were also obtained from public sources. The results showed that water consumption decreased even *before* fines had been set up, presumably as a result of stimulus control (media coverage and appeals).

From the examples above, measures of behavioral product, by virtue of their unobtrusiveness, can be powerful observational tools. Further evidence for the potential of these methods is the fact that they can be misused. Some examples mentioned may have raised ethical concerns in the reader. The reader may wonder whether it is an ethical breach, for instance, to count the number of beer cans in a family's garbage. Webb *et al.* (1981) devoted an entire book chapter to such ethical concerns. As a rule, the researcher should attempt to perform measurements in such a way that identification of specific subjects is minimized. This proviso is particularly important for behaviors considered culturally "undignified."

Observations in Standardized Settings, Including Behavioral Tasks

The behavioral observations outlined above assess subjects in their natural environment. However, if the task is to observe behaviors that are of low frequency, behavioral observations in the natural environment are ineffective. If a patient has a fear of snakes, for example, it would be a rare event to observe him or her facing a snake during normal daily activities. For this reason, analogue situations have been designed in which subjects are required to engage in the behavior of interest. Two such situations, to be discussed later, are the role-play test for social skills assessment and the behavioral avoidance test to assess phobic avoidance behavior.

Another problem with observations in the natural environment is that much "noise" is introduced by uncontrolled changes in the environment. By standardizing the environment, the phenomena of interest can be isolated. In the study by Ekman *et al.* (1990) of the Duchenne smile referred to earlier, the situation was standardized by having the subjects watch movies. The psychiatric or behavioral interview represents another standard situation in which behavioral observations are possible. For example, recording of *speech characteristics* during the Type A interview have been used to assess Type A behavior (Chesney *et al.*, 1990). Type A's differed from Type B's with respect to speaking rate, "hard voice," syllabic emphasis, loudness, and a number of other variables related to hostility and competitiveness.

Expressed Emotion (EE) is another measure based on behavioral observations of psychiatric interviews, in this case with the relatives of psychiatric patients (Leff & Vaughn, 1985). The interviews are observed for "critical comments," "hostility," "emotional overinvolvement," "warmth," and "positive remarks." An overall measure of expressed emotion is derived as a composite of critical comments, hostility, and overinvolvement. High EE has been found to predict relapse in schizophrenia and depression (Hooley & Teasdale, 1989; Leff & Vaughn, 1985). The study by Hooley and Teasdale (1989), however, also illustrates the fact that complex observational procedures are not automatically the most efficient types of assessments. The depressed patient's response to the simple question, "How critical is your spouse of you?" was better than the EE interview scores in predicting relapse of depression!

For socially sanctioned low-frequency behaviors, such as stealing or firesetting, a situation may have to be set up to increase the rate of these behaviors. Such an "entrapment" method was used by Switzer, Deal, and Bailey (1977) in order to measure stealing behavior in elementary school children. A specified number of objects, such as bright-colored marking pens, nickels, and erasers, were placed in the classroom at the beginning of each school day. The number of objects missing at the end of the day represented their measure of *stealing*.

Behavioral Role-Play Test

The *behavioral role-play test* refers to an assessment procedure in which an individual's social skills are evaluated by presenting a series of problematic interpersonal situations. Behavioral samples are collected when the individual responds as if he or she were in the natural environment. In its most basic format, a behavioral role-play test is comprised of: (1) a descriptive narrative of the problematic situation (script); (2) prompt lines; (3) actors (the research participant and a significant other, peer, or staff confederate); and (4) an audio- or videotaping device to record the interaction.

The particular social skills evaluated vary according to the coding system employed by the researcher. Typically, observations are made of conversational content, paralinguistics, nonverbal behavior, and social perception. Thus, speech content may be rated for global measures of appropriateness, effectiveness, and "rewardingness" (i.e., ability to reinforce others in the natural environment). Speech also may be rated for measures of response latency, number of pauses, and duration. Paralinguistic elements, including volume, tone, and pacing, may be rated. Similarly, facial expression, gaze, gesture frequency, posture, and proximal distance may be rated as nonverbal elements (Trower, Bryant, & Argyle, 1978). Finally, under the rubric of social perception, assessment can be made of an individual's ability to express interest without conveying a sense of "threat," to decode verbal and nonverbal cues of others, and to understand cultural mores and modify behavior accordingly (Morrison & Bellack, 1981).

Social skills assessments have been used for a variety of research questions. For example, Liberman, DeRisi, and Mueser (1989) have used social skills assessments as an outcome measure for behaviorally oriented interventions with schizophrenia. Morrison, Bellack, and Manuck (1985) used a role-play test to explore psychosomatic hypotheses concerning aggression in hypertensives. They found deficits in both the "unassertive" and "overassertive" directions. Other assessment applications have been conducted in the areas of affective disorder, substance abuse, and impulse control problems (Bellack, Morrison, Mueser, & Wade, 1989; Eriksen, Bjornstad, & Gotestam, 1986; Morrison & Bellack, 1987; Morrison, Van Hasselt, & Bellack, 1987).

Investigators who are considering using a role-play test to pursue a research question can construct such tests from scratch or adopt a standardized test published in the literature. For adult populations, these include the Behavioral Assertiveness Test-Revised (BAT-R), which presents 10 interpersonal situations evaluating positive and negative assertion within a multiple-response format (Eisler, Hersen, Miller, & Blanchard, 1975). The Simulated Social Interaction Test (SSIT) (Curran, 1984) also may be employed for evaluating global measures of social skills in a brief interaction format. The SSIT is comprised of eight scenarios assessing social competence for positive assertion (e.g., expressing appreciation and warmth, receiving compliments, dating initiation) and negative assertion (e.g., responding to confrontation, disapproval, and conflict with family members). Several specialized formats have also been developed. For example, the Dating Situation Test (DST) (Twentyman, Boland, & McFall, 1981) measures heterosocial competence. Subsequent review of the recorded role-play assessment with the subject may be considered for possible inclusion into the treatment strategy (Liberman et al., 1989). Thus, reviewing the performance with the patient may be a useful therapeutic adjunct to promote positive behavioral change. Additional discussion of critical conceptual and psychometric issues may be found in the following reviews: Arkowitz, 1981; Becker and Heimberg (1988); Curran, Farrell, and Grunberger (1984); Eisler and Frederiksen (1980); Hollin and Trower (1986), Matson and Ollendick (1988), and Schlundt and McFall (1985).

Behavioral Avoidance Tests

A behavioral avoidance test (BAT) is an assessment procedure in which an individual is instructed to approach a feared or avoided object or situation. In the simplest format, the BAT is used in the assessment of simple phobia, such as fear of snakes, needles, or insects. (Emmelkamp & Felton, 1985; Lang & Lazovik, 1963; Ost & Hugdahl, 1985). In this test, subjects are simply asked to approach the feared object. Measurements include the minimum distance from the feared object or total duration of contact. This test may be elaborated with psychophysiological measures.

Depending on the demands placed on the patient, the BAT exists in two different forms: the modal format and the heroic format. In the *modal* format, "typical" performance is assessed by instructing subjects to approach only until they experience anxiety or other discomfort. In the *heroic* format, "maximal" performance is assessed by instructing participants to maximize the duration of exposure or proximity to the feared stimulus (Nietzel, Bernstein, & Russell, 1988).

The BAT as applied to *agoraphobics* can also be a simple test; the patient can be instructed to walk outside along a specified path, and the distance walked can be measured (S. Agras, Leitenberg, & Barlow, 1968). However, current studies employ more elaborate strategies (Marchione, Michelson, Greenwald, & Dancu, 1987; Mavissakalian & Michelson, 1982; Michelson, 1987; Michelson et al., 1985, 1990). Subjects are asked to enter specific situations along a standardized course. Often, they wear an ambulatory physiological monitor measuring heart rate. At specific stations in the course, subjects are asked to provide a self-report fear rating, such as subjective units of distress (SUDS). In the test's most elaborate form, subjects also may carry a portable tape recorder in which they verbalize their ongoing thoughts; content analysis is applied to the tapes to codify different classes of "cognitions" (R. Schwartz & Michelson, 1987).

Design considerations of behavioral avoidance tests have been reviewed extensively elsewhere (Barlow, 1988; Jacob & Lilienfeld, 1991; Kern, 1984; Nietzel *et al.*, 1988; Rowland & Canavan, 1983).

SUMMARY

In this chapter, we have provided a catalog of physiological and behavioral assessment methods, all having the common characteristic that they do not rely on subject self-report. Obviously, our selection of examples reflects our own experiences, preferences, and interests. As we mentioned in the introduction, these methods should not be adopted without proper consideration of specific methodological issues and sources of error. References have been provided for further study in this regard. The novice investigator is urged to pursue deeper study of a method before embarking on a project in which it is used.

Our approach to discussing measurements has been to focus on one assessment variable at a time. By providing examples of hypothetical processes for which the measured variable might be an index, we may have created the impression that a one-to-one relationship frequently exists between a variable and an underlying construct. As pointed out by Cacioppo and Tassinary (1990), however, a change in a measured variable can be a reflection of many different underlying processes. For example, heart rate increases in response to imagining a fear-producing scene are not only related to the fearfulness of the scene, but are also affected by the cognitive effort involved in the act of imagining (e.g., Lang *et al.*, 1983). The elevated heart rates in the surgeons in the operation room mentioned earlier may not only have been due to "stress," but also to physical activity and exposure to anesthetic agents. The controversy over whether it is possible to detect lies with psychophysiological measures (see Furedy, 1986) is another index of the problem of multiple determinants of change in a variable.

One way of narrowing down the number of plausible alternative hypotheses is to obtain measures in multiple channels, all of which tap into the underlying construct. Thus, more precise information of underlying constructs can be obtained by *combining* different measures. This is not to say that multiple measures are *always* preferred. In fact, Kramer, Pruyn, Gibbons, Greenhouse, Grochoncinski, Vaternaux, and Kupfer (1987) pointed out that multiple measures can present the researcher with too many choices and require complicated statistical analyses. Furthermore, measures of multiple variables might tempt investigators after the fact to "pick" those measures that confirm their hypotheses. Nevertheless, the measures described in this chapter can be combined with the self-report measures in the previous chapter, as well as the biochemical measures of the next chapter. For example, anxiety is typically measured along the behavioral, self-report, and physiological dimensions.

For some research questions it may even be necessary to gather data from multiple individuals. In a study for which we have much admiration, Levenson and Gottman (1983) obtained measures from multiple physiological, behavioral, and self-report channels simultaneously from two different individuals (in this case married couples). The investigators tested their hypothesis that in high-conflict situations, distressed couples would have greater "physiological link-age." For example, the heart rates of the members of these dyads might increase simultaneously—perhaps because they both "got angry" at the same time. The investigators measured the following variables in both spouses concomitantly: interbeat intervals, pulse transit time, skin conductance, and general somatic activity (the latter via an electromechanical transducer attached to a platform under each subject's chair). In addition, the interactions were recorded on videotape. Subjects also rated their affects during the interaction. The investigators indeed found that marital dissatisfaction was positively related to physiological linkage. Furthermore, dissatisfied wives had increased tendencies to reciprocate their husbands' negative affect, whereas dissatisfied husbands had less tendencies to reciprocate their wives' positive affects.

Through the example above and the others described in this chapter, we hope that our readers now have a preliminary appreciation of the equipment available in the researcher's "toolbox" of assessment methods. We also hope that you have developed an appreciation for the considerable care, creativity, and ingenuity involved in developing new assessment methods. By keeping up with the literature, you can now begin the process of upgrading and adding to your collection of assessment tools.

Acknowledgments.   Rolf G. Jacob was supported in part by grant HL-40962 from the National Heart, Lung, and Blood Institute and grant MH-40757 from the National Institute for Mental Health. Duncan B. Clark was supported in part by grant AA06267 from the National Institute on Alcohol Abuse and Alcoholism. The authors would like to thank Sue Russell Gelburd for her editorial advice and Richard Jennings, William Pelham, Lisa Tamres, and Jacqueline Dunbar-Jacob for their feedback on previous versions of this manuscript.

REFERENCES

Abel, G., Blanchard, E. B., Barlow, D. H., & Mavissakalian, M. (1975). Identifying specific erotic cues in sexual deviations by audiotaped descriptions. *Journal of Applied Behavior Analysis, 8,* 247–260.

Abramczyk, R. R., Jordan, D. E., & Hegel, M. (1983). "Reverse" Stroop effect in the performance of schizophrenics. *Perceptual and Motor Skills, 56,* 99–106.

Agras, S., Leitenberg, H., & Barlow, D. H. (1968). Social reinforcement in the modification of agoraphobia. *Archives of General Psychiatry, 19,* 423–427.

Agras, W. S., Jacob, R. G., & Ledebeck, M. (1980). The California drought: A quasi-experimental study of social policy. *Journal of Applied Behavior Analysis, 13,* 561–570.

Allen, M. T., & Crowell, M. D. (1989). Patterns of autonomic response during laboratory stressors. *Psychophysiology, 26,* 603–614.

American Psychiatric Association. (1987). *Diagnostic and statistical manual of mental disorders* (3rd ed., rev.). Washington, DC: Author.

Anastasiades, P., & Johnston, D. W. (1990). A simple activity measure for use with ambulatory subjects. *Psychophysiology, 27,* 87–93.

Anderson, K. J. (1990). Arousal and the inverted U relationship: A critique of Neiss's "reconceptualizing arousal." *Psychological Bulletin, 107,* 96–100.

Andreassi, J. L. (1989). *Psychophysiology: Human behavior and physiological response*. Hillsdale, NJ: Lawrence Erlbaum.

Arkowitz, H. (1981). Assessment of social skills. In A. S. Bellack & M. Hersen (Eds.), *Behavioral assessment: A practical handbook* (2nd ed., pp. 296–327). New York: Pergamon Press.

Asperinsky, E., Lynch, J. A., Mack, M. E., Tzankoff, S. P., & Hurn, E. (1985). Comparison of eye motion in wakefulness and REM sleep. *Psychophysiology, 22*, 1–10.

Astrand, P. O., & Rodahl, L. (1986). *Textbook of work physiology* (3rd ed.). New York: McGraw-Hill.

Atkins, M. S., Pelham, W. E., & Licht, M. H. (1988). The development and validation of objective classroom measures for conduct and attention deficit disorders. In R. J. Prinz, *Advances in behavioral assessment of children and families, Vol. 4* (pp. 3–31). Greenwich, CT: JAI Press.

Ax, A. F. (1953). The physiological differentiation between fear and anger in humans. *Psychosomatic Medicine, 15*, 433–442.

Bakeman, R., & Gottman, J. M. (1986). *Observing interaction: An introduction to sequential analysis*. New York: Cambridge University Press.

Barlow, D. H. (1988). *Anxiety and its disorders*. New York: Guilford Press.

Barry, R. J. (1990). Scoring criteria for response latency and habituation in electrodermal research: A study in the context of the orienting response. *Psychophysiology, 27*, 94–100.

Barthell, C. N., & Holmes, D. S. (1968). High school yearbooks: A non-reactive measure of social isolation in graduates who later become schizophrenic. *Journal of Abnormal Psychology, 73*, 313–316.

Basmajian, J. V. (1978). *Muscles alive—Their functions revealed by electromyography*. Baltimore: Williams & Wilkins.

Becker, R. E., & Heimberg, R. G. (1988). Assessment of social skills. In A. S. Bellack & M. Hersen (Eds.). *Behavioral assessment: A practical handbook* (3rd ed., pp. 365–395). New York: Pergamon Press.

Beidel, D. C., Turner, S. M., Jacob, R. G., & Cooley, M. R. (1989). Assessment of social phobia: Reliability of an impromptu speech task. *Journal of Anxiety Disorders, 3*, 149–158.

Bellack, A. S., Morrison, R. L., Mueser, K. T., & Wade, J. (1989). Social competence in schizoaffective disorder, bipolar disorder, and negative and non-negative schizophrenia. *Schizophrenia Research, 2*, 391–401.

Berger, R. D., Akselrod, S., Gordon, D., & Cohen, R. J. (1986). An efficient algorithm for spectral analysis of heart rate variability. *IEEE Transactions of Biomedical Engineering, BME-33*, 901–904.

Berlin, C. I., & McNeil, M. R. (1976). Dichotic listening. In *Contemporary issues in experimental phonetics* (pp. 327–357). New York: Academic Press.

Blumenthal, T. D., & Levey, B. J. (1989). Prepulse rise time and startle reflex modification: Different effects for discrete and continuous prepulses. *Psychophysiology, 26*(2), 158–165.

Bouhuys, A. L., Schutte, H. K., Beersma, D. G. M., and Nieboer, G. L. (1990). Relationship between depressed mood and vocal parameters before, during and after sleep deprivation: A circadian rhythm study. *Journal of Affective Disorders, 19*, 249–258.

Boukadoum, A. M., & Kontas, P. Y. (1986). EOG-based recording and automated detection of sleep rapid eye movements: A critical review. *Psychophysiology, 22*, 598–611.

Bradley, M. M., Cuthbert, B. N., & Lang, P. J. (1990). Startle reflex modification: Emotion or attention? *Psychophysiology, 27*, 513–522.

Bradshaw, J. L., & Burden, V. (1986). Dichotic and dichaptic techniques. *Neuropsychologia, 24*, 79–90.

Bruder, G. E. (1983). Cerebral laterality and psychopathology: A review of dichotic listening studies. *Schizophrenia Bulletin, 9*, 134–151.

Buss, D. M., Block, J. H., & Block, J. (1980). Preschool activity level: Personality correlates and developmental implications. *Child Development, 51*, 401–408.

Cacioppo, J. T., & Tassinary, L. G. (1990). Inferring psychological significance from physiological signals. *American Psychologist, 45*, 16–28.

Carrol, D., Turner, R. R., & Hellawell, J. C. (1986). Heart rate and oxygen consumption during active psychological challenge: The effects of level of difficulty. *Psychophysiology, 23*, 174–181.

Charney, D. S., & Heninger, G. R. (1986). Abnormal regulation of noradrenergic function in panic disorders. *Archives of General Psychiatry, 43*, 1042–1054.

Chesney, M. A., Ekman, P., Friesen, W. V., Black, G. W., & Hecker, M. H. L. (1990). Type A behavior pattern: Facial behavior and speech components. *Psychosomatic Medicine, 53*, 307–319.

Chirico, A. M., & Stunkard, A. J. (1960). Physical activity and human obesity. *New England Journal of Medicine, 263*, 935–940.

Clark, D. B., Taylor, C. B., Hayward, C., King, R., Margraf, J., Ehlers, A., Roth, W. T., & Agras, W. S. (1990). Motor activity and tonic heart rate in panic disorder. *Psychiatry Research, 32*, 45–53.

Clark, D. B., Taylor, C. B., & Hayward, C. (1990). Naturalistic assessment of panic episodes. In J. Ballenger (Ed.), *The clinical aspects of panic disorder* (pp. 83–97). New York: Alan R. Liss.

Clark, D. C., & Agras, W. S. (1991). The assessment and treatment of performance anxiety in musicians. *American Journal of Psychiatry, 148*, 598–605.

Clementz, B. A., & Sweeney, J. A. (1990). Is eye movement dysfunction a biological marker for schizophrenia?—A methodological review. *Psychological Bulletin, 108*, 77–92.

Cohen, A. S., Barlow, D. H., & Blanchard, E. B. (1985). Psychophysiology of relaxation-associated panic attacks. *Journal of Abnormal Psychology, 94*, 96–101.

Coles, G. H., Donchin, E., & Porges, S. W. (1986). *Psychophysiology: Systems, processes, and applications.* New York: Guilford Press.

Corby, J. C., Roth, W. T., Zarcone, W. P., Jr., & Kopell, B. S. (1977). Psychophysiological correlates of the practice of tantric yoga meditation. *Archives of General Psychiatry, 35*, 571–577.

Cramer, J. A., Mattson, R. H., Prevey, M. L., Scheier, R. D., & Ouellette, V. L. (1989). How often is medication taken as prescribed? *Journal of the American Medical Association, 261*, 3273–3277.

Curran, J. P. (1984). A procedure for the assessment of social skills: The simulated social interaction test. In J. P. Curran & P. M. Monti (Eds.), *Radical approaches to social skills training* (pp. 16–47). London: Croon Helm.

Curran, J. P., Farrell, A. D., & Grunberger, A. J. (1984). Social skills: A critique and a rapprochement. In P. Trower (Ed.), *Radical approaches to social skills training* (pp. 16–47). London: Croon Helm.

Dalgleish, T., & Watts, F. N. (1990). Biases of attention and memory in disorders of anxiety and depression. *Clinical Psychology Review, 10*, 589–604.

Davidson, R. J., Ekman, P., Saron, C. D., Senulis, J. A., & Friesen, W. V. (1990). Approach-withdrawal and cerebral asymmetry: Emotional expression and brain physiology: I. *Journal of Personality and Social Psychology, 58*(2), 330–341.

Dimberg, U. (1990). Facial electromyography and emotional reactions. *Psychophysiology, 27*, 481–494.

Donchin, E., Karis, D., Bashore, T. R., Coles, M. G. H., & Gratton, G. (1986). Cognitive psychophysiology and human information processing. In M. G. H. Coles, E. Donchin, & S. W. Porges (Eds.), *Psychophysiology: Systems, processes, and applications* (pp. 244–267). New York: Guilford Press.

Dunbar, J., Dunning, E. J., & Dwyer, K. (1989). Compliance measurement with arthritis regimen. *Arthritis Care and Research, 2*(3), S8–S16.

Dunner, D. (1985). Anxiety and panic: Relationship to depression and cardiac disorders. *Psychosomatics, 26*, 18–22.

Dyer, F. N. (1973). The Stroop phenomenon and its use in the study of perceptual, cognitive, and response processes. *Memory and Cognition, 1*, 106–120.

Eisler, R. M., & Frederiksen, L. W. (1980). *Perfecting social skills: A guide to interpersonal behavioral development.* New York: Plenum Press.

Eisler, R. M., Hersen, M., Miller, P. M., & Blanchard, E. B. (1975). Situational determinants of assertive behaviors. *Journal of Consulting and Clinical Psychology, 43*, 330–340.

Ekman, P., & Friesen, W. V. (1978). *Facial Action Coding System: A technique for the measurement of facial movement.* Palo Alto: Consulting Psychologists Press. (Quoted by Chesney, 1990).

Ekman, P., Levenson, R. W., & Friesen, W. V. (1983). Autonomic nervous system activity distinguishes among emotions. *Science, 221*, 1208–1210.

Ekman, P., Davidson, R. J., & Friesen, W. V. (1990). The Duchenne smile: Emotional expression and brain physiology: II. *Journal of Personality and Social Psychology, 38*(2), 343–353.

Emmelkamp, P. M. G., & Felton, M. (1985). The process of exposure in vivo: Cognitive and physiological changes during treatment of acrophobia. *Behaviour Research and Therapy, 23*, 219–224.

Eriksen, L., Bjornstad, S., & Gotestam, K. (1986). Social skills training for alcoholism: One year treatment outcome for groups and individuals. *Addictive Behaviors, 11,* 309–329.

Falk, J. R., Halmi, K. A., & Tryon, W. W. (1985). Activity measures in anorexia nervosa. *Archives of General Psychiatry, 42,* 811–814.

Foster, G. E., Evans, D. F., & Hardcastle, J. D. (1978). Heart rates of surgeons during operations and other clinical activities and their modification by oxprenol. *Lancet, No. 8078,* 1323–1325.

Fowles, D. C. (1982). Heart rate as an index of anxiety: Failure of a hypothesis. In J. T. Cacioppo & R. E. Petty (Eds.), *Perspectives in cardiovascular psychophysiology.* New York: Guilford Press.

Fowles, D. C. (1986). The eccrine system and electrodermal activity. In G. H. Coles, E. Donchin, & S. W. Porges (Eds.), *Psychophysiology: Systems, processes, and applications* (pp. 51–87). New York: Guilford Press.

Fowles, D. C., Christie, M. J., Edelberg, R., Grings, W. W., Lykken, D. T., & Venables, P. H. (1981). Committee report: Publication recommendations for electrodermal measurements. *Psychophysiology, 18,* 232–239.

Freedman, R. B., Ianni, P., Ettedgui, E., & Puthezhath, N. (1985). Ambulatory monitoring of panic disorder. *Archives of General psychiatry, 42,* 244–248.

Fridlund, A. J., & Cacioppo, J.T. (1986). Guidelines for human electromyographic research. *Psychophysiology, 23,* 567–589.

Fried, L. A., Kenardy, J. A., Ironson, G. H., & Taylor, C. B. (1989). Are there spontaneous panic attacks? Paper presented at the meeting of the American Psychological Association. New Orleans, LA.

Furedy, J. J. (1986). Lie detection as psychophysiological differentiation: Some fine lines. In G. H. Coles, E. Donchin, & S. W. Porges (Eds.), *Psychophysiology: Systems, processes, and applications* (pp. 683–701). New York: Guilford Press.

Gaffney, F. A., Fenton, B. J., Lane, L. D., & Lake, R. (1988). Hemodynamic, ventilatory, and biochemical responses of panic patients and normal controls with sodium lactate infusion and spontaneous panic attacks. *Archives of General Psychiatry, 45,* 53–60.

Geer, J. H., O'Donohue, W. T., & Schorman, R. H. (1986). Sexuality. In G. H. Coles, E. Donchin, & S. W. Porges (Eds.), *Psychophysiology: Systems, processes, and applications* (pp. 407–430). New York: Guilford Press.

George, D. T., Nutt, D. J., Walker, W. V., Porges, S. W., Adinoff, B., & Linnoila, M. (1989). Lactate and hyperventilation substantially attenuate vagal tone in normal volunteers: A possible mechanism of panic provocation? *Archives of General Psychiatry, 46,* 153–156.

Golden, C. (1978). *The Stroop Color and Word Test: A manual for clinical and experimental uses.* Chicago: Stoelting.

Gorman, J. M., Fyer, M. R., Goetz, R., Askanazi, J., Liebowitz, M. R., Fyer, A. J., Kinney, J., & Klein, D. F. (1988). Ventilatory physiology of patients with panic disorder. *Archives of General Psychiatry, 45,* 31–39.

Gotlib, I. H., & McCann, C. D. (1984). Construct accessibility and depression: An examination of cognitive and affective factors. *Journal of Personality and Social Psychology, 47,* 427–439.

Grady, C. L., Grimes, A. M., Patronas, N., Sunderland, T., Foster, N. L., & Rapoport, S. I. (1989). Divided attention, as measured by dichotic speech performance, in dementia of the Alzheimer type. *Archives of Neurology, 46,* 317–320.

Graves, R., & Bradley, R. (1987). Millisecond interval timer and auditory reaction time programs for the IBM PC. *Behavior Research Methods and Instrumentation, 19,* 30–35.

Hassett, J., & Danforth, D. (1982). An introduction to the cardiovascular system. In J. T. Cacioppo & R. E. Petty (Eds.). *Perspectives in cardiovascular psychophysiology* (pp. 4–18). New York: Guilford Press.

Hibbert, G., & Pilsbury, D. (1988). Hyperventilation in panic attacks: Ambulant monitoring of transcutaneous carbon dioxide. *British Journal of Psychiatry, 153,* 76–80.

Hollin, C. R., & Trower, P. (1986). Social skills training: Critique and future development. In C. R. Hollin & P. Trower (Eds.), *Handbook of social skills training: clinical applications and new directions* (pp. 237–257). Oxford: Pergamon Press.

Holzman, P. S., Levy, D.L., & Proctor, L. R. (1976). Smooth pursuit eye movements, attention and schizophrenia. *Archives of General Psychiatry, 33,* 1415–1420.

Hooley, J. M., & Teasdale, J. D. (1989). Predictors of relapse in unipolar depressives: expressed emotion, marital distress, and perceived criticism. *Journal of Abnormal Psychology, 98*, 229–235.

House, A. E., House, B. J., & Campbell, M. B. (1981). Measure of interobserver agreement: Calculation formulas and distribution effects. *Journal of Behavioral Assessment, 3*, 37–57.

Jacob, R. G. (1988). Panic disorder and the vestibular system. *Psychiatric Clinics of North America, 11*, 361–374.

Jacob, R. G., & Rapport, M. (1984). Panic disorder. In S. M. Turner (Ed.), *Behavioral treatment of anxiety disorders* (pp. 187–237). New York: Plenum Press.

Jacob, R. G., & Turner, S. M., (1984). Somatoform disorders. In S. M. Turner & M. Hersen (Eds.), *Adult Psychopathology* (pp. 304–328). New York: Wiley.

Jacob, R. G., O'Leary, K. D., & Rosenblad, C. (1978). Formal and informal classroom settings: Effects on hyperactivity. *Journal of Abnormal Child Psychology, 6*, 47–59.

Jacob, R. G., Beidel, D. C., & Shapiro, A. P. (1984). The relaxation word of the day: A simple technique to measure adherence to relaxation. *Journal of Behavioral Assessment, 6*, 159–165.

Jacob, R. G., Moller, M. B., Turner, S. M., & Wall, I. C. (1985). Otoneurological examination of panic disorder and agoraphobia with panic attacks: A pilot study. *American Journal of Psychiatry, 142*, 715–720.

Jacob, R. G., Shapiro, A. P., Reeves, R. A., Johnsen, A. M., McDonald, R. H., & Coburn, P. C. (1986). Comparison of relaxation therapy for hypertension with placebo, diuretics or betablockers. *Archives of Internal Medicine, 146*, 2335–2350.

Jacob, R. G., Simons, A. D., Rohay, J., Manuck, S., & Waldstein, S. R. (1989). The circular mood scale: A new technique of measuring ambulatory mood. *Journal of Psychopathology and Behavioral Assessment, 11*, 697–716.

Jacob, R. G., Lilienfeld, S. O., Furman, J. M. R., & Turner, S. M. (1989). Space and motion phobia in panic disorder with vestibular dysfunction. *Journal of Anxiety Disorders, 3*, 117–130.

Jacob, R. G., & Lilienfeld, S. O. (1991). Panic disorder: Diagnosis, medical assessment, and psychological assessment. In J. R. Walker, G. R. Norton, & C. A. Ross (Eds.), *Panic disorder and agoraphobia: A comprehensive guide for the practitioner* (pp. 16–103). Pacific Grove, CA: Brooks/Cole.

Jacob, R. G., Chesney, M. A., Williams, D. M., Ding, Y., & Shapiro, A. P. (1991). Relaxation therapy for hypertension: Design effects and treatment effects. Annals of Behavioral Medicine, *13*, 5–17.

Jacob, R. G., Shapiro, A. P., O'Hara, P., Portser, S., Kruger, A., Gatsonis, C., & Ding, Y. (1992). Relaxation therapy for hypertension: Setting-specific effects. *Psychosomatic Medicine, 54*, 87–101.

Jennings, J. R. (1986). Bodily changes during attending. In G. H. Coles, E. Donchin, & S. W. Porges (Eds.), *Psychophysiology: Systems, processes, and applications* (pp. 268–289). New York: Guilford Press.

Jennings, J.R ., Tahmoush, A. J., & Redmond, D. P. (1980). Non-reactive measurement of peripheral vascular activity. In I. Martin & P. H. Venables (Eds.), *Techniques in Psychophysiology*. New York: Wiley.

Johnston, W. A., & Dark, V. J. (1986). Selective attention. *Annual Review of Psychology, 37*, 43–75.

Kass, M. A., Meltzer, D. W., & Gordon, M. (1984). A miniature monitor for eyedrop medication. *Archives of Ophthalmology, 102*, 1550–1554.

Kazdin, A. E. (1979). Unobtrusive measures in behavioral assessment. *Journal of Applied Behavior Analysis, 12*, 713–724.

Keele, S. W. (1986). Motor control. In L. Boff & J. P. Kaufman (Eds.), *Handbook of perception and human performance, Volume 2* (pp. 1–60). New York: Wiley.

Kenardy, J. A., Evans, L., & Oei, T. (1988). The importance of cognitions in panic attacks. *Behavior Therapy, 19*, 471–483.

Kenardy, J. A., Taylor, C. B., & Fried, L. A. (1989).Circadian cosine model predicts anxiety in panic. Paper presented at the meeting of the American Psychiatric Association, San Francisco, CA.

Kern, J. M. (1984). Relationship between obtrusive laboratory and unobtrusive naturalistic behavioral fear assessments: Treated and untreated subjects. *Behavioral Assessment, 6*, 45–60.

King, R., Bayon, E. P., Clark, D. B., & Taylor, C. B. (1988). Tonic arousal and activity: Relationships to personality and personality disorder traits in panic patients. *Psychiatry Research, 25*, 65–72.

Kitsch, W. (1982). *Memory and cognition*. Malabar, FL: R. E. Krieger.

Korff, J., & Geer, J. H. (1983). Relationship between subjective sexual arousal experience and genital responses. *Psychophysiology, 20,* 121–127.

Korner, A. F., Zeenah, C. H., Linden, J., Berkowitz, R. I., Kraemer, H. C., & Agras, W. S. (1985). The relation between neonatal and later activity and temperament. *Child Development, 56,* 38–42.

Kramer, H. C., Pruyn, J. P., Gibbons, R. D., Greenhouse, J. B., Grochoncinski, V. J., Vaternaux, C., &Kupfer, D. J. (1987). Methodology in psychiatric research. *Archives in General Psychiatry, 44*(12), 1100–1106.

Kruse, W., & Weber, E. (1990). Dynamics of drug regimen compliance—its assessment by microprocessor-based monitoring. *European Journal of Clinical Pharmacology, 38,* 561–565.

Kupfer, D. J., Weiss, B. L., Foster, G., Detre, T. P., Delgado, J., & McPartland, R. (1974). Psychomotor activity in affective states. *Archives of General Psychiatry, 30,* 765–768.

Kutcher, S. P., Blackwood, H.R ., St. Clair, D., Gaskell, D. F., & Muir, W. J. (1987). Auditory P300 in borderline personality disorder and schizophrenia. *Archives of General Psychiatry, 44,* 645–650.

Lane, D. J., Greenstadt, L., Shapiro, D., & Rubinstein, E. (1983). Pulse transit time and blood pressure: An intensive analysis. *Psychophysiology, 20,* 45–49.

Lang, P. J. (1968). Fear reduction and fear behavior: Problems in treating a construct. In J. M. Shlien (Ed.), *Research in psychotherapy (Vol. 3).* Washington, DC: American Psychological Association.

Lang, P. J., & Lazovik, A. D. (1963). Experimental desensitization of a phobia. *Journal of Abnormal and Social Psychology, 66,* 519–525.

Lang, P. J. Levin, D. N., Miller, G. A., & Kozak, M. J. (1983). Fear behavior, fear imagery, and the psychophysiology of emotion: The problem of affective response integration. *Journal of Abnormal Psychology, 92,* 276–306.

Lang, P. J., Bradley, M. M., & Cuthbert, B. N. (1990). Emotion, attention, and the startle reflex. *Psychological Review, 97*(3), 377–395.

Larsen, P. B.,Schneiderman, N., & DeCarlo-Pasin, R. (1986). Physiological bases of cardiovascular psychophysiology. In G. H. Coles, E. Donchin, & S. W. Porges (Eds.), *Psychophysiology: Systems, processes, and applications* (pp. 122–165). New York: Guilford Press.

Leff, J. P., & Vaughn, C. (Eds.). (1985). *Expressed emotion in families: Its significance of mental illness.* New York: Guilford Press.

Leroy, R. F., & Ebersole, J. S. (1983). An evaluation of ambulatory, cassette EEG monitoring. *Neurology, 33,* 1–7.

Levenson, R. W., & Gottman, J. M. (1983). Marital interaction: Physiological linkage and affective exchange. *Journal of Personality and Social Psychology, 45*(3), 587–597.

Levenson, R. W., Ekman, P., & Friesen, W. (1990). Voluntary facial action generates emotion-specific autonomic nervous system activity. *Psychophysiology, 27,* 363–384.

Ley, R. (1985). Agoraphobia, the panic attack and hyperventilation syndrome. *Behaviour Research and Therapy, 23,* 79–81.

Liberman, R. P., DeRisi, W. J., & Mueser, K. T. (1989). *Social skills training for psychiatric patients.* New York: Pergamon Press.

Maarse, F. J., Mulder, L. J. M., Sjouw, W. P. B., & Akkerman, A. E. (1988). *Computers in psychology: Methods, instrumentation, and psychodiagnostics.* Amsterdam: Swets and Zeitlinger.

Mahon, M. L., & Iacono, W. G. (1987). Another look at the relationship of electrodermal activity to electrode contact area. *Psychophysiology, 24,* 216–222.

Marchione, K. E., Michelson, L., Greenwald, M., & Dancu, C. (1987). Cognitive behavioral treatment of agoraphobia. *Behaviour Research and Therapy, 25,* 319–328.

Margraf, J., Ehlers, A., & Roth, W. T. (1986). Lactate infusions and panic attacks: A review and critique. *Psychosomatic Medicine, 48,* 23–51.

Marler, M., Jacob, R. G., Lehoczky, J. L., & Shapiro, A. P. (1988). The statistical analysis of treatment effects in 24-h ambulatory blood pressure recordings. *Statistics in Medicine, 7,* 697–716.

Martin, I., & Venables, P. H. (1980). *Techniques in Psychophysiology.* New York: Wiley.

Mathews, A., & MacLeod, D. (1985). Selective processing of threat cues in anxiety states. *Behaviour Research and Therapy, 23,* 563–569.

Mathews, A., & MacLeod, C. (1986). Discrimination of threat cues without awareness in anxiety states. *Behaviour Research and Therapy, 23,* 563–569.

Mathews, A., May, J., Mogg, K., & Eysenck, M. (1990). Attentional bias in anxiety: Selective search or defective filtering? *Journal of Abnormal Psychology, 99*, 166–173.

Matson, J. L., & Ollendick, T. H. (1988). *Enhancing children's social skills: Assessment and training.* New York: Pergamon Press.

Mavissakalian, M., & Michelson, L. (1982). Patterns of psychophysiological change in the treatment of agoraphobia. *Behaviour Research and Therapy, 20*, 347–356.

Michelson, L. (1987). Cognitive-behavioral assessment of agoraphobia. In L. Michelson & L. M. Ascher (Eds.), *Anxiety and Stress Disorders* (pp. 213–279). New York: Guilford Press.

Michelson, L., Mavissakalian, M., & Marchione, K. (1985). Cognitive and behavioral treatments of agoraphobia: Clinical, behavioral and psychophysiological outcomes. *Journal of Consulting and Clinical Psychology, 53*, 913–925.

Michelson, L., Mavissakalian, M., Marchione, K., Ulrich, R. F., Marchione, N., & Testa, S. (1990). Psychophysiological outcome of cognitive, behavioral and psychophysiologically-based treatments of agoraphobia. *Behaviour Research and Therapy, 28*, 127–139.

Michie, P. T., Fox, A. M., Ward, P. B., Catts, S. V., & McConaghy, N. (1990). Event-related potential indices of selective attention and cortical lateralization in schizophrenia. *Psychophysiology, 27*, 209–227.

Miller, R. E. (1987). Method to study anhedonia in hospitalized psychiatric patients. *Journal of Abnormal Psychology, 96*(1), 41–45.

Miran, M., & Miran, E. (1984). Cerebral asymmetries: Neuropsychological measurement and theoretical issues. *Biological Psychology, 19*, 295–304.

Mogg, K., Mathews, A., & Weinman, J. (1987). Memory bias in clinical anxiety. *Journal of Abnormal Psychology, 96*, 94–98.

Morrison, R., & Bellack, A. S. (1981). The role of social perception in social skills. *Behavior Therapy, 12*, 69–79.

Morrison, R., & Bellack, A. S. (1987). Social functioning of schizophrenic patients: Clinical and research issue. *Schizophrenia Bulletin, 13*, 715–725.

Morrison, R. L., Bellack, A. S., & Manuck, S. B. (1985). Role of social competence in borderline essential hypertension. *Journal of Consulting and Clinical Psychology, 53*(2), 248–255.

Morrison, R. L., Van Hasselt, V. B., & Bellack, A. S. (1987). Assessment of assertion and problem-solving skills in wife abusers and their spouses. *Journal of Family Violence, 2*, 227–238.

Naatanen, R., & Picton, T. (1987). The N! wave of the human electric and magnetic response to sound: A review and analysis of the component structure. *Psychophysiology, 24*, 375–425.

Neiss, R. (1988). Reconceptualizing arousal: Psychobiological states in motor performance. *Psychological Bulletin, 103*, 345–366.

Neiss, R. (1990). Ending arousal's reign of error: A reply to Anderson. *Psychological Bulletin, 107*, 101–105.

Nesse, R. M., Cameron, O. G., Curtis, G. C., McCann, D. S., & Huber-Smith, M. J. (1984). Adrenergic function in patients with panic anxiety. *Archives of General Psychiatry, 41*, 771–776.

Newton, J. E., Paige, S. R., Angel, C., & Reese, W. (1988). Heart rate and activity in response to natural stimuli in nervous and normal pointer dogs. *Biological Psychiatry, 23*, 829–833.

Nietzel, M. T., Bernstein, D. A., & Russell, R. L. (1988). Assessment of anxiety and fear. In A. S. Bellack & M. Hersen (Eds.), *Behavioral assessment: A practical handbook* (3rd ed., pp. 280–312). New York: Pergamon Press.

Obrist, P. A. (1982). Cardiac-behavioral interactions: A critical appraisal. In J. T. Cacioppo & R. E. Petty (Eds.), *Perspectives in cardiovascular psychophysiology.* New York: Guilford Press.

Ogilvie, R. D., McDonagh, D. M., Stone, S. N., & Wilkinson, R. T. (1988). Eye movements and the detection of sleep onset. *Psychophysiology, 26*, 81–90.

Ornitz, E. M., & Guthrie, D. (1989). Long-term habituation and sensitization of the acoustic startle response in the normal adult human. *Psychophysiology, 26*(2), 166–173.

Ost, L., & Hugdahl, K. (1985). Acquisition of blood and dental phobia and anxiety response patterns in clinical patients. *Behaviour Research and Therapy, 23*, 27–34.

Ost, L. G., Sterner, U., & Lindahl, I. L. (1984). Physiological responses in blood phobics. *Behaviour Research and Therapy, 22*(2), 109–117.

Pagano, R. R., Rose, R. M., Stivers, R. M., & Warrenburg, S. (1976). Sleep during transcendental meditation. *Science*, *191*, 308–310.

Paul, G. L. (Ed.). (1986). *Assessment in residential treatment settings*. Champaign, IL: Research Press.

Paul, G. L. (Ed.). (1987a). *The staff-resident interaction chronograph*. Champaign, IL: Research Press.

Paul, G. L. (Ed.). (1987b). *The time-sample behavioral checklist*. Champaign, IL: Research Press.

Paul, G. L., & Lentz, R. J. (1977). *Psychosocial treatment of chronic mental patients: Milieu versus social-learning programs*. Cambridge: Harvard University Press.

Paul, G.L., Mariotto, M. J., &Redfield, J. P. (1986). Sources and methods for gathering information in formal assessment. In G. L. Paul (Ed.), *Assessment in residential treatment settings* (pp. 27–62). Champaign, IL: Research Press.

Pelham, W. E., & Milich, R. (1991). Individual differences in response to ritalin in classwork and social behavior. In L. Greenhill & B. P. Osman (Eds.), *Ritalin: Theory and patient management* (pp. 203–221). New York: MaryAnn Liebert.

Pelham, W. E., Jr., McBurnett, K., Harper, G. W., Milich, R., Murphy, D. A., Clinton, J. C., & Thiele, C. (1990). Methylphenidate and baseball playing in ADHD children: Who's on first? *Journal of Consulting and Clinical Psychology*, *58*, 130–133.

Pilsbury, D., & Hibbert, G. (1987). An ambulatory system for long-term continuous monitoring of transcutaneous pCO2. *Bulletin of European Physiopathological Respiration*, *23*, 9–13.

Porcino, L. J., Rapoport, J. L., Behar, D., Sceery, W., Ismond, D. R., & Bunney, W. E., Jr. (1983). A naturalistic assessment of the motor activity of hyperactive boys: I. Comparison with normal controls. *Archives of General Psychiatry*, *40*, 681–687.

Porges, S. W., McCabe, P. M., & Youngue, B. G. (1982). Respiratory heart rate interactions: Psychophysiological implications for pathophysiology and behavior. In J. T. Cacioppo & R. E. Petty (Eds.), *Perspectives in cardiovascular psychophysiology*. New York: Guilford press.

Pritchard, W. S. (1986). Cognitive event-related correlates of schizophrenia. *Psychological Bulletin*, *100*, 43–66.

Raine, A., & Venables, P. H. (1987). Contingent negative variation, P3 evoked potentials, and antisocial behavior. *Psychophysiology*, *24*, 191–199.

Raine, A., & Venables, P. H. (1988). Enhanced P3 evoked potentials and longer P3 recovery times in psychopaths. *Psychophysiology*, *25*, 30–38.

Rowland, L. A., & Canavan, A. G. (1983). Is a B.A.T. therapeutic? *Behavioral Psychotherapy*, *11*, 139–146.

Roy-Byrne, P. P., Cowley, D. S., Greenblatt, D. J., Shader, R. I., & Hommer, D. (1990). Reduced benzodiazepine sensitivity in panic disorder. *Archives of General Psychiatry*, *47*, 534–538.

Scherer, K. R. (1987). Vocal assessment of affective disorders. In J. D. Maser (Ed.), *Depression and expressive behavior* (pp. 57–82). Hillsdale, NJ: Lawrence Erlbaum.

Schlundt, D. G., & McFall, R. M. (1985). New directions in the assessment of social competence and social skills. In L. L'Abate & M. A. Milan (Eds.), *Handbook of social skills training and research* (pp. 22–49). New York: Wiley.

Schneider, W. (1988). Micro experimental laboratory: An integrated system for IBM PC compatibles. *Behaviour Research Methods, Instruments, and Computers*, *20*, 206–217.

Schwartz, G. E. (1986). Emotion and psychophysiological organization: A system approach. In M. G. H. Coles, E. Donchin, & S. W. Porges (Eds.), *Psychophysiology: Systems, processes and applications* (pp. 354–377). New York: Guilford Press.

Schwartz, R., & Michelson, L. (1987). States of mind model: Cognitive balance in the treatment of agoraphobia. *Journal of Consulting and Clinical Psychology*, *55* 557–565.

Servais, S. B., Webster, J. G., & Montoye, H. J. (1984). Estimating human energy expenditure using an accelerometer device. *Journal of Clinical Engineering*, *9*, 159–170.

Shapiro, D. H., Jr., & Walsh, R. N. (1984). *Meditation: Classic and contemporary perspectives*. New York: Aldine.

Shear, M. K., & Fyer, M. R. (1988). Biological and psychophysiologic findings in panic disorder. In A. J. France & R. E. Hales (Eds.), *American psychiatric press review of psychiatry, Volume 7* (pp. 29–53). Washington, DC: American Psychiatric Press.

Shear, M. K., Harshfield, G. A., Polan, J., Mann, J., & Frances, A. (1983). Autonomic function in panic disorder patients (abstract). *Psychophysiology, 20,* 470.

Sherwood, A., Allen, M. T., Fahrenberg, J., Kelsey, R. M., Lovallo, W. R., & van Doornen, L. J. P. (1990). Committee report: Methodological guidelines for impedance cardiography. *Psychophysiology, 27,* 1–23.

Siever, L. J., Keefe, R., Bernstein, D. P. O., Coccaro, E. F., Klar, H. M., Zemishlany, Z., Peterson, A. E., Davidson, M., Mahon, T., Torvath, T., & Mohs, R. (1990). Eye tracking impairment in clinically identified patients with schizotypal personality disorder. *American Journal of Psychiatry, 147*(6), 740–745.

Simpson, A., & Turpin, G. (1983). A device for ambulatory skin conductance monitoring. *Psychophysiology, 20*(2), 225–229.

Smith, G. R., Monson, R. A., & Ray, D. C. (1986). Psychiatric consultation in somatization disorder: A randomized study. *New England Journal of Medicine, 22*(22), 1407–1413.

Stemmler, G. (1989). The autonomic differentiation of emotions revisited: Convergent and discriminant validation. *Psychophysiology, 26*(6), 617–632.

Stevens, J. R., Bigelow, L., Denny, D., Lipkin, J., Livermore, A. H., Rauscher, F., & Wyatt, R. J. (1979). Telemetered EEG-EOG during psychotic behaviors of schizophrenia. *Archives of General Psychiatry, 36,* 251–262.

Suen, H. K., & Ary, D. (1989). *Analyzing quantitative behavioral observation data.* Hillsdale, NJ: Lawrence Erlbaum.

Switzer, E. B., Deal, T. E., & Bailey, J. S. (1977). The reduction of stealing in second graders using a group contingency. *Journal of Applied Behavior Analysis, 10,* 267–272.

Tart, C. (1969). (Ed.) *Altered states of consciousness.* New York: Wiley.

Tassinary, L. G., Cacioppo, J. T., & Green, T. R. (1989). A psychometric study of surface electrode placements for facial electromyographic recording: I. The brow and cheek muscles. *Psychophysiology, 26*(1), 1–16.

Taylor, C. B., Agras, W. S., Schneider, J. A., & Allen, R. A. (1983). Adherence to instructions to practice relaxation exercises. *Journal of Consulting and Clinical Psychology, 51,* 952–953.

Taylor, C. B., Telch, M. J., & Havvik, D. (1983). Ambulatory heart rate changes during panic attacks. *Journal of Psychiatric Research, 17,* 261–266.

Taylor, C. B., Sheikh, J., Agras, W. S., Roth, W. T., Margraf, J., Ehlers, A., Maddock, R. J., & Gossard, D. (1986). Ambulatory heart rate changes in patients with panic attacks. *American Journal of Psychiatry, 143,* 478–482.

Taylor, C. B., Fried, L., & Klein, J. (1990). The use of real-time computer diary for acquisition and processing. *Behaviour Research and Therapy, 28,* 93–97.

Thakor, N. V., Yang, M., Amaresan, M., Reiter, E., Hoen-Saric, R., & McLeod, D. R. (in press). A microcomputer-based ambulatory monitor for anxiety disorders. *Journal of Ambulatory Monitoring.*

Torsvall, L., Akerstedt, T., Gillander, K., & Knutsson, A. (1989). Sleep on the night shift: 24-hour EEG monitoring of spontaneous sleep/wake behavior. *Psychophysiology, 26*(3), 352–358.

Trandel, D. V., & McNally, R. J. (1987). Perception of threat cues in post-traumatic stress disorder: Semantic processing without awareness. *Behaviour Research and Therapy, 25,* 469–476.

Trower, P., Bryant, B., & Argyle, M. (1978). *Social skills and mental health.* Pittsburgh: University of Pittsburgh Press.

Turner, S. M., Beidel, D. C., & Epstein, L. H. (1991). Vulnerability and risk for anxiety disorders. *Journal of Anxiety Disorders, 5,* 151–166.

Turpin, G., Shin, P., & Lader, M. (1983). Ambulatory electrodermal monitoring: Effects of ambient temperature, general activity, electrolyte media and length of recording. *Psychophysiology, 20,* 219–224.

Turpin, G. (1986). Effects of stimulus intensity on autonomic responding: The problem of differentiating orienting and defense reflexes. *Psychophysiology, 23*(1),1–14.

Tursky, B. R., & Jamner, L. D. (1982). Measurement of cardiovascular functioning. In J. T. Cacioppo & R. E. Petty (Eds.), *Perspectives in cardiovascular psychophysiology.* New York: Guilford Press.

Twentyman, C., Boland, T., & McFall, R. M. (1981). Heterosocial avoidance in college males: Four studies. *Behavior Modification, 5*, 523–552.

Vrana, S. R., Cuthbert, B. N., & Lang, P. J. (1986). Fear imagery and text processing. *Psychophysiology, 23*(3), 247–253.

Vrana, S. R., Cuthbert, B. N., & Lang, P. J. (1989). Processing fearful and neutral sentences: Memory and heart rate change. *Cognition and Emotion, 3*, 179–195.

Watson, D., Clark, L. A., & Tellegen, A. (1988). Development and validation of brief measures of positive and negative affect: The PANAS scales. *Journal of Personality and Social Psychology, 54*, 1063–1070.

Webb, E. J., Campbell, D. T., Schwartz, R. D., Sechrest, L., & Grove, J. B. (1981). *Non-reactive measures in the social sciences* (2nd ed.). Boston: Houghton Mifflin.

Weiss, B. L., Foster, G., Reynolds, C. F., & Kupfer, D. J. (1974). Psychomotor activity in mania. *Archives of General Psychiatry, 31*, 379–383.

Weiss, R. L., & Summers, K. J. (1983). Marital interaction coding system III. In E. E. Filsinger (Ed.), *Marriage and family assessment* (pp. 85–116). Beverly Hills: Sage.

Weiss, T., del Bo, A., Reichek, N., & Engelman, K. (1980). Pulse transit time in the analysis of autonomic nervous system effects on the cardiovascular system. *Psychophysiology, 17*, 202–207.

Westall, R., Perksey, M. N., & Chute, D. L. (1986). Accurate millisecond timing on Apple's Macintosh using Drexel's MilliTimer. *Behaviour Research Methods and Instrumentation, 18*, 307–311.

White, W. B., & Baker, L. H. (1987). Ambulatory blood pressure monitoring in patients with panic disorder. *Archives of Internal Medicine, 147*, 1973–1975.

White, W. B., & Baker, L. H. (1986). Episodic hypertension secondary to panic disorder. *Archives of Internal Medicine, 146*, 1129–1130.

Wielgus, M. S., & Harvey, P. D. (1988). Dichotic listening and recall in schizophrenia and mania. *Schizophrenia Bulletin, 14*, 689–700.

Williams, J. M., & Broadbent, K. (1986). Distraction by emotional stimuli: Use of a Stroop task with suicide attempters. *British Journal of Clinical Psychology, 8*, 14–18.

Williams, R. B., Jr. (1984). Measurement of local blood flow during behavioral experiments: Principles and practice. In J. A. Herd, A. M. Gotto, P. G. Kaufmann, & S. M. Weiss (Eds.), *Cardiovascular instrumentation. Proceedings of the working conference on applicability of new technology to biobehavioral research* (pp. 207–218). (NIH Publication No. 84-1654). Washington, DC: U.S. Dept. of Health and Human Services: National Institutes of Health.

Williams, R. B., Bittker, T. E., Buchsbaum, M. S., & Wynne, L. C. (1975). Cardiovascular and neurophysiologic correlates of sensory intake and rejection: I. Effect of cognitive tasks. *Psychophysiology, 12*, 427–433.

Zahn, T. P. (1986). Psychophysiological approaches to psychopathology. In G. H. Coles, E. Donchin, & S. W. Porges (Eds.), *Psychophysiology: Systems, processes, and applications* (pp. 508–611). New York: Guilford Press.

CHAPTER 9

Biological Markers

Stephen D. Samuelson and George Winokur

INTRODUCTION

A biological finding which discriminates between psychiatric diseases or disease subtypes, or which predicts treatment response or relapse, would be useful in research and clinical efforts alike. A biologic test which predicts genetic vulnerability would also be useful to those who are interested in studying heritable forms of illness. Trait markers identify vulnerability to a disease and are present regardless of whether the individual is actually ill. Alternatively, state markers are found only in currently affected patients, and might help with diagnostic, prognostic, and therapeutic decisions.

A true biological (trait or state) marker must be relatively specific if it is to serve as a confirmatory test. It should have sufficient positive predictive value and sensitivity to be used to screen for an illness. If the marker is to be used to predict vulnerability to disease, it must be shown to persist after remission, and to be present more often among high-risk groups than the general population.

Currently, there are no biological findings for a mental illness that meet these criteria ideally. Instead, we are left with a series of biological *correlates* with psychiatric diseases. In this chapter, we will focus on these putative biological markers. A plethora of studies have looked at reasonable marker candidates in virtually every psychiatric syndrome, but only a few lines of investigation have

Stephen D. Samuelson • Department of Psychiatry, The University of Texas Health Science Center at San Antonio, San Antonio, Texas 78284-7729.   **George Winokur** • Department of Psychiatry, College of Medicine, University of Iowa, Iowa City, Iowa 52242.
Research in Psychiatry: Issues, Strategies, and Methods, edited by L. K. George Hsu and Michel Hersen. Plenum Press, New York, 1992.

stood up to the test of replication. An attempt will be made to comment, where possible, on the utility of the assay as a vulnerability (trait) or diagnostic (state) marker. Furthermore, this chapter will be restricted to consideration of relatively well-established findings pertaining to *nongenetic* markers for illness; a discussion of population or molecular genetics and linkage markers is beyond the scope of this chapter.

Finally, the difference between a biological marker and a biological *etiology* should be kept in mind. Evidence from animal studies or genetics may suggest causality in some cases. However, it is likely that many of these correlates are neither necessary nor sufficient for the production of illness.

PUTATIVE MARKERS FOR AFFECTIVE ILLNESS

Sleep Studies and Electroencephalography

Polysomnography

Rapid eye movement (REM) sleep occurs rhythmically throughout the night, about once every 90 minutes. Reduction in the interval from the onset of sleep until the beginning of the first REM period (REM latency) has been found to distinguish depressed from control subjects (Gillin, Duncan, Murphy, Post, Wehr, Goodwin, Wyatt, & Bunney, 1981; Kupfer & Foster, 1972; Kupfer, Foster, Coble *et al.*, 1978), and is more prominent in endogenous depressions (Giles, Roffwarg, Schlesser, & Rush, 1986; Giles, Schlesser, Rush, Orsulak, Fulton, & Roffwarg, 1987; Rush, Giles, Roffwarg, & Parker, 1982).

As reduced REM latency may continue to be present after clinical remission of depression (Rush, Erman, Giles, Schlesser, Carpenter, Vasavada, & Roffwarg, 1986), it could be a trait marker for certain kinds of depression. This finding is consistent with studies of sleep patterns among monozygotic and dizygotic twins demonstrating genetic control of REM latency (Webb & Campbell, 1983). Furthermore, REM latency is concordant among endogenously depressed family members (Giles, Roffwarg, & Rush, 1987), and relatives of depressed patients with reduced REM latency have significantly shorter REM latency than relatives of depressed patients with nonreduced REM latency (Giles, Kupfer, Roffwarg, Ruth, Biggs, & Etzel, 1989). These findings taken together strongly suggest that decreased REM latency may reflect vulnerability to certain types of depression.

Other polysomnographic findings in depression include disrupted sleep continuity, decreased Stage 3 and Stage 4 sleep, altered distribution of REM sleep (increased total REM time especially during the first half of the night), and decreased slow-wave sleep (Reynolds & Kupfer, 1987; Reynolds, Kupfer, & Taska, 1985). However, these abnormalities are not strongly concordant among relatives of depressed subjects (Giles *et al.*, 1989), and we know of no studies showing them to be stable after clinical remission.

Muscarinic Cholinergic Induction of REM Sleep

A cholinergic hypothesis for affective disorder was proposed by Janowsky, El-Yousef, and Davis (1972) nearly two decades ago. A line of evidence which has been highly replicated in support of this view is abnormal muscarinic cholinergic induction of REM sleep among depressed patients (M. Berger, Riemann, Hoechli, & Spiegel, 1989; Sitaram, Nurnberger, Gershon, & Gillin, 1980; Sitaram, Nurnberger, Gershon, & Gillin, 1982; Sitaram, Dube, Jones, Bell, Gurevich, & Gershon, 1984). This test has at least partial specificity for depression versus illnesses such as alcoholism, eating disorders, and personality disorders (Berger et al., 1989; Lauer, Zulley, Krieg, Riemann, & Berger, 1988; Overstreet, Janowsky, & Rezvani, 1989). Although earlier reports suggested that abnormal REM induction may be a vulnerability marker for major depression, more recent results with remitted patients have been inconsistent (Riemann & Berger, 1989; Steiger, von Bardeleben, Herth, & Holsboer, 1989).

Quantitative Electroencephalography

The amplitudes of voltage potentials occurring at different frequencies in an electroencephalogram (EEG) are measured simultaneously at several locations on the scalp. The frequency bands usually recorded include *delta* (1 to 4 cycles per second [cps]), *theta* (4 to 8 cps), *alpha* (8 to 12 cps), and *beta* (12 to 30 cps) waves. Information regarding scalp position, frequency band, and amplitude can be correlated to produce topographic maps of brain electrical activity.

Such qualitative EEG findings are often disturbed in depressed patients relative to normals, and some investigators have used multivariate analytic methods to correctly identify up to 85% of depressed patients from control, alcoholic, and demented subjects (John, Prichep, Fridman, & Easton, 1988). A study by Lieber and Newbury (1988a) found that unipolar depressives ($N = 111$) had excessive alpha activity and deficient beta activity, whereas the pattern was reversed among bipolar depressives ($N = 41$). In another study by Lieber and Newbury (1988b), deficient beta activity combined with excessive theta activity seemed to be related to the presence of endogenous symptoms. As discussed in a recent review by Schneider (1990), these findings have been replicated among elderly patients, are different from EEG changes observed in normal aging and in dementia, and have been shown to persist in clinically recovered depressed patients compared with age-matched controls.

Imaging Studies

The relationship between regional cerebral blood flow (RCBF) as measured by xenon 133 inhalation and oxidative metabolism (Raichle, Grubb, Gado, Eichling, & Ter-Pogossian, 1976) has led to the use of this method to search for alterations in brain activity among psychiatric patients. Investigations have sought to describe global as well as topographic differences. Although there have been some reports of decreased RCBF (Sackeim, Prohovnik, Moeller, Brown, Apter, Prudic, Devanand, & Mukherjee, 1990) among unipolar depressed patients compared with controls, the evidence has been conflicting, with some studies showing no difference (Silfverskiold & Risberg, 1989), and others indicating actually increased RCBF (Rosenberg, Vostrup, Andersen, & Bolwig, 1988).

Positron emission tomography, which is a more sophisticated and perhaps more direct measure of metabolic activity in the brain, has also been used to study psychiatric patients. Abnormalities of the rate of glucose metabolism have been described among bipolar and unipolar depressed patients, as well as recovered depressed patients, with the predominant disturbance occurring in the anterolateral prefrontal cortices (Baxter, Phelps, Mazziotta, Schwartz, Gerner, Selin, & Sumida, 1985; Baxter, Schwartz, Phelps, Mazziotta, Guze, Selin, Gerner, & Sumida, 1989; Schwartz, Baxter, Mazziotta, Gerner, & Phelps, 1987). Although further replication and refinement of these data are needed, the findings are particularly interesting in that some measures have little overlap between primary (bipolar or unipolar) depression and normals or nondepressed psychiatric controls (Baxter *et al.*, 1989). Also, the observation that abnormal metabolism may persist after clinical remission is suggestive of a potential trait marker.

Dupont, Jernigan, and Butters (1990) discovered subcortical hyperintense regions using magnetic resonance imaging (MRI) which differentiated groups of otherwise healthy bipolar depressed patients younger than 55 years old from normals. Such regions continued to be present without change one year later, and were positively correlated with number of hospitalizations. This observation is consistent with other work on bipolar illness suggesting that acquired and genetic forms of illness might be discernible on the basis of EEG findings (Cook, Shukla, & Hoff, 1986).

Neuroendocrine Findings

Dexamethasone Suppression Test

Corticotropin-releasing hormone (CRH) is released by the hypothalamus into the portal circulation leading to the anterior lobe of the pituitary gland, where it stimulates the release of adrenocorticotropic hormone (ACTH) into the general circulation. This agent, in turn, stimulates the secretion of cortisol from the adrenal cortex. Adrenal corticoids exercise negative feedback onto the release of both ACTH and CRH.

Dexamethasone is an adrenal corticoid distinct from cortisol, but it nonetheless activates pituitary and hypothalamic negative feedback mechanisms for cortisol. Because dexamethasone and cortisol are chemically distinct, serum cortisol can be measured accurately following ingestion of dexamethasone. A single 1 mg dose of dexamethasone administered at night results in suppression of serum cortisol measured the following morning or afternoon in most normal subjects.

The dexamethasone suppression test (DST), as the aforementioned protocol is known, became a very popular research tool in psychiatry during the late 1970s when it was demonstrated that many depressed patients fail to suppress serum cortisol following dexamethasone (Carroll, Curtis, & Mendels, 1976).

However, it was soon discovered that although DST-nonsuppression frequently occurs in hospitalized depressed patients, other psychiatric illnesses can also have high incidences of nonsuppression (Coryell, 1984). In addition, the DST has an overall sensitivity in major depression of only about 44% (Arana, Baldessarini, & Ornsteen, 1985), which effectively precludes its use as a screening test for this illness. Furthermore, DST status contributes little to predictions about treatment response, although there have been reports that DST-nonsuppressors are less likely to respond to placebo than normal suppressors (APA Task Force, 1987).

Nonetheless, the test has been demonstrated to be abnormal more frequently among certain subtypes of depression. Approximately half of endogenously depressed patients are abnormal suppressors, whereas only 6% to 23% of neurotic or minor depressives escape suppression (Kasper & Beckman, 1983). A novel experimental design was employed by Winokur, Black, and Nasrallah (1987) to study the phenomenology of DST-suppressors and DST-nonsuppressors. Only the two extremes of the suppression–nonsuppression continuum were considered, based on postdexamethasone cortisol results. Over 400 patients with major depressive disorder were given DST: 163 "suppressors" had a postdexamethasone cortisol level less than 1.5 µg/dL, and 164 "nonsuppressors" had a postdexamethasone cortisol greater than 6.0µg/dL. Normal suppressor status was related to early age of onset, absence of delusions or melancholia, presence of a diagnosis of secondary depression, and family history of alcoholism.

The distinction between primary and secondary depression (Coryell, 1988; Feighner, Robins, Guze, & Goodwin, 1972) by DST had previously been described by Schlesser, Winokur, and Sherman (1980). They found 65 of 146 primary depressives with dexamethasone nonsuppression, but every one of 42 secondary depressives and 109 nondepressed controls suppressed normally. The association of normal DST results with family history of alcoholism is consistent with other studies suggesting that "depressive spectrum disorder" (Winokur, Behar, Van Valkenburg, & Lowry, 1978) is associated with normal DST results (Coryell, Gaffney, & Burkhardt, 1982; Schlesser et al., 1980). The presence of psychosis or a diagnosis of bipolar illness is also associated with DST-nonsuppression (Asnis, Halbreich, Nathan, Ostrow, Novacenko, Endicott, & Sachar, 1982; Schlesser et al., 1980).

At present, the only practical application for the DST derives from evidence that patients who are DST nonsuppressors when ill are more likely to relapse if they continue to exhibit abnormal suppression following treatment (even if they are by then asymptomatic) than patients that were nonsuppressors but revert to normal suppression after treatment (Ariana, Baldessarini, & Ornsteen, 1985). An argument can also be made for using the DST to aid with differential diagnosis of unusual phenocopies of depression (e.g., discriminating somatization disorder with secondary depression versus primary affective disorder with somatic features).

Thus, although the DST may be of limited clinical utility, the association of abnormal results with endogenous, primary, psychotic unipolar depression, and with bipolar depression makes it an intriguing biological finding. Also, DST status has been associated with familial subtypes of unipolar depression (Coryell *et al.*, 1982; Schlesser *et al.*, 1980), suggesting etiologic significance. However, DST normalizes with clinical remission in most patients (APA Task Force, 1987), and thus is not a trait marker. It is also not known whether DST status during episodes of illness breeds true, although the relationship between DST results and familial subtypes would be consistent with such.

Urinary Free Cortisol Determination

The failure of depressed patients to suppress serum cortisol after dexamethasone reflects excessive hypothalamic-pituitary-adrenal (HPA) axis drive (Kathol, Jaeckle, Lopez, & Meller, 1989). In fact, the hypercortisolism which often accompanies depression is occasionally so pronounced that it can be difficult to distinguish from Cushing's disease (Gold & Chrousos, 1985).

One measure of overall HPA activity is the amount of unconjugated cortisol present in a 24-hour urine collection. In a study by Kathol (1985a,b), urinary free cortisol (UFC) samples were obtained on recovered depressive patients who had been DST-nonsuppressors and control subjects every two to four weeks through an entire year. Mean UFC levels from the recovered patients were higher throughout the year, especially during summer and fall, compared with controls.

One patient in the aforementioned study relapsed during the study period. Interestingly, this patient's UFC measures rose steadily prior to the appearance of clinical depression, remained elevated during hospitalization, and returned to previously low levels following clinical improvement (Kathol, 1985b).

Urinary free cortisol measurement reflects gross HPA axis function, and the elevation of such in some individuals may constitute a vulnerability marker for major depressive disorder.

Cosyntropin Stimulation, Corticotropin-Releasing Hormone Stimulation, and Insulin Tolerance Testing

In order to understand the nature of the HPA axis abnormalities in affective illness more completely, artificial stimulation of the axis at different points has been performed. Such experiments seek to observe and at times functionally isolate particular aspects of the axis, thus circumventing the confusion which can result from the presence of highly interrelated mechanisms.

For example, treatment with synthetic ACTH (Cosyntropin) demonstrated hyperresponsiveness of cortisol release among depressed versus control subjects (Amsterdam, Maislin, Gold, & Winokur, 1989; Jaeckle, Kathol, & Lopez, 1987). This finding is consistent with adrenal hypertrophy in depressed subjects observed by abdominal MRI (Amsterdam *et al.*, 1989) and autopsy (Dorovini-Zis & Zis, 1987).

When the pituitary gland is stimulated with exogenous (ovine) CRH, or when the hypothalamus is stimulated by insulin-induced hypoglycemia to release CRH endogenously, a prompt rise in serum ACTH level is observed, with corresponding increase in cortisol secretion. Studies of CRH-stimulation test (CRHST) and insulin tolerance test (ITT) in depressed subjects have demonstrated attenuated pituitary ACTH response (contrary to the *increased* ACTH release observed in Cushing's disease), presumably due to CRH-receptor downregulation at the level of the pituitary resulting from chronic suprahypophyseal drive (Amsterdam *et al.*, 1989; Gold & Chrousos, 1985; Kathol *et al.*, 1989). Placing the site of the HPA abnormality in depression above the level of the pituitary is also consistent with evidence reported by Nemeroff, Owens, Bissette, Andorn, and Stanley (1988) of CRH receptor downregulation in the brains of suicide victims.

Although patients with major depression often have baseline hypercortisolemia (Jaeckle *et al.*, 1987; Lopez, Kathol, & Jaeckle, 1987), the net cortisol response to the CRHST or ITT is often decreased compared to controls (Amsterdam *et al.*, 1989; Gold & Chrousos, 1985; Kathol *et al.*, 1989), perhaps due to short-loop feedback as well as to blunted ACTH secretion.

Thyrotropin-Releasing Hormone Stimulation Test

The mean thyroid-stimulating hormone (TSH) response to thyrotropin-releasing hormone (TRH) is deficient among groups of depressed patients compared to controls (Prang, Wilson, Lara, Alltop, & Breese, 1972), but there is considerable overlap in TSH values, and the disturbance normalizes with recovery (Kirkegaard, Norlein, Lauridsen, Bjorum, & Christiansen, 1975). The utility of this test as a marker for depression is therefore limited, as is the utility of CRHST and ITT. Interestingly, some have found that many patients improve following treatment with T_3 (Cytomel), and these individuals seem to have an *increased* TSH response to TRH (Targum, Greenberg, Harmon, Kessler, Salerian, & Fram, 1984), but this has not been replicated (see Gitlin, Weiner, & Fairbanks, 1987). Thus, the role of the hypothalamic-pituitary-thyroid (HPT) axis in depression may have some prognostic utility, although replication of this research is needed.

Some correlations between HPT and HPA axis functioning have been observed in depressed patients, such as positively correlated blunting of both TSH and ACTH following CRHST (Lesch, Muller, Kruse, & Schulte, 1989), which is thought to reflect a common suprapituitary disturbance. Others, however, have found a dissociation between TRHST and DST results (Kirkegaard & Carroll, 1980). Therefore, although a common aberrancy proximal to the pituitary gland is implicated for these two endocrine systems, complex and independently modulated central and peripheral mechanisms may distort the expression at the level of the adrenal and thyroid glands in depressive illness.

Growth Hormone Response to Clonidine

Growth hormone (GH) is secreted from the anterior lobe of the pituitary gland in response to alpha$_2$-adrenergic stimulation or growth hormone-releasing hormone (GHRH). This response has been found by several investigators to be blunted in depressed patients versus controls (Checkley, Slade, & Shur, 1981; Lesch et al., 1989; Matussek, Ackenheil, Hippius, Muller, Schroder, Schultes, & Wasilewski, 1980), although some negative studies exist (Eriksson, Balldin, Lindstedt, & Modigh, 1988; Siever, Uhde, Jimmerson, Post, Lake, & Murphy, 1984).

This finding is in accord with increased alpha$_2$-adrenergic activity in depressed patients, a hypothesis also supported by platelet binding studies (see below). In fact, recent work in this area suggests that the decreased responses of pituitary hormones (e.g., GH, TSH, ACTH) reflect a more general suprahypophyseal abnormality (Lesch et al., 1989; Thomas, Beer, Harris, John, & Scanlon, 1989), perhaps related to a disturbance in alpha$_2$-adrenergic activity (Amsterdam, Maislin, Skolnick, Berwish, & Winokur, 1989).

Blunting of GH response seems to have a degree of specificity for endogenous depression over neurotic or secondary depression (Ansseau, Scheyvaerts, Doumont, Poirrier, Legros, & Frank, 1984; Ansseau, Von Frenckell, Cerfontaine, Papart, Frank, Timsit-Berthier, Geenen, & Legros, 1988; Matussek et al., 1980). Patients with eating disorders (Brambilla, Ferrari, Invitti, Zanoboni, Massironi, Catalano, Cocchi, & Muller, 1989) and schizophrenia (Matussek et al., 1980) also have a normal GH response. However, blunted secretion has been observed in panic disorder (Uhde, Vittone, Siever, Kaye, & Post, 1986) and obsessive compulsive disorder (Siever & Uhde, 1985). Findings with alcoholism are inconsistent, although an association between breath alcohol level and GH response has been observed (Muller, Hoehe, Klein, Nieberle, Kapfhammer, May, Muller, & Fichter, 1989).

Although the test lacks specificity for affective disorders, the abnormal findings in depression, panic disorder, and obsessive-compulsive disorder have led some to speculate that this abnormality might be a nonspecific marker for tricyclic-responsive illnesses (Uhde et al., 1986). The blunted response seems to continue in drug-free patients after recovery from major depression (Mitchell, Bearn, Corn, & Checkley, 1988; Steiger et al., 1989), so this finding might be a trait phenomenon.

Monoamines and Their Metabolites in Body Fluids

The study of monoamines and their metabolites in plasma, urine, and cerebrospinal fluid has been of interest since the 1950s. Although some findings are fairly well-replicated, many conflicting studies exist, and although this work supports a general view that biological correlates do occur in affective disorder, no particular hypothesis has been consistently supported (Henn, 1986).

Adrenergic Neurotransmitters and Their Metabolites

Observations of increased catecholamine content of the urine of manic patients and decreased content in that of depressed patients were among the first findings in the study of monoamines (Strom-Olsen & Weil-Malherbe, 1964). More recent findings suggest that depressed patients excrete more epinephrine and norepinephrine than controls, with increased excretion of catecholamine metabolites. Decreased plasma 3-methoxy-4-hydroxyphenylglycol (MHPG), however, has been observed in melancholic versus nonmelancholic depressives, bipolar versus unipolar depressives, and in dexamethasone nonsuppressors versus normal suppressors (Roy, Jimmerson, Pickar, 1986; Roy, Pickar, DeJong, Karoum, & Linnoila, 1988). Some, but not all, studies of cerebrospinal fluid support these findings (reviewed by Davis, Koslow, Gibbons, Maas, Bowden, Casper, Hanin, Javaid, Chang, & Stokes, 1988; Maas, Koslow, Davis, Katz, Frazer, Bowden, Berman, Gibbons, Stokes, & Landis, 1987). Such findings suggest that many patients with depression have *hyper*adrenergic activity, perhaps in association with increased cholinergic activity (Janowsky, Risch, Ziegler, Gillin, Huey, & Rausch, 1986).

Serotonin and 5-HIAA

Decreased cerebrospinal fluid (CSF) 5-hydroxyindoleacetic acid (5-HIAA), the major metabolite of serotonin, has been associated with violent suicide and major depressive disorder (Coppen & Doogan, 1988; Gibbons & Davis, 1986). Challenge tests of serotonergic responsivity (as indicated by prolactin or growth hormone secretion) also have associated decreased serotonergic activity with suicidality (Coccaro, Siever, Klar, Maurer, Cochrane, Cooper, Mohs, & Davis, 1989; Coppen & Doogan, 1988).

Dopamine and HVA

Studies of homovanillic acid (HVA) content in the CSF have provided conflicting results (P. A. Berger, Faull, Kilkowski, Anderson, Kraemer, Davis, & Barchas, 1980; Davis *et al.*, 1988). Low HVA has been related, along with low 5-HIAA, to increased likelihood of suicidal behavior (Roy, DeJong, & Linnoila, 1989).

Gamma-Aminobutyric Acid (GABA)

Plasma and CSF GABA levels seem to be decreased in affective illness, although the significance of this is uncertain (Berrettini, Nurnberger, Hare, Gershon, & Post, 1982).

Peripheral Tissue Models for CNS Activity in Affective Illness

Platelet Serotonin Uptake

Platelets have uptake sites in their membrane which are saturable and carrier-mediated, and demonstrate structural specificity for serotonin (Stahl, 1977; Stahl & Meltzer, 1978). Because of these pharmacologic similarities between platelet and brain uptake of serotonin, as well as evidence implicating serotonergic mechanisms in depression, platelets were proposed as models for serotonergic activity in affective illnesses (Pletscher, 1968; Shaw, Camps, & Eccleston, 1967; Sneddon, 1973). A review of the literature by Rausch, Janowsky, Risch, and Huey (1986) indicated that 18 studies of platelet serotonin uptake in affective disorders had been carried out, 8 of which included kinetics analysis (i.e., determination of density and affinity of uptake sites). All eight studies found decreased uptake, usually due to decreased receptor density (V_{max}) rather than change in affinity (K_m). Since then, decreased platelet serotonin uptake (with findings of decreased V_{max} but normal K_m when kinetics parameters are determined) among depressed patients have been replicated numerous times (Butler & Leonard, 1988; Quitana, 1989; Rausch et al., 1986; Rausch, Rich, & Risch, 1988; Slotkin, Whitmore, Barnes, 1989). The abnormal uptake has been observed to persist after clinical improvement although it may revert to control levels after 1 year of lithium treatment (Coppen, Swade, & Wood, 1980).

Interestingly, treatment with tricyclic antidepressants has been shown to normalize the uptake rate (Quitana, 1989), but such seems to be mediated by an increase in the K_m and may have little effect on V_{max} (Meltzer, Aurora, Baber, & Tricou, 1981). However, a recent study by Rausch et al. (1988) found that *electroconvulsive therapy* produces normalization of V_{max}.

Although decreased platelet serotonin uptake does not seem to differentiate between bipolar depression, schizoaffective disorder, and unipolar depression (Meltzer et al., 1981), nonaffective illnesses, such as schizophrenia (Lingjaerde, 1983), anorexia nervosa (Zemishlany, Modai, Apter, Jerushalmi, Samuel, & Tyano, 1987), and obsessive-compulsive disorder (Weizman, Carmi, Hermesch, Shahar, Apter, Tyano, & Rehavi, 1986) do not have decreased serotonin uptake.

Meltzer and Aurora (1988) found that monozygous twins have significantly greater concordance of serotonin uptake rate than dizygous twins or nontwin siblings. These results implicate a degree of genetic control in platelet serotonin uptake rate, and these findings together provide evidence that this might represent a vulnerability marker for affective illness.

The main impediment to the clinical utility of serotonin uptake is the large overlap which is typically found between patients and controls in even the most positive of data sets. In addition, decreased serotonin uptake among other psychiatric illnesses, such as panic disorder and alcoholism, has been observed, calling into question the specificity of this test.

Platelet Imipramine Binding

Another putative biological marker which has been studied extensively in affective illness is the platelet [^{3}H]-imipramine binding site. Animal and autopsy studies have demonstrated that imipramine binding sites in the brain correspond with regions of serotonergic neuronal activity. Furthermore, the platelet imipramine binding site is allosterically related to the serotonin uptake site, and it noncompetitively inhibits serotonin uptake (for a review, see Wagner, Aberg-Wistedt, Asberg, Ekqvist, Martensson, & Montero, 1985).

Imipramine binding to platelets is specific and saturable, although the kinetics of such are complicated somewhat by the presence of both high- and low-affinity binding (Ieni, Zukin, & Van Praag, 1984). Currently, only the high-affinity binding site has been linked to Na+K+-ATPase and serotonin uptake, and this site in particular is disturbed in certain psychiatric illnesses (Hrdina, 1989).

The binding of imipramine to platelet membranes from depressed patients versus controls has been found in most studies to differ in the density of binding sites (B_{max}), but not in the affinity of imipramine for such (K_a) (Baron, Barkai, Gruen, Peslow, Fieve, & Quitkin, 1986; Briley, Langer, Raizman, Sechter, & Zarifian, 1980; Langer, Galzin, Poirier, Loo, Sechter, & Zarifian, 1987; Slotkin et al., 1989). Both tricyclic antidepressants and electroconvulsive therapy increase binding, particularly the B_{max} (Cowen, Geaney, Schachter, Green, & Elliot, 1984; Langer, Sechter, Loo, Raisman, & Zarifian, 1986), a fact which has probably confounded studies seeking to address the trait versus state question. In a study by Wagner, Aberg-Wistedt, Asberg, Bertilsson, Martensson, and Montero (1987), patients ($N = 51$) with severe depression in whom decreased B_{max} reverted to control levels after starting tricyclic antidepressant or electroconvulsive therapy were followed up 2 years later. Those who were clinically remitted and off medications had persistently decreased B_{max} compared with controls.

There is also some suggestion that this finding has a genetic component. Lewis and McChesney (1985) found decreased B_{max} among unipolar as well as bipolar patients, but among unipolar patients this difference was due mostly to patients with a family history of depressive disorder without histories of alcoholism or sociopathy. Patients without a family history for psychiatric illness, and those with alcoholism or sociopathy among first degree relatives (sporadic depressive disorder and depressive spectrum disorder), did not differ from controls in imipramine binding or density of binding sites. This finding was replicated among geriatric patients with depression (Schneider, Fredrickson, Severson, & Sloan, 1986).

Because abnormalities in imipramine binding occur in other psychiatric illnesses, such as panic disorder, obsessive-compulsive disorder, eating disorders, and enuresis (Lewis, Noyes, Coryell, & Clancy, 1985; Weizman et al., 1986), and because of the overlap between normals and patients, this test has little clinical utility. Nonetheless, the possibility that it identifies a subgroup of genically predisposed patients suggests that it may be useful in establishing greater homogeneity among experimental groups in molecular genetic, outcome, or biological marker studies.

Lymphocyte Beta-Adrenergic Receptors

Beta-adrenergic receptors exist on lymphocytes and mediate intracellular mechanisms with the second messenger cyclic adenosine monophosphate (cAMP) by modulating adenylate cyclase activity (Coffee and Hadden, 1985).

If lymphocytes are treated with the adrenergic agonist isoproterenol, adenylate cyclase is stimulated, and increased levels of cAMP result. Although the density and also the affinity of this receptor are unchanged, the isoproterenol-stimulated increase in cAMP is blunted in depressed patients compared with controls (Extein, Tallman, Smith, and Goodwin, 1979; Halper, Brown, Sweeney, Kocsis, Peters, & Mann, 1988; Mann, Brown, Halper, Sweeney, Kocsis, Stokes, & Bilezikian, 1985). These findings are thought to represent a defect possibly affecting events distal to receptor binding *per se*, such as adenylate cyclase activity.

Platelet Alpha-Adrenergic Receptors

Platelet alpha-adrenoceptors are predominantly of the Type 2 subgroup and are involved in platelet aggregation (Campbell, 1981; Kafka & Paul, 1986). In the brain, presynaptic inhibitory $alpha_2$-adrenoceptors negatively modulate norepinephrine release into the synaptic cleft. If some affective illnesses involve decreased adrenergic activity as certain monoamine hypotheses of depression suggest, increased $alpha_2$-adrenoceptor activity would be a putative mechanism for such.

There is evidence from ^{3}H-clonidine, ^{3}H-para-amino-clonidine, or ^{3}H-yohimbine binding studies that platelet $alpha_2$-adrenergic receptors are increased in depressed patients versus controls (Garcia-Sevilla, Zis, Hollingsworth, Greden, & Smith, 1981; Garcia-Sevilla, Guimon, Garcia-Vallejo, & Fuster, 1986). Furthermore, tricyclic and monoamine oxidase inhibiting antidepressants, lithium, and electroconvulsive therapy result in decreased alpha-adrenoceptor density (reviewed in Garcia-Sevilla *et al.*, 1986), although a recent study found no differences in receptor binding following 4 to 6 weeks of imipramine, tyrosine, or placebo in depressed patients (Wolfe, Gelenberg, & Lydiard, 1989). Some studies have demonstrated that receptor density rather than the affinity for ligand is higher in patients than in controls (Pandey, Janicak, Javaid, & Davis, 1989), but in others both affinity and density are increased (Takeda, Harada, & Otsuki, 1989).

The specificity of this measurement for depression is questionable since there have been reports of increased receptor density in schizophrenia, schizoaffective disorder, anorexia nervosa, generalized anxiety disorder, essential hypertension, and drug withdrawal (Kafka & Paul, 1986; Pandey *et al.*, 1989; Sevy, Papadimitriou, Surmont, Goldman, & Mendlewicz, 1989).

PUTATIVE MARKERS FOR SCHIZOPHRENIA

Brain Imaging Studies

Computerized Tomography

Using computed tomographic (CT) scanning, certain patients with schizophrenia have been shown to have a degree of ventricular and/or sulcal enlargement (Okasha and Madikur, 1982; Rieder, Mann, Weinberger, van Kammen, & Post, 1983; Weinberger, Bigelow, Klein, Rosenblatt, & Wyatt, 1980). Pandurangi, Dewan, and Boucher (1986) studied patients with enlarged versus nonenlarged ventricles and controls, and found that ventricular enlargement was associated with abnormal EEG and impaired neuropsychiatric testing (Halstead-Reitan battery). Several other studies have investigated neurobehavioral function in relation to CT findings, but these have yielded conflicting results that are often due to small sample size, idiosyncratic CT measurement techniques, and insensitive cognitive techniques (Zec & Weinberger, 1986). An association between enlarged ventricles and longer duration of illness and severity of negative symptoms has been described (Kemali, Maj, Galderisi, Salvati, Starace, Valente, & Pirozzi, 1987), although others have found the enlargement of sulcul and ventricular spaces to be diffuse and not related to disease severity or negative symptoms (Pfefferbaum, Zipursky, Lim, Zatz, Stahl, & Jernigan, (1988).

Magnetic Resonance Imaging

Magnetic resonance imaging (MRI) has several advantages over CT in the study of intracranial structures. Recent studies of schizophrenic patients and controls matched for educational achievement replicated former studies which found enlarged ventricular volume among patients (Andreasen, Ehrhardt, Swayze, Alliger, Yuh, Cohen, & Ziebell, 1990; Gur, Mozley, Resnick, Shtasel, Kohn, Zimmerman, Herman, Atlas, Grossman, Erwin, & Gur, 1991).

These structural findings have not been related to family history of schizophrenia or "schizophrenia-spectrum" disorders, nor has there been investigation into a possible genetic role in the development of such (e.g., twin studies). However, offspring of schizophrenic mothers who go on to develop the illness have larger ventricles and also are more likely to have a history of birth complication than control children (Schulsinger, Parnas, Petersen, Schulsinger, Teasdale, Mednick, Moller, & Silverton, 1984).

Positron Emission Tomography

Positron emission tomography (PET) scanning is an interesting technology which is still in its infancy with regard to applications in psychiatric research. Early studies indicated possible qualitative differences in brain metabolic activity (e.g., hypofrontality, decreased basal ganglia activity, cortical laterality effects) among schizophrenic patients compared to controls (see review in Cohen, Semple, & Gross, 1986). More recent studies, however, have suggested increased frontal and reduced parietal glucose metabolism in acutely ill, drug-naive patients (Cleghorn, Garnett, Nahmias, Firnau, Brown, Kaplan, Szechtman, & Szechtman, 1989), as well as increased temporal lobe glucose use in chronic schizophrenia (DeLisi, Buchsbaum, Holcomb, Langston, King, Kessler, Pickar, Carpenter, Morihisa, Margolin et al., 1989).

A particularly exciting application of PET scanning in schizophrenia is quantitation of dopamine receptor density. In accord with a dopaminergic hypothesis for schizophrenia, significantly increased dopamine receptor density specific to the Type 2 (D_2) receptor has been found by one group, and a second study identified nonsignificant decreases in D_2 receptor density (Andreasen, Carson, Evans, Farde, Gjedde, Hakim, Lal, Nair, Sedvall, Tune, & Wong, 1988). One criticism of this work has been that if patients are not drug-naive, then findings of increased receptor density might be a drug effect (i.e., due to upregulation in response to inhibition of dopamine binding). In fact, a recent study of 18 patients with schizophrenia who had never received treatment and 20 normal controls found no difference in D_2 receptor density or affinity in the putamen or caudate nucleus (Farde, Wiesel, Stone-Elander, Halldin, Nordstrom, Hall, & Sedvall, 1990).

Cerebrospinal Fluid Studies

The search for cerebrospinal fluid characteristics in schizophrenia has focused on the measurement of neurotransmitters and their metabolites. Currently, there exists a sizable literature on the subject, with several conflicting and negative studies (see review in van Kammen, Peters, & van Kammen, 1986).

The only finding from CSF studies that seems to distinguish patients with schizophrenia from normals is increased mean norepinephrine (NE) content (Kemali, DelVecchio, & Maj, 1982; Lake, Sternberg, van Kammen, Ballenger, Ziegler, Post, Kopin, & Bunney, 1980). Elevated NE also has been correlated with relapse following withdrawal from haloperidol (van Kammen, Peters, van Kammen, Nugent, Goetz, Yao, & Linnoila, 1989). Degradation products of neurotransmitters, such as homovanillic acid (HVA), 5-hydroxyindoleacetic acid (5-HIAA), and 3-methoxy-4-hydroxyphenylglycol (MHPG) have been studied, but few have found differences between patients and controls. Interestingly, decreased HVA (van Kammen et al., 1986) as well as decreased 5-HIAA (Potkin, Weinberger, Linnoila, & Wyatt, 1983) have been associated with increased cortical atrophy (5-HIAA has also been related to ventricular enlargement) in schizophrenic patients.

Platelet Monoamine Oxidase Activity

Monoamine oxidase Type B comprises 80% of brain MAO, and is present in blood platelets. Early findings suggested that platelet MAO activity is decreased in schizophrenia (Campbell, 1981; Reveley, Glover, Sandler, & Spokes, 1981; Wyatt, Potkin, & Murphy, 1979).

More recent studies have also reported low platelet MAO activity among schizophrenics (Ivanovic & Majkic-Singh, 1988; Meltzer & Zureick, 1987; Rose, Castellani, Boeringa, Boeringa, Malek-Ahmadi, Lankford, Bessman, Fritz, Denney, Denney, & Abell, 1986), but other large, well-controlled studies have found no difference between platelet MAO activity of patients and normals (Fleissner, Seiffert, Schneider *et al.*, 1987), and there is evidence that it may be an artifact of treatment with antipsychotic medications (Maj, Arena, Galderisi, Starace, & Kemali, 1987). Furthermore, although some autopsy studies of brain MAO activity indicate selectively decreased activity in frontal and limbic regions of schizophrenics (Owen, Crow, Frith, Johnson, Johnstone, Lofhouse, Owens, & Poulter, 1987), other reports have been negative in this regard (Mann, Kaplan, & Bird, 1986; Wyatt *et al.*, 1979). Finally, MAO activity does not seem to be related to enlarged ventricles in schizophrenic patients (Pandurangi *et al.*, 1986).

All considered, there are enough conflicting reports regarding platelet MAO activity in schizophrenia to call into doubt its usefulness as a diagnostic or vulnerability marker for that disease.

Eye-Tracking Studies

Schizophrenia has been associated with abnormalities of eye movement, especially inappropriate saccadic movements during smooth-pursuit eye tracking. The prevalence of abnormal eye tracking in the general population is only 8%, compared to over half of schizophrenic patients (Holzman, Proctor, & Hughes, 1973; Holzman, Proctor, Levy, Yasillo, Meltzer, & Hurt, 1974; Shagass, Amadeo, & Overton, 1974). This increased prevalence cannot be attributed to antipsychotic medications (Spohn, Coyne, & Spray, 1988), to acute psychosis (vandenBosch & Rozendaal, 1988), or to inattention (Holzman, Levy, & Proctor, 1976).

The principal difficulty in identifying abnormal eye tracking as a biologic marker for schizophrenia is one of specificity, since patients with other psychiatric illnesses (e.g., mania) also frequently manifest abnormalities of eye tracking (Shagass *et al.*, 1974).

However, there is a strong genetic component within families of schizophrenics, but possibly not those of other disorders. Forty-five percent of psychiatrically well first-degree relatives of schizophrenic probands have abnormal eye tracking (Holzman, Kringlen, Levy, & Haberman, 1980). This is in contrast to relatives of patients with affective disorders, who do not appear to have eye-tracking abnormalities more often than the general population (Levy, Yasillo, Dorus, Shaughnessy, Gibbons, Peterson, Janicak, Gaviria, & Davis, 1983). Other evidence from twin studies also implicates a genetic component within families of schizophrenics (Holzman *et al.*, 1980), but not in families with bipolar illness or reactive psychosis (Holzman, Kringlen, Matthysse, Flanagan, Lipton, Cramer, Levin, Lange, & Levy, 1988). Furthermore, one group has been able to support an autosomal dominant model for the transmission of abnormal eye tracking and/or schizophrenia (Holzman *et al.*, 1988).

This evidence suggests that abnormalities of smooth pursuit eye tracking might constitute a state marker for illnesses such as bipolar disorder, but a trait marker for schizophrenia.

PUTATIVE MARKERS FOR ANXIETY DISORDERS

Lactate Infusion

The intravenous infusion of lactic acid results in panic attacks among 60% to 80% of patients with panic disorder, and only 0% to 20% of normals (Balon, Pohl, Yeragani, Rainey, & Weinberg, 1988; Gaffney, Fenton, Lane, & Lake, 1988; Liebowitz, Gorman, Fyer, Dillon, Levitt, & Klein, 1986; Pitts & McClure, 1967). The panic attacks produced by lactate infusion are of the same quality as spontaneous panic attacks (Balon, Yergani, & Pohl, 1988). And this response has relative specificity for panic disorder versus major depressive disorder (Cowley, Dager, & Dunner, 1987), although patients with panic attacks in the context of major depression cannot be distinguished from panic disorder patients without major depression by lactate infusion (Cowley, Dager, & Dunner, 1986). Furthermore, alcoholic patients with panic disorder do not panic as frequently with lactate infusion as nonalcoholic panic disorder patients (George, Nutt, Waxman, & Linnoila, 1989).

The pathophysiology of lactate-induced panic attacks is related to hyperventilation-induced hypocapnia and low inorganic phosphorus (Gorman, Cohen, Liebowitz, Fyer, Ross, Davies, & Klein, 1986). This is consistent with the inducibility of panic attacks by breathing carbon dioxide-enriched air (Sanderson, Rapee, & Barlow, 1989). Also, susceptibility to panic attacks has been associated with baseline anxiety (Cowley, Hyde, Dager, & Dunner, 1987; Dillon, Gorman, Liebowitz, Fyer, & Klein, 1987), basal prolactin levels in males (Hollander, Liebowitz, Cohen, Gorman, Fyer, Papp, & Klein, 1989), and serum cortisol levels among those who have delayed panic attacks following lactate infusion (Hollander, Liebowitz, Gorman, Cohen, Fyer, & Klein, 1989).

There is also evidence suggesting that lactate infusion may be a vulnerability marker for panic disorder. Panic disorder is known to cluster in families, and a recent study by Balon, Jordan, Pohl *et al.* (1989) found that family history of panic disorder is predicted by response to lactate infusion among normal subjects.

Mitral Valve Prolapse

Up to 10% of the general population has a usually benign condition known as prolapsing mitral valve leaflet syndrome, floppy-valve syndrome, systolic click-murmur syndrome, or simply mitral valve prolapse. There is a definite female preponderance, with familial clustering suggestive of autosomal dominant transmission (Braunwald, 1983). Some studies have described an excess of mitral valve prolapse (about 30%) among patients with panic disorder (Goodwin, 1986). Mitral valve prolapse in these cases is usually mild, and has not been related to inducibility of panic attacks by lactate infusion (Gorman, Goetz, Fyer, King, Fyer, Liebowitz, & Klein, 1988).

Some serious questions exist, however, regarding the validity of these findings. In a study by Hartman, Kramer, Brown, and Devereux (1982), 38 (27%) of 140 patients with mitral valve prolapse had a history of panic attacks, and 22 (16%) of these met DSM-III criteria for panic disorder. However, among 103 first degree relatives of probands with mitral valve prolapse, 33 relatives also had prolapse, and only one (3%) of these relatives was found to have panic disorder. Similarly, of the remaining 70 relatives without mitral valve prolapse, two (3%) were found to have panic disorder. This lack of familial association between panic disorder and mitral valve prolapse has been replicated (Bowen, Orchard, Keegan, & D'Arcy, 1985; Devereux, Kramer-Fox, & Shear, 1986), and suggests that the excess of panic disorder among patients with prolapse is possibly due to a selection bias which favors more highly symptomatic patients. In addition, recent findings (Dager, Comess, Saal, Sisk, Beach, & Dunner, 1989) indicate that M-mode echocardiography, one of the techniques frequently employed in studies of mitral valve prolapse and panic disorder, may not be sufficiently reliable for diagnosing mitral valve prolapse (interrater reliability, *kappa* = 0.11 to 0.45).

PUTATIVE MARKERS FOR ALCOHOLISM

Several biochemical indices can be used to identify heavy alcohol intake. Moreover, a variety of putative biological correlates with alcoholism have been proposed. Although the search for biological markers in alcoholism is complicated by the direct effects of ethanol itself, indirect approaches which study high-risk groups circumvent this problem to some degree.

Several state markers for alcohol *intake* exist. These are related to hepatocellular injury, the induction of liver enzymes, and other metabolic disturbances following heavy ethanol intake. Serum gamma-glutamyl transpeptidase (GGTP) is disproportionately elevated with respect to other liver enzymes in this context. Serum measures of osmolality, uric acid, glutamic-oxaloacetic transaminase (SGOT), glutamic-pyruvic transaminase (SGPT), alkaline phosphatase, bilirubin, and triglycerides, as well as mean erythrocyte cell volume, also tend to be increased by alcohol ingestion. Of course, blood alcohol level (% wt/vol) above 300% at any time, or above 100% on routine examination indicates heavy ethanol intake, and a level greater than 150% without other signs of intoxication indicates tolerance to ethanol from chronic exposure (see review in Wallach, 1986).

Abnormal thyroid-stimulating hormone (TSH) response to thyroid-releasing hormone (TRH) has been observed among a third of abstinent alcoholics (Loosen, Prange, & Wilson, 1983; Muller, Hoehe, Klein, Nieberle, Kapfhammer, May, Muller, & Fichter, 1989) and 30% to 50% of acutely withdrawn alcoholics (Loosen, Wilson, Dew et al., 1979; Muller et al., 1989). Platelet MAO activity (Fleissner et al., 1987; Tabekoff, Hoffman, Lee, Saito, Willard, & Leon-Jones, 1988) and serotonin uptake among alcoholics (Boismare, Lhuintre, Daoust, Moore, Saligaut, & Hillemand, 1987) are decreased, as is adenosine receptor-stimulated adenylate cyclase activity in lymphocytes (Diamond, Wrubel, Estrin, & Gordon, 1987). Some have also found decreased erythrocyte membrane fluidity associated with selectively decreased surface carbohydrate content (Beauge, Stibler, & Borg, 1985). The degree to which these disturbances are primary to alcoholism, or merely effects of chronic ethanol exposure, has not been established.

None of these findings has been identified as vulnerability markers, nor are they sufficiently specific to serve as diagnostic markers for this illness.

In the case of alcoholism, evidence of a vulnerability marker must include demonstration of the abnormality among groups at high risk for the illness. This approach circumvents the problem of ethanol exposure, and has been used with some success in a few studies. Nonalcoholic sons of alcoholics were found to have decreased serum cortisol following ethanol ingestion compared to controls (Schuckit, Gold, & Risch, 1987). It is interesting that urinary excretion of epinephrine following alcohol ingestion was lower in first degree relatives of alcoholics than in subjects with negative family histories for alcoholism (Swartz, Drews, & Cadoret, 1987), especially since the hypothalamic-pituitary-adrenal axis may be modulated by central adrenergic activity (Tilders, Berkenbosch, & Smelik, 1982). Likewise, subjective responses to ethanol in individuals with a first degree relative with alcoholism are less intense than in individuals with a negative family history (Schuckit, 1984). Furthermore, when cortisol response, prolactin response, and subjective reports are considered together, the majority of individuals with positive or negative family histories of alcoholism can be correctly identified (Schuckit & Gold, 1988).

Finally, an interesting biological "invulnerability marker" for alcoholism has been observed among Oriental populations. Approximately half of Orientals lack mitochondrial (Type 2) aldehyde dehydrogenase ($ALDH_2$). Alcohol intolerance among Orientals may be related to this deficiency. The genes for normal (Caucasian type) and abnormal (Oriental type) $ALDH_2$ have been identified (Shibuya & Yoshida, 1988b), and a recent study demonstrated that persons of

Oriental descent who have the Caucasian form of the gene have a much higher risk for developing alcoholic liver diseases (Shibuya & Yoshida, 1988a).

SUMMARY

The increasing popularity of defining psychiatric illnesses according to a biological and medical model has been accompanied by an enormous proliferation of biological marker studies. We have presented the material according to diagnosis and have included findings in affective illness (bipolar and unipolar), schizophrenia, anxiety disorders, and alcoholism. Studies of markers in these illnesses range from sleep and electrophysiological studies through receptor studies, biogenic amine studies, and neuroendocrinological studies, to brain-imaging studies. This review, however, merely scratches the surface of the current body of literature. The entire area of molecular and epidemiologic genetics was left untouched, and several other lines of research were also not mentioned. Further discussion might also have taken up the search for biological markers among such diagnoses as obsessive-compulsive disorder, dementia, anorexia nervosa, bulimia, antisocial personality, and other personality disorders, not to mention the numerous psychiatric illnesses which affect children (e.g., conduct disorder, attention deficit hyperactivity disorder, infantile autism, and Gilles de la Tourette syndrome to name a few).

In view of the vast literature on the subject, it is reasonable that we come up with some principles for the study of biological markers in psychiatric illness. First, it is necessary that there be replication of findings. As an example, if 10 studies have been done and 8 are in favor of the finding, we might consider the finding more important than if the breakdown were 5 and 5. Moreover, appropriate reasons for the two negative studies would also make the finding more convincing. A criterion of three positive studies in separate laboratories and no negative studies might be a useful way to define appropriate replication.

There should be internal consistency. If an individual reports association between an illness and a particular biological marker, and another person reports association with a second marker, it would be valuable to see if the two studies are consistent with each other. Often biological variables are inter-related, and it is of interest to know if their association with a particular illness is in the same direction. Appropriate discussion and further replication is needed where findings involving different but interrelated biological indices seem to be mutually exclusive.

There should be consistency between clinical and biological variables. For example, if a low amount of cerebrospinal fluid 5-hydroxyindoleacetic acid were associated with an endogenous depression and also with suicide attempts and delinquent behavior, then there might be some question about the specificity of the finding or the consistency thereof. (Endogenous depressives are rarely delinquent although they do make suicide attempts, and sociopathic men are often depressed, but these depressions are generally not of the endogenous type.) The clinical implications of the biological findings should make sense.

Finally, studies of biological markers in psychiatric illness should take cognizance of the reliability in appropriate psychiatric diagnosis. Systematic criteria should be used, and an effort should be made to attach the findings to a very specific illness or subcategory of illness. These methodological improvements should enable us to come up with better biological markers for more specific illnesses.

REFERENCES

Amsterdam, J. D., Maislin, G., Gold, P., & Winokur, A. (1989). The assessment of abnormalities in hormonal responsiveness at multiple levels of the HPA axis in depressive illness. *Psychoneuroendocrinology, 14,* 43–62.

Amsterdam, J. D., Maislin, G., Skolnick, B., Berwish, N., & Winokur, A. (1989). Multiple hormone responses to clonidine administration in depressed patients and healthy volunteers. *Biological Psychiatry, 26,* 265–278.

Andreasen, N., Carson, R., Evans, A., Farde, L., Gjedde, A., Hakim, A., Lal, S., Nair, N., Sedvall, G., Tune, L., & Wong, D. (1988). Workshop on schizophrenia, PET, and dopamine D_2 receptors in the human neostriatum. *Schizophrenia Bulletin, 3,* 471–484.

Andreasen, N. C., Ehrhardt, J. C., Swayze, V. W., Alliger, R. J., Yuh, W. T. C., Cohen, G., & Ziebell, S. (1990). Magnetic resonance imaging of the brain in schizophrenia: The pathophysiologic significance of structural abnormalities. *Archives of General Psychiatry, 47,* 35–44.

Ansseau, M., Scheyvaerts, M., Doumont, A., Poirrier, R., Legros, J. J., & Frank, G. (1984). Concurrent use of REM latency, dexamethasone suppression, clonidine and apomorphine tests as biological markers of endogenous depression: A pilot study. *Psychiatry Research, 12,* 261–272.

Ansseau, M., Von Frenckell, R., Cerfontaine, J. L., Papart, P., Frank, S., Timsit-Berthier, M., Geenen, V., & Legros, J. J. (1988). Blunted response of growth hormone to clonidine and apomorphine in endogenous depression. *British Journal of Psychiatry, 153,* 65–71.

APA Task Force on Laboratory Tests in Psychiatry. (1987). The dexamethasone suppression test: An overview of its current status in psychiatry. *American Journal of Psychiatry, 114,* 1253–1262.

Arana, G. W., Baldessarini, R. J., & Ornsteen, M. (1985). The dexamethasone suppression test for diagnosis and prognosis in psychiatry. *Archives of General Psychiatry, 42,* 1193–1204.

Asnis, G. M., Halbreich, U., Nathan, R. S., Ostrow, L., Novacenko, H., Endicott, J., & Sachar, E. J. (1982). The dexamethasone suppression test in depressive illness: Clinical correlates. *Psychoneuroendocrinology, 7,* 295–301.

Balon, R., Pohl, R., Yeragani, V. K., Rainey, J. M., & Weinberg, P. (1988). Lactate- and isoproterenol-induced panic attacks in panic disorder patients. *Psychiatry Research, 23,* 153–160.

Balon, R., Yergani, V. K., & Pohl, R. (1988). Phenomenological comparison of dextrose-, lactate-, and isoproterenol-associated panic attacks. *Psychiatry Research, 26,* 43–50.

Balon, R., Jordan, M., Pohl, R., *et al.* (1989). Family history of anxiety disorders in control subjects with lactate-induced panic attacks. *American Journal of Psychiatry, 146,* 1304–1306.

Baron, M., Barkai, A., Gruen, R., Peslow, E., Fieve, R., & Quitkin, F. (1986). Platelet [3H]imipramine binding in affective disorders: Trait versus state characteristics. *American Journal of Psychiatry, 143,* 711–717.

Baxter, L. R., Phelps, M. E., Mazziotta, J. C., Schwartz, J. M., Gerner, R. H., Selin, C. E., & Sumida, R. M. (1985). Cerebral metabolic rates for glucose in mood disorders: Studies with positron emission tomography and fluorodeoxyglucose F18. *Archives of General Psychiatry, 42,* 441–447.

Baxter, L. R., Schwartz, J. M., Phelps, M. E., Mazziotta, J. C., Guze, B. H., Selin, C. E., Gerner,

R. H., & Sumida, R. M. (1989). Reduction of prefrontal cortex glucose metabolism common to three types of depression. *Archives of General Psychiatry, 46,* 243–250.

Beauge, F., Stibler, H., & Borg, S. (1985). Abnormal fluidity and surface carbohydrate content of the erythrocyte membrane in alcoholic patients. *Alcohol Clinical Experimental Research, 9,* 322–327.

Berger, M., Riemann, D., Hoechli, D., & Spiegel, R. (1989). The cholinergic rapid eye movement sleep induction test with RS-86. *Archives of General Psychiatry, 46,* 412–428.

Berger, P. A., Faull, K. F., Kilkowski, J., Anderson, P. J., Kraemer, H., Davis, K. L., & Barchas, J. D. (1980). CSF monoamine metabolites in depression and schizophrenia. *American Journal of Psychiatry, 137,* 174–180.

Berrettini, W. H., Nurnberger, J. I., Jr., Hare, T., Gershon, E. S., & Post, R. M., (1982). Plasma and CSF GABA in affective illness. *British Journal of Psychiatry, 141,* 483–488.

Boismare, F., Lhuintre, J. P., Daoust, M., Moore, N., Saligaut, C., & Hillemand, B. (1987). Platelet affinity for serotonin is increased in alcoholics and former alcoholics: A biological marker for dependence? *Alcohol & Alcoholism, 22,* 155–159.

Bowen, R. C., Orchard, R. C., Keegan, D. L., & D'Arcy, C. (1985). Mitral valve prolapse and psychiatric disorders. *Psychosomatics, 26,* 926–932.

Brambilla, F., Ferrari, E., Invitti, C., Zanoboni, A., Massironi, R., Catalano, M., Cocchi, D., & Muller, E. E. (1989). Alpha$_2$-adrenoceptor sensitivity in anorexia nervosa: GH response to clonidine or GHRH stimulation. *Biological Psychiatry, 25,* 256–264.

Braunwald, E. (1983). Valvular heart disease. In R. D. Petersdorf, H. E. Adams, E. Braunwald, K. J. Isselbacher, J. B. Martin, & J. D. Wilson (Eds.), *Harrison's principles of internal medicine* (10th ed., pp. 1402–1417). New York: McGraw-Hill.

Briley, M. S., Langer, S. Z., Raizman, R., Sechter, D., & Zarifian, E. (1980). Tritiated imipramine binding sites are decreased in platelets of untreated depressed patients. *Science, 209,* 303–305.

Butler, J., & Leonard, B. E. (1988). The platelet serotonergic system in depression and following sertraline treatment. *International Clinical Psychopharmacology, 3,* 343–347.

Campbell, I. C. (1981). Blood platelets in psychiatry. *British Journal of Psychiatry, 138,* 78–80.

Carroll, B. J., Curtis, G. C., & Mendels, J. (1976). Neuroendocrine regulation in depression. II. *Archives of General Psychiatry, 33,* 1051–1058.

Checkley, S. A., Slade, A. P., & Shur, E. (1981). Growth hormone and other responses to clonidine in patients with endogenous depression. *British Journal of Psychiatry, 138,* 51–55.

Cleghorn, J. M., Garnett, E. S., Nahmias, C., Firnau, G., Brown, G. M., Kaplan, R., Szechtman, H., & Szechtman, B. (1989). Increased frontal and reduced parietal glucose metabolism in acute untreated schizophrenia. *Psychiatry Research, 28,* 119–133.

Coccaro, E. F., Siever, L. J., Klar, H. M., Maurer, G., Cochrane, K., Cooper, T. B., Mohs, R. C., & Davis, K. L. (1989). Serotonergic studies in patients with affective and personality disorders. *Archives of General Psychiatry, 46,* 587–599.

Coffee, R. G., & Hadden, J. W. (1985). Neurotransmitters, hormones, and cyclic nucleotides in lymphocyte regulation. *Federation of American Societies for Experimental Biology Proceedings, 44,* 112–117.

Cohen, R. M., Semple, W. E., & Gross, M. G. (1986). Positron emission tomography. *Psychiatric Clinics of North America, 9,* 63–79.

Cook, B. L., Shukla, S., & Hoff, A.L. (1986). EEG abnormalities in bipolar affective disorder. *Journal of Affective Disorders, 11,* 147–149.

Coppen, A., Swade, C., & Wood, K. (1980). Lithium restores abnormal platelet 5-HT transport in patients with affective disorders. *British Journal of Psychiatry, 136,* 235–238.

Coppen, A. J., & Doogan, D. P. (1988). Serotonin and its place in the pathogenesis of depression. *Journal of Clinical Psychiatry, 49,* 4s–11s.

Coryell, W. (1984). The use of laboratory tests in psychiatric diagnosis: The DST as an example. *Psychiatric Development, 3,* 139–159.

Coryell, W. (1988). Secondary depression. In J. O. Cavenar, Jr. (Ed.), *Psychiatry* (pp. 1–9). Philadelphia: J. B. Lippencott.

Coryell, W., Gaffney, G., & Burkhardt, P. E. (1982). The dexamethasone suppression test and familial subtypes of depression—a naturalistic replication. *Biological Psychiatry, 17,* 33–39.

Cowen, P. J., Geaney, D. P., Schachter, M., Green, A. R., & Elliot, J. M. (1984). Desipramine treatment in normal subjects. *Archives of General Psychiatry, 43*, 61–67.

Cowley, D. S., Dager, S. R., & Dunner, D. L. (1986). Lactate-induced panic in primary affective disorder. *American Journal of Psychiatry, 143*, 646–648.

Cowley, D. S., Dager, S. R., & Dunner, D. L., (1987). Lactate infusions in major depression without panic attacks. *Journal of Psychiatric Research, 21*, 243–248.

Cowley, D. S., Hyde, T. S., Dager, S. R., & Dunner, D. L. (1987). Lactate infusions: The role of baseline anxiety. *Psychiatry Research, 21*, 169–179.

Dager, S. R., Comess, K. A., Saal, A. K., Sisk, E. J., Beach, K. W., & Dunner, D. L. (1989). Diagnostic reliability of M-mode echocardiography for detecting mitral valve prolapse in 50 consecutive panic patients. *Comprehensive Psychiatry, 30*, 369–375.

Davis, J. M., Koslow, S. H., Gibbons, R. D., Maas, J. W., Bowden, C. L., Casper, R., Hanin, I., Javaid, J. I., Chang, S. S., & Stokes, P. E. (1988). Cerebrospinal fluid and urinary biogenic amines in depressed and healthy controls. *Archives of General Psychiatry, 45*, 705–717.

DeLisi, L. E., Buchsbaum, M. S., Holcomb, H. H., Langston, K. C., King, A. C., Kessler, R., Pickar, D., Carpenter, W. T., Morihisa, J. M., Margolin, R. *et al.* (1989). Increased temporal lobe glucose use in chronic schizophrenic patients. *Biological Psychiatry, 25*, 835–851.

Devereux, R. B., Kramer-Fox, R., & Shear, M. K. (1986). Prevalence of panic disorder in relatives [letter]. *Psychosomatics, 27*, 797.

Diamond, I., Wrubel, B., Estrin, W., & Gordon, A. (1987). Basal and adenosine receptor-stimulated levels of cAMP are reduced in lymphocytes from alcoholic patients. *Proceedings of the National Academy of Sciences of the United States of America, 84*, 1413–1416.

Dillon, D. J., Gorman, J. M., Liebowitz, M. R., Fyer, A. J., and Klein, D. F. (1987). Measurement of lactate-induced panic and anxiety. *Psychiatry Research, 20*, 97–105.

Dorovini-Zis, K., & Zis, A. P. (1987). Increased adrenal weight in victims of violent suicide. *American Journal of Psychiatry, 144*, 1214–1215.

Dupont, R. M., Jernigan, T. L., & Butters, N. (1990). Subcortical abnormalities detected in bipolar affective disorder using MRI. *Archives of General Psychiatry, 47*, 55–59.

Eriksson, E., Balldin, J., Lindstedt, G., & Modigh, K. (1988). Growth hormone responses to the alpha$_2$-adrenoceptor agonist guanfacine and to growth hormone releasing hormone in depressed patients and controls. *Psychiatry Research, 26*, 59–67.

Extein, I., Tallman, J., Smith, C. C., & Goodwin, F. K. (1979). Changes in lymphocyte beta-adrenergic receptors in depression and mania. *Psychiatry Research, 1*, 191–197.

Farde, L., Wiesel, F., Stone-Elander, S., Halldin, C., Nordstrom, A., Hall, H., & Sedvall, G. (1990). D$_2$ dopamine receptors in neuroleptic-naive schizophrenic patients. *Archives of General Psychiatry, 47*, 213–219.

Feighner, J. P., Robins, E., Guze, S. B., & Goodwin, F. K. (1972). Diagnostic criteria for use in psychiatric research. *Archives of General Psychiatry, 26*, 57–63.

Fleissner, A., Seiffert, R., Schneider, K. *et al.* (1987). Platelet monoamine oxidase activity and schizophrenia—a myth that refuses to die? *European Archives of Psychiatry and Neurology, 237*, 8–15.

Gaffney, F. A., Fenton, B. J., Lane, C. R., & Lake, C. R. (1988). Hemodynamic, ventilatory, and biochemical responses of panic patients and normal controls with sodium lactate infusion. *Archives of General Psychiatry, 45*, 53–60.

Garcia-Sevilla, J. A., Zis, A. P., Hollingsworth, P. J., Greden, J. F., & Smith, C. B. (1981). Platelet alpha$_2$-adrenergic receptors in major depressive disorder: Binding of tritiated clonidine before and after tricyclic antidepressant drug treatment. *Archives of General Psychiatry, 38*, 1327–1333.

Garcia-Sevilla, J. A., Guimon, J., Garcia-Vallejo, P., & Fuster, M. J. (1986). Biochemical and functional evidence of supersensitive platelet alpha$_2$-adrenoceptors in major affective disorder. *Archives of General Psychiatry, 43*, 51–57.

George, D. T., Nutt, D. J., Waxman, R. P., & Linnoila, M. (1989). Panic response to lactate administration in alcoholic and nonalcoholic patients with panic disorder. *American Journal of Psychiatry, 146*, 1161–1165.

Gibbons, R. D., & Davis, J. M. (1986). Consistent evidence for a biological subtype of depression characterized by low CSF 5-HIAA monoamine levels. *Acta Psychiatrica Scandinavica, 74*, 8–12.

Giles, D. E., Roffwarg, H. P., Schlesser, M. A., & Rush, A. J. (1986). Which endogenous depressive symptoms relate to REM latency reduction? *Biological Psychiatry, 21*, 473–482.

Giles, D. E., Roffwarg, H. P., & Rush, A. J. (1987). REM latency concordance in depressed family members. *Biological Psychiatry, 22*, 910–914.

Giles, D. E., Schlesser, M. A., Rush, A. J., Orsulak, P. J., Fulton, C. L., & Roffwarg, H. P. (1987). Polysomnographic findings and dexamethasone nonsuppression in unipolar depression: A replication and extension. *Biological Psychiatry, 22*, 872–882.

Giles, D. E., Kupfer, D. J., Roffwarg, H. P., Rush, A. J., Biggs, M. M., & Etzel, B. A. (1989). Polysomnographic parameters in first-degree relatives of unipolar probands. *Psychiatry Research, 27*, 127–136.

Gillin, J. C., Duncan, W. C., Murphy, D. L., Post, R. M., Wehr, T. A., Goodwin, F. K., Wyatt, R. J., & Bunney, W. E., Jr. (1981). Age-related changes in sleep in depressed and normal subjects. *Psychiatry Research, 4*, 72–78.

Gitlin, M., Weiner, H., Fairbanks, L. (1987). Failure of T3 to potentiate tricyclic antidepressant response. *Journal of Affective Disorders, 13*, 267–272.

Gold, P. W., & Chrousos, G. P. (1985). Clinical studies with corticotropin releasing factor: Implications for the diagnosis and pathophysiology of depression, Cushing's disease, and adrenal insufficiency. *Psychoneuroendocrinology, 10*, 401–419.

Goodwin, D. W. (1986). *Anxiety.* New York: Oxford University Press.

Gorman, J. M., Cohen, B. S., Liebowitz, M. R., Fyer, A. J., Ross, D., Davies, S. O., & Klein, D. F. (1986). Blood gas changes and hypophosphatemia in lactate-induced panic. *Archives of General Psychiatry, 43*, 1067–1071.

Gorman, J. M., Goetz, R. R., Fyer, M., King, D. L., Fyer, A. J., Liebowitz, M. R., & Klein, D. F. (1988). The mitral valve prolapse connection. *Psychosomatic Medicine, 50*, 114–122.

Gur, R. E., Mozley, P. D., Resnick, S. M., Shtasel, D., Kohn, M., Zimmerman, R., Herman, G., Atlas, S., Grossman, R., Erwin, R., & Gur, R. C. (1991). Magnetic resonance imaging in schizophrenia: I. Volumetric analysis of brain and cerebrospinal fluid. *Archives of General Psychiatry, 48*, 407–412.

Halper, J. P., Brown, R. P., Sweeney, J. A., Kocsis, J. H., Peters, A., Mann, J. J. (1988). Blunted beta-adrenergic responsivity of peripheral blood mononuclear cells in endogenous depression. *Archives of General Psychiatry, 45*, 241–246.

Hartman, N., Kramer, R., Brown, W. T., & Devereux, R. B. (1982). Panic disorder in patients with mitral valve prolapse. *American Journal of Psychiatry, 139*, 669–670.

Henn, F. A. (1986). The neurobiologic basis of psychiatric illnesses. In G. Winokur & P. Clayton (Eds.), *The medical basis of psychiatry* (pp. 461–485). Philadelphia: W. B. Saunders.

Hollander, E., Liebowitz, M. R., Cohen, B., Gorman, J. M., Fyer, A. J., Papp, L. A., & Klein, D. F. (1989). Prolactin and sodium lactate-induced panic. *Psychiatry Research, 28*, 181–191.

Hollander, E., Liebowitz, M. R., Gorman, J. M., Cohen, B., Fyer, A., & Klein, D. F. (1989). Cortisol and sodium lactate-induced panic. *Archives of General Psychiatry, 46*, 135–140.

Holzman, P. S., Proctor, L. R., & Hughes, D. W. (1973). Eye-tracking patterns in schizophrenia. *Science, 181*, 179–180.

Holzman, P. S., Proctor, L. R., Levy, D. L., Yasillo, N. J., Meltzer, H. Y., & Hurt, S. W. (1974). Eye-tracking dysfunctions in schizophrenic patients and their relatives. *Archives of General Psychiatry, 31*, 143–151.

Holzman, P. S., Levy, D. L., & Proctor, L. R. (1976). Smooth pursuit eye movements, attention and schizophrenia. *Archives of General Psychiatry, 33*, 1415–1420.

Holzman, P. S., Kringlen, E., Levy, D. L., & Haberman, S. (1980). Deviant eye tracking in twins discordant for psychosis: A replication. *Archives of General Psychiatry, 37*, 627–631.

Holzman, P. S., Kringlen, E., Matthysse, S., Flanagan, S. D., Lipton, R. B., Cramer, G., Levin, S., Lange, K., & Levy, D. L. (1988). A single dominant gene can account for eye tracking dysfunctions and schizophrenia in offspring of discordant twins. *Archives of General Psychiatry, 45*, 641–647.

Hrdina, P. D. (1989). Imipramine binding sites in brain and platelets: Role in affective disorders. *International Journal of Clinical Pharmacological Research, 9*, 119–122.

Ieni, J. R., Zukin, S. R., & Van Praag, H. M. (1984). Human platelets possess multiple [3H]-imipramine binding sites. *European Journal of Pharmacology, 106*, 669–672.

Ivanovic, I. D., & Majkic-Singh, N. (1988). Determination of platelet monoamine oxidase by new continuous spectrophotometric method. *Journal of Clinical Chemistry and Clinical Biochemistry, 26*, 447–451.

Jaeckle, R., Kathol, R. G., & Lopez, J. (1987). Enhanced adrenal sensitivity to exogenous cosyntropin stimulation in major depression. *Archives of General Psychiatry, 44*, 233–240.

Janowsky, D. S., El-Yousef, M. K., & Davis, J. M. (1972). Cholinergic-adrenergic hypothesis of mania and depression. *Lancet, 2*, 632.

Janowsky, D. S., Risch, S. C., Ziegler, M. G., Gillin, J. C., Huey, L., & Rausch, J. (1986). Physostigmine-induced epinephrine release in patients with affective disorder. *American Journal of Psychiatry, 143*, 919–921.

John, E. R., Prichep, L. S., Fridman, J., & Easton, P. (1988). Neurometrics: computer-assisted differential diagnosis of brain dysfunctions. *Science, 239*, 162–169.

Kafka, M. S., & Paul, S. (1986). Platelet alpha$_2$-adrenergic receptors in depression. *Archives of General Psychiatry, 43*, 91–95.

Kasper, S., & Beckman, H. (1983). Dexamethasone suppression test in a pluridiagnostic approach: Its relationship to psychopathological and clinical variables. *Acta Psychiatrica Scandinavica, 68*, 31–37.

Kathol, R. G. (1985a). Circadian rhythm and peak frequency of corticosteroid excretion: Relationship to affective disorder. *Psychiatry Medicine, 3*, 53–63.

Kathol, R. G. (1985b). Persistent elevation of urinary free cortisol and loss of circannual periodicity in recovered depressive patients. *Journal of Affective Disorders, 8*, 137–145.

Kathol, R. G., Jaeckle, R. S., Lopez, J. F., & Meller, W. H. (1989). Pathophysiology of HPA axis abnormalities in patients with major depression: An update. *American Journal of Psychiatry, 146*, 311–317.

Kemali, D., DelVecchio, M., & Maj, M. (1982). Increased noradrenaline levels in CSF and plasma of schizophrenics. *Biological Psychiatry, 17*, 711–717.

Kemali, D., Maj, M., Galderisi, S., Salvati, A., Starace, F., Valente, A., & Pirozzi, R. (1987). Clinical, biological, and neuropsychological features associated with lateral ventricular enlargement in DSM-III schizophrenic disorder. *Psychiatry Research, 21*, 137–149.

Kirkegaard, C., & Carroll, B. J. (1980). Dissociation of TSH and adrenocortical disturbances in endogenous depression. *Psychiatry Research, 3*, 253–264.

Kirkegaard, C., Norlein, N., Lauridsen, U. B., Bjorum, N., & Christiansen, C. (1975). Protirelin stimulation test and thyroid function during treatment of depression. *Archives of General Psychiatry, 32*, 1115–1118.

Kupfer, D. J., & Foster, F. G. (1972). Interval between onset of sleep and rapid eye movement sleep as an indicator of depression. *Lancet, 11*, 684–686.

Kupfer, D. J., Foster, F. G., Coble, P. *et al.* (1978). The application of EEG sleep for the differential diagnosis of affective disorders. *American Journal of Psychiatry, 135*, 69–74.

Lake, C. R., Sternberg, D. E., van Kammen, D. P., Ballenger, J. C., Ziegler, M. G., Post, R. M., Kopin, I. J., & Bunney, W. E. (1980). Schizophrenia: Elevated cerebrospinal fluid norepinephrine. *Science, 207*, 331–333.

Langer, S. Z., Sechter, D., Loo, H., Raisman, R., & Zarifian, E. (1986). Electroconvulsive shock therapy and maximum binding of platelet tritiated imipramine binding in depression. *Archives of General Psychiatry, 43*, 949–952.

Langer, S. Z., Galzin, A. M., Poirier, M. F., Loo, H., Sechter, D., & Zarifian, E. (1987). Association of 3H-imipramine and 3H-paroxetine binding with the 5HT transporter in brain and platelets: Relevance to studies in depression. *Journal of Receptor Research, 7*, 499–521.

Lauer, C., Zulley, J., Krieg, J. C., Riemann, D., & Berger, M. (1988). EEG and thee cholinergic REM induction test in anorexic and bulimic patients. *Psychiatry Research, 26*, 171–181.

Lesch, K. P., Muller, U., Kruse, K., & Schulte, H. M. (1989). Endocrine responses to growth hormone-releasing hormone, thyrotropin-releasing hormone and corticotropin-releasing hormone in depression. *Acta Psychiatrica Scandinavica, 79*, 597–602.

Levy, D. L., Yasillo, N. J., Dorus, E., Shaughnessy, R., Gibbons, R. D., Peterson, J., Janicak, P. G., Gaviria, M., & Davis, J. M. (1983). Relatives of unipolar and bipolar patients have normal pursuit. *Psychiatry Research, 10*, 285–293.

Lewis, D. A., & McChesney, C. (1985). Tritiated imipramine binding distinguishes between subtypes of depression. *Archives of General Psychiatry, 42*, 485–488.

Lewis, D. A., Noyes, R., Coryell, W., & Clancy, J. (1985). Tritiated imipramine binding to platelets is decreased in patients with agoraphobia. *Psychiatry Research, 16*, 1–9.

Lieber, A. L., & Newbury, N. D. (1988a). Diagnosis and subtyping of depressive disorders by quantitative electroencephalography: III. Discriminating unipolar from bipolar depression. *Hillside Journal of Clinical Psychiatry, 10*, 165–172.

Lieber, A. L., & Newbury, N. D. (1988b). Diagnosis and subtyping of depressive disorders by quantitative electroencephalography: IV. Discriminating subtypes of unipolar depression. *Hillside Journal of Clinical Psychiatry, 10*, 173–182.

Liebowitz, M. R., Gorman, J. M., Fyer, A., Dillon, D., Levitt, M., & Klein, D. F. (1986). Possible mechanisms for lactate's induction of panic. *American Journal of Psychiatry, 143*, 495–500.

Lingjaerde, O. (1983). Serotonin uptake and efflux in blood platelets from untreated and neuroleptic-treated schizophrenics. *Biological Psychiatry, 18*, 1345–1356.

Loosen, P. T., Wilson, J. C., Dew, B. W. et al. (1979). Thyrotropin-releasing hormone (TRH) in abstinent alcoholic men. *American Journal of Psychiatry, 136*, 540–547.

Loosen, P. T., Prange, A. J., Jr., & Wilson, J. C. (1983). TRH (Protirelin) in depressed alcoholic men: Behavioral and endocrine response. *American Journal of Psychiatry, 140*, 1145–1149.

Lopez, J., Kathol, R. G., & Jaeckle, R. S. (1987). The HPA axis response to insulin hypoglycemia in depression. *Biological Psychiatry, 22*, 153–166.

Maas, J. W., Koslow, S. H., Davis, J., Katz, M., Frazer, A., Bowden, C. L., Berman, N., Gibbons, R., Stokes, P., & Landis, H. (1987). Catecholamine metabolism and disposition in healthy subjects. *Archives of General Psychiatry, 44*, 337–344.

Maj, M., Arena, F., Galderisi, S., Starace, F., & Kemali, D. (1987). Factors associated with decreased platelet MAO activity in chronic schizophrenics. *Progress in Neuropsychopharmacology and Biological Psychiatry, 11*, 79–86.

Mann, J. J., Brown, R. P., Halper, J. P., Sweeney, J. A., Kocsis, J. H., Stokes, P. E., & Bilezikian, J. P. (1985). Reduced sensitivity of lymphocyte beta-adrenergic receptors in patients with endogenous depression and psychomotor agitation. *New England Journal of Medicine, 313*, 715–720.

Mann, J. J., Kaplan, R. D., & Bird, E. D. (1986). Elevated postmortem monoamine oxidase B activity in the caudate nucleus of Huntington's disease compared to schizophrenics and controls. *Journal of Neural Transmission, 65*, 277–283.

Matussek, N., Ackenheil, M., Hippius, H., Muller, F., Schroder, H., Schultes, H., & Wasilewski, B. (1980). Effect of clonidine on growth hormone release in psychiatric patients and controls. *Psychiatry Research, 2*, 25–36.

Meltzer, H. Y., & Zureick, J. K. (1987). Relationship of auditory hallucinations and paranoia to platelet MAO activity in schizophrenics: Sex and race interactions. *Psychiatry Research, 11*, 79–86.

Meltzer, H. Y., & Aurora, R. C. (1988). Genetic control of serotonin uptake in blood platelets: A twin study. *Psychiatry Research, 24*, 263–269.

Meltzer, H. Y., Aurora, R. C., Baber, R., & Tricou, B. J. (1981). Serotonin uptake in blood platelets of psychiatry. *Archives of General Psychiatry, 38*, 1322–1326.

Mitchell, P. B., Bearn, J. A., Corn, T. H., & Checkley, S. A. (1988). Growth hormone response to clonidine after recovery in patients with endogenous depression. *British Journal of Psychiatry, 152*, 34–38.

Muller, N., Hoehe, M., Klein, H. E., Nieberle, G., Kapfhammer, H. P., May, F., Muller, O. A., & Fichter, M. (1989). Endocrinological studies in alcoholics during withdrawal and after abstinence. *Psychoneuroendocrinology, 14*, 113–123.

Nemeroff, C. B., Owens, M. J., Bissette, G., Andorn, A. C., & Stanley, M. (1988). Reduced corticotropin releasing factor binding sites in the frontal cortex of suicide victims. *Archives of General Psychiatry, 45,* 577–580.

Okasha, A., & Madikur, O. (1982). Cortical and central atrophy in chronic schizophrenia: A controlled study. *Acta Psychiatrica Scandinavica, 65,* 29–34.

Overstreet, D. H., Janowsky, D. S., & Rezvani, A. H. (1989). Alcoholism and depressive disorders: Is cholinergic sensitivity a biological marker? *Alcohol, 24,* 253–255.

Owen, F., Crow, T. J., Frith, C. D., Johnsson, J. A., Johnstone, E. C., Lofhouse, R., Owens, G. C., & Poulter, M. (1987). Selective decreases in MAO-B activity in postmortem brains from schizophrenic patients with type II syndrome. *British Journal of Psychiatry, 151,* 514–519.

Pandey, G. N., Janicak, P. G., Javaid, J. I., & Davis, J. M. (1989). Increased ^{3}H-clonidine binding in the platelets of patients with depressive and schizophrenic disorders. *Psychiatry Research, 28,* 73–88.

Pandurangi, A. K., Dewan, M. J., & Boucher, M. (1986). A comprehensive study of schizophrenic patients: II. biological, neuropsychological, and clinical correlates of CT abnormality. *Acta Psychiatrica Scandinavica, 73,* 161–171.

Pfefferbaum, A., Zipursky, R. B., Lim, K. O., Katz, L. M., Stahl, S. M., & Jernigan, T. L. (1988). Computed tomographic evidence for generalized sulcal and ventricular enlargement in schizophrenia. *Archives of General Psychiatry, 45,* 633–640.

Pitts, F. N., & McClure, J. N. (1967). Lactate metabolism in anxiety neurosis. *New England Journal of Medicine, 277,* 1329–1336.

Pletscher, A. (1968). Metabolism transfer and storage of 5HT in blood platelets. *British Journal of Pharmacology, 32,* 1–16.

Potkin, S. G., Weinberger, D. R., Linnoila, M., & Wyatt, R. J. (1983). Low CSF 5-HIAA in schizophrenic patients with enlarged cerebral ventricles. *American Journal of Psychiatry, 140,* 21–25.

Prang, A. J., Wilson, I. C., Lara, P. P., Alltop, L. B., & Breese, G. R. (1972). Effects of thyrotropin releasing hormone in depression. *Lancet, 11,* 999.

Quitana, J. (1989). Platelet serotonin uptake dynamic changes in depression: Effects of long-term imipramine treatment and clinical recovery. *Journal of Affective Disorders, 16,* 233–242.

Raichle, M. E., Grubb, R. L., Gado, M. H., Eichling, J. O., & Ter-Pogossian, M. P. (1976). Correlation between regional cerebral blood flow and oxidative metabolism. *Archives of Neurology, 8,* 523–526.

Rausch, J. L., Janowsky, D. S., Risch, S. C., & Huey, L. Y. (1986). A kinetic analysis and replication of decreased platelet serotonin uptake in depressed patients. *Psychiatry Research, 19,* 105–112.

Rausch, J. L., Rich, C. L., & Risch, S. C. (1988). Platelet serotonin transport after a single ECT. *Psychopharmacology, 95,* 139–141.

Reveley, M. A., Glover, V., Sandler, M., & Spokes, E. G. (1981). Brain monoamine oxidase activity in schizophrenics and controls. *Archives of General Psychiatry, 38,* 663–665.

Reynolds, C. F., & Kupfer, D. J. (1987). Sleep research in affective illness: State-of-the-art circa 1987. *Sleep, 10,* 199–215.

Reynolds, C. F., Kupfer, D. J., & Taska, L. S. (1985). EEG sleep in healthy elderly, depressed, and demented subjects. *Biological Psychiatry, 20,* 431–442.

Rieder, R. O., Mann, L. S., Weinberger, D. R., van Kammen, D. P., & Post, R. M. (1983). Computed tomographic scans in patients with schizophrenia, schizoaffective disorder, and bipolar disorder. *Archives of General Psychiatry, 40,* 735–739.

Riemann, D., & Berger, M. (1989). EEG sleep in depression and in remission and the REM sleep response to the cholinergic agonist RS-86. *Neuropsychopharmacology, 2,* 145–152.

Rose, R. M., Castellani, S., Boeringa, J. A., Boeringa, A., Malek-Ahmadi, P., Lankford, A., Bessman, J. D., Fritz, R. R., Denney, C. B., Denney, R. M., & Abell, C. W. (1986). Platelet MAO concentration and molecular activity: II. Comparison of normal and schizophrenic populations. *Psychiatry Research, 17,* 141–151.

Rosenberg, R., Vostrup, S., Andersen, A., & Bolwig, T. (1988). Effect of ECT on cerebral blood flow in melancholia assessed with SPECT. *Convulsive Therapy, 4,* 62–73.

Roy, A., Jimmerson, D. C., Pickar, D., (1986). Plasma 3-methoxy-4-hydroxyphenylglycol (MHPG) in depressive disorders: Relationship to the dexamethasone suppression test. *American Journal of Psychiatry, 143*, 846–851.

Roy, A., Pickar, D., DeJong, J., Karoum, F., & Linnoila, M. (1988). Norepinephrine and its metabolites in cerebrospinal fluid, plasma, and urine: Relationship to hypothalamic-pituitary-adrenal axis function in depression. *Archives of General Psychiatry, 45*, 849–857.

Roy, A., DeJong, J., & Linnoila, M. (1989). Cerebrospinal fluid monoamine metabolites and suicidal behavior in depressed patients: A five-year follow-up study. *Archives of General Psychiatry, 46*, 609–612.

Rush, A. J., Giles, D. E., Roffwarg, H. P., & Parker, C. R. (1982). Sleep EEG and dexamethasone suppression test findings in outpatients with unipolar major depressive disorders. *Biological Psychiatry, 17*, 327–341.

Rush, A. J., Erman, M. K., Giles, D. E., Schlesser, M. A., Carpenter, M. A., Vasavada, N., & Roffwarg, H. P. (1986). Polysomnographic findings in recently drug-free and clinically remitted depressed patients. *Archives of General Psychiatry, 43*, 878–884.

Sackeim, H. A., Prohovnik, I., Moeller, J. R., Brown, R. P., Apter, S., Prudic, J., Devanand D. P., & Mukherjee, S. (1990). Regional cerebral blood flow in mood disorders. *Archives of General Psychiatry, 47*, 60–70.

Sanderson, W. C., Rapee, R. M., & Barlow, D. H. (1989). The influence of an illusion of control on panic attacks induced via inhalation of 5.5% carbon dioxide-enriched air. *Archives of General Psychiatry, 46*, 157–164.

Schlesser, M. A., Winokur, G., & Sherman, B. M. (1980). Hypothalamic-pituitary-adrenal axis activity in depressive illness. *Archives of General Psychiatry, 37*, 737–743.

Schneider, L. S. (1990). Biological markers in geriatric depression. *Psychiatric Annals, 20*, 83–91.

Schneider, L. S., Fredrickson, E., Severson, J., & Sloan, R. B. (1986). 3H-imipramine binding in depressed elderly: Relationship to family history and clinical response. *Psychiatry Research, 19*, 257–266.

Schuckit, M. A. (1984). Subjective responses to alcohol in sons of alcoholics and controls. *Archives of General Psychiatry, 41*, 879–884.

Schuckit, M. A., & Gold, E. O. (1988). A simultaneous evaluation of multiple markers of ethanol/placebo challenges in sons of alcoholics and controls. *Archives of General Psychiatry, 45*, 211–216.

Schuckit, M. A., Gold, E., & Risch, C. (1987). Plasma cortisol levels following ethanol in sons of alcoholics and controls. *Archives of General Psychiatry, 44*, 942–945.

Schulsinger, F., Parnas, J., Petersen, E. T., Schulsinger, H. T., Teasdale, T. W., Mednick, S. A., Moller, L., & Silverton, L. (1984). Cerebral ventricular size in the offspring of schizophrenic mothers. *Archives of General Psychiatry, 41*, 602–606.

Schwartz, J. M., Baxter, L. R., Mazziotta, J. C., Gerner, R. H., & Phelps, M. E. (1987). The differential diagnosis of depression: Relevance of positron emission tomography studies of cerebral glucose metabolism to the bipolar-unipolar dichotomy. *Journal of the American Medical Association, 258*, 1368–1374.

Sevy, S., Papadimitriou, G. N., Surmont, D. W., Goldman, S., & Mendlewicz, J. (1989). Noradrenergic function in generalized anxiety disorder, major depressive disorder, and healthy subjects. *Biological Psychiatry, 25*, 141–152.

Shaw, D. M., Camps, F. E., & Eccleston, E. G. (1967). 5-hydroxytryptamine in the hindbrain of depressive suicides. *British Journal of Psychiatry, 113*, 1407–1411.

Shagass, C., Amadeo, M., & Overton, D. A. (1974). Eye-tracking performance in psychiatric patients. *Biological Psychiatry, 9*, 245–260.

Shibuya, A., & Yoshida, A. (1988a). Frequency of the atypical aldehyde dehydrogenase-2 gene in Japanese and Caucasians. *American Journal of Human Genetics, 43*, 741–743.

Shibuya, A., & Yoshida, A. (1988b). Genotypes of alcohol-metabolizing enzymes in Japanese with alcohol liver diseases: a strong association of the usual Caucasian-type, aldehydedehydrogenase gene (ALD½) with the disease. *American Journal of Human Genetics, 43*, 744–748.

Siever, L. J., & Uhde, T. W. (1985). New studies and perspectives on the noradrenergic receptor system in depression: Effects of the alph-2-adrenergic agonist clonidine. *Biological Psychiatry, 19*, 131–156.

Siever, L. J., Uhde, T. W., Jimmerson, D. C., Post, R. M., Lake, C. R., & Murphy, D. L. (1984). Plasma cortisol responses to clonidine in depressed patients and controls. *Archives of General Psychiatry, 41*, 63–68.

Silfverskiold, P., & Risberg, J. (1989). Regional cerebral blood flow in depression and mania. *Archives of General Psychiatry, 46*, 253–259.

Sitaram, N., Nurnberger, J. I., Jr., Gershon, E. S., & Gillin, J. C. (1980). Faster cholinergic REM sleep induction in euthymic patients with primary affective illness. *Science, 208*, 200–202.

Sitaram, N., Nurnberger, J. I., Jr., Gershon, E. S., & Gillin, J. C. (1982). Cholinergic regulation of mood and REM sleep: Potential model and marker of vulnerability to affective disorder. *American Journal of Psychiatry, 139*, 571–576.

Sitaram, N., Dube, S., Jones, D., Bell, J., Gurevich, D., & Gershon, E. S. (1984). Cholinergic REM-induction response as a state and possible genetic vulnerability marker of depression. *Clinical Neuropharmacology, 7*, 966–967.

Slotkin, T. A., Whitmore, W. L., & Barnes, S. A. (1989). Reduced inhibitory effect of imipramine on radiolabeled serotonin uptake into platelets in geriatric depression. *Biological Psychiatry, 25*, 687–689.

Sneddon, J. M. (1973). Blood platelets as a model for monoamine-containing neurones. *Progress in Neurobiology, 1*, 151–187.

Spohn, H. E., Coyne, L., & Spray, J. (1988). The effect of neuroleptics and tardive dyskinesia on smooth-pursuit eye movement in chronic schizophrenics. *Archives of General Psychiatry, 45*, 833–840.

Stahl, S. M. (1977). The human platelet. *Archives of General Psychiatry, 34*, 509–516.

Stahl, S. M., & Meltzer, H. Y. (1978). A kinetic and pharmacologic analysis of 5-hydroxytryptamine transport by human platelets and platelet storage granules: Comparison with central serotonergic neurones. *Journal of Pharmacological Experimental Therapy, 205*, 118–132.

Steiger, A., von Bardeleben, U., Herth, T., & Holsboer, F. (1989). Sleep EEG and nocturnal secretion of cortisol and growth hormone in male patients with endogenous depression before treatment and after recovery. *Journal of Affective Disorders, 16*, 189–195.

Strom-Olsen, R., & Weil-Malherbe, H. (1964). Humoral changes in manic-depressive psychosis with particular reference to the excretion of catecholamines in urine. *Journal of Mental Science, 104*, 696–704.

Swartz, C. M., Drews, V., & Cadoret, R. (1987). Decreased epinephrine in familial alcoholism. *Archives of General Psychiatry, 44*, 938–941.

Tabekoff, B., Hoffman, P. L., Lee, J. M., Saito, T., Willard, B., & Leon-Jones, F. D. (1988). Differences in platelet enzyme activity between alcoholics and controls. *New England Journal of Medicine, 318*, 134–139.

Takeda, T., Harada, T., & Otsuki, S. (1989). Platelet ^{3}H-clonidine and ^{3}H-imipramine binding and plasma cortisol level in depression. *Biological Psychiatry, 26*, 52–60.

Targum, F. D., Greenberg, R. D. Harmon, R. H., Kessler, K., Salerian, A. J., & Fram, D. H. (1984). Thyroid hormone and TRH stimulation in refractory depression. *Journal of Clinical Psychiatry, 45*, 345–346.

Thomas, R., Beer, R., Harris, B., John, R., & Scanlon, M. (1989). GH responses to growth hormone releasing factor in depression. *Journal of Affective Disorders, 16*, 133–137.

Tilders, F. J. H., Berkenbosch, F. & Smelik, P. G. (1982). Adrenergic mechanisms involved in the control of pituitary-adrenal activity in the rat: A beta-adrenergic stimulatory mechanism. *Endocrinology, 110*, 114–120.

Uhde, T. W., Vittone, B. J., Siever, L. J., Kaye, W. H., & Post, R. M. (1986). Blunted growth hormone response to clonidine in panic disorder patients. *Biological Psychiatry, 21*, 1077–1081.

vandenBosch, R., & Rozendaal, N. (1988). Subjective cognitive dysfunction, eye tracking, and slow brain potentials in schizophrenia and schizoaffective patients. *Biological Psychiatry, 24*, 741–746.

van Kammen, D. P., Peters, J., & van Kammen, W. B. (1986). Cerebrospinal fluid studies of monoamine metabolism in schizophrenia. *Psychiatric Clinics of North America, 9*, 81–97.

van Kammen, D. P., Peters, J., van Kammen, W. B., Nugent, A., Goetz, K. L., Yao, J., & Linnoila, M.

(1989). CSF norepinephrine in schizophrenia is elevated prior to relapse after haloperidol withdrawal. *Biological Psychiatry*, *26*, 176–188.

Wagner, A., Aberg-Wistedt, A., Asberg, M., Ekqvist, B., Martensson, B., & Montero, D. (1985). Lower 3H-imipramine binding in platelets from untreated depressed patients compared to healthy controls. *Psychiatry Research*, *16*, 131–139.

Wagner, A., Aberg-Wistedt, A., Asberg, M., Bertilsson, L., Martensson, B., & Montero, D. (1987). Effects of antidepressant treatments on platelet tritiated imipramine binding in major depressive disorder. *Archives of General Psychiatry*, *44*, 870–877.

Wallach, J. (1986). *Interpretations of diagnostic tests* (pp. 644–646). Boston: Little, Brown.

Webb, W. B., & Campbell, S. C. (1983). Relationships in sleep characteristics of identical and fraternal twins. *Archives of General Psychiatry*, *40*, 1093–1095.

Weinberger, D. R., Bigelow, L. B. Klein, S. T., Rosenblatt, J. E., & Wyatt, R. J. (1980). Cerebral ventricular enlargement in chronic schizophrenia: An association with poor response to therapy. *Archives of General Psychiatry*, *37*, 11–13.

Weizman, A., Carmi, M., Hermesh, H., Shahar, A., Apter, A., Tyano, S., & Rehavi, M. (1986). High-affinity imipramine binding and serotonin uptake in platelets of eight adolescent and ten adult obsessive-compulsive patients. *American Journal of Psychiatry*, *143*, 335–339.

Winokur, G., Behar, D., Van Valkenburg, C., & Lowry, M. (1978). Is a familial definition of depression both feasible and valid? *Journal of Nervous and Mental Disease*, *166*, 764–768.

Winokur, G., Black, D. W., & Nasrallah, A. (1987). DST nonsuppressor status: Relationship to specific aspects of the depressive syndrome. *Biological Psychiatry*, *22*, 360–368.

Wolfe, N., Gelenberg, A. J., & Lydiard, R. B. (1989). Alpha$_2$-adrenergic receptor sensitivity in depressed patients: Relation between 3H-yohimbine binding to platelet membranes and clonidine-induced hypotension. *Biological Psychiatry*, *25*, 382–392.

Wyatt, R. J., Potkin, S. G., & Murphy, D. L. (1979). Platelet monoamine oxidase activity in schizophrenia: A review of the data. *American Journal of Psychiatry*, *136*, 377–385.

Zec, R. F., & Weinberger, D. R. (1986). Relationship between CT scan findings and neuropsychological performance in chronic schizophrenia. *Psychiatric Clinics of North America*, *9*, 49–62.

Zemishlany, Z., Modai, I., Apter, A., Jerushalmi, Z., Samuel, E., & Tyano, S. (1987). Serotonin uptake by blood platelets in anorexia nervosa. *Acta Psychiatrica Scandinavica*, *75*, 127–130.

PART IV

RESEARCH TOPICS

CHAPTER 10

Diagnostic Issues

JAMES W. THOMPSON

INTRODUCTION

Nosology, or the science of disease classification, is one of the basic sciences of medicine. Whether the physician is engaged in clinical work, research, or administration, the accurate classification of a patient's syndrome, disease, or other pathological state is the key to effectiveness. Clinically, medicine relies heavily upon the categorization of patients to determine appropriate treatment and prognosis. Sometimes a change in nosology precedes changes in treatment. For example, until the separation of diabetes into diabetes insipidus and diabetes mellitus (Garrison, 1929), the advent of appropriate treatment was not possible. In other cases, the nosologic changes reflect a new understanding of a disorder. An example of this is the separation of schizophreniform disorder from schizophrenia (Andreasen, 1987; Helzer, Kendell, & Brockington, 1983), categories which reflect a particular view of prognosis.

The researcher is no less dependent on accurate classification. Well-designed methodology and sophisticated statistics yield little of value if the study groups are not valid and reliable clinical groups. As an example, much psychotherapy research has suffered because of the tendency to include persons with any mental disorder, as though their pathology was identical (APA Commission on Psychotherapies, 1982).

Even the physician engaged in administration is greatly handicapped if the

James W. Thompson • Department of Psychiatry, University of Maryland School of Medicine, Baltimore, Maryland 21201.

Research in Psychiatry: Issues, Strategies, and Methods, edited by L. K. George Hsu and Michel Hersen. Plenum Press, New York, 1992.

data used for decision making do not reflect clinical reality. For example, a category of "severely mentally ill" in a management information system calls for a different approach, depending on whether it does or does not include patients with organic mental disorders.

My purpose in this chapter is to provide a brief history of nosology in medicine and in psychiatry in particular; to illustrate several issues in psychiatric nosology; and to present the areas of nosologic research and some of the approaches utilized in each.

HISTORY OF NOSOLOGY

The development of psychiatric nosology has been synonymous with the development of nosology in general medicine throughout most of recorded history. Perhaps the earliest written evidence of attempts to characterize specific conditions is from Chinese medicine of 2600 B.C. (Howells, 1975). In Egyptian writings of the sixteenth century B.C., a "handbook" of surgical diagnosis and procedures has been discovered (Garrison, 1929). Howells (1975) indicated that both the ancient Chinese and Egyptians demonstrated a concern for the interactions between psyche and soma, as have numerous cultures throughout history.

Western theories of medical classification began with the Greeks. There were numerous descriptions of "madness" in Greek plays (Simon, 1978). Plato "discovered" the mind and its disorders, equating sickness with injustice and conflict (Simon, 1978). In the fourth century A.D., Hippocrates was instrumental in determining the boundaries of medicine, as he dissociated medicine from theurgy (i.e., cure by divine intervention) and philosophy. He also crystallized the scattered medical knowledge of the time into systematic science (Garrison, 1929). Importantly, he formulated the theory of the four humors. All illnesses were seen as resulting from imbalances in these humors. A group of personality types was also formulated using these four humors. An excess of blood led to a *sanguine* personality (courageous, hopeful, and confident). An excess of yellow bile led to a *choleric* personality (angry and irascible). Too much black bile caused a *melancholic* personality (a person who is depressed and gloomy). And excessive phlegm led to a *phlegmatic* personality (unenthusiastic, dull, cold, and apathetic).

Galen (A.D. 130–200) elaborated a system of pathology which combined the humoral theory of Hippocrates with the four elements of Pythagoras. His ideas were held as the final authority in medicine until the time of Vesalius (1514–1564). He also described paranoia, phantasies (i.e., delusions), and dysthymia (Mora, 1980a).

The middle ages were a time of slow movement in medical science (including in nosology) (Garrison, 1929). Mora (1980a), however, pointed out that some progress was made. Avicenna (980–1037) described four types kinds of *melancholia* (a term which was used to describe various mental disorders), basing his ideas on temperaments. This classification anticipated the constitutional dimension of psychopathology. Mora also indicated that melancholia came to be attributed not to noxious humors but to the damaged faculties of the mind. Along these lines, Thomas Aquinas and Albert the Great in the thirteenth century argued that somatic disturbances caused insanity.

Later thinkers such as Fernel (sixteen century) described the symptoms of each disease in medicine, tried to localize various fevers in different organs of the body, and also made reference to pathogenesis. For example, Fernel separated infections that were due to lues (syphilis) from those that were due to gonorrhea (Garrison, 1929; Mora, 1987). Platter published the first classification of diseases in 1602, including a classification of mental disorders. His classification consisted of the three categories of "mentis imbecillitas," "consternation," and "defatigatio" (Mora, 1987). Later in that century, Thomas Sydenham characterized diseases by unique descriptive signs and symptoms, as well as by the likely natural course and eventual outcome (Garrison, 1929; Osler, 1972). Although his primary interest was not mental disorder, Sydenham described the details of neurotic and hysterical symptoms, perhaps for the first time describing symptoms of mental disorder which were not psychotic or psychopathic.

It should also be noted that the sixteenth century also witnessed the development of modern pathology (through Vesalius), which led to the correlation of clinical disease entities with an anatomical basis for classification. This was the first of many later discoveries which led to the classification of diseases on the basis of specific causal mechanisms, such as the discovery by Snow that microorganisms could cause disease and be prevented by sanitary measures (MacMahon & Pugh, 1970), the discovery of immunization by Pasteur (Garrison, 1929), and the discovery of specific antibiotics by Flemming (Bordley & Harvey, 1976).

Mora (1987) indicated that it was early in the seventeenth century that Descartes laid the groundwork for the mind–body split. By distinguishing between body and soul, Descartes opened up the "scientific" study of the body, but in doing so also opened the door to the mind–body dualism which still profoundly affects medical practice (including nosology). Howells (1975) claimed that this ushered in the "somatic era," which abandoned the holistic approach to the sick.

It is with the work of Chairugi and Pinel that an identifiable field of psychiatric nosology began to emerge. Pinel believed that mental life consisted of an integration of the psychological analysis of ideas with the emotional drives. He listed five forms of insanity: melancholia, mania with and without delirium, dementia, and idiocy (Mora, 1980a).

Bleuler, known for his detailed descriptions of schizophrenia (Bleuler, 1950), also elucidated what is perhaps the first "criteria set" with his "four A's" of schizophrenia (autism, ambivalence, disordered affect, and disordered associations). Using etiology as the key concept in classification, Freud conceptualized diagnostic categories that were based on inferences about unconscious conflict as an etiological mechanism (Menninger, Mayman, & Pruyser, 1963). Kraepelin is often called the "father" of descriptive psychiatry (although, as we have seen, there were many workers in descriptive classification before him). Perhaps more important was Kraepelin's insistence on the collection of data to support his classifications. Using this technique, for example, he clearly differentiated manic-depressive psychosis from dementia praecox (schizophrenia).

The evolution of psychiatric nosology in the United States can be dated to publication of the first American textbook on psychiatry by Benjamin Rush in 1812 (Rush, 1962). At first, nosologies in the United States were very European. Later, in the United States psychiatrists were strongly influenced by the psycho-biological theories of mental disorder etiology of Adolph Meyer (Mora, 1980b). Also, psychoanalytic theory, which taught that conflict was the etiology of mental disorder, led away from concerns about distinguishing discrete disorders on the basis of description. This gave rise to a system that combined all persons with mental disorders into very few categories. (This is perhaps analogous to the four humors, where a limited number of very broad concepts were held to represent the etiologic roots of all disorders.) This "lumping" approach to psychiatric nosology was reflected in the 1840 census of mental hospitals, which had but one psychiatric category of mental disorders, "insane and idiotic" (Redick, Manderscheid, Witkin, & Rosenstein, 1983). Seven diagnostic categories were used in the 1880 census.

In 1917, the forerunner of the American Psychiatric Association (APA) adopted a plan of uniform statistics for mental hospitals, but it was limited as a nosology (American Psychiatric Association, 1952). In 1933, a revised APA system was incorporated into the first edition of the American Medical Association's Standard and Classified Nomenclature of Disease (American Psychiatric Association, 1952). The inadequacies of this classification system became apparent during World War II when the classification was only able to account for 10% of the wartime psychopathological conditions. After the war, three different nomenclatures were developed. This situation led to the development of the first edition of the *Diagnostic and Statistical Manual of Mental Disorders* (DSM-I) (American Psychiatric Association, 1952).

Ten years later, the United States National Committee on Vital and Health Statistics appointed a subcommittee on mental disorders which proposed a revision of the nosology; it became the first draft of ICD-8 and DSM-II, which were almost identical (American Psychiatric Association, 1968; World Health Organization, 1967).

The publication of DSM-III in 1980 (American Psychiatric Association, 1980) was a major departure for nosology in psychiatry as well as for the entire health field (Thompson & Regier, 1985). Much of the etiological inference was removed, except where there was clear evidence of etiology (e.g., multi-infarct dementia). The addition of operational criteria was another advance. Psychiatry was the first medical specialty to develop a system of operational criteria. One of the few general conditions for which formal criteria are used in diagnosis is rheumatic fever (Krupp, Chatton, & Werdegar, 1985). Although there are many informal criteria for making general medical diagnoses, the diagnosis of most illnesses still is the subject of intense discussion (e.g., Modan, Harris, & Halkin, 1989).

ISSUES IN PSYCHIATRIC NOSOLOGY

The Usefulness of Psychiatric Nosology

Psychiatric symptoms and disorders have long been considered by non-psychiatrists to be vague and difficult to understand. Even psychiatrists, so this argument goes, cannot use these diagnoses reliably. This is thought to be in contrast to the rest of medicine, where symptoms and diagnostic entities are considered to be specific, reliable, valid, and easily understood. To some extent psychiatry has deserved this reputation. For many analytically oriented psychiatrists, the dynamic formulation is more important than the diagnosis. This was appropriate when psychotherapy was the major treatment modality which the psychiatrist had to offer. But as the possibilities for treatment have grown, so has the necessity to develop diagnostic entities which describe conditions amenable to specific therapies. (For example, "panic disorder" calls for a specific set of interventions, unlike a "hysterical reaction," as this phenomenon was often called in the recent past.)

In the general medical sector, psychiatric diagnosis is especially suspect, in part because of the above reputation, but also because of the particular difficulties primary care physicians have in making these diagnoses (Goldberg, 1983). Whether these difficulties arise from inadequate training, differences in practice patterns, or attitudinal or other factors is not clear (Kessler, Amick, & Thompson, 1985). But one effect is that primary care physicians see psychiatric diagnosis as a mystery and assume that this is due to the nature of psychiatry rather than to themselves.

Another reason that psychiatric nosology is often seen as "soft" is that as conditions are found to have an "organic" basis, or an effective treatment is developed, they are automatically regarded as nonpsychiatric. One writer has indicated that "biomedical psychiatry has traditionally been associated with the search for additional conditions to be turned over to colleagues in internal medicine or neurology" (Baldessarini, 1983, p. 1), a theme echoed by other authors (Goodwin & Guze, 1979; Klerman, 1984). Examples are general paresis, the encephalitides, epilepsy, and vitamin deficiency syndromes.

Related to this phenomenon is the belief in our society (and also in general medicine) that psychiatric disorders are not "real," and are "just in the patient's head." Naturally, this trivializing of mental disorder leads to the trivializing of psychiatric diagnosis. If mental disorders are not real, then trying to name them so is an exercise in futility.

Finally, the entry into "mental health" practice of numerous nonphysicians in the middle twentieth century has led to a deemphasis on nosology. Many persons in these groups were philosophically opposed to the sociological concept of "labeling," which they confused with diagnosis (Fisher, Mehr, & Truckenbrod, 1974; Loeb; Wolf, Rosen, & Rutman, 1968). Others saw the use of nosologies as "medical," and not appropriate for their mental health "clients" (Walder, Cohen, Breiter, Warman, Orme-Johnson, & Pavey, 1972). Only as it has become necessary to use a diagnosis for reimbursement have these groups apparently reversed their stance with regard to nosology. Even so, it is not uncommon to encounter in the nonmedical literature the oxymoron "mental health diagnosis" (as though diagnosis is a way to delineate aspects of health rather than illness).

This is part of the backdrop for the rapid progress in recent years in psychiatric nosology, culminating in DSM-III. Psychiatric diagnosis had the long-standing reputation of being invalid, unreliable, and of dubious value. Since World War II, however, new modes of treatment and new understandings of mental disorder have arisen, and psychiatry has found it increasingly necessary to justify reimbursement for psychiatric treatment (Rodriquez, 1988; Sharfstein, 1987). (After all, why would a third-party payor choose to pay for treatment for disorders which are not "real," and cannot be described?) The DSM series, culminating with DSM-III and DSM-III-R (American Psychiatric Association, 1987) was in part a response to these pressures.

Other Issues in Nosology

There are many general issues in nosology which are not specific to any particular symptom or syndrome. Some of these issues revolve around the character of psychopathology. Do psychopathological entities represent a continuum or discrete entities? (For example, is major depression a distinct syndrome from dysthymia, or does one entity gradually merge into the other?) Vaillant and Schnurr (1988) put this in terms of whether mental disorders are dimensional or categorical. They also asked whether we are identifying diatheses and symptoms rather than discrete syndromes. Recently, another related issue has arisen, that of whether mental disorders tend to coexist with one another, and whether the presence of one should rule out another in a hierarchical system (Boyd, Burke, Gruenberg, Holzer, Rae, George, Karno, Stoltzman, McEvoy, & Nestadt, 1984; Stewart, McGrath, Liebowitz, Harrison, Quitkin, & Rabkin, 1985).

Other issues concern the course of mental disorder. Are some mental disorders episodic, such as an upper respiratory infection or pneumonia? Are others chronic, such as congestive heart failure or diabetes? If some are chronic, are they progressive or cyclic, or do they follow some other reoccurring pattern?

Also, there are issues of dimensionality (popularized in DSM-III as "axes"). Are the five axes of DSM-III the proper ones? Are there others that should be considered, such as axes to measure the dimensions of culture, psychodynamics, etiology, defense mechanisms, severity, etc. (Mezzich, 1980; Mezzich, Fabrega, & Mezzich, 1987; Spitzer & Williams, 1980)? As a related topic, there is the issue of defining the boundaries between mental disorder and social problems.

Should there be an axis to measure quality of life or socioeconomic status in a similar way that DSM-III-R Axis IV measures severity of psychosocial stressors (American Psychiatric Association, 1987), since these interrelate with a person's mental well-being?

With regard to the use of criteria, there are a host of issues. These include the use of monothetic systems (wherein a group of criteria are all necessary to make a diagnosis) versus polythetic systems (wherein the patient must meet a criterion level for a given number of signs and symptoms from a list) (Skodol & Spitzer, 1987). There is the question of whether to "weight" criteria (i.e., whether some should count for more than others in arriving at a diagnosis). And there is the issue as to what should constitute the burden of proof necessary in order to include a particular criterion for a particular disorder.

It is in this context of rapid growth in psychiatric nosological research, with many important and interesting questions awaiting inquiry, that this chapter is written. There are enormous opportunities to substantially contribute to the field, and the approaches to nosologic research are so broad as to be of interest to a wide variety of investigators. Some of these opportunities and approaches are discussed next.

AREAS OF NOSOLOGIC RESEARCH

Overview

As noted, there are many areas of research in nosology, and many approaches to research in these areas. A useful categorization is provided by Klerman and colleagues (Klerman, Hirschfeld, Andreasen, Coryell, Endicott, Fawcett, Keller, & Scheftner, 1987), who divided research into studies concerned with reliability, internal validity, external validity, and boundary problems. They also listed several approaches to these areas. Using this or other categorizations allows the researcher to conceptualize more clearly the area of inquiry, the hypotheses to be tested, and the approaches to be used. Often, there is a temptation to try to arrive at answers to a myriad of questions in a single study, using a variety of approaches. This is almost certainly doomed to failure, however, since a proper approach to one question may be precisely the wrong approach for another question. Also, if the hypothesis is not clear, it will be difficult to interpret the results of the study. The researcher who attempts to answer many questions often ends up answering none.

Validity

The Area

Validity is the most important and the most difficult area in nosology. It concerns whether a diagnostic entity describes what it purports to describe, that is, a group of patients who are alike in some important way.

The Problems

The first major problem in the study of validity is defining what should be the focus of such studies.[2] Is it a group of psychodynamics, a biological substrate, a level of functioning, a commonly agreed upon description of symptoms, etc.? Underlying this problem is the question of etiology—What are the causes of mental disorders? The DSM-III-R indicates that it is atheoretical with regard to this question, but clearly the DSM-III-R weighs in heavily on the side of symptom description as the most important way to group disorders. This may well be the best approach, given the relative absence of knowledge about etiology in most disorders. But this approach involves a calculated risk that diverse conditions may be grouped together based on superficial description. This has often led to confusion in medicine. For example, diabetes insipidus and diabetes mellitus, scarlatina and measles, and lues and gonorrhea were put together on the basis of such superficialities (Garrison, 1929). Such errors are not benign ones, as the search for etiologic agents and effective treatments can be stymied by diversity in the group being investigated.

In any research project, the investigator must decide what he or she believes to be most important (whether this be description, genetics, psychodynamics, etc.), and be able to defend that decision. The investigator also must assess his or her "audience." Testing the validity of a diagnostic category for researchers may be quite different from testing the validity of a diagnosis to be used for international data collection.

A second major problem has to do with the standard by which a particular diagnostic entity is to be measured. This is also related to etiology. Other specialties in medicine often rely on laboratory examinations (e.g., thyroid function tests), physical signs and symptoms (e.g., those of congestive heart failure), or other measures (e.g., blood pressure determination) as their measure of "truth." Psychiatry has few of these "objective" measures. Spitzer (1983) proposed that instead of a "gold standard," psychiatry must rely on a "LEAD standard," or longitudinal assessments by experts of all the data (i.e., concurrent validity).

Vaillant and Schnurr (1988) also suggested that a concurrent validity strategy, using various approaches simultaneously, is the best way to define a "case" (in epidemiologic terminology). And they agreed with Kendell (1975) and with Wing, Bebbington, and Robins (1981) that predictive validity (i.e., predicting the risk of poor outcome over time) is the best single index, although this alone is not enough to establish validity.

It should be noted that the problem of the gold standard is not unique to psychiatric nosology. One only has to look at the problems in defining hypertension or obesity, or the often conflicting systems of cancer staging, to see the

---

[2]There is no attempt here or in subsequent sections of this chapter to provide an exhaustive list of problems or approaches. Rather, the attempt is to identify some of the major problems and review selected approaches which have been taken in attempting to solve these problems.

same problems in general medicine. Here, also, there is a heavy reliance on LEAD standards to assess validity (if, indeed, validity has been assessed at all). To use the hypertension example, does one define this diagnostic category by using only diastolic blood pressure, or by using both systolic and diastolic pressures? What numerical cutoffs are necessary to meet criteria? Is course of illness also important? Is renal pathology to be considered?

It is key for the researcher to decide what will serve as the standard for the "true" diagnosis. A good choice or choices will allow results to be readily interpreted. A poor choice will allow for little more than guesses about the interpretation of results.

The Questions

1. What is the most important parameter in studying validity? Is it psychodynamics, symptom description, biology, psychosocial factors, genetics, or some other factor?
2. What is the best standard of "truth?"
3. Is the diagnostic category, subcategory, or criterion being studied a valid measure of pathology?

The Approaches

Overview. One way of categorizing approaches to validity testing is offered by Spitzer and Williams (1980). They divide validity into the classic types of validity. *Face validity* is "the extent to which the description of a particular category seems, on the face of it, to describe accurately the characteristic features of persons with a particular disorder" (p. 1037). That is, does it make sense to persons educated in clinical assessment? *Descriptive validity* is "the extent to which the characteristic features of a particular mental disorder are unique to that category, relative to other mental disorders and conditions" (p. 1037). *Predictive validity* is whether the category predicts something of importance for patients with the disorder (e.g., clinical outcome, course, prognosis). And *construct validity* is "the extent to which evidence supports a theory that is helpful in explaining the etiology of a disorder or the nature of the pathophysiological process" (p. 1039). That is, is the category consistent with biological factors, genetics, environmental factors, etc.? Spitzer and Williams (1980) pointed out that although the etiology of most mental disorders is not known, there is some construct validity for many psychiatric diagnostic categories.

Another way of classifying validity testing is to distinguish between internal and external validity. Feinstein (1977) described this distinction by noting that in internal validity we do not go beyond the observed evidence (i.e., the category itself). For example, validity can be assessed by using agreement between experts, comparing several nondefinitive diagnostic systems (or instruments), or by mathematical means. In external validity, we check the diagnostic category or criterion against something that is outside of the observed evidence.

That is, we compare the category against a standard which we consider to represent "truth." Clearly, this is the strongest form of validity testing. In the text that follows, several approaches to internal and external validity determination will be discussed.

An example of assessing the validity of specific diagnostic categories is given by Klerman *et al.* (1987) in their discussion of major depression and related affective disorders. They reviewed internal validity studies which use statistics, such as factor analysis and cluster analysis, correlations of symptoms with one another (e.g., delusions with suicidal intent in major depression with psychotic features), and clinician agreement as to the existence of a particular disorder. With regard to external validity, they reviewed epidemiologic research, as well as research on genetics, psychosocial factors, response to treatment, and clinical course and outcome.

Epidemiology. Incidence and prevalence studies are largely useful for internal validation, and then only when there is a comparison of cases with a second diagnostic method. In the Epidemiologic Catchment Area studies (Regier & Burke, 1987), these comparisons or "clinical reappraisals" were done by various means (Eaton & Kessler, 1985). These included comparing the diagnostic instrument used in the study with another instrument, and assessing a sample of cases identified in the community with a psychiatric interview. Another method utilized was reassessing a sample of cases identified by lay interviewers with the same instrument given by a clinician (Eaton & Kessler, 1985), but this is more of a reliability than a validity study.

The field of epidemiology is concerned in the final analysis with etiology (Kleinbaum, Kupper, & Morgenstern, 1982), and some of its techniques are therefore useful for external validation. These include studies of risk factors (Kleinbaum *et al.*, 1982) and longitudinal studies of the course of illness (Srole & Fischer, 1980).

Family Aggregation and Genetic Transmission. These studies can lead to external validation, since, by definition, they are an attempt to correlate a diagnosis with outside evidence (with that evidence presumed to represent an etiologic factor). Several methods are used to make this correlation. In family aggregation studies (e.g., Guze, Cloninger, Martin, & Clayton, 1983), the families of persons with a disorder are sought out, and the risk of the disorder in the family is determined. In twin studies (Kendler, 1983), several types of comparisons are possible. Often, identical twins who have been reared together or apart are identified, with their complete sibships and the sibships of their parents compared.

Another method utilized in genetics research is adoption studies (Merikangas, 1987). These usually consist of comparing psychopathology in adopted children whose biological parents have a mental disorder, with those children whose parents do not have a mental disorder, or of comparing the biologic and adoptive parents of affected children (Rainer, 1980). Finally, there is the search for genetic markers, association, and linkage (Rainer, 1980).

Psychosocial Factors. According to Klerman *et al.* (1987), these are studies of personality correlates, social support, and life events. To the extent that these are thought to be etiologic, they are studies of external validity. In the DSM-II era, the nosology strongly implied that many mental disorders were "reactions" to life events. This reflected the influence of Adolph Meyer (Mora, 1980b), and the experience with the stress-related illnesses of World War II (American Psychiatric Association, 1968). In actual studies, however, even when psychosocial factors have shown correlations with the presence of mental disorders, the evidence for etiology has been poor (Schwab & Schwab, 1978). Personality factors have been disappointing (e.g., Hirschfeld & Klerman, 1979), as have social support and life events (Henderson, 1988). A major problem with the use of social support and life events as standards by which to measure the validity of a diagnostic category is that it is often not clear whether these are causes or results of mental disorders. Also, with regard to life events, the patient or other informant may retrospectively link symptoms with particular life events in an attempt to "explain" the symptoms. Finally, there is the problem of remembering life changes *per se* (Jenkins, Hurst, & Rose, 1979). The researcher using this approach must not only show correlations but also demonstrate proper sequencing (i.e., the disorder occurring after the event in question), and a connection between the event and the development of the disorder.

Response to Treatment In some ways, a clinical trial is a study in external validity of the diagnostic category involved, if the treatment is of known efficacy. (The treatment is therefore the measure of "truth".) Kendell (1982), however, observed that disorders responding to the same treatment may not have the same etiology. Nevertheless, if a treatment modality has a specific and exclusive effect on a particular disorder, this is a form of external validation for the category. Perhaps the closest psychiatric medicine has come to this is the response of bipolar disorder, manic to lithium carbonate.

Clinical Course and Outcome. Goodwin and Guze (1979) claimed that classification has two functions: communication and prediction. They indicated that a diagnostic entity has a predictable life history—it stays the same, or, if it changes, the change must be routine. Similarly, a valid diagnostic entity should have a predictable outcome with treatment and without treatment. It follows that studies of clinical course and outcome can inform us about external validity. A classic example is Kraepelin's distinction between manic depression and dementia praecox that was based on the differential course of these illnesses (Mora, 1980a).

The basic approach in this area of research is the follow-up study. Because it is expensive and difficult to mount long-term follow-up studies, there are few of these. Kendell, Brockington, and Leff (1979) studied patients from the United States/United Kingdom Diagnostic Project which used six operational definitions of schizophrenia, and reported that all six definitions predicted poor symptomatic outcome after 6 years. A 5-year follow-up of patients from the Washington International Pilot Study of Schizophrenia showed that the Schneiderian first-rank symptoms had poor predictive value (Hawk, Carpenter, & Strauss, 1975; Strauss & Carpenter, 1977). Srole and Fischer (1980) reported on the Midtown Manhattan Longitudinal Study, and Vaillant and Schnurr (1988) reported on a long-term follow-up of college students. Unfortunately, no diagnostic instruments were utilized in the latter two studies. The NIMH Collaborative Program on the Psychobiology of Depression is a longitudinal prospective study of affective disorders (Katz, Secunda, Hirschfeld, & Koslow, 1979).

Biochemical and Neurophysiological Studies Basically, these studies are searches for biologic or other "markers" that either would be pathognomonic of or strong evidence for, or that would point to vulnerability to a particular illness. If found, such markers might be a gold standard to use in external validity determination. A recent, widely studied attempt to define such a marker for depression was the Dexamethasone Suppression Test (DST) (Arana, Baldessarini, & Ornsteen, 1985). Quantification of studies on the brain and special senses is another approach. For example, Shagass, Roemer, and Straumanis (1982) studied the relationships between psychiatric diagnosis and quantitative EEG variables. Pursuit eye movement (i.e., tracking) dysfunction has been linked to vulnerability for schizophrenia (Holzman, Proctor, & Hughes, 1973). Such techniques as computerized tomography have also been used to search for markers related to schizophrenia and its subtypes (Jaskiw, Andreasen, & Weinberger, 1987; Nasrallah, Jacoby, McCalley-Whitters, & Kuperman, 1982).

In this approach to research, it should be remembered that very few markers in medicine are indeed pathognomonic of a single disease, or can distinguish in all cases between normals and affected individuals. Also, very few diseases can be defined on the basis of a single marker. Even normal and abnormal values for basic laboratory tests are based on a mathematical distribution which optimizes specificity and sensitivity, rather than demonstrating a direct one-to-one linkage between a value on the test and an illness. The hope for a single test, such as the DST, to diagnose a particular mental disorder is to expect more than has been possible elsewhere in medicine. A more realistic expectation is to find markers which can serve as indicators as to the presence or absence of a particular disorder. Such indicators are but one piece of the diagnostic puzzle.

Comparison of Systems. Comparison between diagnostic systems can be useful in internal validity studies. For example, Kendell *et al.* (1979) compared the diagnosis of schizophrenia in six diagnostic systems, and McGlashan (1983) compared three diagnostic systems to separate patients with borderline personality disorder from those with schizotypal personality disorder. Thompson, Green, and Savitt (1983) and Thompson and Pincus (1989) compared the systems in DSM-III and DSM-III-R to ICD-9-CM using an expert consensus method.

Expert Consensus. To some extent, internal validity can be demonstrated by asking a large number of users of a classification how they make diagnoses in every day practice (e.g., Lipkowitz & Idupaganti, 1983). This is a relatively weak method, however, since the biases of those surveyed usually cannot be controlled. This method also tends to reinforce the status quo, since clinicians will tend to answer in light of how they were trained and how they practice, rather than in light of possible innovations in the classification.

Cross-Cultural and Cross-National Studies. Related to the internal validation strategy of comparing diagnostic systems is the comparison of a single system across cultural or national boundaries. If the same pathology is found in two or more cultures or countries, this is presumptive evidence that a single entity is being measured. Westermeyer (1985) discussed the use of diagnosis cross-culturally. Shore, Manson, Bloom, Keepers, and Neligh (1987) demonstrated that standard instruments appear to be useful for the diagnosis of depression in some American Indians. Martinez (1986) noted that rates of illness appear to be similar in Hispanics and Anglos, although the expression of illness may differ. Cannon and Locke (1977) made the important point that apparent differences in syndromes between racial groups may reflect stereotyping of the minority population. The so-called culture bound syndromes are also a fertile area for study, as they may represent unique syndromes or different presentations of western syndromes (Simons & Hughes, 1985). In perhaps the most famous cross-national study (see Kramer, 1969; Cooper, Kendell, Gurland, Sharpe, Copeland, & Simon, 1972), it was demonstrated that schizophrenia rates in the United States and the United Kingdom were similar, and that apparent differences were the result of differential coding practices.

Statistics. Statistical methods are useful in the determination of internal validity. Andreasen and Grove (1982) discussed these methods as compared to other methods and showed that cluster analysis supports the Research Diagnostic Criteria (RDC) and the DSM-III categorization of depression. Other authors have used factor analysis (Livesley & Jackson, 1986). A newer method is grade of membership analysis (Blazer, Swartz, Woodbury, Manton, Hughes, & George, 1988). Other techniques are also useful, and the researcher should be familiar with their possibilities (Cohen & Cohen, 1983; Kleinbaum & Kupper, 1978).

Philosophy. An important tool in the validation of nosology is the production by nosological experts of "think pieces" about nosology in general, or about categories in particular. It is from such writings that many ideas for research arise. The logical treatment of a nosological problem can sometimes shed more light on a category than the approaches described above. In closing this section of the chapter, it is important to recognize some of these writers, and encourage the researcher to pursue their writings. They include Akiskal (1983); Goodwin & Guze (1979); Kendell (1975, 1982); Mezzich (1980); Spitzer (1983); and Spitzer & Williams (1980) among others.

Reliability

The Area

Reliability is whether a diagnostic entity is reproducible time after time, in various contexts, by many raters. As noted above, this is an area which has been a source of criticism against psychiatry (Colby & Spar, 1984). However, with the advent of DSM-III and its field trials (Spitzer, Forman, & Nee, 1979), psychiatry became the first medical specialty to subject its diagnoses to an investigation of reliability (Klerman, 1984). Although it remains the only specialty to do so, calls for reliability testing of psychiatric diagnoses continue.

The Problems

The major problem in reliability testing is that its value is directly proportional to the degree of validity which has been demonstrated. If a set of criteria are well operationalized, they may be very reliable, but a different set of criteria for the same disorder may be equally as reliable.

A second major problem, discussed below, is how to operationalize diagnostic criteria. There are various ways of eliciting history, signs, and symptoms from patients, and each one may carry a different level of reliability. Related to this is the need to decide whether unreliability has to do with the criteria *per se*, with the instrument being used to elicit the criteria, or with the way the instrument is being applied. It is very important to appreciate that a seemingly small change can lead to large differences in reliability. These can be changes in the instrument, the raters, the training for the raters, or the patient (or other) group chosen for study.

The Questions

1. Is each criterion (e.g., delusions of worthlessness) reproducible time after time, in various contexts, by many raters?
2. Is each diagnostic category (e.g., major depression with mood congruent psychotic features) reproducible time after time, in various contexts, by many raters?
3. Is each major diagnostic grouping (e.g., affective disorders) reproducible time after time, in various contexts, by many raters?

The Approaches

Instruments. Various approaches to reliability testing have been used. Most involve the translation of a diagnostic entity into a standard format (instrument), and the application of this instrument by many raters to many patients. A primary part of such research then is instrument development (Burke, 1987; Robins, 1987). A primary task is to introduce as little bias as possible into these instruments, and clearly identify the bias which is introduced.

There will be no attempt here to review the extensive literature on psychiatric survey instruments. Suggestions for the interested reader include work on the Renard Diagnostic Interview (Helzer, Robins, Croughan, & Welner, 1981), the Schedule for Affective Disorders and Schizophrenia (SADS) (Endicott & Spitzer, 1978), the Present State Exam (PSE) (Wing, Cooper, & Sartorius, 1974), the NIMH Diagnostic Interview Schedule (DIS) (Robins, Helzer, Croughan, Williams, & Spitzer, 1981), the Composite International Diagnostic Interview (CIDI) (Robins, Wing, Wittchen, Helzer, Babor, Burke, Farmer, Jablenski, Pickens, Regier, Sartorius, & Towle, 1988), and the Structured Clinical Interview for DSM-III-R (Spitzer, Williams, Gibbon, & First, 1990).

These instruments range from semistructured interviews, which provide specific questions to be asked but also allow leeway in the interview, to highly structured instruments, which proscribe each word that is to be said by the interviewer. It is also possible to do an open-ended interview using a simple checklist of criteria or symptoms, but this is not standardized enough to use in reliability testing.

A structured interview done by a nonclinician suffers from validity (and therefore reliability) problems, since the nonclinician has no way to evaluate the answers to technical questions (e.g., whether the patient is describing a true delusion or a hallucination). A totally structured interview done by a clinician will be more valid, but if the clinician is not allowed to stray from the instrument, there is little gained over a nonclinician interview. Use of a clinical vignette suffers from another validity (and therefore reliability) problem, that of whether it is possible to give a valid picture of a patient in such a format. The use of audiotape as a standard stimulus for reliability rating also suffers from this problem, but less so; the use of videotape suffers still less, although the issue could still be raised. Importantly, the rater cannot ask a videotape, audiotape, or vignette a question. The beauty of these methods, however, is that they do not change between ratings, and therefore offer the most standardized stimulus.

Selecting Patients. The ideal would be to randomly select people from the community in large numbers, but this would be extremely expensive. Short of this, patients can be selected from treatment settings. In each method of selection, however, bias is introduced. Choosing treated individuals clearly shifts the sample toward the more severe end of the psychopathology continuum. The shift would be more extreme if only inpatient settings were sampled. For illnesses which very often end up in treatment (e.g., psychotic disorders), this is not a severe problem. For mild disorders (e.g., adjustment disorders), few will be picked up in such a sample, and these cases may be unusual in some way. The bias introduced by studying a population under treatment is known as *Berkson's bias* (Kleinbaum *et al.*, 1982).

There are several ways to go about choosing a sample of patients under treatment. In the DSM-III field trials (Spitzer *et al.*, 1979), clinicians were asked to diagnose consecutive patients in their practice, or "catch-as-catch-can," to approximate the method of random sampling. The problems were that the clinicians were volunteers and, by definition, were not randomly chosen. Since they only participated in groups, there was no control over their interaction (although they were asked to make independent ratings). Unless there is a random start to taking sequential patients, randomness is compromised. Furthermore, "catch-as-catch-can" is almost by definition *not* random, since this leaves the choice of the patients entirely up to the clinician, who may choose who he or she feels will cooperate most fully.

Another way of approaching patient selection is not to randomize patients at all but rather to choose them with a known bias, and then control for the bias in the data interpretation phase. Patients could be chosen who meet specific guidelines; for example, males with schizophrenic disorder who are within two weeks of acute inpatient admission. The reliability ratings could be generalized only to this group of patients.

Selecting Raters. Another variable in the reliability equation is in the choosing of raters. Again, the best way would be to select psychiatrists (and other raters) randomly from a full universe of such persons. Another approach, however, would be to determine the rater variables which are to be varied (e.g., age, sex, race, practice setting), and choose raters in such a way that these variables are representative.

One important source of bias is related to how the raters are recruited. For example, if raters are chosen from persons who are attending professional meetings, those who do not go to meetings would not be represented. To correct for this, subsamples might be chosen from such underrepresented groups. Other bias can arise from the circumstances of data collection. For example, if raters are to work in groups, someone must be present to ensure that there is no exchange of information until after the ratings are made.

Study Methodology. There are many methodologies which can be used: one interviewer can interview the same patient more than once; several interviewers can interview the same patient; one interviewer can audiotape or videotape an interview, with the second raters listening or watching; one interviewer can watch an interview done by a second interviewer, and rate the instrument with or without the opportunity to ask additional questions of the patient; or a written clinical vignette can be rated by several independent raters.

Each methodology has its own difficulties. The ideal situation might seem to be two raters doing a separate interview with the same patient. However, the two interviews will not be standardized, since the interview style will be somewhat different; the first interview may stimulate recall (or repression) of some facts, and key facts may be given to one, but not to the other, interviewer. The argument in favor of such a process is that if reliability is demonstrated in spite of all this, the finding is robust.

An important issue is interviewer and rater training, since efforts must to be made to standardize the process of applying the instrument and rating the interview. If the study is ongoing, periodic checks as to how the instrument is being applied will also be necessary. If the methodology involves asking raters to score another person's interview (e.g., from a videotape), there is the question of whether each rater should be specially trained, and if so, how he or she is to be trained.

Statistics. The usual statistic for measuring reliability between raters is the *kappa statistic* (Fleiss, 1981). A weighted kappa statistic is also in use in order to weight disagreements of varying importance (Cohen, 1968). Spitznagel and Helzer (1975) proposed the *Y statistic* for quantification of agreement, which corrects for some of the problems of the kappa statistic. A discussion of several alternatives can be found in Light (1971).

Boundary Issues

The Area

Much validity research is implicitly concerned with boundaries. If a category is valid, this indicates that it is a relatively homogenous group with definable boundaries between it and other conditions, and between it and normality. In this section, however, the focus will be on studies addressing an explicit boundary question.

The Problems

The important boundaries to be considered are boundaries between disorders (i.e., between psychiatric disorders *per se* and between psychiatric and other medical disorders), and between pathology and normality. In each case, the distinction is important clinically. If the boundary between disorders is incorrectly defined, some patients will be inappropriately treated (if treatment between the two conditions differs). For example, from a treatment point of view the boundary between bipolar disorder and schizophrenic disorder, and the boundary between depression and hypothyroidism are important ones. On the other hand, given the treatment approaches presently available, the boundary between the various subtypes of schizophrenia is not as important. (Of course, if the point of view taken relates not to clinical treatment, but to prognosis, course of illness, or other factors, the boundary issues of importance may also change.) The abnormal/normal boundary is also clinically important, especially when the treatment carries potential adverse effects (as most do), or when the prognosis is better for one condition than for another.

Another boundary issue has to do with atypical cases. No matter how well designed a nosological system is, there will be patients who do not fit neatly into the categories. The challenge for the nosologic researcher is to determine whether those cases actually represent additional syndromes, or whether they represent "outliers." For example, is there a distinct entity of "schizoaffective disorder," or are these cases the overlapping outliers of schizophrenic and affective disorders?

Kendell (1982) also reminded us that having made boundary distinctions, we should not close our eyes to further evidence which argues against the boundaries we have drawn. He pointed out that in other branches of medicine, many conditions that once appeared to be discrete diseases, such as hypertension and diabetes, have proved on detailed investigation to consist of groups of related disorders involving complicated interactions among a number of different genes and a variety of environmental agents (Sowers & Zemel, 1990).

The Questions

1. Does the diagnostic category clearly distinguish normality from pathology?
2. Does the diagnostic category represent a syndrome which is distinct, or does it overlap with other syndromes?
3. Do atypical cases represent additional syndromes, or outliers of known syndromes?

The Approaches

Epidemiology. Epidemiologic studies can help distinguish the normal from the pathological. For example, if the prevalence of a particular disorder is extremely high, it brings up the question of whether many normals are being included in the category (i.e., the criteria are too broad, or are being too broadly applied) (e.g.,Thompson, Burns, Bartko, Boyd, Taube, & Bourdon, 1988). Epidemiologic studies can also help in distinguishing between disorders, or in pointing out where symptoms of disorders appear to greatly overlap. The amount of co-morbidity within a community setting is one method of doing this (Boyd *et al.*, 1984). Also, atypical cases can be studied by examining "cases" which do not meet threshold for a diagnosis and yet are clearly symptomatic. The use of interview instruments in the clinical setting can also be useful in determining boundaries, in a similar way to their use in field epidemiology (e.g., Zanarini, Gunderson, Frankenburg, & Chauncey, 1990).

Family Aggregation and Genetic Transmission. The aim of many genetics studies is to discover genetically based illnesses which are by definition separate from other illnesses. There is much work in this direction, with one of the most studied problems being the distinction between schizophrenic disorder and schizoaffective disorder (Coryell & Zimmerman, 1988). Family studies are also quite useful in separating disorders from each other. For example, Guze *et al.* (1983) found that in the great majority of cases, schizophrenia and primary affective disorder can be distinguished by follow-up and the study of first-degree relatives.

Psychosocial Factors. These issues are often not useful when correlated with variables derived from a treated population, since admission into particular types of treatment facilities are strongly correlated with psychosocial factors (e.g., admissions to a state mental hospital are likely to be of low socioeconomic status). However, they can be useful in boundary determination when correlated with community prevalence and incidence rates.

Response to Treatment. When new syndromes are identified, these studies are often the source. A group of patients who do not respond to treatment may be the first step at defining a new condition, or in clarifying a boundary between two disorders (Sargant, 1962). Two disorders which appear to respond to the same treatment may point toward the identity of (or overlap between) the two disorders. A recent example is the work of Hudson and Pope (1990) in which they reviewed the literature on antidepressant response and proposed a grouping of several disorders into an "affective spectrum disorder." The investigator must be aware, however, that response to a similar treatment may *not* signify the identity of two disorders, and that some patients with the same disorder may respond to different treatments, depending on other factors (such as individual characteristics of the patient, environment, etc.).

Clinical Course and Outcome. By observing course of illness, Kraepelin was able to distinguish between manic depression and dementia praecox (Mora, 1980a). More recently, work in separating schizophrenic disorder from schizophreniform disorder has been based on course (Helzer *et al.*, 1983). Course and outcome studies to answer boundary questions, like those to study validity, require a follow-up period (or at least an attempt to retrospectively gather longitudinal data).

Biochemical and Neurophysiological Studies. Work here is directed toward finding common markers between two illnesses which may suggest a relationship between them. One example is the work on schizotypal personality disorder and schizophrenic disorder which "suggests that many schizotypal individuals share psychobiological abnormalities with schizophrenic individuals" (Siever & Kendler, 1987, p. 313).

Statistics. Kendell (1982) illustrated a statistical approach to boundary problems, although he believed that statistical methods should be used along with other methods. He indicated that in psychiatry it is difficult to decide on boundaries because we have seldom demonstrated "discontinuities or 'points of rarity'" between related syndromes (p. 1336). He suggested that in an attempt to do this, cluster analysis is one option. Kendell also suggested the method of demonstrating "a nonlinear relationship between symptomatology and some other independent variable" (p. 1336)—a biochemical abnormality, performance on a physiologic or psychologic test, or proportion of patients with a family history of disease.

Other multivariate techniques are also useful in boundary determination. Factor analysis can assist in identifying groups of variables (criteria) which predict some independent variable, and the overlap between factors can be compared (Kleinbaum & Kupper, 1978). A newer analytic technique which shows promise is the grade of membership (GOM) analysis (Blazer *et al.*, 1988), which presents a picture of how closely a variable (criterion) is related to a particular group.

Philosophy. As in validity studies, the importance of careful thought cannot be underestimated in the search for boundaries. Medical research has become more and more quantitative, many times to its own detriment. A poorly formed hypothesis or questionable data can often be covered up with complicated methodology and sophisticated statistics. But in the qualitative "think pieces" which appear in book chapters, and occasionally in journals, there are no tables, statistics, or intricate procedures to fall back upon. The author's arguments rise or fall of their own weight. And it is often through such writing that the important hypotheses are formulated.

THE PRESENT AND THE FUTURE

The present international classification of mental disorders is contained in ICD-9 (World Health Organization, 1978), which has been modified for use in the United States as ICD-9-CM (National Center for Health Statistics, 1980). DSM-III-R is very similar to ICD-9-CM (Thompson & Pincus, 1989), although the latter contains no diagnostic criteria. (ICD-9-CM does contain a glossary of mental disorder terminology.) The new revision of the international classification, ICD-10 (World Health Organization, in press), will be substantially different from its predecessor. It will contain clinical criteria for mental disorders and also research criteria, and, in this sense, will be closer to a nosology than has been the case previously. At this writing, ICD-10 is due for implementation in January, 1993.

The DSM-IV process is also well under way and is timed to coincide with ICD-10 development. There is much collaboration between the two. DSM-IV process (Frances, Widiger, & Pincus, 1989) has involved extensive literature reviews, with field trials on focused issues and a general reliability field trial planned. As the DSM-IV and ICD-10 processes unfold, there will be increased opportunities for nosologic research in the United States and internationally.

SUMMARY

This chapter begins with a review of the history of psychiatric nosology. Some perceive the specialty as a particularly problematic area in nosology while others consider it to be in the forefront of the field of medical nosology. Whether either or both of these perceptions are true, the issues of validity, reliability, and boundaries are very much the same in psychiatry as in other specialties, as this chapter indicates. It is true that some terms in psychiatry have proven difficult to define and standardize. Indeed, it may be because of the necessity to introduce better definition and standardization that psychiatry has moved farther than the field as a whole in operationalizing and standardizing diagnostic criteria. This experience allows those involved with psychiatric nosology and statistics to be optimistic about the potential of such efforts, while simultaneously being aware of the many pitfalls involved.

Every researcher in psychiatry will touch on issues of nosology, regardless of the substance of his or her research. Thus, it behooves him or her to be aware of the promise and problems of the field. For the researcher specifically interested in nosology, the immediate future will be filled with opportunities to profoundly influence psychiatry and all of medicine. The problem for nosologic researchers will not be to find interesting questions, but to force themselves to focus on a small enough portion of this enormous field to allow for careful hypothesis formulation and attention to the detail which is necessary to achieve valid results.

REFERENCES

Akiskal, H. S. (1983). Dysthymic disorder: Psychopathology of proposed chronic depressive subtypes. *American Journal of Psychiatry, 140*, 11–20.

American Psychiatric Association. (1952). *Diagnostic and statistical manual of mental disorders.* Washington, DC: Author.

American Psychiatric Association. (1968). *Diagnostic and statistical manual of mental disorders* (2nd ed.). Washington, DC: Author.

American Psychiatric Association. (1980). *Diagnostic and statistical manual of mental disorders* (3rd ed.). Washington, DC: Author.

American Psychiatric Association. (1987). *Diagnostic and statistical manual of mental disorders* (3rd ed., rev.). Washington, DC: Author.

Andreasen, N. C. (1987). Schizophrenia and schizophreniform disorders. In G. L. Tischler (Ed.), *Diagnosis and classification in psychiatry: A critical appraisal of DSM-III* (pp. 103–123). Cambridge: Cambridge University Press.

Andreasen, N. C., & Grove, W. M. (1982). The classification of depression: Traditional versus mathematical approaches. *American Journal of Psychiatry, 139*, 45–52.

APA Commission on Psychotherapies. (1982). *Psychotherapy research: Methodological and efficacy issues.* Washington: American Psychiatric Association.

Arana, G. W., Baldessarini, R. J., & Ornsteen, M. (1985). The Dexamethasone Suppression Test for diagnosis and prognosis in psychiatry. *Archives of General Psychiatry, 42*, 1193–1204.

Baldessarini, R. J. (1983). *Biomedical aspects of depression and its treatment.* Washington: American Psychiatric Press.

Blazer, D., Swartz, M., Woodbury, M., Manton, K. G., Hughes, D., & George, L. K. (1988). Depressive symptoms and depressive diagnoses in a community population. *Archives of General Psychiatry, 45,* 1078–1084.

Bleuler, E. (1950). *Dementia praecox or the group of schizophrenias.* New York: International Universities Press.

Bordley, J., III, & Harvey, A. M. (1976). *Two centuries of American medicine: 1776–1976.* Philadelphia: W.B. Saunders.

Boyd, J. H., Burke, J. D., Gruenberg, E., Holzer, C. E., Rae, D. S., George, L. K., Karno, M., Stoltzman, R., McEvoy, L., & Nestadt, G. (1984). The exclusion criteria of DSM-III: A study of the co-occurrence of hierarchy-free syndromes. *Archives of General Psychiatry, 41,* 983–989.

Burke, J. D., Jr. (1987). Diagnostic assessment. In A. E. Skodol & R. L. Spitzer, *An annotated bibliography of DSM-III* (pp. 13–22). Washington, DC: American Psychiatric Press.

Cannon, M. S., & Lock, B. Z. (1977). Being black is detrimental to one's mental health: Myth or reality? *Phylon, 38,* 408–428.

Cohen, J. (1968). Weighted kappa: Nominal scale agreement with provision for scaled disagreement or partial credit. *Psychological Bulletin, 70,* 213–220.

Cohen, J., & Cohen, P. (1983). *Applied multiple regression/correlation analysis for the behavioral sciences* (2nd ed.). Hillsdale, NJ: Lawrence Erlbaum.

Colby, K. M., & Spar, J. E. (1984). *The fundamental crisis in psychiatry: Unreliability of diagnosis.* Springfield, IL: Charles C Thomas.

Cooper, J. E., Kendell, R. E., Gurland, B. J., Sharpe, L., Copeland, J. R. M., & Simon, R. (1972). *Psychiatric diagnosis in New York and London.* London: Oxford University Press.

Coryell, W., & Zimmerman, M. (1988). The heritability of schizophrenia and schizoaffective disorder. *Archives of General Psychiatry, 45,* 323–327.

Eaton, W. W., & Kessler, L. G. (Eds.). (1985). *Epidemiology field methods in psychiatry: The NIMH Epidemiology Catchment Area Program.* Orlando: Academic Press.

Endicott, J., & Spitzer, R. L. (1978). A diagnostic interview: The schedule for affective disorders and schizophrenia. *Archives of General Psychiatry, 35,* 837–844.

Feinstein, A. R. (1977). A critical overview of diagnosis in psychiatry. In V. M. Rakoff, H. C. Stancer, & H. B. Kedward (Eds.), *Psychiatric diagnosis* (pp. 189–206). New York: Brunner/Mazel.

Fisher, W., Mehr, J., & Truckenbrod, P. (1974). *Human services: The third mental health revolution.* New York: Alfred Publishing.

Fleiss, J. L. (1981). *Statistical methods for rates and proportions* (2nd ed.). New York: Wiley-Interscience.

Frances, A. J., Widiger, T. A., & Pincus, H. A. (1989). The development of DSM-IV. *Archives of General Psychiatry, 46,* 373–375.

Garrison, F. H. (1929). *An introduction to the history of medicine* (4th ed.). Philadelphia: W.B. Saunders.

Goldberg, D. (1983). Training family physicians in mental health skills: Implications of recent research findings. In D. L. Parron & F. Solomon (Eds.), *Mental health services in primary care settings: Report of a conference April 2–3, 1979, Washington, D.C.* (pp. 70–87). (U.S. Department of Health and Human Services, DHHS Publication No. ADM 83-995). Washington, DC: National Institute of Mental Health.

Goodwin, D. W., & Guze, S. B. (1979). *Psychiatric diagnosis* (2nd ed.). New York: Oxford University Press.

Guze, S. B., Cloninger, C. R., Martin, R. L., & Clayton, P. J. (1983). A follow-up and family study of schizophrenia. *Archives of General Psychiatry, 40,* 1273–1280.

Hawk, A. B., Carpenter, W. T., & Strauss, J. S. (1975). Diagnostic criteria and five year outcome in schizophrenia. *Archives of General Psychiatry, 32,* 343–347.

Helzer, J. E., Robins, L. N., Croughan, J. L., & Welner, A. (1981). Renard Diagnostic Interview: Its reliability and procedural validity with physicians and lay interviewers. *Archives of General Psychiatry, 38,* 393–398.

Helzer, J. E., Kendell, R. E., & Brockington, I. F. (1983). Contribution of the six-month criterion to the predictive validity of the DSM-III definition of schizophrenia. *Archives of General Psychiatry, 40,* 1277–1280.

Henderson, A. S. (1988). *An introduction to social psychiatry.* Oxford: Oxford University Press.

Hirschfeld, R. M. A., & Klerman, G. L. (1979). Personality attributes and affective disorders. *American Journal of Psychiatry, 136*, 67–70.

Holzman, P. S., Proctor, L. R., & Hughes, D. W. (1973). Eye tracking patterns in schizophrenia. *Science, 181*, 179–181.

Howells, J. G. (1975). Introduction. In J. G. Howells (Ed.), *World history of psychiatry* (pp. vii–xviii). New York: Brunner/Mazel.

Hudson, J. I., & Pope, H. G., Jr. (1990). Affective spectrum disorder: Does antidepressant response identify a family of disorders with a common pathology? *American Journal of Psychiatry, 147*, 552–564.

Jaskiw, G. E., Andreasen, N. C., & Weinberger, D. R. (1987). X-Ray computed tomography and magnetic resonance imaging in psychiatry. In R. E. Hales & A. J. Frances (Eds.), *American Psychiatry Association annual review, Vol. 6* (pp. 260–299). Washington, DC: American Psychiatric Press.

Jenkins, C. D., Hurst, M. W., & Rose, R. M. (1979). Life changes: Do people really remember? *Archives of General Psychiatry, 36*, 379–384.

Katz, M. M., Secunda, S. K., Hirschfeld, R. M. A., & Koslow, S. H. (1979). NIMH Clinical Research Branch Collaborative Program on the Psychobiology of Depression. *Archives of General Psychiatry, 36*, 765–777.

Kendell, R. E. (1975). *The role of diagnosis in psychiatry*. Boston: Blackwell Scientific Publications.

Kendell, R. E. (1982). The choice of diagnostic criteria for biological research. *Archives of General Psychiatry, 39*, 1334–1339.

Kendell, R. E., Brockington, I. F., & Leff, J. P. (1979). Prognostic implications of six alternative definitions of schizophrenia. *Archives of General Psychiatry, 36*, 25–31.

Kendler, K. S. (1983). Overview: A current perspective on twin studies of schizophrenia. *American Journal of Psychiatry, 140*, 1413–1425.

Kessler, L. G., Amick, B. C., III, & Thompson, J. (1985). Factors influencing the diagnosis of mental disorder among primary care patients. *Medical Care, 23*, 50–62.

Kleinbaum, D. G., & Kupper, L. L. (1978). *Applied regression analysis and other multivariable methods*. North Scituate, MA: Duxbury Press.

Kleinbaum, D. G., Kupper, L. L., & Morgenstern, H. (1982). *Epidemiologic research: Principles and quantitative methods*. Belmont, CA: Lifetime Learning Publications.

Klerman, G. L. (1984). The advantages of DSM-III. *American Journal of Psychiatry, 141*, 539–542.

Klerman, G. L., Hirschfeld, R. M. A., Andreasen, N. C., Coryell, W., Endicott, J., Fawcett, J., Keller, M. B., & Scheftner, W. A. (1987). Major depression and related affective disorders. In G. L. Tischler (Ed.), *Diagnosis and classification in psychiatry: A critical appraisal of DSM-III* (pp. 3–31). Cambridge: Cambridge University Press.

Kramer, M. (1969). Cross-national study of diagnosis of the mental disorders: Origins of the problem. *American Journal of Psychiatry, 125* (Supplement), I–II.

Krupp, M. A., Chatton, M. J., & Werdegar, D. (1985). *Current medical diagnosis and treatment, 1985*. Los Altos, CA: Lange Medical Publications.

Light, R. J. (1971). Measures of response agreement for qualitative data: Some generalizations and alternatives. *Psychological Bulletin, 76*, 465–477.

Lipkowitz, M. H., & Idupaganti, S. (1983). Diagnosing schizophrenia in 1980: A survey of U.S. psychiatrists. *American Journal of Psychiatry, 140*, 52–55.

Livesley, W. J., & Jackson, D. N. (1986). The internal consistency and factorial structure of behaviors judged to be associated with DSM-III personality disorders. *American Journal of Psychiatry, 143*, 1473–1474.

Loeb, A., Wolf, A., Rosen, M., & Rutman, I. D. (1968). The influence of diagnostic label and degree of abnormality on attitudes toward former mental patients. *Community Mental Health Journal, 4*, 334–339.

MacMahon, B., & Pugh, T. F. (1970). *Epidemiology: Principles and methods*. Boston: Little, Brown.

Martinez, C., Jr. (1986). Hispanics: Psychiatric issues. In C. B. Wilkinson (Ed.), *Ethnic psychiatry* (pp. 61–88). New York: Plenum Press.

McGlashan, T. H. (1983). The borderline syndrome: I. Testing three diagnostic systems. *Archives of General Psychiatry, 40*, 1311–1318.

Menninger, K., Mayman, M., & Pruyser, P. (1963). *The vital balance: The life process in mental health and illness.* New York: Viking Press.

Merikangas, K. R. (1987). Genetic epidemiology of psychiatric disorders. In R. E. Hales & A. J. Frances, *American Psychiatric Association annual review, Vol. 6* (pp. 625–646). Washington, DC: American Psychiatric Press.

Mezzich, J. E. (1980). Multiaxial diagnostic systems in psychiatry. In H. I. Kaplan, A. M. Freedman, & B. J. Sadock (Eds.), *Comprehensive textbook of psychiatry/III* (3rd ed., pp. 1072–1079). Baltimore: Williams & Wilkins.

Mezzich, J. E., Fabrega, H., & Mezzich, A. C. (1987). On the clinical utility of multiaxial diagnosis. In G. L. Tischler (Ed.), *Diagnosis and classification in psychiatry: A critical appraisal of DSM-III* (pp. 449–463). Cambridge: Cambridge University Press.

Modan, M., Harris, M. I., & Halkin, H. (1989). Evaluation of WHO and NDDG criteria for impaired glucose tolerance: Results from two national samples. *Diabetes, 38,* 1630–1635.

Mora, G. (1980a). Historical and theoretical trends in psychiatry. In A. I. Kaplan, A. M. Freedman, & B. J. Sadock (Eds.), *Comprehensive textbook of psychiatry/III* (3rd ed., pp. 4–98). Baltimore: Williams & Wilkins.

Mora, G. (1980b). Theories of personality and psychopathology: Adolph Meyer. In A.I. Kaplan, A. M. Freedman, & B. J. Sadock (Eds.), *Comprehensive textbook of psychiatry/III* (3rd ed., pp. 805–812). Baltimore: Williams & Wilkins.

Mora, G. (1987). Introduction. In V. Chiarugi, *On insanity and its classification* (pp. xiii–cxli). Canton, MA: Science History Publications.

Nasrallah, H. A., Jacoby, C. G., McCalley-Whitters, M., & Kuperman, S. (1982). Cerebral ventricular enlargement in subtypes of chronic schizophrenia. *Archives of General Psychiatry, 39,* 774–777.

National Center for Health Statistics. (1980). *International classification of diseases, 9th revision, clinical modification* (Vol. 1). (DHHS Publication No. DHHS 80-1260). Washington, DC: Department of Health and Human Services.

Osler, W. (1972). *The evolution of modern medicine.* New York: Arno Press.

Rainer, J. D. (1980). Genetics and psychiatry. In A. I. Kaplan, A. M. Freedman, B. J. Sadock (Eds.), *Comprehensive textbook of psychiatry/III* (3rd ed., pp. 135–154). Baltimore: Williams & Wilkins.

Redick, R. W., Manderscheid, R. W., Witkin, M. J., & Rosenstein, M. J. (1983). *A history of the U.S. national reporting program for mental health statistics: 1840–1983.* (DHHS Publication No. ADM 83-1296). Washington, DC: Department of Health and Human Services.

Regier, D. A., & Burke, J. D. (1987). Psychiatric disorders in the community: The Epidemiologic Catchment Area Program. In R. E. Hales & A. J. Frances (Eds.), *American Psychiatry Association annual review, Vol. 6* (pp. 610–624). Washington, DC: American Psychiatric Press.

Robins, L. N. (1987). The assessment of psychiatric diagnosis in epidemiological studies. In R. E. Hales & A. J. Frances, *American Psychiatric Association annual review, Vol. 6* (pp. 589–609). Washington, DC: American Psychiatric Press.

Robins, L. N., Helzer, J. E., Croughan, J., Williams, J. B. W., & Spitzer, R. L. (1981). The NIMH Diagnostic Interview Schedule: Its history, characteristics, and validity. *Archives of General Psychiatry, 38,* 381–389.

Robins, L. N., Wing, J., Wittchen, H. U., Helzer, J. E., Babor, T. F., Burke, J., Farmer, A., Jablenski, A., Pickens, R., Regier, D. A., Sartorius, N., & Towle, L. H. (1988). The Composite International Diagnostic Interview. *Archives of General Psychiatry, 45,* 1069–1077.

Rodriquez, A. R. (1988). An introduction to quality assurance in mental health. In G. Stricker & A. R. Rodriquez (Eds.), *Handbook of quality assurance in mental health* (pp. 3–36). New York: Plenum Press.

Rush, B. (1962). *Medical inquiries and observations upon the diseases of the mind.* New York: Hafner Press.

Sargant, W. (1962). The treatment of anxiety states and atypical depressions by the monoamine oxidase inhibitor drugs. *Journal of Neuropsychiatry, 3 (Suppl 1),* 96–103.

Schwab, J. J., & Schwab, M. E. (1978). *Sociocultural roots of mental illness: An epidemiologic survey.* New York: Plenum Press.

Shagass, C., Roemer, R. A., & Straumanis, J. J. (1982). Relationships between psychiatric diagnosis and some quantitative EEG variables. *Archives of General Psychiatry, 39,* 1423–1435.

Sharfstein, S. S. (1987). Third-party payments, cost containment, and DSM-III. In G. L. Tischler (Ed.), *Diagnosis and classification in psychiatry: A critical appraisal of DSM-III* (pp. 530–538). Cambridge: Cambridge University Press.

Shore, J. H., Manson, S. M., Bloom, J. D., Keepers, G., & Neligh, G. (1987). A pilot study of depression among American Indian patients with Research Diagnostic Criteria. *American Indian and Alaska Native Mental Health Research, 1,* 4–15.

Siever, L. J., & Kendler, K. S. (1987). An evaluation of the DSM-III categories of paranoid, schizoid, and schizotypal personality disorders. In G. L. Tischler (Ed.), *Diagnosis and classification in psychiatry: A critical appraisal of DSM-III* (pp. 300–320). Cambridge: Cambridge University Press.

Simon, B. (1978). *Mind and madness in ancient Greece: The classical roots of modern psychiatry.* Ithaca, NY: Cornell University Press.

Simons, R. C., & Hughes, C. C. (Eds.). (1985). *The culture-bound syndromes: Folk illnesses of psychiatric and anthropological interest.* Dordrecht, Netherlands: D. Reidel.

Skodol, A. E., & Spitzer, R. L. (Eds.). (1987). *An annotated bibliography of DSM-III.* Washington, DC: American Psychiatric Press.

Sowers, J. R., & Zemel, M. B. (1990). Clinical implications of hypertension in the diabetic patient. *American Journal of Hypertension, 3(5 Pt. 1),* 415–424.

Spitzer, R. L. (1983). Psychiatric diagnosis: Are clinicians still necessary? *Comprehensive Psychiatry, 24,* 399–411.

Spitzer, R. L., & Williams, J. B. W. (1980). Classification of mental disorders. In H. I. Kaplan, A. M. Freedman, & B. J. Sadock (Eds.), *Comprehensive textbook of psychiatry/III* (3rd ed., pp. 1035–1072). Baltimore: Williams & Wilkins.

Spitzer, R. L., Forman, J. B. W., & Nee, J. (1979). DSM-III field trials: I. Initial interrater diagnostic reliability. *American Journal of Psychiatry, 136,* 815–817.

Spitzer, R. L., Williams, J. B. W., Gibbon, M., & First, M. B. (1990). *User's guide for the Structured Clinical Interview of DSM-III-R (SCID).* Washington, DC: American Psychiatric Press.

Spitznagel, E. L., & Helzer, J. E. (1975). A proposed solution to the base rate problem in the kappa statistic. *Archives of General Psychiatry, 42,* 725–728.

Srole, L., & Fischer, A. K. (1980). The Midtown Manhattan Longitudinal Study vs 'the mental paradise lost' doctrine: A controversy joined. *Archives of General Psychiatry, 37,* 209–221.

Stewart, J. W., McGrath, P. J., Liebowitz, M. R., Harrison, W., Quitkin, F., & Rabkin, J. (1985). Treatment outcome validation of DSM-III depressive subtypes. *Archives of General Psychiatry, 42,* 1148–1153.

Strauss, J. S., & Carpenter, W. T. (1977). Prediction of outcome in schizophrenia. *Archives of General Psychiatry, 34,* 159–163.

Thompson, J. W., & Pincus, H. (1989). A crosswalk from DSM-III-R to ICD-9-CM. *American Journal of Psychiatry, 146,* 1315–1319.

Thompson, J. W., & Regier, D. A. (1985). The coding of diagnostic criteria for mental disorders and its integration into the general disease classification. In R. A. Cote, D. J. Protti, & J. R. Scherrer (Eds.), *Role of informatics in health data coding and classification systems* (pp. 271–288). Amsterdam: North-Holland.

Thompson, J. W., Green, D., & Savitt, H. L. (1983). Preliminary report on a crosswalk from DSM-III to ICD-9-CM. *American Journal of Psychiatry, 140,* 176–180.

Thompson, J. W., Burns, B. J., Bartko, J., Boyd, J. H., Taube, C. A., & Bourdon, K. A. (1988). The use of services by persons with and without phobia. *Medical Care, 26,* 183–198.

Vaillant, G. E., & Schnurr, P. (1988). What is a case? A 45-year study of psychiatric impairment within a college sample selected for mental health. *Archives of General Psychiatry, 45,* 313–319.

Walder, L. O., Cohen, S. I., Breiter, D. E., Warman, F. C., Orme-Johnson, D., & Pavey, S. (1972). Parents as agents of behavior change. In S. E. Golann & C. Eisendorfer, *Handbook of community mental health* (pp. 595–616). New York: Appleton-Century-Crofts.

Westermeyer, J. (1985). Psychiatric diagnosis across cultural boundaries. *American Journal of Psychiatry, 142,* 798–805.

Wing, J. K., Cooper, J. E., & Sartorius, N. (1974). *Measurement and classification of psychiatric symptoms.* New York: Cambridge University Press.

Wing, J. K., Bebbington, P., & Robins, L. N. (1981). Testing theories of psychiatric disorders in the community. In J. K. Wing, P. Bebbington, & L. N. Robins (Eds.), *What is a Case?* (p. 217). New York: Grant McIntyre Medical Books.

World Health Organization. (1967). *International classification of diseases, 8th revision*. Geneva: World Health Organization.

World Health Organization. (1978). *International classification of diseases, 9th revision*. Geneva: World Health Organization.

World Health Organization. (in press). *International classification of diseases and related health problems, 10th revision*. Geneva: World Health Organization.

Zanarini, M. C., Gunderson, J. G., Frankenburg, F. R., & Chauncey, D. L. (1990). Discriminating borderline personality disorder from other Axis II disorders. *American Journal of Psychiatry, 147,* 161–167.

CHAPTER 11

Epidemiology

NANCY L. DAY

INTRODUCTION

Although most reviews of psychiatric epidemiology trace the beginnings of the field to much more recent times (Grob, 1985; Weissman & Klerman, 1978), early reports of mortality from psychiatric disorders can be found in the seventeenth-century observations that were made by John Graunt (1662/1939), one of the first investigators to systematize data collection and hence one of the first epidemiologists. In 1632, in the 122 parishes in the vicinity of London, England, Graunt observed that of the 9,535 deaths, 5 died of "lunatique," 15 people "made away themselves," 1 was "affrighted," and 11 died of grief. In addition, 7 were "murthered" and 18 were "executed or prest to death" (p. 24), clearly non-psychiatric diagnoses, but areas of interest to modern psychiatric epidemiology. Further, he went on to note that these causes of death, unlike the plague, remained relatively constant from year to year.

Graunt also differentiated mortality among "lunaticks," by separating those who died from their madness from those who were mad but who died of other afflictions, estimating that the probability was approximately 1 out of 1,500 that a man would die a lunatick in Bedlam. This, probably was the first approximation of a prevalence rate in psychiatric epidemiology.

Graunt also framed the essential question of all epidemiological investigations when he asked, "to what purpose tends all this laborious buzzing and

Nancy L. Day • Western Psychiatric Institute and Clinic, 3811 O'Hara Street, Pittsburgh, Pennsylvania 15213.

Research in Psychiatry: Issues, Strategies, and Methods, edited by L. K. George Hsu and Michel Hersen. Plenum Press, New York, 1992.

groping?" to which he answered, "those who cannot apprehend the reason of these Enquiries, are unfit to trouble themselves to ask them" (p. 77). However, he continued more helpfully to define the philosophical underpinning for epidemiology by demonstrating the necessity of collecting data for governing, planning, and for the proper allocation of resources (i.e., the essential public health aspects of epidemiology).

A more modern definition of epidemiology is the study of the distribution of disease and the determinants of disease within the population (MacMahon & Pugh, 1970). The basic parameters of epidemiology are measures of disease frequency, incidence, and prevalence, and the focus for study is a population rather than individual cases. The comparison of the distribution and frequency of disease across different populations allows the epidemiologist to identify potential etiological agents.

John Snow (1855/1936) studied the incidence of cholera among people who were exposed to two different sources of water and was able to identify the relationship between water source and disease incidence. James Lind (1753/1953) observed that there was a relationship between the availability of fresh fruit and/or wine on sea cruises and the occurrence of scurvy among the sailors. Both of these historic epidemiologic studies were instrumental in identifying potential mechanisms for averting further disease, although neither scientist understood the etiology of the disease. Thus, although epidemiology is a science involved in studying etiology, it has practical implications for intervention and prevention, sometimes in the absence of understanding the cause of the disease.

In this chapter, I will first address methodological issues of study design as they specifically apply to the exploration of psychiatric disorders. Then I will explore the development of psychiatric epidemiology, describe some of the large epidemiological projects that have been conducted, and discuss some of the findings with respect to the prevalence of psychiatric disorders in the United States.

METHODOLOGICAL ISSUES

Causal Models

Epidemiology developed from the study of infectious diseases which were described by a single cause/single disease model. However, as sanitation became widespread and vaccination became available, the rates of infectious disease decreased. People lived longer, and other causes of morbidity and mortality became more prominent. These disorders, the chronic diseases such as mental illness, heart disease, and cancer, could not be explained by a single-cause etiological hypothesis. It became clear that one agent could cause a multitude of diseases. Alcohol use is associated with psychiatric morbidity

(American Psychiatric Association, 1987) as well as cancer and heart disease (U.S. Department of Health and Human Services, 1990). Conversely, it was also clear that one disease, depression, for example, may result from psychosocial (Ilfeld, 1977) or biological effects (Thase, Frank, & Kupfer, 1985), or a combination of these factors (Charney & Weissman, 1988). Thus, for chronic diseases, the study of etiology moved from the concept of a single agent's causing a single disease to the much more complex idea of risk factors, that is, factors known to increase the probability of disease, and vulnerability, or the characteristics within individuals that make them more susceptible to disease.

To address this issue, multifactorial models that allow the investigator to assess the impact of all of the risk factors at the same time must be used which required the development of sophisticated statistical techniques and more complex models of the relationship between variables. For example, in some cases, the presence or the level of one variable may change the relationship between another variable and the outcome. These variables are called *moderating* or *buffering variables*, or sometimes *vulnerability factors* (Cleary & Kessler, 1982; Finney, Mitchell, Cronkite, & Moos, 1984). In the exploration of the relationship between life events, depression, and social support, the relationship between life events and depression is thought to be modified by the level of social support available to the subject (Cleary & Kessler, 1982).

In addition to multiple-risk factors and interactions between variables, factors can be linked sequentially as part of a causal chain. For example, one could posit that a family situation causes depression which, in turn, causes suicide. The mediating variable (depression) is affected by the independent variable (family situation), which in turn, affects the dependent variable (suicide): an A causes B causes C pattern.

It is important also to consider factors that are not part of the causal sequence but that may affect the conclusions drawn from an analysis. These confounding factors can bias the conclusions from the study. *Confounds* are defined as factors or characteristics that are causally related to the disorder being studied. They are also associated with the risk factor that is being studied, although they are not causally related to the risk factor (Kelsey, Thompson, & Evans, 1986). For example, when we are interested in the relationship between prenatal alcohol exposure and the subsequent development of cognitive deficits, illicit drug use must be considered as a potential confounder.

Study Design

Research in epidemiology also required the development of new study designs. The experimental paradigm cannot be easily applied to human populations, and the wide range of variability among and between human populations makes comparisons very difficult. Two broad strategies for research can be defined: descriptive studies and analytic studies.

Descriptive studies are hypothesis generating and are undertaken when there is little information on the pattern of disease in the population. Descriptive data on the distribution of the disease within age, sex, social class, or occupational groups, in addition to the geographic pattern and the distribution over time, all provide information that can then be used to formulate hypotheses.

Analytic studies test the hypotheses that are generated. During World War II, it was noted that mental illness was distributed differently between soldiers who were exposed to stressful conditions on the battlefield and those who were not (Weissman & Klerman, 1978), leading to the hypothesis that stress caused mental illness. Analytic studies, such as the one conducted by Leighton, Harding, Macklin, Hughes, and Leighton (1963), were designed to test this hypothesis. In a rural Canadian county, these researchers compared rates of psychiatric morbidity between subjects who lived in socially organized settings versus those who lived in disorganized environments. They documented a relationship between social disorganization and increased rates of mental illness.

The aforementioned studies follow a general sequence in the exploration and proof of the etiology of disease (cf. Kelsey et al., 1986). The first step is a clinical observation of a potential relationship between a disease and some factor. A descriptive epidemiologic study would then explore this association on a population level followed by an analytic study that would test the relationship. In some cases, it is possible to move this sequence of causal proof one step further by demonstrating that exposure to the hypothesized cause increases the probability of disease, and that removal of the factor decreases the probability of disease. For example, researchers have assessed the impact of a disaster as a stressor on the psychiatric status of a population (Bromet & Schulberg, 1987). On the other hand, prohibition was an experiment on the effect on the subsequent morbidity and mortality after removal of a factor (Terris, 1967). Thus, intervention and prevention not only have public health meaning, but they also can provide proof of causality.

Analytic studies can be divided into three general groups: cohort or prospective studies, case-control or retrospective studies, and cross-sectional studies. Prospective studies identify a group of people (a cohort) on the basis of an exposure and represent natural experiments. Within the cohort design, etiology is explored by the comparison of the incidence of disease between the exposed and the nonexposed and the concordance of disease and risk factors. An example of a prospective study is the work by Brown, Bifulco, and Harris (1987). They interviewed 435 working-class women and single mothers from inner-city London to assess the level of their investment in multiple areas of their lives. One year later, they assessed the relationship between commitment to life roles, life events in the intervening year, and the presence of depression at follow-up and found a relationship between life events and subsequent depression. This relationship, however, was modified by the context of the event. In our own research (Day, Robles, Richardson, Geva, Taylor, Scher, Stoffer, Cornelius, & Goldschmidt, 1991), we have interviewed women who used alcohol and drugs during their pregnancy and have followed their offspring over time. This study has enabled us to evaluate the long-term consequences of prenatal toxic exposure on subsequent behavioral, cognitive, and physical development.

The *historical prospective study* is a variant of the prospective study. In this design, data that were collected at an earlier time point are used to describe the current status of a cohort. Robins (1974) found records from a child psychiatric clinic where children had been treated 30 years earlier. This investigator tracked the subjects and evaluated their current mental health status, demonstrating that children who had psychiatric problems, particularly those who were antisocial, grew up to be adults with mental health problems.

Clinical trials are prospective studies and are the closest that epidemiology gets to the true experimental design. In a clinical trial, patients are selected and are then sorted, usually randomly, into groups that will receive different treatments. A good example of this design is the National Institute of Mental Health (NIMH) Treatment of Depression Collaborative Research Program (Elkin, Shea, Watkins, Imber, Sotsky, Collins, Glass, Pilkonis, Leber, Doeherty, Fiester, & Parloff, 1989). In this program, 250 patients with major depressive disorder were randomly assigned to four treatment groups: interpersonal psychotherapy, cognitive behavior therapy, imipramine hydrochloride plus clinical management, and placebo plus clinical management. Patients in all four groups showed improvement after 16 weeks, but there was a clear ordering of improvement: the patients with imipramine plus clinical management did best whereas those with placebo and clinical management did worst. There was also an interaction with the severity of illness. Patients with the most severe symptomatology and the greatest impairment in functioning were the most likely to respond to imipramine plus clinical management. Among patients with less severe disease, there were no significant differences among the four treatments.

Case-control studies identify the study population on the basis of the presence or absence of the specific disease under study. The investigator then assesses the relative occurrence of hypothesized risk factors in the cases and controls. This method is often used in studies of the heritability of disorders. The Yale–NIMH study, for example, compared psychiatric illness in families of psychiatric patients with the rate of psychiatric illness in families of normal controls and found that there was a two- to threefold increase in major depression in the first-degree relatives of patients with affective disorder (Weissman, Gershon, Kidd, Prusoff, Leckman, Dibble, Hamovit, Thompson, Pauls, & Guroff, 1984).

Cross-sectional studies investigate the relationship between the risk factor and disease at one point in time. A good example of the use of cross-sectional design was a study by Costello, Costello, Edelbrock, Burns, Dulcan, Brent, and Janiszewski (1988). These investigators screened children, aged 7 to 11, who were attending a Health Maintenance Organization (HMO) for primary care. Children who scored high on the screening instrument were subsequently administered a diagnostic interview. It is reported that 22% of the children attending the HMO had a DSM-III diagnosis.

Incidence and Prevalence Rates

Incidence and prevalence are two rates that are used within descriptive and analytic studies. *Incidence* is defined as the number of new cases of disease in a population at risk within a defined period of time. It can only be measured in a prospective study, where the population is chosen to be disease free at the beginning of the study. The development of new cases over the period of observation allows the investigator to explore the relationship between the occurrence of disease and the hypothesized risk factor.

Obviously, this statistic is easier to determine in a study of an infectious disease where a relatively clear time of onset can be ascertained. In chronic diseases and in psychiatric disorders, the definition of a new case is problematic. In general, studies use the point of diagnosis of the disorder to define the time when the subject became a case. However, psychiatric illness may have existed for some time before the actual diagnosis, and this represents, at best, an approximation of the time of onset.

This problem of onset is of concern for several reasons. First, given that the time of onset is likely to have been considerably earlier than the diagnosis, there is a probability that risk factors that were present at onset may no longer be there. Therefore, there is a chance of missing a real relationship. Furthermore, there is a chance of mistaking variables that are the consequence of the disease for risk factors. Psychiatric epidemiologists have spent considerable time exploring whether the fact that schizophrenic patients have lower social class is a risk factor for the disease or a consequence of the disorder. In one case, social class may be etiological; in the other, schizophrenics may acquire lower social class as a result of their illness—the social drift hypothesis.

The second major statistic used in epidemiology is the *prevalence rate*. This rate is defined as the number of cases that exist at a given point in time (point prevalence) or over a period of time (period prevalence) in the population. Since all cases are counted, there is no consideration of whether they are new or old, and there is no concern whether each member of the population is actually at risk. Although this rate is useful for planning and for public health projections, it is not a useful rate for etiological studies.

Prevalence is the product of the incidence and duration of a disorder. Disorders of short duration will have a lower prevalence than those of longer duration if the incidence is equal. Therefore, the prevalence of a disorder in the population is susceptible to interventions that affect duration, such as changes in treatment, whereas incidence is affected only by prevention.

This relationship is illustrated in the research that was conducted by Hollingshead and Redlich in New Haven, Connecticut (1958). In addition to enumerating the individuals who were receiving psychiatric care, the study had as its goal an examination of the relationship between social class and the prevalence and distribution of psychiatric disorders and the characteristics of treatment. All patients who were in treatment with a psychiatrist or who attended a psychiatric clinic or mental hospital between May 31 and December 1,

1950, and who were residents of the New Haven area were counted. Data on the patients were obtained from the psychiatrists and from medical records. A classification scheme from the Veterans Administration was used to standardize the diagnoses. Control data for this study were provided by sampling households in the area. Social class was defined by area of residence, occupation, and education (i.e., the Hollingshead Index of Social Position).

The investigators found that incidence and duration of schizophrenia were directly related to social class. The prevalence of schizophrenia among the lower social classes was higher than among patients of upper social status. For neuroses, however, the reverse was found. Although there was no difference among social classes in the incidence of neurosis, the duration of treatment was greater for the upper social classes, and, therefore, the prevalence of neurosis was much higher among patients in this group.

Sampling

Study subjects can be sampled from a number of different sources for epidemiologic studies. One could sample psychiatric cases from a clinical or hospital sample, or from a general population sample. Subjects could be recruited from a general medical clinic or from a mental health facility. To the extent that the sample is drawn from a population that is representative of all other comparable populations, then the findings can be extrapolated. If the sample is taken from a very unique population, then the generalizability will be extremely limited.

However, where the sample is drawn does make a difference. Inpatients will be more severely ill than outpatients, and the distribution of diagnoses is likely to be very different. Berkson (1946) demonstrated mathematically that the probability of being admitted to the hospital is greater for each additional diagnosis. Therefore, if a sample is selected from an institution, the probability is greater that the patients will have multiple problems. Unless this is corrected, the data from the institutional sample would lead to an erroneous conclusion about the rate of co-morbidity.

HISTORY OF PSYCHIATRIC EPIDEMIOLOGY

Early studies of psychiatric illness were generally concerned with administrative issues, and research was focused on counting the number of people who were institutionalized (Grob, 1985). As the field developed, two kinds of studies were commonly found. The first explored the distribution of psychiatric disorders, accepting the diagnosis given by the institution. The second type of study used symptom scales as the assessment. These two types of studies represented two differing views of psychiatric illness. Studies that were diagnostically based were grounded in the belief that there were separate and distinct disorders: this is the *biomedical view*. The research that involved symptom scales, on the other hand, represented a belief that mental health and mental illness were on a continuum and that the categories of disease were not distinct: this is the *psychosocial view*.

Among the first type of studies were the surveys that were conducted in Baltimore (Lemkau, Tietze, & Cooper, 1942) and in Tennessee (Roth & Luton, 1943), both during the 1930s. Also in that decade, Faris and Dunham (1939) explored the relationship between the residence of patients, the rate of hospitalization for psychiatric disorders, and the level of social disorganization by geographic location. The latter study demonstrated that the highest rates of admission to mental hospitals occurred in areas with the highest levels of social disorganization, confirming their hypothesis that social disorganization was a risk factor for mental illness.

These early studies were criticized for their definition of psychiatric disorder (Weissman & Klerman, 1978). Studies that used medical records were justifiably criticized for the lack of reliability in the diagnoses. On the other hand, studies that used symptom lists were equally criticized for their inability to make diagnoses.

The time during World War II and the immediate postwar period provided opportunities for change in the field of psychiatric epidemiology (Weissman & Klerman, 1978). During the war, psychiatric disorders accounted for the largest number of rejections for military service. Among the recruits who were accepted and who were considered to be mentally sound, however, investigators noted that the rates of psychoneuroses and personality reactions fluctuated in response to combat and other wartime experiences. Researchers concluded from this observation that stress was a major risk factor in the development of these particular psychiatric disorders (Weissman & Klerman, 1978). Thus, stress became an important concept in postwar psychiatric epidemiology.

Although stress was introduced as a new finding, it was, in fact, a further progression from the earlier theories of environmentalism. Thus, once again research in civilian populations turned to the environment for postwar equivalents of stress and investigated urbanization, anomie, poverty, rapid social change, and lower social status. A number of studies also examined the relationship between psychiatric disorders and stress; examples of these included the Midtown Manhattan study (Srole, 1978) and the research performed in Stirling County, Nova Scotia (Leighton *et al.*, 1963).

DIAGNOSTIC CLASSIFICATION

In postwar psychiatric epidemiology, the focus changed from the assessment of symptoms lists to a concern with diagnosis. Rather than deal with a continuum of mental health, investigators focused instead on the questions of *caseness*. Psychiatric disorders, in general, cannot be identified by lesions, anatomical changes, or physiological measures. Therefore, the question of what constitutes a case is difficult and is subject to differences across clinicians, research protocols, and cultures.

It was necessary to have agreed-upon criteria so that clinical data and research data could be comparable. Standardized and reliable assessments and criteria needed to be developed so that the instruments could be used across many different populations by clinicians with varying levels of training. This requirement led to a focus by researchers in the field of psychiatric epidemiology on diagnostic categorization.

Although the scales that were developed for assessment during World War II provided a basis for a more standardized measurement of psychiatric illness, these instruments were used only to measure levels of health and illness rather than to generate specific diagnoses. After this period, instruments were developed that focused primarily on the measurement of depression. The instruments that were developed by Zung (1965), Hamilton (1960), and Beck (1969) measured the symptoms that were associated with depression. Some of these tests were self-report measures and others were clinician administered. These tools had the advantage that they were standardized, relatively quick, and easy to administer; but they had the disadvantage that they did not provide a diagnosis.

The data from these and other measures formed the bases for the Feighner Criteria (Feighner, Robins, Guze, Woodruff, Winokur, & Munoz, 1972). Subsequently, a structured interview, the Renard Diagnostic Interview (Helzer, Robins, Croughan, & Welner, 1981), was developed to elicit the information that was required to make diagnoses using these criteria. The Feighner Criteria provided the basis for the Research Diagnostic Criteria (Spitzer, Endicott, & Robins, 1978) which, in turn, were used to formulate the DSM-III (American Psychiatric Association, 1980). Concurrently, the Psychiatric Status Schedule (PSS) was developed (Spitzer & Endicott, 1968), and this instrument, in turn, formed the basis for the SADS (Schedule for Affective Disorder and Schizophrenia) and the SADS-L—the lifetime version (Spitzer & Endicott, 1968).

Another interview that covered a broad spectrum of diagnoses was designed for use in the Epidemiological Catchment Area studies (Robins, Helzer, Orvaschel, Anthony, Blazer, Burnam, & Burke, 1985). This instrument, the Diagnostic Interview Schedule (DIS), incorporated the Feighner, the RDC, and the DSM-III criteria. The DIS assesses the presence, duration, and severity of symptoms. It determines whether the symptoms occurred and severity of the particular symptom (defined as to whether it limited activity or required physician consultation), and whether medication was taken. Symptoms that meet the severity criteria and that cannot be explained by medical phenomena are then used as "building blocks" for diagnoses (Regier, Myers, Kramer, Robins, Blazer, Hough, Eaton, & Locke, 1985).

When children are the focus of interest, the problem becomes even more complex, as the diagnosis may be made from information provided by the child or by the parent. Studies conducted by Costello (1989b) and by Offord, Boyle, and Racine (1989) demonstrated that reported symptoms and even diagnoses vary substantially, depending on whether the child's report or the parent's report is used to make the diagnosis. For example, in a random household sample of children in Ontario, Canada, the rate of conduct disorder among boys who were 12 to 16 years old was a 4.0% in the parental reports, compared to 7.2% in the youths' reports (Offord *et al.*, 1989). In the Costello (1989b) sample, in the cases where either the parent or the child reported problems, there was agreement on the disorder in only 10% of the cases.

RELIABILITY AND VALIDITY

Two parameters are used in evaluating the usefulness of a diagnostic instrument. *Reliability* is defined as the reproducibility of a measurement, that is, the ability of the interview to measure the same thing in the same way every time (Bartko & Carpenter, 1976). Shrout, Spitzer, and Fleiss (1987) have added an extra dimension to this definition by specifying that the instrument must also distinguish between groups in a reproducible manner. Reliability can be affected by mistaken information, changes in clinical practice, and the use of different criteria for diagnosis. Sources of error in information include temporal or seasonal changes in the expression of the disorder and the incorrect reporting of the timing of symptoms. Since diagnoses in the DSM-III and the DSM-III-R systems are constructed from algorithms that consider the presence, time, and severity of symptoms, mistakes in reporting can clearly affect the accuracy of a diagnosis.

There are a number of ways to measure reliability experimentally; these include the use of case vignettes, videotapes of interviews, the assessment of interrater agreement, and test–retest studies (Grove, Andreasen, McDonald-Scott, Keller, & Shapiro, 1981). With regard to the DIS, the findings have been mixed, with studies indicating only modest reliability for most diagnoses (Anthony, Folstein, Romanoski, Von Korff, Nestadt, Chahal, Merchant, Brown, Shapiro, Kramer, & Gruenberg, 1985; Helzer, Robins, McEvoy, Spitznagel, Stoltzman, Farmer, & Brockington, 1985).

Validity is an even more difficult concept to define with respect to psychiatric diagnoses. *Validity* is a measure of whether the construct that is being measured is actually the real construct. A valid diagnosis measures a disorder that is unique and that can be differentiated from other diagnostic categories on the basis of such factors as symptoms, biological variables, long-term outcome, and treatment response (Bartko & Carpenter, 1976; Rutter, 1981). As an example, Costello (1989a), in a comparison of five studies of psychopathology in children, noted the remarkable consistency in correlates of the psychiatric diagnoses. Older children, boys, and lower social class children were more likely to exhibit psychiatric disorder. Correlates of specific disorders were found consistently, even though the actual rates of these disorders varied across studies.

EPIDEMIOLOGIC STUDIES OF THE PREVALENCE
OF PSYCHIATRIC DISORDERS

As Robins (1990) has pointed out, the major role of epidemiology in general and psychiatric epidemiology in particular is to estimate the overall prevalence of psychiatric disorders in the population. Thus, in this section, a few of the larger, general population studies that were conducted in psychiatric epidemiology will be reviewed briefly.

The Midtown Manhattan study was conducted between November, 1953 and July, 1954. A total of 1,660 people were interviewed, representing a probability sample of 16/1,000 individuals in the age range of 20 to 59. The authors argued that, because of the difficulty of making correct diagnoses, the problems with accuracy of diagnosis in the early stages of illness, the low rates of diagnostic reliability, and the high probability that a diagnosis will be changed during an episode, a symptom scale was a more reasonable assessment of psychiatric morbidity. Of the individuals interviewed in the study, 18.5% were found to be well or symptom free; 23.4% were reported to have marked or severe symptom formation or to be incapacitated or impaired. These latter categories reflected the psychiatric judgment that these individuals were not able to carry out their daily life roles and were considered to be the equivalent of patients in treatment populations (Srole, 1978). Among the subjects with serious morbidity, 73.3% reported that they had never received treatment, 21% had received care in the past, and 5.4% were currently being treated. Almost half of those who had never received treatment indicated that they would be unlikely to use mental health services.

In a study conducted by the Joint Commission on Mental Illness and Health a household sample of 2,460 Americans over the age of 21 was interviewed. They reported that 20% of those interviewed had felt that they were going to experience a nervous breakdown, and nearly half of those had consulted some professional source for help (Gurin, Veroff, & Feld, 1960).

Leighton et al. (1963) studied a random sample of 1,010 adults who were living in Stirling County, Nova Scotia. Like the Midtown Manhattan study, only 17% of the sample was rated as symptom free, whereas 32% of the total sample (31% of the men and 33% of the women) was rated as significantly impaired. At least 20% of the population, it was felt, was in need of psychiatric treatment. Overall, women showed more psychiatric morbidity than men, although the proportions with significant morbidity were the same. Older people had higher rates than younger people; higher social class was associated with better mental health.

More recently, the NIMH funded a multicenter collaborative effort to explore the prevalence of psychiatric disorders in the general population. The Epidemiologic Catchment Area (ECA) study was the first multisite assessment of prevalence, and the first large epidemiological study to use the DSM-III criteria. Also, as discussed earlier, the DIS was developed to allow researchers to assess the prevalence of specific symptoms that are required to meet the criteria for each diagnosis in the DSM-III. Because of logistic and cost concerns, the DIS was also developed specifically to allow the use of lay interviewers. Conceptually, the DIS was used to measure the symptoms of psychiatric disorders. These separate symptoms could be assorted and reassorted to make up different diagnoses.

A combined report from the multiple sites of the ECA studies found that 32% of Americans had experienced at least one psychiatric disorder in their lifetime and that 20% of the population had an active or current disorder (Robins, Locke, & Regier, 1991). These rates fall in the middle of the earlier population studies. The Stirling County study found that 24% of the population had significant impairment, whereas 11% of the subjects in the Baltimore study were found to have a DSM-I diagnosis. The Midtown Manhattan study did not use specific diagnostic categories but found that 23% of the sample was significantly impaired. Thus, the rates are within the same range, even though different methods were used for diagnosis.

In the ECA study (Robins *et al.*, 1991), the most common disorder was phobia, with a lifetime prevalence of 14.3% and a current prevalence of 8.8%. The next in line was alcohol abuse/dependence, with lifetime and current prevalences of 13.8% and 6.3%, respectively. These diagnoses were followed by anxiety disorder, major depressive episodes, and drug abuse/dependence.

The median age for the appearance of the first symptoms was 16 in the ECA study; 90% of the population had experienced the first symptoms of the diagnosis by age 38. Antisocial personality was the disorder with the earliest onset at 8 years of age. Ninety percent of the subjects who had antisocial personality had symptom onset by age 12. In contrast, depressive episodes had the latest onset (age 25), and the widest age range for presentation, with 90% of those diagnosed presenting symptoms by age 52.

Young subjects in the study were more likely to have both a current and a lifetime psychiatric diagnosis than older people, a finding that was at variance with the earlier studies. The specific diagnoses that lead to higher rates in younger people were antisocial personality, drug abuse/dependence, and manic episodes. Remission was also age related and was lowest in the under 30 age group.

Sociodemographic factors were clear predictors of the prevalence of psychiatric disorder. African Americans had higher rates of psychiatric morbidity than did Hispanics or whites. People who had completed high school or more education had lower rates compared to those who had not completed high school. Individuals who were separated or divorced and those who were cohabiting and had never been married had the highest rates of illness. However, these findings on education and marital status must be interpreted with caution. Since these were cross-sectional data, the direction of the relationships cannot be determined, and, as discussed earlier, it is not clear whether these factors which correlate with the prevalence of disorder are causes or consequences of the disorder.

One of the most striking findings from the ECA studies was the low rate of treatment received by those individuals with current diagnoses. Only 19% of the subjects with current diagnoses reported that they had received inpatient treatment in the past year or outpatient treatment in the past 6 months. Those most likely to receive treatment were unmarried females with a high school education or greater (27%), and the least likely to receive treatment were married men with less than a high school education (11%). The probability of treatment also varied with the type of diagnosis. Patients with somatization disorder, panic disorder, and schizophrenia were more likely to receive mental health care, whereas those with antisocial personality, cognitive deficits, alcohol and drug abuse, or dependence were least likely. Therefore, the picture of mental illness in a community population is substantially different than what would be found in a clinical population.

The ECA studies of a general population sample have demonstrated that subjects with psychiatric disorders are younger, unmarried, and of lower social class. There were no differences in prevalence rates between men and women, diagnoses varied by age, sex, education, and the extent of co-morbidity. Further, the probability of receiving treatment, while generally low, also varied by demographic characteristics, diagnostic categories, and co-morbidity. The differences found between clinical and general population samples and the high proportion of individuals with psychiatric illness who did not receive care, highlight the usefulness of epidemiological data in describing the correlates of psychiatric disorders more accurately.

SUMMARY

Epidemiology is a methodology and a framework for organizing ideas about etiology and for conducting research into these hypotheses. It is, however, dependent on the field of psychiatry to produce definitions of the outcome measures and to explicate the specific criteria that will be used to measure the occurrence of disorders. Therefore, the focus of psychiatric epidemiology as a field of research has been toward the development of reliable, valid, and standardized diagnoses and instruments. In the absence of these basic tools, little forward progress could be made in the field.

Psychiatric epidemiology has now reached what Dohrenwend (1990) has termed the third generation of studies: studies that use standardized diagnostic criteria and standard instruments for data collection. The development of the DSM system, and particularly the DSM-III and its subsequent revisions, as well as the information provided by the ECA project, will enable researchers to begin to make more accurate estimates of the actual prevalence of psychiatric morbidity in the general population. The development of standardized criteria and instruments has now made it possible for researchers to compare data in a reliable way across different populations. To return to John Graunt, although the task is not complete, we have moved past the stage of "laborious buzzing and groping" into a systematic diagnostic framework. With new tools developed, psychiatric epidemiology can move forward to investigate questions of etiology.

REFERENCES

American Psychiatric Association. (1980). *Diagnostic and statistical manual of mental disorders* (3rd ed.). Washington, DC: Author.

American Psychiatric Association. (1987). *Diagnostic and statistical manual of mental disorders* (3rd ed., rev.). Washington, DC: Author.

Anthony, J. C., Folstein, M., Romanoski, A. J., Von Korff, M. R., Nestadt, G. R., Chahal, R., Merchant, A., Brown, H., Shapiro, S., Kramer, M., & Gruenberg, E. M. (1985). Comparison of the lay diagnostic interview schedule and a standardized psychiatric diagnosis. *Archives of General Psychiatry, 42,* 667–675.

Bartko, J. J., & Carpenter, W. T. (1976). On the methods and theory of reliability. *Journal of Nervous and Mental Disease, 163,* 307–317.

Beck, A. T. (1969). *Depression: Clinical experimental and theoretical aspects.* New York: Harper & Row.

Berkson, J. (1946). Limitations of the application of four-fold tables to hospital data. *Biometric Bulletin, 2,* 47–53.

Bromet, E. J., & Schulberg, H. C. (1987). Epidemiologic findings from disaster research. In R. E. Hales & A. J. Francis (Eds.), *American Psychiatric Association Annual Review, Volume 6* (pp. 676–689). Washington, DC: American Psychiatric Press.

Brown, G. W., Bifulco, A., & Harris, T. O. (1987). Life events, vulnerability and onset of depression: Some refinements. *British Journal of Psychiatry, 150,* 30–42.

Charney, E. A., & Weissman, M. M. (1988). Epidemiology of depressive illness. In J. J. Mann (Ed.), *Phenomenology of depressive illness* (pp. 45–74). New York: Human Sciences Press.

Cleary, P.D., & Kessler, R. C. (1982). The estimation and interpretation of modifier effects. *Journal of Health and Social Behavior, 23,* 159–169.

Costello, E. J. (1989a). Developments in child psychiatric epidemiology. *Journal of Child and Adolescent Psychiatry, 28,* 836–841.

Costello, E. J. (1989b). Child psychiatric disorders and their correlates: A primary care pediatric sample. *Journal of the American Academy of Child and Adolescent Psychiatry, 28,* 851–855.

Costello, E. J., Costello, A. J., Edelbrock, C., Burns, B. J., Dulcan, M. K., Brent, D., & Janiszewski, S. (1988). Psychiatric disorders in pediatric primary care. *Archives of General Psychiatry, 45,* 1107–1116.

Day, N. L., Robles, N., Richardson, G., Geva, D., Taylor, P., Scher, M., Stoffer, D., Cornelius, M., & Goldschmidt, L. (1991). The effects of prenatal alcohol use on the growth of children at three years of age. *Alcoholism: Clinical and Experimental Research, 15,* 67–71.

Dohrenwend, B. P. (1990). The problem of validity in field studies of psychological disorders revisited. *Psychological Medicine, 20,* 195–208.

Elkin, I., Shea, S., Watkins, J. T., Imber, S. D., Sotsky, S. M., Collins, J. F., Glass, D. R., Pilkonis, P. A., Leber, W. R., Doeherty, J. P., Fiester, S. J., & Parloff, M. B. (1989). National Institute of Mental Health treatment of depression collaborative research program. General effectiveness of treatments. *Archives of General Psychiatry, 46,* 971–982.

Faris, R., & Dunham, H. (1939). *Mental disorders in urban areas: An empirical study of schizophrenia and other disorders.* Chicago: University of Chicago Press.

Feighner, J. P., Robins, E., Guze, S. B., Woodruff, R. A., Winokur, B., & Munoz, R. (1972). Diagnostic criteria for use in psychiatric research. *Archives of General Psychiatry, 26,* 57–63.

Finney, J. W., Mitchell, R. E., Cronkite, R. C., & Moos, R. H. (1984). Methodological issues in estimating main and interactive effects: Examples from copying/social support and stress field. *Journal of Health and Social Behavior, 25,* 85–98.

Graunt, J. (1939). *Natural and political observations made upon the bills of mortality* (W. F. Willcox, Ed.). Baltimore: Johns Hopkins Press. (Original work published 1662).

Grob, G. N. (1985). The origins of American psychiatric epidemiology. *American Journal of Public Health, 75*, 229–236.

Grove, W. M., Andreasen, N. C., McDonald-Scott, P., Keller, M. B., & Shapiro, R. W. (1981). Reliability studies of psychiatric diagnosis: Theory and practice. *Archives of General Psychiatry, 38*, 408–413.

Gurin, G., Veroff, J., & Feld, S. (1960). *Americans view their mental health. A nationwide interview survey.* (Monograph Series No. 4, Joint Commission on Mental Illness and Health). New York: Basic Books.

Hamilton, M. (1960). A rating scale for depression. *Journal of Neurology and Neurosurgical Psychiatry, 23*, 56–62.

Helzer, J. E., Robins, L. N., Croughan, J. L., & Welner, A. (1981). Renard Diagnostic Interview: Its reliability and procedural validity with physicians and lay interviewers. *Archives of General Psychiatry, 38*, 393–398.

Helzer, J. E., Robins, L. N., McEvoy, L. T., Spitznagel, E. L., Stoltzman, R. K., Farmer, A., & Brockington, I. F. (1985). A comparison of clinical and diagnostic interview schedule diagnoses. *Archives of General Psychiatry, 42*, 657–666.

Hollingshead, A., & Redlich, F. (1958). *Social class and mental illness.* New York: Wiley.

Ilfeld, F. W. (1977). Current social stressors and symptoms of depression. *American Journal of Psychiatry, 134*, 161–166.

Kelsey, J. L., Thompson, W. D., & Evans, A. S. (1986). *Methods in observational epidemiology.* New York: Oxford University Press.

Leighton, D. C., Harding, J. S., Macklin, M. A., Hughes, C. C., & Leighton, A. H. (1963). Psychiatric findings of the Stirling County study. *American Journal of Psychiatry, 119*, 1021–1026.

Lemkau, P., Tietze, C., & Cooper, H. (1942). Complaint of nervousness and the psychoneuroses. *American Journal of Orthopsychiatry, 12*, 214–223.

Lind, J., (1953). *A treatise of the scurvy.* In C. P. Steward & D. Guthrie (Eds.), *Lind's treatise on scurvy.* Edinburgh: University Press. (Original work published 1753).

MacMahon, B., & Pugh, T. (1970). *Epidemiology: Principles and methods.* Boston: Little, Brown.

Offord, D. R., Boyle, M. H., & Racine, Y. (1989). Ontario child health study: Correlates of disorder. *Journal of the American Academy of Child and Adolescent Psychiatry, 28*, 856–860.

Regier, D. A., Myers, J. K., Kramer, M., Robins, L. N., Blazer, D. G., Hough, R. L., Eaton, W. W., & Locke, B. Z. (1985). Historical context, major objectives and study design. In W. W. Eaton & L. G. Kessler (Eds.), *Epidemiologic field methods in psychiatry* (pp. 3–19). New York: Academic Press.

Robins, L. N. (1974). *Deviant children grown up: A sociological and psychiatric study of sociopathic personality.* Huntington, NY: Robert E. Krieger.

Robins, L. N. (1990). Psychiatric epidemiology: A historic review. *Social Psychiatry and Psychiatric Epidemiology, 25*, 16–26.

Robins, L. N., Helzer, J. E., Orvaschel, H., Anthony, J. C., Blazer, D. G., Burnam, A., & Burke, J. D. (1985). In W. W. Eaton & L. G. Kessler (Eds.), *Epidemiologic field methods in psychiatry. The NIMH epidemiologic catchment area program* (pp. 143–168). New York: Academic Press.

Robins, L. N., Locke, B. Z., & Regier, D. A. (1991). An overview of psychiatric disorders in America. In L. N. Robins & D. A. Regier (Eds.), *Psychiatric disorders in America: The epidemiologic catchment area study* (pp. 328–366). New York: Free Press.

Roth, W. F., & Luton, F. H. (1943). The mental health program in Tennessee. *American Journal of Psychiatry, 99*, 662–673.

Rutter, M. (1981). Longitudinal studies: A psychiatric perspective. In S. Mednick, A. Baert, & B. Bachmann (Eds.), *Prospective longitudinal research* (pp. 326–336). Oxford: Oxford University Press.

Shrout, P. E., Spitzer, R. L., & Fleiss, J. L. (1987). Quantification of agreement in psychiatric diagnosis revisited. *Archives of General Psychiatry, 44*, 172–177.

Snow, J. (1936). *Snow on cholera.* New York: Commonwealth Fund.

Spitzer, R. L., & Endicott, J. (1968). *Schedule for affective disorders and schizophrenia.* New York: New York State Psychiatric Institute.

Spitzer, R. L., Endicott, J., & Robins, E. (1978). Research diagnostic criteria: Rationale and reliability. *Archives of General Psychiatry, 35*, 773–782.

Srole, L. (1978). Midtown and several other populations. In L. Srole & A. Fischer (Eds.), *Mental health in the metropolis: The midtown Manhattan study* (pp. 183–217). New York: New York University Press.

Terris, M. (1967). The epidemiology of cirrhosis of the liver. National mortality rate. *American Journal of Public Health, 57*, 2076–2088.

Thase, M. E., Frank, E., & Kupfer, D. J. (1985). Biological processes in major depression. In E. E. Beckham & W. R. Leber (Eds.), *Handbook of depression: Treatment, assessment and research* (pp. 816–913). Homewood, IL: Dorsey Press.

U.S. Department of Health and Human Services. (1990). *Alcohol and Health.* Seventh Special Report to the U.S. Congress (pp. 107–128). Rockville, MD: Author.

Weissman, M. W., & Klerman, G.L. (1978). Epidemiology of mental disorders: Emerging trends in the United States. *Archives of General Psychiatry, 35*, 705–712.

Weissman, M. W., Gershon, E. S., Kidd, K. K., Prusoff, B. A., Leckman, J. F., Dibble, E., Hamovit, J., Thompson, W. D., Pauls, D. L., & Guroff, J. J. (1984). Psychiatric disorders in relatives of probands with affective disorders. *Archives of General Psychiatry, 41*, 13–21.

Zung, W. W. (1965). A self-rating depression scale. *Archives of General Psychiatry, 12*, 63–70.

CHAPTER 12

Psychopharmacology

SILVIA S. GRATZ AND GEORGE M. SIMPSON

INTRODUCTION

Research in psychopharmacology is both blessed and plagued by its history. In 1949, the psychiatrist John Cade discovered the antimanic properties of lithium when he hypothesized that manic-depressive illness is analogous to thyrotoxicosis-myxedema. Eventually, he determined that lithium made guinea pigs lethargic and manic patients calm. Within a 2-year span (1950–1951), this discovery generated three Australian and three French studies. Despite this initial enthusiasm with lithium, this event did not launch psychopharmacology as an important therapeutic field. The French surgeon Henri Laborit's keen observation that chlorpromazine (CPZ) nullified preoperative anxiety, mitigated surgical stress, and thereby eliminated its postoperative consequences, led him with dynamic persuasion to convince early psychiatrists to give CPZ for psychotic states. Colonel Paraire, a psychiatrist and Laborit's colleague, has been credited with the first report and publication on the therapeutic effects of intravenous (IV) CPZ in a manic patient; this article appeared in the Annales Médico-Psycholigiques in March, 1952. Delay and Deniker's study of 38 subjects, although totally lacking in methodological rigor by modern day standards (an open study with mixed diagnoses without controls and rating scales), nevertheless, resulted in one of the notable therapeutic advances of the century, provoked research throughout the world, and stirred the ambitions of pharmaceutical

Silvia S. Gratz and George M. Simpson • Department of Psychiatry, Medical College of Pennsylvania, Eastern Pennsylvania Psychiatric Institute, Philadelphia, Pennsylvania 19129.

Research in Psychiatry: Issues, Strategies, and Methods, edited by L. K. George Hsu and Michel Hersen. Plenum Press, New York, 1992.

manufacturers. Delay and Deniker (1952) not only recognized the astonishing efficacy of CPZ, but also announced that this was a unique therapeutic agent with unique unwanted side effects. Although earlier psychiatric usage of CPZ has been attributed to Sigwald, he did not report his observations and experience with CPZ in 48 psychiatric patients until April 25, 1953. It should be emphasized that this report was presented in the form of case histories of 5 psychotics and 43 neurotics (Caldwell, 1978). The stage was set for a large number of ambitious but unsophisticated studies throughout the world which soon resulted in the serendipitous discovery of imipramine, the first tricyclic antidepressant, by Kuhn in 1957. For more than a century, psychiatrists had been somewhat indiscriminate in their usage of drugs. Today there exists a reasonable probability that it would be quite difficult to persuade an experienced clinician/researcher to evaluate any agent in such an open fashion without methodological and ethical concerns—a factor related in part to legal and ethical constraints as well as exaggerated claims in open trials which are frequently never confirmed.

ANIMAL MODELS

A direct result of these early experimental efforts was the development of animal models to predict similar activity to the prototypical agents. Efforts in this direction had a tendency to produce pharmacological agents that were entirely too similar to the prototypical drugs. In effect, psychopharmacology research, for some 20 years after the initial important discoveries, focused on the evaluation of a large series of agents that differed but little in their side effect profile and not at all in their therapeutic outcome. Only a rigorously designed controlled study with adequate evaluation procedures and sufficient sample size could answer questions of a drug–drug difference. Therefore, in drug discovery, animal models may produce information on the behavioral and biochemical changes which suggest potential efficacy in certain specific forms of psychopathology, but it is important to realize that various species of animals react differently to the same drug. A drug that lacks toxicity in animals and is suggestive of some therapeutic effect will require subsequent studies in humans that will attempt to corroborate or reject suggestive data from animal models.

PHARMACOKINETICS AND PHARMACODYNAMICS

Pharmacokinetics links the application of *kinetics* (rate of change in a system) to *pharmakon* (Greek word for drugs). Specifically, *pharmacokinetics* refers to the rate of change in drug concentration within a biological system: anatomical organs, body tissues, and fluids. In practice, pharmacokinetics describes the relationships between drug dose and drug concentration in blood, plasma, or other body components (i.e., the concentration of drug in body components over time). The associated science of *pharmacodynamics* describes the relationships between drug concentration and drug response (i.e., how an organism responds to a specific concentration of the drug). It is essential to recognize that the relationship between a drug dose and the effect it produces varies among patients, and even at times within the same patient under different conditions. Variability, therefore, can be categorized either according to pharmacokinetic factors or pharmacodynamic factors. Figure 1 demonstrates the interrelationship among these terms.

In the past, the solutions to many pharmacotherapy issues were answered by trial and error. The clinical investigator arbitrarily chose a dose, the interval between doses, the route of administration, and then followed the patient's progress. After assessment of the desired effect and signs of toxicity, the dosage regimen was adjusted empirically. This empirical approach had a tendency to leave many questions unanswered. Why, for example, do many of the benzodi-azepines require a dosing regimen of every 6 to 8 hours to be effective for anxiolysis, whereas most of the antipsychotics can be given once daily? Gener-ally, an empirical approach offers at best an awkward method to establish a safe and effective dosage regimen of another drug. Once the therapeutic phases of pharmacokinetics and pharmacodynamics have been defined for a given drug, a therapeutic dosage regimen can be designed to achieve a therapeutic re-sponse. Knowledge of the pharmacokinetics of a particular drug aids the clini-cians in anticipating the optimal dosage regimen for a given patient and in making a prediction when a specific dosage regimen is altered. The magnitudes of both the desired response and toxicity are functions of the drug concentration at the site(s) of action—a basic tenet of pharmacokinetics. Therapeutic failure results when either the drug concentration is too low (ineffective therapy), or is too high (unacceptable toxicity). Between the limits of concentration lies a region known as a *therapeutic window*. It is rare that the concentration of a drug can be measured directly at the site of action; however, the concentration can be measured at an alternative site—the plasma (Rowland & Tozer, 1989). An

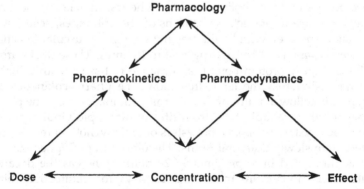

Figure 1. The interrelationships between pharmacokinetic and pharmacodynamic factors.

optimal dosage regimen, therefore, would take into consideration all these foregoing factors and maintain the plasma concentration of a drug within a therapeutic window. A target area or therapeutic window has been established for nortriptyline (NT) (50–150 ng/mL plasma)—a widely used antidepressant. It should be emphasized that control on a dosage basis alone is most difficult. Optimal drug therapy is achieved when plasma drug concentration data and the pharmacokinetics of the drug are known. For the majority of patients, knowledge of a drug's therapeutic window and pharmacokinetics should theoretically lead to a more rapid establishment of a safe and effective dosage range. The narrower this dosage range, the more difficult is the maintenance of values within it. The upper limit of a drug's plasma concentration may be either like NT, a result of diminishing efficacy at higher concentrations without noticeable signs of toxicity, or like lithium, a result of the possibility of life-threatening toxicity.

The association between benzodiazepine plasma concentrations and pharmacodynamics is controversial (Baird & Hailey, 1972; Greenblatt, Shader, & MacLeod, 1978; Hillestad, Hansen, & Melsom, 1974; Kyriakopouloss, Greenblatt, & Shader, 1978). The onset and initial intensity of the neuropharmacological actions of benzodiazepines tend to approximate the rate of rise and peak concentrations of the drugs in plasma after a single dose. During the gradual decline of plasma levels in the elimination phase of a single dose and during chronic therapy, however, the relationships between plasma levels and pharmacological effects are less apparent. The multitude of neuropharmacological effects of benzodiazepines complicates the identification of relationships of drug concentrations to pharmacodynamics. There are few studies that have demonstrated the plasma concentration threshold for specific effects of benzodiazepines (Pry-Roberts & Hug, 1984). Ghoneim, Korttila, and Chiang (1981) have attempted to associate certain tests of mental and psychomotor function with kinetic data. Digit recall (a measure of amnestic effects) and plasma drug levels after an intravenous injection of diazepam (0.2 mg/kg) in Caucasians resulted in a peak effect on recall that was found 30 minutes after administration and was still evident 2 hours after administration.

Few conclusions with clinical relevance can be elicited from the study of the pharmacokinetics and metabolism of antipsychotics. In general, most antipsychotics tend to have unpredictable patterns of absorption, especially with oral administration and even with liquid preparations. Intramuscular injections can increase the availability of active drug by 4 to 10 times. These drugs are highly lipid soluble, highly protein bound, accumulate in tissues with a high blood supply, and easily cross the fetal circulation. The pharmacokinetics of these agents typically follow a multiphasic patterns. Elimination from the plasma has a tendency to be more rapid than from sites of high lipid binding such as the central nervous system (CNS). Depot esters of antipsychotics are absorbed and eliminated more slowly than oral forms. The oral form of fluphenazine hydrochloride is eliminated in approximately 20 hours, whereas the decanoate or enanthate ester can require more than 20 days for elimination (Simpson, Yadalam, Stephanos, Lo, & Cooper, 1990). Although we currently have techniques available which permit monitoring of antipsychotic drug plasma levels, there is a need for more detailed information on kinetics as well as the significance of therapeutic and toxic levels.

THE FOOD AND DRUG ADMINISTRATION (FDA)

At the turn of the century, conditions were unfavorable in the United States food and drug industries. Food processing and handling were often unsanitary and spoiled foods were treated with chemicals and sold. The approach of the FDA has undergone a radical transformation in the 75 years since the old Bureau of Chemistry was charged with implementing the Pure Food and Drugs Act of 1906 (Marwick, 1985; Ziporyn, 1985). The activity of the FDA is to monitor and review the results of clinical trials and to assure that biotechnology products are safe and effective for their intended use. Sponsors of research on new drugs or alternative therapeutic uses of approved drugs file a Notice of Claimed Investigational Exemption for a New Drug (IND) application to conduct clinical trials. The type and spectrum of clinical trials under the IND are crucial to producing the scientific evidence for the safety and effectiveness determinations that are required for approval of the drug for marketing (Miller & Young, 1989). Generally, the evidence is obtained in the following phases which in practice may overlap and occur simultaneously.

METHODOLOGY OF CLINICAL TRIALS

Study Protocol

A study protocol is the first major milestone to be reached and is essential for the success of any drug trial whether it be for multicenter studies or limited to the use by a single investigator. The study protocol embraces every aspect of management and assessment of patients (e.g., inclusion/exclusion criteria, consent, patient registration, trial design, safety monitoring), copies of forms and rating measures, instructions for their completion and scoring, as well as a summary of the data collected and the methods of analysis. We should never lose sight of the primary objective of any drug trial—an estimation of the difference(s) between randomized treatments on some chosen measure of efficacy (Freeman & Tyrer, 1989).

Phase 1

Typically, these clinical trials are tolerance studies in normal volunteers in an effort to render an idea about safety, toxicity, and side effects and to predict what the animal model has suggested for the drug's usage. The first objective is to determine an acceptable single drug dosage (i.e., how much of this drug can be administered without causing serious side effects). This information is obtained from dose escalation experiments in which the healthy volunteer is subjected to incremental dosages of the drug according to a predetermined schedule. In addition, Phase 1 clinical trials will frequently incorporate studies of drug metabolism and bioavailability and, ultimately, studies of multiple doses will be undertaken to determine the appropriate dose schedule for usage in Phase 2. Although Phase 1 clinical trials may render information on the toxicity of the drug, it is often difficult to extrapolate dosage from normals to psychiatric patients.

Phase 2

This phase consists of controlled clinical trials, usually on a small scale (frequently 100 to 200 subjects) and dose-ranging investigations into the drug's efficacy while continuing to learn more about the drug's safety in patients with a specific disease or symptom for which the drug is indicated. The first important question is, what is the dosage? For example, a drug like CPZ given in 50- or 100-mg dosages to normal subjects will invariably produce intense sedation and higher dosages would not be tolerated. This would also be true of drugs like amitriptyline in similar dosages. Nevertheless, in patients with diagnosed schizophrenia or depression (who are treated with CPZ and amitriptyline, respectively), dosages of at least 3 times that amount might be required and are most often well tolerated. A Phase 2 clinical trial could be conducted openly with an experienced clinician to evaluate incremental dosages of the drug and its effect on the patient's illness (psychopathology) and also to evaluate behavioral side effects as well as organ toxicity. The conclusion of such a study would lead to the development of a controlled comparison study to determine definitively whether or not the drug is active in the condition and to be followed by or concomitantly with a comparison with existing treatments. The proof of efficacy is a *sine qua non* for FDA approval and is also a requirement before general testing in females. Females who are pregnant, nursing, or are at risk of becoming pregnant should be excluded from all trials. Until efficacy has been demonstrated, however, women would be excluded, unless they were postmenopausal or surgically sterilized. A major requirement for drug development progress is that patients be exposed to the least possible risk consistent with anticipated benefit (Burlington & Gubish, 1987).

Phase 3

Phase 3 studies may overlap with late Phase 2 studies and are expanded controlled trials that include long-term toxicity studies. These studies are conducted in the field by a variety of clinicians who are not employed by the pharmaceutical companies, but rather are associated with university medical centers, teaching hospitals, state hospitals, Veterans Administration Medical Centers, or who are in private practice. These expanded controlled trials (typically lasting several months) need not be comparative (i.e., they may or may not need a placebo or comparison to a standard treatment) and proceed if data give reasonable assurance of safety (Spriet & Simon, 1985). If, however, one of the aims is to determine further a drug's therapeutic effect or potential value outweighing potential risks, a comparison will be necessary.

Phase 4

Phase 4 studies entail postmarketing clinical trials which may be of several varieties, including additional studies that elucidate the presence and frequency of less frequent adverse effects; large-scale, long-term studies to determine the effect of the drug on morbidity and mortality; or trials in categories of patients (e.g., children or nursing mothers) who are not adequately studied during other premarketing phases (Miller & Young, 1989).

Much of the methodology to be detailed for a new agent will apply to the establishment of new indications for an existing therapeutic agent that is indicated in one condition for a possible new indication. Since this involves a condition outside the language of the approved labeling, these studies require an IND procedure (e.g., the study of carbamazepine, an established therapy for seizure disorders and trigeminal neuralgia employed in the treatment of mania). The use of carbamazepine in patients with affective disorder is ill-defined and does not have FDA approval for its usage in the treatment of mood disorders (e.g., bipolar disorder) and is still experimental in this patient population. Jefferson, Greist, Ackerman, and Carroll (1987) have pointed out that further clinical research is needed to identify carbamazepine's range of clinical effects and the risks associated with this agent's long-term usage. Four double-blind controlled studies have suggested that carbamazepine may be a potential prophylactic treatment for bipolar disorder (Lusznat, Murphy, & Nunn, 1988; Okuma, Inanga, Otsuki, Keisuke, Takahashi, Hazama, Mori, & Watanabe, 1981; Placidi, Lenzi, Lazzerini, Cassano, & Akiskal, 1986; Watkins, Callender, Thomas, Tidmarsh, & Shaw, 1987). Even with evidence for such optimism surrounding carbamazepine as a useful psychotropic, there is still a need for carefully designed, double-blind, prospective studies to establish the efficacy of this agent for the prophylaxis of bipolar disorder (Prien & Gelenberg, 1989).

DRUG STUDY DESIGNS

Drug–placebo and drug–drug designs are the rule in the evaluation of psychopharmacological agents (whether new, old, or in combination with drugs or psychosocial treatments). It is often useful to give at least a 1-week period of placebo to all patients prior to beginning the evaluation proper of the drug agent under study. This period tends to eliminate patients from the study (e.g., rapid remitters), those who have a self-limiting illness, or those who respond to nonspecific factors and thus tend to diminish the number of positive results in both the drug and placebo groups. This introductory placebo period, however, ultimately makes it easier to prove efficacy. Following the placebo period, the double-blind study may begin with appropriate initial evaluations. The double-blind paradigm (considered indispensable in the evaluation of new drug treatment) requires that neither the investigator nor the patient be aware of the treatment assignment. Ideally, everyone who has contact with the patient should be blind; the minimal requirement, however, is that both the patient and the rater be blind. The researcher must have confidence that the reaction of the subject is changed by the drug being studied. Although this may be easily accomplished by splitting the sample into 2 groups—the experimental group (those being given the drug) and the control group (those being treated similarly but without the active drug)—such nonrandom assignment of subjects into experimental and control groups may produce differences that are a function of selection bias rather than to the drug's effect. If assignment is done in a random fashion, there is some assurance that the groups (experimental and control) at least start the same. It is important to emphasize, however, that subsequent differential treatment of groups may produce differences which are not related to the drug effect. Thus, if one group is monitored and given pills, while the control group has no intervention, the apparent differences may be a reflection of this process and not of the drug. Even in a study where each group receives a pill, differential side effects (i.e., the presence or absence of side effects) could influence the study. In some cases, this has led to the use of an "active" placebo (i.e., an agent with side effects similar to the study drug but with a known therapeutic effect), such as small doses of atropine to mimic the anticholinergic side effects of tricyclic antidepressants (TCAs).

Drug–Placebo Designs

In the event that a specific drug treatment is thought to be effective for a particular illness, a randomized double-blind experiment can be initiated in which each subject would be given either the active drug or a placebo for a specified time interval. Significant factors in response or nonresponse may include effects of cognitive expectations, drug-use experience, and individual versus group setting strategies. Although this method has been viewed as a definitive way to establish drug activity, it has been demonstrated that subjects who are more sophisticated may have a rather good idea of what they are supposed to experience and, therefore, may tend to give expected answers unless elaborate measures are taken to control for this (see above). However, despite such possibilities, placebo-controlled studies are in general valid and indispensable, and their random assignment is crucial.

Drug–Drug Designs

If a known dosage of a drug has been established (e.g., haloperidol 5–20 mg), this may be compared to an investigational Drug X which has been shown to be efficacious from previous dosing schedules. These 2 drugs may be evaluated in a direct comparison on a similar population (i.e., schizophrenic patients). It should be recognized, however, that an optimal dose of a drug may not always be determined. Another way of defining activity would be to utilize multiple dose studies of the investigational drug and look for a dose-response relationship. For example, there would be 3 dosages of the experimental drug that is, a straightforward dose-response study where the prediction would be a therapeutic gradient and similarly for side effects. This is a technique widely used in animal studies and, until recently, to a lesser extent in humans. This technique, however, is of great importance in strictly defining the effective dose of a drug or in using the same design in an attempt to establish a plasma drug-level response range. At the very least, there would be the notion that one or two of the dosages would be superior to the lower dosages of the drug (e.g., 300 mg of imipramine has been demonstrated to be superior to 150 mg of imipramine in nondeluded depressives) (Simpson, Lee, Cuculic, & Kellner, 1976). This, in effect, demonstrates that imipramine is therapeutically effective. One must demonstrate that the investigational drug is equal to or more active than the standard drug or that it produces fewer or less severe side effects (e.g., extrapyramidal symptoms in an investigational antipsychotic). This strategy can also be combined with a known active drug which enhances the study, by contrasting both the efficacy and the side effects. The further addition of placebo-producing 5 cells makes the study even more rigorous.

Other Related Problems

Associated issues facing clinical psychopharmacology include: (1) Is one therapy superior to another? (2) Is efficacy enhanced by combination therapy? (3) Does dose improve efficacy (e.g., are side effects the limiting factor?) (4) Are risks of increasing dose and efficacy countered by risks of increasing the side-effect profile? Our study (Simpson *et al.*, 1976) which demonstrated that 300 mg of imipramine was more effective than 150 mg of imipramine may help the clinician to define who is really the treatment-resistant patient.

IMPLEMENTING TECHNIQUE

Once a drug has been claimed to be effective for particular symptoms of a disease state (Phase 2), it may or may not be compared to a placebo. Nevertheless, use of a placebo improves a study design. In Phase 3, in which clinical trials are extended to a larger and more varied population, one may take the dose that was effective in Phase 2 and compare it to a standard treatment in a double-blind study (drug A versus drug B). It is often unknown, however, what the most effective dose is in Phase 3; therefore, the most effective dose needs to be defined in Phase 3 testing. This study may be implemented, as previously mentioned, by having a group of randomly assigned patients receive 3 different dosages of the drug (hypothetical drug A—75 mg, 150 mg, 300 mg) and determining which is the most effective dose with an acceptable side-effect profile. This procedure may be combined with that of another group of patients who are randomly assigned to receive an effective dose of a standard drug currently available (e.g., haloperidol or CPZ, if the new treatment were for psychosis). One may also have a placebo group in almost any study to reaffirm the effectiveness of the therapy (drug A versus drug B versus placebo). In this example, therefore, 5 groups would be randomly assigned.

SPECIAL ISSUES

As already mentioned, if an agent is thought to have, for example, anti-depressant properties and is well tolerated in normal controls (Phase 1), then evaluation in patients suffering from the disorder follows next (Phase 2). Ideally, the design of such a study should be a comparison of the "active" treatment against an inactive treatment in order to establish that there is some degree of efficacy. Phases 2 and 3 are often combined to accelerate approval of the drug. In the United States, one must establish one pivotal study (typically Phase 3) (not specifically stated by the FDA, but rather implied) and that study preferably should be multicenter for labeling (e.g. indications, side effects, etc.) with enough patients to establish safety issues and superiority of the experimental drug over a comparative drug. Phase 3 clinical trials may compare the drug with placebo or the current standard treatment (e.g., imipramine—a prototypical antidepressant).

Even in Phase 3 clinical trials, the problems are very complicated, since at this stage in the study, precise dosages are unknown. Also, one must make decisions in the study, whether the populations should be inpatients or out-patients. Antidepressants may be considered a special case, since depressions are often episodic, tending toward spontaneous remissions and exacerbations. Assessment of treatment effectiveness may be limited by inadequacies of depressive nosology (see the section below on Advances in Psychopharmacology). One of the benefits of an inpatient study is that the patients are under continual surveillance and, therefore, their compliance with taking medication is much better assured and the evaluation of side effects is carried out much more intensively. On the other hand, the number of inpatient depressions compared to outpatient depressions is very small. They are more likely to be very severe major depressions with a higher percentage of psychotic depres-sions. There are data which indicate that psychotic depressions respond less well to conventional pharmacotherapy than do nonpsychotic depressions. Also, if a placebo condition is employed, there are conceivably potential inherent fiscal and ethical dilemmas. For example, insurance companies may not pay for pla-cebo studies (even though they may be warranted) when there are active treat-ments available. Therefore, ideally, there should be a 1-week no-treatment period, a 1-week placebo period, and a 6-week active medication treatment compared to a placebo condition. This ideal situation is almost impossible to execute in an inpatient setting; thus, placebo-controlled studies tend to be carried out more in outpatient populations. In general, it would appear that in outpatient studies, nonspecific factors play an even greater role, and, therefore, a much larger sample size and possibly several sites will be needed in order to show differences. There is also the problem with drop outs and medication compliance and the medicolegal considerations of using a placebo for a serious condition. The rationale for using a placebo is that in all of the outpatient studies of depression, more than one-third of the patients responded to the attention they received during a clinical trial and thus were prevented from the possible short-term and long-term side effects of the agents, the cost, etc.

In all these conditions, it is imperative that subjects be systematically defined as required for a specific study (see the section above on Study Protocol). Normally, this would include a diagnosis that is translatable to other studies, plus specific criteria that would include the length of the illness, the number of previous episodes, age, sex, previous drug responsivity, and so forth, plus criteria that are associated with severity. Inclusion criteria establish the broad category of patients intended to be treated, whereas exclusion criteria establish contraindications (an example appears in Table 1). For subjects who meet the DSM-III-R criteria for Major Affective Disorder in an outpatient setting, there should be a qualification as to how this information was obtained, such as by a structured clinical interview (SCID), from a history by an experienced clinician or, preferably, by two experienced clinicians, plus a severity item which might be a Hamilton Rating Scale (e.g., a total score of 18). Even in this situation, however, one would need to qualify which Hamilton Rating Scale is used, since the original Hamilton is seldom used and various people have different modifications of this scale. In addition, one needs to consider other aspects of the type of depression, such as is this a primary or secondary depression or is this another subcategory of Major Affective Disorder (e.g., a major depressive episode with psychotic features, dysthymia)? Thus, there is a range of inclusion and exclusion criteria. In any new drug studies, these factors can be of dramatic influence. On the other hand, females who are capable of becoming pregnant may not participate in any type of study to establish the efficacy of a drug agent; this prohibition is according to law in the United States. Yet the male to female ratio is equal to 1:2; women become depressed more frequently than do men. Therefore, if women are not inclusionary subjects for any experimental protocol, the study may become a bit more difficult.

Patients who meet inclusion and exclusion criteria are then randomly assigned to active medication or placebo and are seen usually at weekly intervals throughout the 4- or 6-week phase of the study. During these weekly intervals, time is devoted to completion of patient self-rating scales, clinician-rating scales, side-effects assessments, evaluations, and laboratory studies. With a reasonably homogeneous population and well-defined inclusion and exclusion criteria, a small sample size may be adequate to show a beneficial effect from a new agent. For example, this might be carried out at one site with some 40 patients divided

Table 1.   Example of Entry Criteria from a Recent Clinical Trial

INCLUSION CRITERIA

1. DSM-III-R diagnosis of schizophrenia in sufficient clinical remission to have allowed the patient to achieve at least 2 months of outpatient or day hospital therapy.
2. Age range: 18 or older.
3. Sex: males and nonpregnant, nonlactating females, providing that the females of childbearing potential are using an adequate method of contraception.
4. At both the beginning and the end of the washout phase: total BPRS (Brief Psychiatric Rating Scale) is less than or equal to 60 points and not more than moderately severe (5) on any item of the scale.
5. Patients with or without (a) previous neuroleptic treatment for schizophrenia, (b) past hospital-ization, or (c) neuroleptic responsiveness, may be included.
6. Patients who fulfil Criterion 1 and are stabilized on the medications.
7. A urine toxicology screen will be performed at baseline and once each year for the duration of the study (3 times) to ensure lack of psychoactive substances.

EXCLUSION CRITERA

1. Patients with clinically significant (i.e., organ system[s] involving a major focus of treatment or incapacitation to the patient) cardiovascular, hepatic, renal, gastrointestinal, metabolic, or other systemic disease.
2. Current probable tardive dyskinesia or a history of tardive dyskinesia or of withdrawal dyskinesia.
3. Patients with concurrent psychiatric or neurological diagnosis including: (a) organic mental disorder (DSM-III-R criteria), (b) seizure disorder, (c) mental retardation (DSM-III-R criteria), (d) DSM-III-R criteria for psychoactive substance dependence (except nicotine dependence) not in full remission, and (e) idiopathic Parkinson's disease.
4. Patients who have received depot medication within the past 2 months.
5. Patients who currently present a danger to themselves or who in the investigator's opinion have demonstrated clinically significant suicidal or homicidal behavior during previous drug-free intervals.
6. Pregnant women and nursing mothers. Women of childbearing potential who are not using an adequate contraceptive method.
7. Patients who test positive on the baseline urine substance-abuse screen.
8. Patients with clinically important abnormalities in ECG, chest X-ray, blood chemistries, or other laboratory parameters.
9. Patients with allergies to several drugs or known hypersensitivity to haloperidol.
10. Patients who are participating in another clinical trial or who have received any experimental therapy or clozapine during the past 1 month.

between a placebo and an active condition. However, the comparison of this "new treatment" to the standard active agent will require a very large study in order that a Type 2 error be avoided. In addition, there is the potential problem that the inability to show differences between putative active treatments does not of necessity imply that one has proven that both treatments are active. This condition could be the result of skewed populations or a badly implemented study. Thus, an ideal study comparison would still contain a placebo condition which, in effect, is the final evaluator of the methodology of the clinical trial.

Subsequently, further studies would be carried out to establish that the drug can be given over a protracted period of time without producing toxicity. In addition, there is a need to establish how long to administer a drug. In studies involved in both schizophrenia and depression, one might employ higher dosages of an active medication to prevent recurrences, if it were determined that patients relapse after withdrawal. Typically, target dosages of a medication are often higher than maintenance dosages.

Maintenance pharmacotherapy, which is aimed at prophylaxis, is frequently studied less adequately than therapy directed to an acute episode. This concept has been recently highlighted in results obtained from a 3-year outcome maintenance study in recurrent depression (Frank, Kupfer, Perel, Cornes, Jarrett, Mallinger, Thase, McEachran, & Grochocinski, 1990). These investigators' findings suggest that active imipramine hydrochloride maintained at an average dose of 200 mg is an effective means of prophylaxis. It should be noted that those patients who chose pharmacotherapy were maintained on higher average daily doses than previous studies have suggested (Prien, Kupfer, Mansky, Small, Tuason, Voss, & Johnson, 1984). In any long-term follow-up study, such issues would need to be addressed in a separate phase of a study design. Since all forms of psychopathology have a tendency to recur, there is a need to investigate such long-term maintenance therapies, preferably in the form of a placebo-controlled study.

The important questions in psychopharmacology are not to say that drug A is similar to drug B, but really to try and delineate new conditions or new diagnostic entities that might be better treated than they are currently. Thus, if we think of diagnosis itself as a hypothesis, we must also realize that there is much less specificity to the current therapeutic agents than their names may suggest. For example, antidepressants work in major depression, minor depression, and work very well in panic disorder. Some antidepressants work in anxiety disorders, some in obsessive-compulsive disorders, and some in the treatment of pain; thus, the term *antidepressant* may be a misnomer. If there are, indeed, further subtypes of depression, it is only by delineating them and evaluating treatments in this population that differences may be seen. For example, in a series of studies of atypical depression (well-defined, but not included in any current diagnostic classification system), Liebowitz, Quitkin, Stewart, McGrath, Harrison, Markowitz, Rabkin, Tricamo, Goetz, and Klein (1988) have shown that phenelzine—a monoamine oxidase inhibitor (MAOI)—is superior to imipramine (a tricyclic) in the treatment of this disorder. This result could be related, at least in part, to subsets in this study's sample of patients who were prospectively judged to have, in addition, a history of spontaneous panic attacks and/or hysteroid dysphoric features. Controlling for this in a further study (Quitkin, McGrath, Stewart, Harrison, Tricamo, Wager, Ocepek-Welikson, Nunes, Rabkin, & Klein, 1990), the same group of investigators demonstrated once again that these operationally defined group of patients responded better to an MAOI than to a tricyclic (phenelzine was consistently superior to imipramine, which was superior to placebo)—a unique finding in psychiatry, since very few studies have demonstrated the superiority of one known active treatment over another proven active treatment.

A further example of this would be the recent multicenter collaborative study of clozapine in treatment-resistant schizophrenia. If clozapine were evaluated in routine studies in newly admitted schizophrenic patients, it is unlikely that any differences in therapeutic outcome would be demonstrated between it and orthodox agents unless an extraordinarily large sample size were used. But in the actual study, in which chart review was followed by a single-blind prospective study in chronic schizophrenia, and treatment resistance was operationalized and only subjects who failed to respond to these four orthodox treatment regimens were included in the final double-blind study, a sample size of less than 300 was sufficient to show that this agent possessed advantages over the prototypical antipsychotic agent CPZ.

MULTICENTER TRIALS

Planning of any clinical trial involves consideration of the number of patients that will be required to provide convincing answers to the research question. The larger the sample size, the more likely it is that a difference between treatments can be determined by a statistical test. Intuitively, we know that we should include as many patients as possible to a study. Clinical trials in psychopharmacology are typically plagued by too small a sample size. Elements that need to be considered simultaneously in thinking about sample size are: (1) Type 1 error (alpha error), (2) Type 2 error (beta error), (3) delta, (4) sample size (N), and (5) variance. In general, low levels of alpha or beta risks, small values of delta, and large variances are all associated with higher sample-size requirements.

Sometimes, it is clear that an investigator needs more patients than are available at one site. The key element in a collaborative or multicenter study is that the study *in toto* is carried out in an identical fashion in more than one place, with the objective of pooling the data obtained—a study which requires greater care and greater specificity than single-site studies (trials conducted at one hospital, clinic, or practice). An advantage of multicenter studies is that the probability is increased of more adequately representing patient characteristics to which the results of the study will be ultimately generalized.

Multicenter studies can be conducted through a central organizational meeting of all the key research personnel from each hospital, or by a training team that goes from site to site. It should be recognized that a special kind of training is required in psychopharmacological research, because of the dependence on psychiatric rating scales. It cannot be assumed that these measures are used uniformly from place to place, as they all require some element of subjective judgment. Some time should be devoted to these measures and to other research data forms to ensure that they will be used properly. It is often necessary to have frequent communication between the monitoring group and each site in an effort to facilitate the scheduling of retraining (i.e., interrater reliability of rating scales, diagnosis, and selection criteria) and troubleshooting visits. Often, it is difficult to sustain motivation in a long-term study on account of the tendency toward a more rapid turnover in personnel.

ADVANCES IN PSYCHOPHARMACOLOGY

Since Kuhn's discovery of the antidepressant properties associated with imipramine in 1957, significant psychopharmacological validation has aided us in the quest for new subtypes of depression based on the response to antidepressants. In a blind controlled study, amitriptyline (a tricyclic antidepressant chemically resembling imipramine and CPZ) was shown to be significantly superior to imipramine in the treatment of females between 30 and 70 years of age who were hospitalized with primary depressive states (Burt, Gordon, Holt, & Hordern, 1962). In a follow-up study of a total sample of 137 females, Hordern, Holt, Burt, and Gordon (1963) instituted a blind inpatient investigation of the phenomenology and treatment of these depressive females and determined that amitriptyline which provided relief in 81% of patients was superior to imipramine, which relieved 54% ($p < .002$). A review of these findings, however, suggests that these drugs were not really different, but rather those who had been treated with imipramine had more psychotic features.

Hammer and Sjoqvist (1967) first demonstrated large plasma steady-state level differences among patients who had received identical oral doses of tricyclic antidepressants. Glassman, Perel, Shostak, Kantor, and Fleiss (1977) addressed the question as to what influence these blood level differences exert on clinical response. In their sample of 60 depressed patients, after a 1-week washout period and 1 week of placebo, these patients received 3.5 mg/kg of imipramine hydrochloride for a 28-day interval. The data demonstrated a statistically and clinically significant relationship between plasma levels and response. Although the sample included unipolars (delusional and nondelusional) and bipolars, only the unipolar delusional patients failed to demonstrate an association between blood level and clinical response. There are other pioneer studies of drug trials that have been successful in suggesting subtypes of depression according to response to antidepressants in nondeluded depressions (Simpson et al., 1976; Spiker, Weiss, Dealy, Griffin, Hanin, Neil, Perel, Rossi, & Soloff, 1985) and in atypical depression (Liebowitz et al., 1988; Quitkin, Stewart, McGrath, Liebowitz, Harrison, Tricamo, Klein, Rabkin, Markowitz, & Wager, 1988; Quitkin, McGrath, Stewart, Harrison, Wager, Nunes, Rabkin, Tricamo, Markowitz, & Klein, 1989; Quitkin et al., 1990). Chronic depression was described as dysthymia in the multiaxial concepts of the DSM-III (Koscis & Frances, 1987; Weissman Leaf, Bruce, & Florio, 1988) and the DSM-III-R (Koscis & Frances, 1987), and differentiation between severe, moderate, and mild depression by drug-response studies have been attempted (Paykel, Freeling, & Hollyman, 1988).

In a double-blind comparison study of 2 dosages of imipramine hydrochloride (150 mg vs. 300 mg daily) on 51 newly admitted hospitalized depressed patients, Simpson et al. (1976) demonstrated that those patients with a psychotic depression responded less well than those patients without psychotic features, and both the physician and patient rating scale data indicated that 300 mg was superior to the 150 mg regimen. Spiker et al. (1985) randomly assigned 51 patients using a prospective double-blind design to study amitriptyline alone, perphenazine alone, or a combination of the two. The results suggested that the combination of amitriptyline and perphenazine was far superior to either of the other two agents alone. It may be hypothesized that those who responded favorably to the combination therapy may actually represent a subset of patients with a delusional depression and that more accurate biological measures are required to define this responsive subset of patients and ultimately refine our current nosology.

In addition, those patients who preferentially respond to MAOIs might help us delineate a clinically useful subtype of depression whose biological diathesis may be distinct. The DSM-III-R does not recognize "atypical depression" as a separate category. Quitkin et al. (1988) studied 60 patients with probable atypical depression and randomly assigned them to phenelzine, imipramine, or placebo. They operationalized their criteria by using Research Diagnostic Criteria (RDC) for depressive illness with a reactive mood and having 1 of 4 associated symptoms (hyperphagia, hypersomnolence, leaden feelings, and sensitivity to rejection). The study results suggested that phenelzine is superior to imipramine and placebo in patients who meet the above defined criteria and they may selectively benefit from MAOIs. A further delineation of mood reactive depressives and a replication study supported the hypothesis of a distinct unipolar depressive subgroup and clearly demonstrated that phenelzine is superior to imipramine for Atypical Depression (Quitkin et al., 1989; Quitkin et al., 1990). It should be emphasized that any of the operationalized criteria which help us to define and categorize clinical syndromes only provide us with a basis to describe various subtypes of psychopathology; in order for these various subtypes to be accorded increased diagnostic recognition, they must be validated by research with psychotropic drugs.

THE FUTURE OF PSYCHOPHARMACOLOGY

Antipsychotic drugs are, to be sure, no panacea for schizophrenia, despite their utility in alleviating many of the associated symptoms of the disorder. In addition, most of the currently available antipsychotics are associated with potential adverse side effects which often limit the patient's ability to function. Remoxipride, a new antipsychotic now under study with perhaps fewer adverse effects, may help patients with schizophrenia who had previously experienced incomplete or no resolution of their symptoms. Remoxipride is a benzamide derivative—a member of a new class of antipsychotic. Similar to the traditional neuroleptics, remoxipride is a dopamine antagonist that blocks dopamine receptors in the brain's limbic and nigrostriatal areas. It is this inactivation of the dopamine receptors in the nigrostriatum that often leads to the development of parkinsonian and other extrapyramidal side effects. Dopamine receptors (D_1 and D_2) are located in both the limbus and nigrostriatum. Unlike other neuroleptics which block dopamine receptors in both the limbic and nigrostriatal areas, remoxipride appears to be a potent D_2 antagonist with preference in the mesolimbic and mesocortical pathways of the brain. Because D_2 receptors predominate in the limbic system, researchers are optimistic that remoxipride will prove to be an effective antipsychotic without causing abnormal involuntary movement disorders typically associated with other neuroleptics.

Another drug that is currently under study is risperidone (R 64766), a benzisoxazole derivative with high specificity for serotonin Type 2 (5-HT$_2$) and dopamine-D_2 receptors which also exhibits binding properties to histamine and noradrenergic receptors. Because of this specificity for serotonin-S_2 and dopamine receptors, risperidone may improve the quality of sleep, reduce negative and affective symptoms in schizophrenia, and may be associated with fewer extrapyramidal side effects than classical neuroleptics. Clinically, risperidone is expected to have antidelusional, antihallucinatory, and antimanic actions because of its central acting D_2 receptor antagonism.

The future of clinical psychopharmacology for schizophrenia depends, to a large extent, on drugs that can treat primarily both positive and negative symptoms of this disorder. Clozapine is one such drug that has been recently marketed. Researchers are currently looking for drugs with benefits similar to clozapine and which lack clozapine's potentially fatal side effect of agranulocytosis. Since early detection and discontinuation of this therapy can often abort the progression of this effect (agranulocytosis), all patients who receive clozapine must have their white blood cell (WBC) counts monitored on a weekly basis. Another approach to treating schizophrenia involves combining neuroleptics with antidepressants. Goff, Brotman, Waites, and McCormick (1990) demonstrated that both negative and positive symptoms of schizophrenia improved in 9 treatment refractory schizophrenic patients who completed a 6-week open label trial of fluoxetine added to their neuroleptics. Although the addition of fluoxetine, a serotonergic agonist, was expected to alleviate negative symptoms (apathy, flat affect) in addition to depressive symptoms, the combination surprisingly improved positive symptoms as well. It is interesting that responders had substantial ratings of depression at baseline; this may reflect, in part, a nonspecific antidepressant effect associated with fluoxetine on this subgroup of schizophrenic patients. Although combinations with different classes of drugs other than antipsychotics may hold promise for schizophrenic patients with unsatisfactory response to conventional neuroleptics, adequate double-blind clinical trials of these combination therapies will ultimately provide the data needed to enhance the heuristic relevance of these treatments.

Antidepressants typically require weeks to produce their therapeutic effects and have been shown to be completely ineffective against some forms of depression. Fluoxetine (Prozac) was the first high-potency serotonin-reuptake blocker introduced in the United States for the treatment of depression. Although claims of greater safety and patient tolerability have been made for new nontricyclic antidepressants, some unpredicted side effects have emerged with widespread usage of Prozac, such as extrapyramidal side effects with and without a combination of neuroleptics (Bouchard, Pourcher, & Vincent, 1989; Brod, 1989; Lipinski, Mallya, Zimmerman, & Pope, 1989; Tate, 1989); inappropriate secretion of antidiuretic hormone (SIADH), and clinically significant drug interactions (Cohen, Mahelsky, & Adler, 1990; Hansen, Dieter, & Keepers, 1990; Hwang & Magraw, 1989). However, fluoxetine as well as other high-potency serotonin reuptake blockers, such as chlomipramine and fluvoxamine, have been shown to be effective in obsessive-compulsive disorder (Perse, Greist, Jefferson, Rosenfeld, & Dar, 1987; Thoren, Asberg, Cronholm, Jornestedt, & Traskman, 1980; Turner, Jacob, Beidel, & Himmelhoch, 1985).

Buspirone (Buspar) is a nonbenzodiazepine anxiolytic which has no significant anticonvulsant properties, does not produce muscle relaxation/sedative hypnotic effects, and does not show potential for physical dependence or abuse in humans (Balster & Woolverton, 1982; Cole, Orzack, Beake, Bird, & Bar-Tal, 1982; Griffith, Jasinski, Casten, & McKinney, 1986; Riblet, Taylor, Eison, & Stanton, 1982; Riblet, Eison, Eison, Taylor, Temple, & VanderMaelen, 1984). Unlike the benzodiazepines, Buspar does not interact significantly with CNS depressants, such as alcohol, shows no significant impairment of psychomotor or cognitive skills, and abrupt discontinuation is not associated with anxiolytic withdrawal effects (Moskowitz & Smiley, 1982). Despite this agent's documented anxiolytic effects, Buspar has been demonstrated to be not significantly superior to placebo in its antipanic or anxiolytic effects in patients with panic disorder (Sheehan, Raj, Sheehan, & Soto, 1990).

To be sure, many of our drug agents are imperfect. Only future efforts toward pursuing more powerful analogues of our currently available agents, while preserving safety profiles, will determine the ultimate therapeutic advantages of these drugs. There are disorders, such as infantile autism and senility, for which we can offer very little. Therefore, it is imperative that we not only improve upon existing pharmacological agents, but also expand the breadth of our pharmacological tools. Although it may seem reasonable that some patients would actually do better without any of our current treatment modalities, there are others who should be treated rapidly and vigorously. Differentiation of this patient population would not only improve treatment, but would also potentially render a much finer incorporation of psychopharmacological agents into treatment approaches involving cooperative efforts from various psychological and sociological disciplines. Beyond that, the question of accurate diagnosis becomes particularly crucial in terms of providing optimal therapeutic response to treatment. Therefore, the precise identification and labeling of clinical syndromes are fundamental to a logical quest for etiology, treatment, and cure.

SUMMARY

Research in psychopharmacology has had a relatively short history, and discoveries of effective agents have usually been serendipitous. This chapter reviewed the concepts of pharmacokinetics and pharmacodynamics as they relate to psychopharmacology and discussed the methodology of clinical trials of psychopharmacologic agents. The design and implementation of drug studies, including multicenter trials were then examined. The chapter ended with an overview of recent advances in psychopharmacology and a discussion of the future of psychopharmacology.

REFERENCES

Baird, E. S., & Hailey, D. M. (1972). Delayed recovery from a sedative: Correlation of the plasma levels of diazepam with clinical effects after oral and intravenous administration. *British Journal of Anesthesia, 44*, 803–807.

Balster, R. L., & Woolverton, W. L. (1982). Intravenous buspirone self-administration in rhesus monkeys. *Journal of Clinical Psychiatry, 43*, 34–37.

Bouchard, R. H., Pourcher, E., & Vincent, P. (1989). Fluoxetine and extrapyramidal side effects [Letter to the editor]. *American Journal of Psychiatry, 146*, 1352–1353.

Brod, T. M. (1989). Fluoxetine and extrapyramidal side effects [Letter to the editor]. *American Journal of Psychiatry, 146*, 1353.

Burlington, D. B., & Gubish, E. R. (1987). Review of investigational biological products by the United States Food and Drug Administration. *Journal of Clinical Research and Drug Development, 1*, 143–152.

Burt, C. G., Gordon, W. F., Holt, N. F., & Hordern, A. (1962). Amitriptyline in depressive states: A controlled trial. *Journal of Mental Science, 108*, 711–730.

Caldwell, A. E. (1978). History of psychopharmacology. In W. G. Clark & J. del Giudice (Eds.), *Principles of psychopharmacology* (pp. 9–40). New York: Academic Press.

Cohen, B. J., Mahelsky, M., & Adler, L. (1990). More cases of SIADH with fluoxetine. *American Journal of Psychiatry, 147*, 948–949.

Cole, J. O., Orzack, M. H., Beake, B., Bird, M., & Bar-Tal, Y. (1982). Assessment of the abuse liability of buspirone in recreational sedative users. *Journal of Clinical Psychiatry, 34*, 69–74.

Delay, J., & Deniker, P. (1952). 38 cas de psychosis traités par la cure prolongée et continué de 4568 R. P. *Annales Médico-Psychologiques, 110*, 364.

Frank, E., Kupfer, D. D. J., Perel, J. M., Cornes, C., Jarrett, D. B., Mallinger, A. G., Thase, M. E., McEachran, A. B., & Grochocinski, V. J. (1990). Three-year outcomes for maintenance therapies in recurrent depression. *Archives of General Psychiatry, 47*, 1093–1099.

Freeman, C., & Tyrer, P. (Eds.). (1989). *Research methods in psychiatry: A beginner's guide.* London: Gaskell.

Ghoneim, M. M., Korttila, K., & Chiang, C. K. (1981). Diazepam effects and kinetics in Caucasians and Orientals. *Clinical Pharmacology and Therapy, 29*, 749–756.

Glassman, A. H., Perel, J. M., Shostak, M., Kantor, S. J., & Fleiss, J. L. (1977). Clinical implications of imipramine plasma levels for depressive illness. *Archives of General Psychiatry, 34*, 197–204.

Goff, D. C., Brotman, A. W., Waites, M., & McCormick, S. (1990). Trial of fluoxetine added to neuroleptics for treatment-resistant schizophrenic patients. *American Journal of Psychiatry, 147*, 492–494.

Greenblatt, D. J., Shader, R. I., & MacLeod, S. M. (1978). Clinical pharmacokinetics of chlordiazepoxide. *Clinical Pharmacokinetics, 3*, 381–394.

Griffith, J. D., Jasinski, D. R., Casten, G. P., & McKinney, G. R. (1986). Investigation of the abuse liability of buspirone in alcohol-dependent patients. *American Journal of Medicine, 80,* 30–35.

Hammer, W., & Sjoqvist, F. (1967). Plasma levels of monomethylated tricyclic antidepressants during treatment with imipramine-like compounds. *Life Science, 6,* 1895–1903.

Hansen, T. E., Dieter, K., & Keepers, G. A. (1990). Interaction of fluoxetine and pentazocine [Letter to the editor]. *American Journal of Psychiatry, 147,* 949–950.

Hillestad, L., Hansen, T., & Melsom, H. (1974). Diazepam metabolism in normal man: Serum concentrations and clinical effects after intravenous, intramuscular, and oral administration. *Clinical Pharmacology and Therapy, 16,* 479–484.

Hordern, A., Holt, N. F., Burt, C. G., & Gordon, W. F. (1963). Amitriptyline in depressive states: Phenomenology and prognostic considerations. *British Journal of Psychiatry, 109,* 815–825.

Hwang, A. S., & Magraw, R. M. (1989). Syndrome of inappropriate secretion of antidiuretic hormone due to fluoxetine [Letter to the editor]. *American Journal of Psychiatry, 146,* 399.

Jefferson, T. W., Greist, J. H., Ackerman, D. L., & Carroll, J. A. (1987). *Lithium encyclopedia for clinical practice* (2nd ed.). Washington, DC: American Psychiatric Press.

Kocsis, J. H., & Frances, A. J. (1987). A critical discussion of DSM-III dysthymic disorder. *American Journal of Psychiatry, 144,* 1534–1542.

Kyriakopoulos, A. A., Greenblatt, D. J., & Shader, R. I. (1978). Clinical pharmacokinetics of lorazepam: A review. *Journal of Clinical Psychiatry, 39,* 16–23.

Liebowitz, M. R., Quitkin, F. M., Stewart, J. W., McGrath, P. J., Harrison, W. M., Markowitz, J. S., Rabkin, J. G., Tricamo, E., Goetz, D. M., & Klein, D. F. (1988). Antidepressant specificity in atypical depression. *Archives of General Psychiatry, 45,* 129–137.

Lipinski, J. F., & Mallya, G., Zimmerman, P., & Pope, H. (1989). Fluoxetine-induced akathisia: Clinical and theoretical implications. *Journal of Clinical Psychiatry, 50,* 339–342.

Lusznat, R. M., Murphy, D. P., & Nunn, C. M. H. (1988). Carbamazepine vs. lithium in the treatment and prophylaxis of mania. *British Journal of Psychiatry, 153,* 198–204.

Marwick, C. (1985). FDA prepares to meet regulatory challenges of the 21st century. *Journal of the American Medical Association, 254,* 2189–2193, 2199–2201.

Miller, H. I., & Young, F. E., (1989). The drug approval process at the Food and Drug Administration. *Archives of Internal Medicine, 149,* 655–657.

Moskowitz, H., & Smiley, A. (1982). Effects of chronically administered buspirone and diazepam in driving-related skills performance. *Journal of Clinical Psychiatry, 34,* 45–55.

Okuma, T., Inanga, K., Otsuki, S., Keisuke, S., Takahashi, R., Hazama, H., Mori, A., & Watanabe, S. (1981). A preliminary double-blind study of the efficacy of carbamazepine in prophylaxis of manic-depressive illness. *Psychopharmacology, 73,* 95–96.

Paykel, E. S., Freeling, P., & Hollyman, J. A. (1988). Are tricyclic antidepressants useful for mild depression? *Pharmacopsychiatry, 21,* 15–18.

Perse, T. L., Greist, J. H., Jefferson, J. W., Rosenfeld, R., & Dar, R. (1987). Fluvoxamine treatment of obsessive-compulsive disorder. *American Journal of Psychiatry, 144,* 1543–1548.

Placidi, G. F., Lenzi, A., Lazzerini, F., Cassano, G. B., & Akiskal, H. S. (1986). The comparative efficacy and safety of carbamazepine versus lithium: A randomized, double-blind 3 year trial in 83 patients. *Journal of Clinical Psychiatry, 47,* 490–494.

Prien, R. F., & Gelenberg, A. J. (1989). Alternatives to lithium for preventive treatment of bipolar disorder. *American Journal of Psychiatry, 146,* 840–848.

Prien, R. F., Kupfer, D. J., Mansky, P. A., Small, J. G., Tuason, V. B., Voss, C. B., & Johnson, W. E. (1984). Drug therapy in the prevention of recurrences in unipolar and bipolar affective disorders: A report of the NIMH collaborative study group comparing lithium carbonate, imipramine, and a lithium carbonate-imipramine combination. *Archives of General Psychiatry, 41,* 1096–1104.

Pry-Roberts, C., & Hug, C. C. (Eds.). (1984). *Pharmacokinetics of anesthesia.* Cambridge, MA: Blackwell Scientific Publications.

Quitkin, F. M., Stewart, J. W., McGrath, P. J., Liebowitz, M. R., Harrison, W. M., Tricamo, E., Klein, D. F., Rabkin, J. G., Markowitz, J. S., & Wager, S. G. (1988). Phenelzine versus imipramine in the treatment of probable atypical depression: Defining syndrome boundaries of selective MAOI responders. *American Journal of Psychiatry, 145,* 306–311.

Quitkin, F. M., McGrath, P. J., Stewart, J. W., Harrison, W., Wager, S. G., Nunes, E., Rabkin, J. G., Tricamo, E., Markowitz, J., & Klein, D. F. (1989). Phenelzine and imipramine in mood reactive depressives. *Archives of General Psychiatry, 46*, 787–793.

Quitkin, F. M., McGrath, P. J., Stewart, J. W., Harrison, W., Tricamo, E., Wager, S. G., Ocepek-Welikson, K., Nunes, E., Rabkin, J. G., & Klein, D. F. (1990). Atypical depression, panic attacks, and response to imipramine and phenelzine. *Archives of General Psychiatry, 47*, 935–941.

Riblet, L. A., Taylor, D. P., Eison, M. S., & Stanton, H. C. (1982). Pharmacology and neurochemistry of buspirone. *Journal of Clinical Psychiatry, 43* (Sec. 2), 11–16.

Riblet, L. A., Eison, A. S., Eison, M. S., Taylor, D. P., Temple, D. L., & VanderMaelan, C. P. (1984). Neuropharmacology of buspirone. *Psychopathology, 17* (Suppl. 3), 69–78.

Rowland, M., & Tozer, T. N. (1989). *Clinical pharmacokinetics*. Philadelphia: Lea & Febiger.

Sheehan, D. V., Raj, A. B., Sheehan, H., & Soto, S. (1990). Is buspirone effective for panic disorder? *Journal of Clinical Psychopharmacology, 10*, 3–11.

Simpson, G. M., Lee, J. H., Cuculic, Z., & Kellner, R. (1976). Two dosages of imipramine in hospitalized endogenous and neurotic depressives. *Archives of General Psychiatry, 33*, 1093–1102.

Simpson, G. M., Yadalam, K. G., Stephanos, M. J., Lo, E. S., & Cooper, T. B. (1990). Single dose pharmacokinetics of fluphenazine after fluphenazine decanoate administration. *Journal of Clinical Psychopharmacology, 10*, 417–421.

Spiker, D. G., Weiss, J. C., Dealy, R. S., Griffin, S. J., Hanin, I., Neil, J. F., Perel, J. M., Rossi, A. J., & Soloff, P. H. (1985). The pharmacological treatment of delusional depression. *American Journal of Psychiatry, 142*, 430–436.

Spriet, A., & Simon, P. (1985). *Methodology of clinical trials*. Paris, France: Karger.

Tate, J. L. (1989). Extrapyramidal symptoms in a patient taking haloperidol and fluoxetine [Letter to the editor]. *American Journal of Psychiatry, 146*, 399–400.

Thoren, P., Asberg, M., Cronholm, B., Jornestedt, L., & Traskman, L. (1980). Clomipramine treatment of obsessive-compulsive disorder: 1. A controlled clinical trial. *Archives of General Psychiatry, 37*, 1281–1285.

Turner, S. M., Jacob, R. G., Beidel, D., & Himmelhoch, J. (1985). Fluoxetine treatment of obsessive-compulsive disorder. *Journal of Clinical Psychopharmacology, 5*, 207–212.

Watkins, S. E., Callender, K., Thomas, D. R., Tidmarsh, S. F., & Shaw, D. M. (1987). The effect of carbamazepine and lithium on remission from affective illness. *British Journal of Psychiatry, 150*, 180–182.

Ziporyn, T. (1985). The Food and Drug Administration: How "those regulations" came to be. *Journal of the American Medical Association, 254*, 2037–2039, 2043–2046.

CHAPTER 13

Psychotherapy Research

Issues to Consider in Planning a Study

JACQUES P. BARBER AND LESTER B. LUBORSKY

INTRODUCTION

Our aim in this chapter is to provide a guide to issues that need to be addressed during the planning of psychotherapy research. Our strategy is to explain the research issues first and then to exemplify them with actual studies of three major therapeutic systems: cognitive therapy, dynamic therapy, and interpersonal psychotherapy. These three systems were chosen because they each are well described and are the focus of much current research activity. Others that might have been selected as examples include: the behavioral, the client-centered, the Gestalt, the family therapy, and the eclectic systems.

The goal of all research is to increase our confidence in our observations, inferences, and conclusions. In other words, as researchers we try to minimize various threats to the validity of our measures and conclusions. Campbell and Stanley (1966) distinguished between *internal validity*—the answer to the question, does the experimental treatment make a different?—and *external validity*—the answer to the question, can this effect be generalized to other populations, settings, treatment variables, and measures? In that regard, at least, psychotherapy research is no different from other domains of research. All the issues to be reviewed in this chapter, therefore, are purported to minimize the various

Jacques P. Barber and Lester B. Luborsky • Center for Psychotherapy Research, Department of Psychiatry, University of Pennsylvania, 3600 Market Street, Philadelphia, Pennsylvania 19104-2648.

Research in Psychiatry: Issues, Strategies, and Methods, edited by L. K. George Hsu and Michel Hersen. Plenum Press, New York, 1992.

threats to validity in psychotherapy research. Owing to space restrictions, we do not review the various general forms of experimental and quasi-experimental designs, nor do we list the various threats to validity. A detailed review of the various designs and threats to validity can be found in Chapters 4 and 5 (in this volume), as well as in Campbell and Stanley (1966).

Because our review is selective and brief, the interested reader is encouraged to turn to the many excellent volumes on psychotherapy research that have been written in the last 20 years. Among these, it is worth mentioning the last two editions of Garfield and Bergin's *Handbook of Psychotherapy and Behavior Change* (1978, 1986). These handbooks not only cover methodological issues in psychotherapy but also provide the reader with an updated summary of the major findings of the field from a variety of perspectives. Other methodological discussions can be found in the American Psychiatric Association Commission on Psychotherapies' (1982) *Psychotherapy Research: Methodological and Efficacy Issues*, in Fiske, Hunt, Luborsky, Orne, Parloff, Reiser, and Tuma (1970), which was recently updated by Luborsky and Fiske (1991). Reviews on more specific topics will be pointed in the text itself.

DESCRIPTION OF PSYCHOTHERAPEUTIC SYSTEMS

In order to be able to describe the planning of research that addresses the process of change of specific therapies, we begin our chapter by briefly describing the assumptions concerning the process of change in three selected major psychotherapies.

Cognitive Therapy

Cognitive therapy (CT) for depression is derived from the premise that depressed patients tend to negatively distort their view of themselves, their ongoing experience, and their future (Beck, Rush, Shaw, & Emery, 1979). The organization of depressive thinking is also characterized by dysfunctional underlying schemata which give rise to spontaneous negative interpretations which Beck calls "automatic thoughts." Finally, depressed people have an idiosyncratic way of processing information. That is, their thinking is subject to several systematic biases that cause them to maintain their belief in the validity of their negative conclusions despite the presence of contradictory evidence.

Cognitive therapy therefore targets the beliefs and cognitive processes underlying depression or any other disorder. But, CT also makes use of a variety of behavioral techniques to induce changes in these cognitions. Cognitive therapists teach their patients to be attentive to automatic negative thoughts and to treat these beliefs as hypotheses to be tested. During work with the client, the therapist demonstrates in various ways the use of these three questions: (1) What is the evidence for or against the belief? (2) What are the alternative interpretations of the event or situation? and (3) What are the implications if the belief is correct?

The answers to these questions are instrumental in helping the patient to evaluate those automatic thoughts, to realize the connections between thoughts and emotions, and to discover rational responses to the *depressotypic* thoughts. As therapy progresses, the client and the therapist begin to look for specific patterns, basic assumptions, or schemata underlying the patient's automatic thinking. In turn, these assumptions are investigated by bringing up evidence "for or against each assumption and belief" (Beck *et al.*, 1979, p. 55). It is this cognitive change that is held responsible for the relief of affective and behavioral symptoms (for more details, see Beck *et al.*, 1979).

Although CT was originally developed for depression, it has been successfully applied to the treatment of panic disorder (Sokol, Beck, Greenberg, Wright, & Berchick, 1989) and opiate addictions (Beck & Emery, 1977). More recent applications include development of manuals for the treatment of personality disorders and cocaine addiction (Beck, Wright, & Newman, 1990), and anxiety disorders (Beck, Emery, & Greenberg, 1985).

The efficacy of cognitive-behavioral therapy in comparison with other forms of therapy is supported by several controlled outcome studies of the treatment of depression (for a detailed review and a meta-analysis, see Dobson, 1989).

Dynamic Psychotherapy

In recent years, new forms and variations on old forms of brief dynamic psychotherapy have emerged (see Crits-Christoph & Barber, 1991, for an extensive review). Among them, two variations have been published in the form of treatment manuals and have been empirically studied: Supportive-Expressive Psychotherapy (SE) (Luborsky, 1984) and Time-Limited Dynamic Psychotherapy (Strupp & Binder, 1984). A third type, Interpersonal Therapy (IPT) (Klerman, Weissman, Rounsaville, & Chevron, 1984) has also receive much research attention, although it is arguable whether dynamic therapists would view IPT as a form of dynamic psychotherapy.

Supportive-Expressive Psychotherapy

In his 1984 book, Luborsky succinctly described the major principles used in psychoanalytic psychotherapy as derived from the works of Freud and of the theorists at the Menninger Foundation. This version of psychoanalytically oriented psychotherapy is named Supportive-Expressive Psychotherapy (SE). Its main characteristics are summarized in terms of two broad categories of techniques: supportiveness and expressiveness (Luborsky, 1984, pp. 10–12).

Supportive Techniques

Supportiveness is inherent in the techniques of almost all psychotherapies. It is derived mainly from nonspecific aspects of the treatment, such as the collaboration of the patient and therapist in trying to help the patient achieve his or her goals. For some patients at some times additional support is needed to foster an alliance and to maintain essential defenses. These techniques do not directly increase understanding but set the stage for it. They help the patient to feel secure enough to venture to try to undo the restrictions in functioning that necessitated the treatment. They are aimed at raising the patient's self-esteem and maintaining the patient's level of functioning.

Expressive Techniques

These techniques were labeled *expressive* from the fact that in SE the therapist facilitates the patient's readiness to express thoughts and feelings and to reflect on them. The therapist's tasks are the successive phases of listening, understanding, responding, and then returning to listening. The therapist's responses include clarifications and interpretations. Interpretations help the patient to understand the symptoms in the context of the relationship conflicts, especially as these are expressed in the transference. The transference reflects the reexperiencing of recurrent early problematic relationships in the present relationship with the therapist.

The Core Conflictual Relationship Theme method (CCRT) (Luborsky & Crits-Christoph, 1990) can help the therapist to formulate the central relationship pattern. The CCRT is inferred from the narratives of interactions of the patient with other people, including the therapist. It has three main components: the wishes, needs, and intentions; the real or expected responses from others (RO); and the responses of the self (RS). The main conflicts among these components typically are between (1) the wishes and responses from others, and (2) the wishes that conflict with other wishes. The CCRT method helps the clinician to find the schema or script or central relationship pattern that is most frequent and conflictual. After recognizing the CCRT, the therapist can use it as a guide in terms of making more accurate interpretations.

As summarized in Luborsky (1984), the theory of psychoanalytic psychotherapy includes three main curative factors: development of the therapeutic alliance, increase in self-understanding, and incorporation of gains.

1. *Building a therapeutic alliance.* The alliance is most basic of all of the aspects of the theory. Four main factors contribute to its development: (a) the inherent aspects of the therapeutic arrangements, such as the regular meetings and the therapist's willingness to help the patient; (b) the therapist's maintenance of an attitude of sympathetic understanding; (c) the degree to which the therapist fits into the patient's concept of a helpful person; and (d) the patient's capacity to establish a positive therapeutic alliance.

2. *Self-understanding.* The theory posits that increased self-understanding is a main prerequisite for the patient's improvement. It is especially helpful for the patient to learn to recognize his or her own central relationship pattern and the conflicts within it and to work through reexperiencing previous conflictual relationships in the current relationship with the therapist. In essence, the patient becomes better able to identify the most maladaptive aspects of the

pattern, including the symptoms and suffering, and to find more adaptive ways of behaving. Nevertheless, even after improved mastery, from time to time the "transference potentials remain recognizable" both in the therapy and thereafter (Luborsky, 1984, p. 23).

3. *Maintaining the therapeutic gains.* Psychodynamic therapists view internalization as a process of incorporating the helpful aspects of the therapy, and, therefore, as a mechanism for maintaining the therapeutic gains. The maintenance is facilitated by the patient's working through of the meanings of termination.

The efficacy of SE has been systematically examined in a comparative study (Woody, Luborsky, McLellan, O'Brien, Beck, Blaine, Herman, & Hole, 1983) of the addition of cognitive therapy or supportive-expressive therapy to drug counseling for opiate addicts in a methadone treatment setting. Both psychotherapies were found to be more effective than the treatment as usual (drug counseling), but not significantly different from each other in effectiveness. Currently, we are evaluating the efficacy of SE for the treatment of patients with a diagnosis of Major Depression (Luborsky, Crits-Christoph, Barber, & Cacciola, 1992).

Interpersonal Therapy for Depression (IPT)

In similar fashion to CT but in contrast to SE, Interpersonal Therapy (Klerman *et al.*, 1984) originally focused on only one disorder—depression. Since then, IPT has been adapted for the treatment of opiate abuse (Rounsaville, Glazer, Wilbur, Weissman, & Kleber, 1983), cocaine abuse (Rounsaville, Gawin, & Kleber, 1985), and there is little doubt that it will be applied to additional disorders in the future. The roots of IPT are mostly with the interpersonal (Sullivanian) school of psychodynamic psychotherapy. IPT focuses on interpersonal functioning, since it assumes that impaired social relationships either cause or perpetuate depression. Its goals are limited to the "symptomatic" and "interpersonal" levels while leaving out the "personality" level.

At first, the symptoms are the center of attention, although no attempt is made to understand all the causes for the onset of depression. The therapist actively keeps the patient focused on the goals of the treatment. In contrast to dynamic therapies, the patient–therapist relationship is not the focus of treatment except when resistance requires it. In contrast to dynamic therapies, the therapist encourages actual practice of the therapeutic skills and even sometimes gives direct advice. The therapist is also more active and less ambitious regarding the range of change to be achieved by the end of treatment than are more traditional psychodynamically oriented psychotherapies. Nevertheless, Rounsaville, Klerman, Weissman, and Chevron (1985) emphasized that IPT differs from cognitive-behavioral therapy (CBT) in its encouraging of the patients' own explorations.

Since IPT has two central goals, managing depressive symptoms and improving interpersonal relationships, Rounsaville, Klerman *et al.* (1985) presented specific techniques relevant to these two domains separately. The interpersonal functioning is explored in the four domains generally relevant to depression: grief, interpersonal disputes, role transitions, and interpersonal deficits (for more details, see Klerman et al., 1984).

The effectiveness of IPT has been examined in the treatment of depression (Elkin et al., 1989), opiate addiction, and alcoholism.

TWO MAJOR ISSUES IN PSYCHOTHERAPY RESEARCH

Now that we have provided a brief account of three major psychotherapies, we turn to the two major issues of psychotherapy research. The first one is concerned with the efficacy of psychotherapy, and the second with the therapeutic processes in terms of how it works. In the following sections, we describe methodological and research issues involved in these two major domains of psychotherapy research. Research findings are presented for the sake of clarifying these issues and not as much to acquaint the reader with recent findings in the field.

ISSUES ABOUT EFFICACY

Thirty years ago, researchers were arguing about whether psychotherapy was effective at all. Since the 1980s, the research issues have become more specific and more specialized. A new consensus emerged supporting the view that (1) psychotherapy is more effective for psychiatric patients than no treatment (Smith, Glass, & Miller, 1980), and (2) there is little evidence to suggest that one psychotherapy is more effective than another (Luborsky, Singer, & Luborsky, 1975; Smith et al., 1980). Researchers are now pursuing more specific issues, such as which kind of psychotherapy (e.g., psychodynamic vs. cognitive) is more effective for which kind of disorder (e.g., depression vs. avoidant personality disorders). Paul (1967) asked this often-quoted question: "What treatment, by whom, is most effective for this individual with that specific problem, and under which set of circumstances?" (p. 111). A preliminary approach to answer these questions can be found in Frances, Clarkin, and Perry (1984).

Patient Selection

An important issue in research on treatment efficacy is the definition of the patient population. There are several reasons for choosing homogenous samples (American Psychiatric Association Commission, 1982). One major reason is that if patients with various diagnoses are treated, then it is possible that some with a particular diagnosis will improve while others will not. Thus, studies on homogeneous samples are more likely to lead to less ambiguous conclusions. Another reason is that only if the sample is homogeneous can the results of different studies be compared. On the other hand, the homogeneity of a sample limits the generalizations that can be derived from a specific study. Psychotherapy researchers differ in their conclusions about these alternatives, but the trend seems to be toward more homogeneous patient samples.

In order to ascertain that samples were homogeneous at least in terms of diagnosis, many new structured and semistructured interviews as well as testing batteries have been developed. A review of these instruments is presented in Chapter 7, in this volume. There are limitations, however, that derive from the selection of patients only on the basis of diagnosis, since they might still present a variety of differences on a wide spectrum of dimensions, such as coping skills and self-esteem.

Measuring Outcome

The issue of the measurement of therapeutic outcome is complex since, like most other scientific measures, it is theory bound. In recent years, most researchers seem to have accepted major measures of the main symptom as adequate outcome measures. Nevertheless, there are other measures of outcome besides symptom checklists, such as personality change, performance in work, mental health, and theoretically relevant measures.

Measures of Specific Symptoms or Syndromes

Measures of symptoms can be divided into two major classes: (1) self-report measures and (2) clinician rating scales. Many studies (i.e., Elkin et al., 1989; Rush, Beck, Kovacs & Hollon, 1977) that examined the efficacy of psychotherapy versus medication for patients with a diagnosis of major depression used as outcome measures self-report measures of depression, such as the Beck Depression Inventory (BDI) (Beck, Ward, Mendelson, Mock, & Erbaugh, 1961) and/or clinician rating scales, such as the 17-item Hamilton Rating Scale for Depression (HRSD) (M. A. Hamilton, 1960, 1967). For example, to be included in the NIMH Depression Collaborative Research Program (Elkin et al., 1989), patients needed to score 14 or higher on the 17-item HRSD.

Measures of General Psychiatric Severity and Psychological Health

In addition to scales measuring only one set of symptoms, psychotherapy outcome researchers use general measures of symptoms, including the 90-item Hopkins Symptom Checklist (SCL-90) (Derogatis, Lipman, & Covi, 1973). The Minnesota Multiphasic Personality Inventory (MMPI) is also used, but less frequently. Measures of general severity or of multidimensional aspects of psychiatric problems not only give researchers an indication of how a specific set of targeted symptoms improved during treatment, but also how the larger picture of psychiatric disturbance has changed as a result of treatment. Both the SCL-90 and the MMPI are self-report scales. But a major difference between the two is that the items on the SCL-90 are transparent to the reader, whereas the items in the MMPI are much less so.

At least for DSM-III-R Axis I disorders (American Psychiatric Association, 1987), there seems to be little disagreement that these symptom checklists are useful measures of outcome. Problems might arise when psychotherapy outcome studies examine the efficacy of psychotherapy for patients with a diagnosis of personality disorder, for whom there is not yet a generally accepted measure of outcome.

Other important measures are clinician rating scales for psychological health. One of the most important is the Luborsky (1975) Health Sickness Rating Scale, from which the Global Assessment Scale (GAS) (Endicott, Spitzer, Fleiss, & Cohen, 1976) was derived.

Presence or Absence of Diagnostic Criteria

Another method to assess the efficacy of treatment is to examine the recovery rate (i.e., the proportion of patients who met a predefined level of clinical recovery). Recovery criteria can be derived either from a continuum scale, such as the BDI or the HRSD, from which cut-off scores are derived, or in a dichotomic division, such as the presence or absence of the inclusion criteria at termination. Use of recovery criteria, however, does not allow for traditional correlational analysis. In addition, the absence of a formal diagnosis does not show whether or not a specific patient has improved more than another when both patients have met the DSM diagnostic criteria for the targeted disorder. Recovery rates, however, give us an indication of how well treatment helps the patients to return to a predetermined level of functioning.

Measures of Performance in the World

Although measures of performance in the world are not used very frequently, they nonetheless are important. Woody et al. (1983) found that the addition of psychotherapy to drug counseling led to a better outcome in work- and income-related variables. There is little doubt that in the case of alcohol and drug addictions, for example, one should be very interested not only in the extent of substance use but also in such variables as work performance and income, since one is interested in relapse prevention and these variables might be related to such issues.

Measures of Relapse and Attrition

For some disorders, not only is the extent of remission an important variable for measuring the efficacy of treatment, but equally important is the attrition rate (in terms of the number of patients who enter, continue, and finish treatment). In the case of cocaine addicts, for example, one of the major difficulties is to keep patients in treatment for a sufficient length of time for them to receive an appropriate dose of treatment.

Another important issue of the patient's response is whether different treatments lead to different rates of relapse. *Relapse* is defined as the return of symptoms associated with the initial episode. In contrast, *recurrence* is the onset of a new episode. In the area of the treatment of depression, for example, there is growing evidence (Barber & DeRubeis, 1989) that cognitive therapy is more effective than antidepressant medication in preventing relapse, although both treatments *do not* differ in their level of efficacy. Hollon, Evans, and DeRubeis (1990) concluded that good evidence exists to suggest that cognitive therapy provides protection from relapse, whereas 12 weeks of imipramine therapy is mainly symptom suppressive. Hollon and co-workers also remind us that there is no evidence yet for the prophylactic role of cognitive therapy (i.e., the prevention of recurrence of depression). Long-term (at least 3 years) follow-up will be needed to assess the issue of prophylaxis. These findings and suggestions indicate that the timing of outcome assessment is and will remain an important issue, and it is not limited to patients' gains at treatment termination. An obvious problem is that to carefully follow patients for an extensive period of time after treatment is an expensive and difficult task.

Effect Size and Clinical Significance

Researchers in the field of psychotherapy as well as in many other fields of psychology and psychiatry have fallen in love with the concept of the significance level. Many studies are accepted for publication if they reported a finding at a significant level, ordinarily a probability value less than or equal to .05 or .01. But significance testing, though important, does not tell us directly about the magnitude of an effect. Significance levels are, among other variables, the consequence of the number of subjects used in a comparison. In order to resolve this problem, many researchers suggested the use and presentation of effect size, that is, "the degree to which the relationship studied differs from zero" (Rosenthal & Rosnow, 1984, p. 22). One major limitation of effect size is that it does not indicate whether an effect is clinically significant. Jacobson and Revenstorf (1988) defined clinically significant change or recovery for a specific patient "as a posttest score that was more likely to belong in the functional than in the dysfunctional population on the variable of interest" (p. 134). Since such criteria require adequate norms which are often unavailable, they suggested to define significant clinical improvement as a score which is two standard deviations beyond the mean of the patient population.

Outcome Measures Tailored to the Patients' Problems

One of the disadvantages of using nomothetic outcome measures is that patients come to treatment for a variety of reasons and are treated for different problems even if they all have the same standard diagnoses. In response to such criticisms, many researchers have turned to the addition or sole use of individualized or case-specific measures that are tailored to a patient's specific criteria of improvement. One widely used individualized measure is the Target Complaints Measure (Battle, Imber, Hoehn-Saric, Stone, Nash, & Frank, 1966) in which the patient is asked to state the three most serious problems he or she wishes to deal with during treatment. Patients are also asked to rate the severity of these problems at intake, termination, and follow-up. In parallel, the therapist and/or independent evaluator can make the same rating.

Theoretically Relevant Measures of Outcome

The measurement of outcome also depends on the theory underlying the therapeutic process. In psychodynamic therapy, for example, one of the major goals of treatment is to provide insight into the unconscious source of the patient's problems and to change disruptive aspects of the core conflicts. Thus, psychodynamic therapists not only strive to achieve symptomatic remission, but also to increase self-awareness, the ability for mature interpersonal relationships, and so on. In consequence, comparing psychodynamic therapy to other forms of treatment on just a measure of symptom improvement does not do justice to the complexity of the dynamic theoretical system. Although these treatment goals may not be relevant to all forms of psychotherapy, such measures are relevant to the comparisons of dynamic therapy to other forms of psychotherapy. Unfortunately, no study that has compared dynamic to other forms of psychotherapy has used dynamically relevant measures of outcome.

Using an example from cognitive therapy, measures of dysfunctional cognitions, such as the Dysfunctional Attitudes Scale (DAS) (Weissman, 1979), might be used as a relevant outcome measure in addition to measures of depression. We will discuss below the role of such theoretically relevant variables as measures of process.

Therapist Effectiveness

Differences in therapists' effectiveness have been explored systematically as part of a study of the efficacy of cognitive therapy, supportive-expressive psychotherapy, and drug counseling (Luborsky, McLellan, Woody, O'Brien, & Auerbach, 1985), where the differences in the therapists' success rates were found to be larger than the differences among the treatments. Recently, Crits-Christoph, Baranackie, Kurcias, Beck, Carroll, Perry, Luborsky, McLellan, Woody, Thompson, Gallagher, and Zitrin (1990) found that the therapist effects were much smaller in the studies in which a detailed manual was used to guide the treatment.

The influence of differences in therapist effectiveness on the results of treatment should be minimized. If one compares two different treatments, one needs to ensure that the therapists do not differ significantly on a variety of dimensions (one of them being effectiveness) across the two conditions. This is often difficult to do because therapist, therapy, and client variables cannot always be cleanly separated. For example, there might be personality differences between therapists of different persuasions, and these differences might have a different impact on distinct groups of patients. In brief, therapist selection is not less important than patient selection.

Randomization

It is standard practice to randomly distribute patients into the different treatment groups in outcome and process research. Randomization is used to solve the problem of systematic differences in patients on significant variables across treatment conditions in *the long run*. On occasions where there is prior knowledge that a variable is relevant to treatment outcome, patients are not only randomly assigned to different treatments but are also stratified according to this variable. For example, we have learned that the addition of psychotherapy to drug counseling for the treatment of opiate addiction is not helpful for those addicts with an additional diagnosis of antisocial personality disorder (ASP) (Woody, McLellan, Luborsky, O'Brien, Blaine, Fox, Herman, & Beck, 1984). Thus, in our view, outcome study of drug addicts should incorporate ASP as a stratifying variable in the randomization process of patients to treatment. In a further analysis of the same data, Woody *et al.* (1984) have shown that drug addicts with ASP, but also with a high level of psychiatric severity, were helped by the addition of either cognitive or supportive psychotherapy to drug counseling (treatment as usual). Thus, it would be worthwhile to control and check for severity level when randomizing patients with substance abuse problems into treatments.

Limitations of Randomization

One of the major limitations of randomization is that a bias can be introduced in the selection of patients. It is likely that patients who agree to be randomly assigned to various forms of treatment (including placebo) differ in important dimensions from patients who approach usual treatment. Furthermore, it is also possible that patients who participate in treatment studies differ from patients who approach regular treatment sources and that some of them will drop out of treatments they do not prefer.

Control Groups

How does one know that a specific treatment is effective? In order to answer this question, one needs to distinguish between two cases: (1) no treatment has been shown to be effective for a specific disorder, or (2) specific treatments have already been shown to be effective. In the first case (e.g., depression), one needs to show that the new treatment versus no treatment (placebo) leads to more reduction of symptoms or to their disappearance. In the case when a specific treatment has already been shown to be effective for a specific disorder, one needs to demonstrate that the new treatment is, at least, as effective as what has become "treatment as usual." Alternatively, the new treatment needs to be compared to a control treatment group, which differs only on the active ingredient to be included in the new treatment condition. Often the control condition is a placebo condition. The rationale as well as the problems of placebo comparison in psychotherapy is similar to the rationale found in medicine in general, although it is more controversial. One source of controversy is that the psychotherapy itself is sometimes viewed as based on a placebo effect. That is, the patient's expectations of benefits, for example, are likely to influence outcome. Thus, the solution has often been to provide patients with an "attention–placebo" treatment, that is, a treatment that has apparent face validity but is not a recognized treatment. The problem, of course, is whether a therapist just speaking with a patient provides an element of psychotherapy. In fact, there is evidence that patients in these intended-to-be control groups show some benefits (American Psychiatric Association Commission, 1982).

In psychotherapy research parlance, the factors causing the placebo effects are referred to as *nonspecific factors*. Among the most important nonspecific factors found in most psychotherapies are the role of a benevolent and helpful listener, the structure provided by the settings of the therapeutic sessions, the provision to patients of a rationale for their troubles and how treatment might be helpful, and the role of the patients' observing and articulating their problems.

In order to control for some of the above nonspecific factors, an alternative for control groups has been the *waiting-list control group* (i.e., patients accepted into a study are randomly assigned to a group where they are informed that they will be seen at a specified point several months later). At the end of the waiting period, patients are assessed again and then accepted into treatment. These control groups provide a sample of patients who are without treatment for the period in which they wait for treatment. Patients in the waiting-list control group often improve during the ensuing period. There have been reports, however, that such patients do not do as well once they are accepted into treatment (Luborsky, Crits-Christoph, Mintz, & Auerbach, 1988). In addition to the ethical issues involved in withholding treatment from patients, an additional drawback of this comparison group is the attrition of such patients during the waiting period.

THE NIMH TREATMENT OF DEPRESSION COLLABORATIVE RESEARCH PROGRAM

We used this multisite study to exemplify and concretize some of the issues mentioned earlier.

During the last decade, Elkin and co-workers (Elkin, Parloff, Hadley, & Autry, 1985; Elkin et al., 1989) have investigated the effectiveness of two forms of brief psychotherapy previously described: cognitive therapy and interpersonal psychotherapy for nonbipolar, nonpsychotic depressed outpatients. This study was the first multisite coordinated study initiated by the NIMH in the field of psychotherapy. Participating in the study were the University of Pittsburgh, George Washington University, and the University of Oklahoma.

In this study, 250 patients were randomly assigned to four 16-week treatment conditions: CT, IPT, imipramine plus clinical management (IMI-CM), and placebo plus clinical management (PLA-CM). Outcome measures included clinician rating scales (HRSD and GAS) and patients' self-reports (BDI and SCL-90 total scores). The main analyses were 3×4 (sites $\times$ treatments) analyses of covariance (ANCOVAs) of mean scores on the four measures. Since marital status was not equally distributed across treatment groups, it was used as a covariate. In addition, pretreatment scores were used as covariates. Each of these considerations and analyses is standard in outcome research of this kind.

Elkin *et al.* (1989) nicely exemplified the impact of the answer to the question of which patients need to be included in statistical analyses. In contrast to other studies that report only on one of these related samples, Elkin *et al.* (1989) reported the same analyses for three samples: the 155 patients who had at least completed 12 sessions and 15 weeks of treatment ("completers") and for whom data were available; 204 patients who completed at least 3.5 weeks of treatment and the latest data point is their termination score; and 239 patients who entered treatment ("intent to treat").

Because of the multitude of statistical analyses and comparisons, the authors used the Bonferroni corrections (for the number of comparisons) to protect against inflation of Type 1 error rate. Thus, results were considered significant when $p < .017$. The general direction of results in all analyses indicated that the PLA-CM group was less effective than either psychotherapy or the IMI-CM. For the 239 patients who *entered* treatment, the IMI-CM patients improved significantly more than the PLA-CM on the SCL-90, and the IMI-CM and the IPT patients were significantly better than the PLA-CM group on the GAS.

For the 155 patients who *completed* treatment, more IPT and IMI-CM patients tended to reach the recovery criteria (HRSD score below 7 or BDI below 10) than PLA-CM patients ($p < .021$ and $p < .020$). Rate of recovery was 57% for IMI-CM, 55% for IPT, and 29% for PLA-CM. Although CT did not differ significantly from other groups, its recovery rate was nevertheless 51%.

Elkin *et al.* (1989) also examined the influence of pretreatment severity (HRSD above 19 and/or GAS below 51 is severe) on outcome. They found that all treatments were similarly effective for less severe patients, but IMI-CM was more effective for the more severe patients on the GAS than the psychotherapies. Using HRSD criteria, IPT was more similar in its effectiveness to IMI-CM.

Elkin *et al.* (1989) concluded from this major study that the psychotherapies, CT and IPT, were about as effective as pharmacotherapy (IMI-CM) at termination on measures of depression and general functioning. Nevertheless, there was some evidence for the specific effectiveness of IPT and no specific effectiveness of CT when compared with PLA-CM. This placebo condition served as "control for regular contact with an experienced and supportive therapist, as well as the more general support provided by the research setting" (Elkin *et al.*, 1989, p. 977).

The meaning of the fact that the psychotherapies were not always significantly better than the placebo condition needs to be examined since the effectiveness of the psychotherapies found in this study was not much different from that found in previous studies. The finding seemed to be due to the "very good performance of the PLA-CM condition" (Elkin *et al.*, 1989, p. 978). Although it is called a placebo condition, the PLA-CM condition consists of clinical management, which includes regular meetings with a trained professional person who discusses with the patient issues related to the medication and other problems. It should also be noted that not much evidence was found for the superiority of IMI-CM over the placebo condition. As an aside, other outcome studies have generally used waiting-list or delayed-treatment groups.

Another important conclusion is that both forms of psychotherapy did not show significant differences from each other. This finding is consistent with the conclusion of Luborsky *et al.* (1975) that psychotherapies show nonsignificant differences in their efficacy.

Despite the relatively weak results obtained in CT, Shea, Elkin, and Collins (1990) recently reported that patients who had been in CT received significantly less further treatment for depression compared to the other groups during the follow-up period.

Uniformity of Treatment Manual Guided Psychotherapies

One of the problems encountered in the earlier outcome study was that there was no check on whether psychotherapists were carrying out their assigned treatments. As a consequence, researchers and theorists began to introduce specific and detailed treatment manuals (Luborsky & DeRubeis, 1984). In these manuals, clinicians provided the main principles of their techniques as well as concrete examples of these principles. The introduction of increasing number of treatment manuals has helped to ensure that researchers engaged in the replication of outcome and process studies were using the same form of treatment. Presently, it is almost impossible to receive a federal grant to conduct an outcome study without providing a treatment manual, and it will also be very difficult to publish such a study in major journals.

Therapists generally find the manuals helpful in learning about the therapy and conducting it, although there are a few problems associated with their use. Introduction of specific treatment manuals did not solve, nor was it intended to solve, the problem of training good therapists (i.e., responsive, empathic, and tactful human beings). Therapists might follow treatment manuals in a rigid way, without taking into account the immediate therapeutic situation or the patient's condition. For example, manuals might recommend that therapists interpret the transference. But no manual will ever be able to detail the exact, tactful wording of an empathic and accurate interpretation or its timing. There-fore, rigid interpretations of the transference might alienate the patients and lead to poorer outcome.

Measures of Adherence and Competence of Therapists

Following the introduction of treatment manuals, researchers developed rating scales for checking therapists' adherence to the manuals. Adherence and competence address different issues. *Adherence* deals with the question of whether the therapists follow the manual's prescriptions. *Competence* addresses the question of whether the therapists follow the therapy prescription in an adequate way. In brief, adherence is related to the measure of frequency of the therapist's congruence with the manual's recommendations, whereas compe-tence is related to the measure of quality of the therapist's behavior.

Woody *et al.* (1983) used a relatively simple measure of adherence to supportive-expressive and cognitive psychotherapies as well as to drug counsel-ing. They have also documented (Luborsky *et al.*, 1985) that with more adher-ence by the therapist to the manual, the patient's outcome was better. One of the problems with such studies is that it is difficult to rule out that high adherence is a function of the difficulty of treating the patient. It may be easier to deliver therapy that is consistent with a manual to patients who are easier to treat. Such patients also are likely to demonstrate better outcome.

The NIMH collaborative study for depression found that adherence to manuals was not at all related to outcome in either IPT or CT (Elkin, 1988). A possible explanation for not replicating the findings of Luborsky *et al.* (1985) could be that their adherence measures have some competence aspects to them as well. However, this conclusion deserves further empirical evaluation.

External Stressors

Ideally, outcome researchers should have a record of the patient's major changes or stressors during treatment, since they obviously could impede or further improvement. In other words, one could easily imagine a patient improv-ing quite satisfactorily during treatment. But when a major negative event, such as a loss in the family, occurs close to the end of treatment, there might be a temporary relapse into depression. Assuming random allocation of patients to treatment groups, one would hope that such occurrences would be randomly distributed across groups, but unfortunately this will not always be the case.

Naturalistic Studies

Some researchers have argued that since patients are not always actually randomized on all variables of interest following assignment to conditions, one should turn to naturalistic studies. Naturalistic studies also mimic real life treatment in clinics. The naturalistic research paradigm has the other advantage of not losing patients because of their unwillingness to be randomly assigned. Although there are many types of naturalistic studies, we will focus our discussion on two general forms: one using groups of patients in noncontrolled settings, and the other using single-case studies.

In our view, the decision whether to use naturalistic studies, controlled clinical trials, and even single-case studies is ultimately a function of what the researcher tries to demonstrate. For example, if one wants to show that psychotherapy X is better at reducing panic attacks than psychotherapy Y, then the study from which the clearest recommendations can be made is the controlled clinical trial. On the other hand, if one wants to study the mechanisms of change in a specific brand of psychotherapy, then the researcher could also use a naturalistic paradigm.

Furthermore, if one accepts the distinction between discovery science and confirmatory science, then naturalistic studies could lead to the generation of hypotheses that could be confirmed or refuted in controlled, experimental studies. In other words, naturalistic studies can provide a descriptive account of what goes on in psychotherapy and can also help us generate hypotheses that could be examined in later empirical studies. In such studies, for example, all patients entering treatment at a specific clinic are assessed at regular intervals on a variety of outcome and process measures.

Single-Case Studies

Often, single-case reports are published to provide readers with evidence of the efficacy of a specific treatment approach and to describe a therapeutic process of change. Recently, Fonagy and Moran (in press) clearly evaluated the many methodological and epistemological issues related to single-case studies, especially as they are relevant to psychoanalysis and dynamic psychotherapy (see also Chapter 3, in this volume). Among the advantages of the empirical study of psychoanalytic hypotheses using single-case studies, Fonagy and Moran mentioned the relative atheoretical approach of single-case studies, the ease with which data can be presented to the general public, the advance of knowledge that can be obtained from such cases, and the parallel between the research method and the actual conduct of psychoanalysis. However, the main problem of single-case studies that still remains concerns the limits on generalization from such evaluations to large samples of patients (Miller, Luborsky, Barber, & Docherty, in press).

Meta-Analysis

In order to derive conclusions from large numbers of studies that sometimes report contradictory results, researchers have developed a quantitative procedure referred to as *meta-analysis*. At the root of this procedure is the computation of effect sizes. *Effect size* is defined as the difference between the means on a specific outcome variable divided by the standard deviation of the pooled groups or the control group. Effect sizes are then the dependent variables to be used in the meta-analysis. The independent variables are the characteristics of the study. The quality of the meta-analysis is directly related to the degree of caution used during the process of choosing the studies and coding their characteristics. If inadequate studies are used or if the characteristics are coded unreliably, then the meta-analysis will yield unreliable conclusions (for a more comprehensive discussion of meta-analysis, see, for example, Kazdin, 1986).

ISSUES ABOUT THE THERAPEUTIC PROCESS

After having shown how researchers go about demonstrating that various forms of treatment are effective, we now turn to the question of how these changes occur and what are the variables that predict the outcome of psychotherapy.

In addition to using naturalistic and controlled random trial studies, investigators interested in understanding how therapeutic change is brought about and in knowing which components of the treatment package are critical have used a special form of controlled research called *dismantling studies*. When a form of therapy has been demonstrated to be effective, researchers, mostly behavior therapists, then break down the treatment into its components and study them individually to see how they bring about the efficacy of the treatment. Kazdin (1986) has also described a "constructive treatment strategy," referring to the development of treatments by *adding* components that may improve their efficacy.

COGNITIVE THERAPY

Hollon, Evans, and DeRubeis (1987) have distinguished between the active components of the therapy and the mechanisms of change. The active components of the therapy refer to those aspects of the treatment (e.g., the use of the three questions) which affect the cognitive mechanisms of change, whereas the mechanisms of change (e.g., a change in schemata) "are defined as patient processes mediating change" in outcome (Hollon & Kriss, 1984, p. 43). An example of an outcome measure is the Beck Depression Inventory (BDI). The active components of the therapy and/or "extra therapy factors" presumably influence the mechanisms of change, which, in turn, cause changes in outcome measures.

In the cognitive therapy literature, such cognitive measures as the Automatic Thought Questionnaire (Hollon & Kendall, 1980) and the Dysfunctional Attitude Scale (DAS) have been developed in the last decade. Often considered a measure of schemata, the DAS is the main instrument available for research on the maladaptive thinking patterns of depressive patients and, therefore, for the mechanism of change of cognitive therapy. The patients are asked how much they agree with such statements as "If I fail at my work, then I am a failure as a person."

No difference between posttreatment DAS scores for patients who received either CT or antidepressant medication (ADM) were found in the research of Simons, Garfield, and Murphy (1984). They also reported no difference on other cognitive measures, such as the Automatic Thought Questionnaires. Since these results were surprising, an additional analysis was performed that showed that the treatment outcome (Did the patient improve?) and not the treatment modality (CT or medication) determined the cognitive changes. DeRubeis, Evans, Hollon, Garvey, Grove, & Tuason (1989) obtained similar results, though they did discover a trend in favor of CT-treated patients when only positive treatment responders were considered. These findings refute the hypothesis that CT has the unique power to affect these cognitive changes, at least as assessed with the above measures.

Dobson and Shaw (1986), Eaves and Ruth (1984), Hollon, Kendall, and Lumry (1986), E. W. Hamilton and Abramson (1983), and Silverman, Silverman, and Eardley (1984) have compared remitted depressives' DAS scores with those of normals. In these studies, the remitted depressives had received a variety of treatments (usually involving pharmacotherapy), but they had not received CT. Barber and DeRubeis (1989) concluded that these studies indicate that the DAS improves to near normal levels with remission from depression irrespective of the kind of treatment.

It is important to realize that the DAS might not be an adequate instrument to assess thinking patterns that predispose one to depression or that are primarily traitlike. Thus, new and different measures of schemata seem urgently required.

Another widely used measure of cognitive change is the Attributional Style Questionnaire (ASQ) developed by Seligman and colleagues (Peterson & Seligman, 1984; Seligman, Abramson, Semmel, von Baeyer, 1979). This measure is derived from the attributional reformulation of the learned helplessness model of depression (Abramson, Seligman, & Teasdale, 1978). According to this model, individuals who habitually explain the causes of bad events in internal terms ("I am at fault"), stable terms ("It will never change"), and global terms ("It's going to undermine everything I do") are at risk for depression following the occurrence of negative events.

DeRubeis *et al.* (1989) found no significant overall difference on the ASQ between ADM-treated and CT-treated patients at the end of treatment. However, restricting the analysis to treatment responders, they found that improved CT-treated patients showed significantly greater change on the ASQ than did improved ADM-treated patients. These results were replicated by Barber, DeRubeis, Beck, Luborsky, and Schweizer (1990). Seligman, Castellon, Cacciola, Schulman, Luborsky, Ollove, and Downing (1988) showed that following CT, unipolar depressives did not differ from controls on the composite score for negative events of the ASQ.

In summary, there is no evidence available to support the hypothesis that change in underlying dysfunctional attitudes (at least as measured by the DAS) is a specific mechanism of change for cognitive therapy. Initial evidence for the role of change in explanatory style as a specific mechanism of change in CT were reported. In their review of the literature on mechanisms of change in CT, Barber and DeRubeis (1989) suggested that instead of focusing on measures of belief changes, future researchers might want to examine what is specifically taught by cognitive therapists during treatment. They recommended focusing more research effort on studying whether patients acquired some of the specific cognitive and behavioral skills specifically taught by cognitive therapist (i.e., the "compensatory skills").

In their recent research, Persons and Miranda (1990) made the very interesting argument that one possible reason for the lack of positive findings with the DAS might be that the underlying and dysfunctional schemata are not activated when patients are remitted. Therefore, they proposed that one needs to activate schemata using a mood induction technique to assess whether patients who have received CT have a similar number of dysfunctional attitudes as patients who have received medication. One of their predictions is that CT-remitted patients induced into a depressive state will show lower levels of dysfunctional attitudes than remitted patients who have received medication.

DYNAMIC THERAPY

In our description of recent findings in dynamic therapy, we should emphasize two important topics of empirical research: the role of the alliance between patients and therapists and role of interpretations. Other topics are reviewed in Luborsky, Barber, and Crits-Christoph (1990) and Miller et al. (in press).

The Role of the Alliance between Patients and Therapists

In the area of early-on treatment factors that predict outcome, we will focus on the relationship between patients and their therapists. Therapists from various schools, including psychoanalysis, have emphasized the role of the relationship between client and therapist, or the therapeutic alliance, as a necessary condition for good outcome in psychotherapy.

There are two different types of therapeutic alliance measures: (1) a questionnaire method in which the patient or the therapist is asked to respond to items describing various facets of the relationship, and (2) a rating method in which independent observers are asked to rate various aspects of the alliance from audio- or videotaped or transcribed sessions. The questionnaires began with that of Barrett-Lennard (1962), followed by more specific alliance measures, such as the Helping Alliance Questionnaire (Luborsky et al., 1985), the Working

Alliance Inventory (Horvath & Greenberg, 1986), and the California Psychotherapy Alliance Scale—Patient Version (CALPAS) (Marmar & Gaston, 1988).

Luborsky (1976) introduced the system of counting of signs as a new
method to rate the level of therapeutic alliance directly from the sessions
(Luborsky, Crits-Christoph, Alexander, Margolis, & Cohen, 1983). Morgan,
Luborsky, Crits-Christoph, Curtis, and Solomon (1982) introduced the global
rating system in which portions of the transcript are rated globally rather than
for specific signs, such as by the helping alliance rating systems. Other global
rating systems were developed by Marmar, Horowitz, Weiss, and Marziali
(1983) (the Therapeutic Alliance Rating System), and by Hartley and Strupp
(1983) (the Vanderbilt Therapeutic Alliance Scale). For a comparison of some of
these measures, see Tichenor and Hill (1989).

Hartley and Strupp (1983), for example, showed that patients who scored
higher on therapeutic alliance measures had a better outcome. Similarly, Marmar, Gaston, Gallagher, and Thompson (1989) demonstrated that the alliance
factors of Patient Commitment and Patient Working Capacity from the CALPAS—
Therapist Version were related to outcome across three treatments (behavioral,
cognitive, and brief dynamic), as was Patient Commitment from the CALPAS—
Patient Version. Luborsky et al. (1988) reviewed eight studies that examined the
relation between therapeutic alliance and outcome, and they found that in each
case therapeutic alliance predicted outcome with a mean correlation of .5. The
same trend was found in a more detailed review (Orlinsky & Howard, 1986). A
recent quantitative review of the many predictive studies again confirmed the
same trend (Horvath, Gaston, & Luborsky, in press).

The Role of Interpretations

A basic tenet of psychodynamic therapy is that the set of feelings and
beliefs that patients come with and transfer to their therapist (the transference)
need to be analyzed and interpreted if treatment is to be successful. Malan
(1976), for example, emphasized the therapist's role in connecting the patient's
pattern of interpersonal relationships, as experienced with the therapist (the
transference), to previous relationships with parental figures ("parent link")
and to relationships with other people.

Studies by Malan (1976) and Marziali (1984) suggested that the frequency of
use of transference interpretations is related to better outcomes. Another version
of transference interpretation, the linkage of the therapist with past significant
persons and with current persons, correlated significantly with outcomes (r
= .57) (McCullough, Winston, Laikin, & Vitolo, 1989). Such results, however,
were not replicated by Piper, Debbane, Bienvenu, de Carufel, and Garant (1986).
Nor did Silberschatz, Fretter, and Curtis (1986) find differences in the patients'
immediate benefits following transference versus nontransference interpretations.

Such lack of replication may not be surprising because other factors than the
frequency of interpretations by itself must influence outcome. McCullough

(1987) found that interpretations followed by affect tended to be associated with better outcome, whereas interventions followed by defensiveness tended to be associated with poorer outcome.

Even these results are surprising, since we know that interpretations may or may not be appropriate. Interestingly, very few studies have addressed the issue of the accuracy of interpretations. One of the main reasons for this lack of scrutiny is the difficulty of finding a criterion against which one could compare the interpretation.

Crits-Christoph, Cooper, and Luborsky (1988) used the patient's Core Conflictual Relationship Theme (CCRT) as a criterion. An independent set of judges identified the CCRT, while another set identified the degree of accuracy in terms of convergence with the therapist's interpretations. The reliabilities (three judges pooled) were high: .84 for accuracy on wishes, .76 for accuracy on responses from other, and .83 for accuracy on responses of self. For 43 patients, the correlation between accuracy on the wish plus response-from-other components of the CCRT with outcomes (a composite measure of ratings of change by therapist and patient) was .44 ($p < .01$). Accuracy on the response-of-self component of the CCRT was not related to outcome, suggesting that it is the focus on the interpersonal aspects of the theme (wish and response-from-other components) which is most important. The predictive strength of accuracy on the wish plus response-from-other components remained even after partialling out the effects of general errors in technique and the quality of the therapeutic alliance. This study also examined whether accurate interpretations had their greatest impact in the context of a positive therapeutic alliance, but no evidence for this clinically appealing proposition was found.

The immediate consequence of interpretations was examined by Silberschatz et al. (1986). Their study is part of a fascinating program of research on therapy process at Mount Zion Hospital in San Francisco to test the theory of therapy of Weiss, Sampson, and the Mount Zion Psychotherapy Research Group (1986). According to this theory, psychopathology is the result of patients' unconscious pathogenic beliefs that interfere with their lives. According to this theory, patients enter treatment with a plan to test out these pathogenic beliefs in order to disconfirm them. The study of Silberschatz et al. (1986) showed that the compatibility of therapists' interventions with an assessment of the patient's unconscious plans seems to coincide with outcome in their sample of three patients.

Crits-Christoph et al. (1988) demonstrated that one could develop a reliable and valid method to measure accuracy and appropriateness of interpretations. Furthermore, they demonstrated that a particular therapist intervention, an accurate interpretation, is related to good outcome. Thus, they have found evidence that "specific" technique factors (active ingredients of therapy) are important to determine outcome, and they have possibly laid down the foundation for refuting the prevalent hypothesis that "general" factors (e.g., warmth and empathy) account for all the effects of psychotherapy.

SUMMARY

In this chapter, we have presented a brief guide for the planning and understanding of psychotherapy research. We have focused on the two major issues of the field: those related to the measurement of the efficacy of psychotherapy and those related to the understanding of the process of psychotherapy. Each of these issues has been presented in terms of actual studies of the three major psychotherapy systems: cognitive, psychodynamic, and interpersonal psychotherapies.

Research addressing the issue of treatment efficacy in psychotherapy does not involve methodological principles that are different from those involved in other biomedical disciplines. In general, researchers in these areas of science use an empirical approach to the scientific method. That is, they use procedures that rely on "objective experience, systematic observation, or experiment to map out the nature of reality" (Rosenthal & Rosnow, 1984, p. 3). In psychotherapy research, this often means that researchers try their best to ascertain that the treatment is delivered as well as possible to at least two well-defined, well-sampled groups of patients, and that the measures of changes are as reliable and valid as possible.

The presence of two different treatment conditions (independent variable) in which the patient's behavior (the dependent variable) is measured before and after the delivery of treatment enables us (when a difference exists between the two groups) to infer that one of the treatment conditions is somehow related to this difference. The use of control, randomization, and all other strategies reviewed in this chapter have the main purpose of helping us to increase the likelihood that no other variable than the treatment has influenced the difference in outcome. In essence, this is the experimental method. But certainty in our conclusion is never achieved. The important lesson that the apprentice scientist reading these lines should remember is that a single study can attempt to answer only a limited set of questions and in no case can answer all questions of interest. The control group (placebo group) used in efficacy studies will determine to a large extent the questions that a specific study can address: Does treatment relieve symptoms or is it more effective than other existing treatments? Does the treatment have additional advantages, such as prevention of relapse? and so on.

To a large extent, studies addressing the question of what are the active mechanisms of change in psychotherapy also follow the same scientific and logical principles applied in other disciplines. But in addition to using the experimental method, process studies can be done using the correlational approach. In short, scientists using this approach examine the correlations between variables in nature and use this knowledge to predict the occurrence of one variable from the other. One major limitation of the correlation approach is that it never tells us much about causality. Again, no single study can answer all questions, since, for example, the issue of a third hypothetical and unmeasured variable explaining the observed change is always possible. Science often advances slowly by refuting each of the successive reasonable alternative explanations and generating new theories that explain new facts. In that sense, this guide specifies in advance some of the issues that a researcher should be attentive to when planning a study or when reading about the results from a new study.

In our chapter, we have emphasized the empirical approach of the scientific method; other approaches (e.g., phenomenological) can also be used depending on the question asked. For example, discovery science (see the section above on Single-Case Study) can be successfully applied to questions related to the process of therapy, whereas we have doubts that it can be applied best to outcome studies. In the last two decades, the field of psychotherapy research has made considerable progress using these approaches. Therefore, we are optimistic that researchers will be able to explore the more ambitious and difficult question of which therapeutic move in which patients and under what conditions will be the most effective.

REFERENCES

Abramson, L. Y., Seligman, M. E. P., & Teasdale, J. (1978). Learned helplessness in humans: Critique and reformulation. *Journal of Abnormal Psychology, 87,* 49–57.

American Psychiatric Association. (1987). *Diagnostic and statistical manual of mental disorders* (3rd ed., rev.). Washington, DC: Author.

American Psychiatric Association Commission on Psychotherapies. (1982). *Psychotherapy research: Methodological and efficacy issues.* Washington, DC: Author.

Barber, J. P., & DeRubeis, R. J. (1989). On second thought: Where the action is in cognitive therapy for depression. *Cognitive Therapy and Research, 13,* 441–457.

Barber, J. P., DeRubeis, R. J., Beck, A. T., Luborsky, L., & Schweizer, E. E. (1990). *Do compensatory skills or attributional style specifically improve during cognitive therapy?* Unpublished manuscript.

Barrett-Lennard, G. T. (1962). Dimensions of therapist response as causal factors in therapeutic change. *Psychological Monographs, 76,* 562.

Battle, C., Imber, S., Hoehn-Saric, R., Stone, A., Nash, E., & Frank, J. (1966). Target complaints as criteria of improvement. *American Journal of Psychotherapy, 20,* 184–192.

Beck, A. T., & Emery, G. (1977). *Cognitive therapy of substance abuse.* Center for Cognitive Therapy, Room 602, 133 South 36th Street, Philadelphia, PA 19104.

Beck, A. T., Ward, C. H., Mendelson, M., Mock, J., & Erbaugh, J. (1961). An inventory for measuring depression. *Archives of General Psychiatry, 4,* 561–571.

Beck, A. T., Rush, A. J., Shaw, B. F., & Emery, G. (1979). *Cognitive therapy of depression.* New York: Guilford Press.

Beck, A. T., Emery, G., & Greenberg, R. L. (1985). *Anxiety disorders and phobias: A cognitive perspective.* New York: Basic Books.

Beck, A. T., Wright, F., & Newman, C. (1990). *Cognitive therapy for cocaine abuse.* Unpublished manuscript. University of Pennsylvania School of Medicine, Center for Cognitive Therapy.

Campbell, D. T., & Stanley, J. C. (1966). *Experimental and quasi-experimental designs for research.* Chicago: Rand McNally.

Crits-Christoph, P., & Barber, J. P. (1991). *Handbook of short-term dynamic psychotherapies.* New York: Basic Books.

Crits-Christoph, P., Cooper, A., & Luborsky, L. (1988). The accuracy of therapists' interpretations and the outcome of dynamic psychotherapy. *Journal of Consulting and Clinical Psychology, 56,* 490–495.

Crits-Christoph, P., Baranackie, K., Kurcias, J. S., Beck, A. T., Carroll, K., Perry, K., Luborsky, L., McLellan, A. T., Woody, G. E., Thompson, L., Gallagher, D., & Zitrin, C. (1990, June). *Meta-analysis of therapist effects in therapy outcome studies*. Paper presented at the meeting of the Society for Psychotherapy Research, Wintergreen, VA.

DeRubeis, R. J., Evans, M. D., Hollon, S. D., Garvey, M. J., Grove, W. M., & Tuason, V. B. (1989). *Active components and mediating mechanisms to cognitive therapy, pharmacotherapy, and combined cognitive-pharmacotherapy for depression: III. Processes of change in the CPT project*. Unpublished manuscript. University of Pennsylvania, Department of Psychology.

Derogatis, L. R., Lipman, R. S., & Covi, L. (1973). SCL-90: An outpatient psychiatric rating scale—preliminary report. *Psychopharmacology Bulletin, 9*, 13–28.

Dobson, K. S. (1989). A meta-analysis of the efficacy of cognitive therapy for depression. *Journal of Consulting and Clinical Psychology, 57*, 414–419.

Dobson, K. S., & Shaw, B. F. (1986). Cognitive assessment with major depressive disorders. *Cognitive Therapy and Research, 10*, 13–29.

Eaves, G., & Rush, A. J. (1984). Cognitive patterns in symptomatic and remitted unipolar major depression. *Journal of Abnormal Psychology, 93*, 31–40.

Elkin, I. (1988, June). *Relationship of therapist's adherence to treatment outcome in the NIMH treatment of depression collaborative research program*. Paper presented at the annual meeting of the Society for Psychotherapy Research in Santa Fe, NM.

Elkin, I., Parloff, M. B., Hadley, S. W., & Autry, J. H. (1985). NIMH treatment of depression collaborative research program: Background and research plan. *Archives of General Psychiatry, 42*, 305–316.

Elkin, I., Shea, S., Watkins, J. T., Imber, S. D., Sotsky, S. M., Collins, J. F., Glass, D. R., Pilkonis, P. A., Leber, W. R., Doeherty, J. P., Fiester, S. J., & Parloff, M. B. (1989). NIMH treatment of depression collaborative research program: General effectiveness of treatments. *Archives of General Psychiatry, 46*, 971–982.

Endicott, J., Spitzer, R., Fleiss, J. L., & Cohen, J. (1976). The Global Assessment Scale. *Archives of General Psychiatry, 33*, 767–771.

Fiske, D. W., Hunt, H. F., Luborsky, L., Orne, M. T., Parloff, M. B., Reiser, M. F., & Tuma, A. H. (1970). The planning of research on effectiveness of psychotherapy. *Archives of General Psychiatry, 22*, 22–32.

Fonagy, P., & Moran, G. (in press). Single case research designs. In N. Miller, L. Luborsky, J. P. Barber, & J. Docherty (Eds.), *Handbook of psychodynamic treatment research and practice: A how-to-do it guide*. New York: Basic Books.

Frances, A., Clarkin, J., & Perry, S. (1984). *Differential therapeutics in psychiatry: The art and science of treatment selection*. New York: Brunner/Mazel.

Garfield, S. L., & Bergin, A. E. (1978). (Eds.). *Handbook of psychotherapy and behavior change: An empirical analysis* (2nd ed.). New York: Wiley.

Garfield, S. L., & Bergin, A. E. (1986). (Eds.). *Handbook of psychotherapy and behavior change: An empirical analysis* (3rd ed.). New York: Wiley.

Hamilton, E. W., & Abramson, L. Y. (1983). Cognitive patterns and major depressive disorder: A longitudinal study in a hospital setting. *Journal of Abnormal Psychology, 92*, 173–184.

Hamilton, M. A. (1960). A rating scale for depression. *Journal of Neurology, Neurosurgery and Psychiatry, 23*, 56–62.

Hamilton, M. A. (1967). Development of a rating scale for primary depressive illness. *British Journal of Social and Clinical Psychology, 6*, 278–296.

Hartley, D., & Strupp, H. (1983). The therapeutic alliance: Its relationship to outcome in brief psychotherapy. In J. Masling (Ed.), *Empirical studies of psychoanalytic theory* (Vol. 1, pp. 1–38). Hillsdale, NJ: Lawrence Erlbaum.

Hollon, S. D., & Kendall, P. C. (1980). Cognitive self-statements in depression: Development of an automatic thoughts questionnaire. *Cognitive Therapy and Research, 4*, 383–395.

Hollon, S. D., & Kriss, M. R. (1984). Cognitive factors in clinical research and practice. *Clinical Psychology Review, 4*, 35–76.

Hollon, S. D., Kendall, P. C., & Lumry, A. (1986). Specificity of depressotypic cognitions in clinical depression. *Journal of Abnormal Psychology, 95*, 52–59.

Hollon, S. D., Evans, M. D., & DeRubeis, R. J. (1987). Causal mediation of change in treatment for depression: Discriminating between nonspecificity and noncausality. *Psychological Bulletin, 102,* 139–149.

Hollon, S. D., Evans, M. D., & DeRubeis, R. J. (1990). Cognitive mediation of relapse prevention following treatment for depression: Implications of differential risks. In R. E. Ingram (Ed.), *Psychological aspects of depression* (pp. 117–136). New York: Plenum Press.

Horvath, A. O., & Greenberg, L. S. (1986). The development of the Working Alliance Inventory. In L. S. Greenberg & W. M. Pinsof (Eds.), *The psychotherapeutic process: A research handbook* (pp. 529–556). New York: Guilford Press.

Horvath, A. O., Gaston, L., & Luborsky, L. (in press). The therapeutic and working alliance. In N. Miller, L. Luborsky, J. P. Barber, & J. Docherty (Eds.), *Handbook of psychodynamic treatment research and practice: A how-to-do it guide.* New York: Basic Books.

Jacobson, N. S., & Revenstorf, D. (1988). Statistics for assessing clinical significance of psychotherapy techniques: Issues, problems, and new developments. *Behavioral Assessment, 10,* 133–145. (See also the entire issue.)

Kazdin, A. E. (1986). The evaluation of psychotherapy: Research design and methodology. In S. L. Garfield & A. E. Bergin (Eds.), *Handbook of psychotherapy and behavior change: An empirical analysis* (3rd ed., pp. 23–68). New York: Wiley.

Klerman, G. L., Weissman, M. M., Rounsaville, B. J., & Chevron, E. S. (1984). *Interpersonal psychotherapy of depression.* New York: Basic Books.

Luborsky, L. (1975). Clinicians' judgments of mental health: Specimen case descriptions and forms for the Health-Sickness Rating Scale. *Bulletin of the Menninger Clinic, 35,* 448–480.

Luborsky, L. (1976). Helping alliances in psychotherapy: The groundwork for a study of their relationship to its outcome. In J. L. Claghorn (Ed.), *Successful psychotherapy* (pp. 92–116). New York: Brunner/Mazel.

Luborsky, L. (1984). *Principles of psychoanalytic psychotherapy: A manual for supportive-expressive (SE) treatment.* New York: Basic Books.

Luborsky, L., Barber, J. P., & Crits-Christoph, P. (1990). Theory based research for understanding the process of dynamic psychotherapy. *Journal of Consulting and Clinical Psychology, 58,* 281–287.

Luborsky, L., & Crits-Christoph, P. (1990). *Understanding transference—the CCRT Method (The Core Conflictual Relationship Theme).* New York: Basic Books.

Luborsky, L., Crits-Christoph, P., Alexander, L., Margolis, M., & Cohen, M. (1983). Two helping alliance methods for predicting outcomes of psychotherapy: A counting signs versus a global rating method. *Journal of Nervous and Mental Disease, 171,* 480–492.

Luborsky, L., Crits-Christoph, P., Mintz, J., & Auerbach, A. (1988). *Who will benefit from psychotherapy? Predicting therapeutic outcomes.* New York: Basic Books.

Luborsky, L., & DeRubeis, R. J. (1984). The use of psychotherapy treatment manuals: A small revolution in psychotherapy research style. *Clinical Psychology Review, 4,* 403–429.

Luborsky, L., & Fiske, D. W. (1991). Principles for designing studies of the process and efficacy of dynamic psychotherapy. Unpublished manuscript. University of Pennsylvania.

Luborsky, L., McLellan, A. T., Woody, G. E., O'Brien, C. P., & Auerbach, A. (1985). Therapist success and its determinants. *Archives of General Psychiatry, 42,* 602–611.

Luborsky, L., Singer, B., & Luborsky, L. (1975). Comparative studies of psychotherapies. *Archives of General Psychiatry, 32,* 995–1008.

Luborsky, L., Crits-Christoph, P., Barber, J., & Cacciola, J. (1992). *Factors influencing outcomes of dynamic psychotherapy for major depression.* Unpublished manuscript.

Malan, D. M. (1976). *Toward the validation of dynamic psychotherapy.* New York: Plenum Press.

Marmar, C. R., & Gaston, L. (1988). *California Psychotherapy Alliance Scales (CALPAS) Manual.* Unpublished manuscript, University of California, San Francisco.

Marmar, C. R., Horowitz, M. J., Weiss, D. S., & Marziali, E. (1986). Development of the Therapeutic Alliance Rating System. In L. S. Greenberg & W. M. Pinsof (Eds.), *The psychotherapeutic process: A research handbook* (pp. 367–390). New York: Guilford Press.

Marmar, C. R., Gaston, L., Gallagher, D., & Thompson, L. W. (1989). *Therapeutic alliance and outcome of behavioral, cognitive and brief dynamic therapy of late-life depression.* Unpublished manuscript.

Marziali, E. (1984). Prediction of outcome of brief psychotherapy from therapist interpretive interventions. *Archives of General Psychiatry, 41,* 301–304.

McCullough, L. (1987, July). *The effects of therapist interventions combined with different patient responses and correlated with outcome at termination of treatment.* Paper presented at the meeting of the Society for Psychotherapy Research, Ulm, Germany.

McCullough, L., Winston, A., Laikin, M., & Vitolo, A. (1989, June). *The effect of robustness of interpretation on patient affective and defensive responding and therapy outcome.* Paper presented at the annual meeting of the Society for Psychotherapy Research, Toronto.

Miller, N., Luborsky, L., Barber, J. P., & Docherty, J. (in press). *Handbook of psychodynamic treatment research and practice: A how-to-do it Guide.* New York: Basic Books.

Morgan, R., Luborsky, L., Crits-Christoph, P., Curtis, H., & Solomon, J. (1982). Predicting the outcomes of psychotherapy by the Penn Helping Alliance Rating Method. *Archives of General Psychiatry, 39,* 397–402.

Orlinsky, D., & Howard, K. (1986). Process and outcome of psychotherapy. In S. Garfield & A. Bergin (Eds.), *Handbook of psychotherapy and behavior change: An empirical analysis* (3rd ed., pp. 311–381). New York: Wiley.

Paul, G. L. (1967). Strategy of outcome research in psychotherapy. *Journal of Consulting Psychology, 31,* 109–118.

Persons, J. B, & Miranda, J. (1990). *Cognitive theories of vulnerability to depression: Reconciling negative evidence.* Unpublished manuscript.

Peterson, C., & Seligman, M. E. P. (1984). Causal explanations as a risk factor for depression: Theory and evidence. *Psychological Review, 91,* 347–374.

Piper, W., Debbane, E., Bienvenu, J., de Carufel, F., & Garant, J. (1986). Relationships between the object of focus of therapist interpretations and outcome in short-term individual psychotherapy. *British Journal of Medical Psychology, 59,* 1–11.

Rosenthal, R., & Rosnow, R. L. (1984). *Essentials of behavioral research: Method and data analysis.* New York: McGraw-Hill.

Rounsaville, B. J., Glazer, W., Wilbur, C. H., Weissman, M. M., & Kleber, H. D. (1983). Short-term interpersonal psychotherapy in methadone maintained opiate addicts. *Archives of General Psychiatry, 40,* 629–636.

Rounsaville, B. J., Gawin, F., & Kleber, H. (1985). Interpersonal psychotherapy adapted for ambulatory cocaine abusers. *American Journal of Drug and Alcohol Abuse, 11,* 171–191.

Rounsaville, B. J., Klerman, G. L., Weissman, M. M., & Chevron, E. S. (1985). Short-term interpersonal psychotherapy for depression. In E. E. Beckham & W. R. Leber (Eds.), *Handbook of depression: Treatment, assessment and research* (pp. 124–150). Homewood, IL: Dorsey Press.

Rush, A. J., Beck, A. T., Kovacs, J. M., & Hollon, S. D. (1977). Comparative efficacy of cognitive therapy vs. pharmacotherapy in outpatient depressives. *Cognitive Therapy and Research, 1,* 17–37.

Seligman, M. E. P., Abramson, L. Y., Semmel, A., & von Baeyer, C. (1979). Depressive attributional style. *Journal of Abnormal Psychology, 88,* 242–247.

Seligman, M. E. P., Castellon, C., Cacciola, J., Schulman, P., Luborsky, L., Ollove, M., & Downing, R. (1988). Explanatory style change during cognitive therapy for unipolar depression. *Journal of Abnormal Psychology, 97,* 13–18.

Shea, T., Elkin, I., & Collins, J. (1990, June). *Follow-up findings from the NIMH TDCRP: Course of depression.* Paper presented at the Annual Meeting of the Society for Psychotherapy Research at Wintergreen, VA.

Silberschatz, G., Fretter, P., & Curtis, J. (1986). How do interpretations influence the process of psychotherapy. *Journal of Consulting and Clinical Psychology, 54,* 646–652.

Silverman, J. S., Silverman, J. A, & Eardley, D. A. (1984). Do maladaptive attitudes cause depression? *Archives of General Psychiatry, 41,* 28–30.

Simons, A. D., Garfield, S. L., & Murphy, G. E. (1984). The process of change in cognitive therapy and pharmacotherapy for depression. *Archives of General Psychiatry, 41,* 45–51.

Smith, M., Glass, C., & Miller, T. (1980). *The benefits of psychotherapy.* Baltimore: Johns Hopkins University Press.

Sokol, L., Beck, A. T., Greenberg, R. L., Wright, F. D., & Berchick, R. J. (1989). Cognitive therapy of panic disorder: A nonpharmacological alternative. *Journal of Nervous and Mental Disease, 177,* 711–716.

Strupp, H. S., & Binder, J. L. (1984). *Psychotherapy in a new key: A guide to time-limited dynamic psychotherapy.* New York: Basic Books.

Tichenor, V., & Hill, C. E. (1989). A comparison of six measures of working alliance. *Psychotherapy, 26,* 195–199.

Weiss, J., Sampson, H., & the Mount Zion Psychotherapy Group (1986). *The psychoanalytic process: Theory, clinical observation & empirical research.* New York: Guilford Press.

Weissman, A. N. (1979). *The Dysfunctional Attitudes Scale: A validation study.* Unpublished manuscript, University of Pennsylvania, Philadelphia.

Woody, G., Luborsky, L., McLellan, A. T., O'Brien, C., Beck, A. T., Blaine, J., Herman, I., & Hole, A. V. (1983). Psychotherapy for opiate addicts: Does it help? *Archives of General Psychiatry, 40,* 639–645.

Woody, G. E., McLellan, A. T., Luborsky, L., O'Brien, C. P., Blaine, J., Fox, S., Herman, I., & Beck, A. T. (1984). Severity of psychiatric symptoms as a predictor of benefits from psychotherapy: The VA-Penn study. *American Journal of Psychiatry, 141,* 1172–1177.

CHAPTER 14

Genetics of Alcoholism

DONALD W. GOODWIN

ISSUES

A Familial Disorder

Alcoholism runs in families. About 20% to 25% of the sons of alcoholics become alcoholics or problem drinkers, and so do about 5% of the daughters (Goodwin, 1979, 1988). These rates are about four or five times greater than the prevalence rate of alcoholism in the general population. Apparently, having two alcoholic parents increases the risk that the children will also become alcoholic, but it is not certain how much the risk is increased. A rough guess would be that children with two parents who are alcoholic have about a 40% chance of becoming alcoholic if they are male and perhaps a 10% to 15% chance if they are female. However, it should be stressed that studies documenting these latter figures are lacking.

Alcoholism, or alcohol dependence, will be the model illness used in this chapter. The observations that are made about alcoholism could just as easily be made about any behavioral disorder that runs in families. Therefore, for the purposes of this chapter, *alcoholism* is defined as a compulsion to drink alcohol, causing harm to the person who drinks or to others.

Donald W. Goodwin • Department of Psychiatry, University of Kansas Medical Center, Kansas City, Kansas 66160.
Research in Psychiatry: Issues, Strategies, and Methods, edited by L. K. George Hsu and Michel Hersen. Plenum Press, New York, 1992.

Nature versus Nurture

Not everything that runs in families is inherited. Languages are an excellent example. Speaking French runs in families but not because of heredity. In dealing with conditions that do run in families, it is important to estimate the relative importance of biological factors and those influences that are broadly called *environmental*. Environmental influences can be more precisely defined as events that produce *learning*—a term designated here to encompass all forms of learning, including conditioning. Separating nature from nurture is not easy. The several strategies that have been employed to accomplish this separation all have various limitations, as will be described in the next section.

Historical Perspective

The fact that alcoholism does run in families has been known for centuries, with the King James Bible alluding to it as well as such classical writers as Aristotle and Plutarch ("Drunkards beget drunkards," said Plutarch some nineteen hundred years ago). Because this familial connection in alcoholism was recognized for such a long period of time, by the end of the nineteenth century, doctors and preachers were unanimous in agreement: alcoholism not only ran in families, it was inherited. At that time, everything that ran in families was believed to be inherited, except perhaps not speaking French or voting Republican. But certainly it was thought that talents and weaknesses were both inherited. Clearly, alcoholism was a weakness, or a vice, or both. Thus, the concept of inheritance was essentially Lamarckian; that is, if the mother took piano lessons, the child might also develop a musical talent. If the father drank, then the sons might become drunkards (Goodwin, 1985).

In the last quarter of the twentieth century, the observation that alcoholism ran in families had developed scientific underpinnings. Drunkard parents did indeed have drunken children: they had them about four or five times more often than did parents who were not alcoholic. Cotton (1979) counted more than 100 studies in the literature that confirmed, beyond any doubt, that alcoholism was a familial disease.

In time, disease, more or less, had replaced weakness. (People still argue about whether alcoholism is a disease like measles; but these arguments are entirely semantic and depend for their persuasiveness on the definition of disease). By the 1920s, the theories of Mendel had replaced those of Larmarck. Actually, in this century, most students who were interested in theories of inheritance were indifferent about which geneticist to give credit. A consensus had formed that inheritance played no part in the development of alcoholism: *environment* explained everything. Children saw what their parents did and they did the same, just like learning French or voting Republican. Blue eyes were inherited; alcoholism was not.

By the 1970s, the pendulum had started to swing back. The old questions were again being raise: Did alcoholism *really* in run in families, perhaps like speaking French, or did it run in families or maybe just a little, like having blue eyes? How do you study such things? Psychologists like Donald Hebb (1958) said you could not. Writing about intelligence, Hebb warned against regarding intelligence as due either to heredity or to environment, or partly to one, partly to the other. "Each is *fully* necessary . . . to ask how much heredity contributes to intelligence is like asking how much the width of a field contributes to its area."

Still, the familial nature of alcoholism was one of the few solid facts about alcoholism upon which investigators could depend. Maybe separating nature from nurture was worth a try. At least some of the relevant dimensions of the field might begin to yield to measurement. Twin and adoption studies were conducted, with each supporting a genetic contribution. Then, in 1990, investigators reported that a gene on chromosome 11 was highly associated with alcoholism (Blum, Noble, Sheridan, Montgomery, Ritchie, Jagadeeswaran, Nogami, Briggs, & Cohn, 1990). This gene was not chosen at random. It was the gene for a receptor for the neurotransmitter *dopamine*. Dopamine is considered to be involved in the so-called reward system of the brain. For example, the effects of cocaine and other addictive substances, including alcohol, are believed to be partly attributable to the differential sensitivity of dopamine neurons.

Identification of a possible gene for alcoholism—an *alcogene*—has since received wide attention. If the study was reproduced in other laboratories, this would provide strong evidence that some people have a genetic predisposition to alcoholism. This is not to deny the importance of learning and psychosocial factors. But, if a gene or genes are identified as promoting alcoholism, they could then function like a switch that can be turned on and off. Lewis Thomas (1979) has often speculated about the possibility that single switches were really responsible for multiorgan or multisystem diseases, such as cancer, and psychiatric conditions, such as alcoholism. In the case of infectious disorders, single switches (infectious organisms) were indeed found. In the case of cancer, oncogenes had been identified, tending to confirm Thomas's hunch.

Whether a single gene or a set of genes will ultimately be shown to be a necessary cause for some forms of alcoholism will require that the findings be reproducible. As will be noted later, the hunt for behavioral disorder genes has produced highly inconsistent findings.

STRATEGIES AND METHODS

Several methods are used for identifying biological factors in a familial disorder, including (1) family studies, (2) twin studies, (3) adoption studies, (4) marker studies, and (5) DNA studies. Each approach will now be examined.

Family Studies

The validity of a medical or psychiatric diagnosis is strongly supported by family studies showing that a particular disorder runs true-to-type in families. Such studies also exist in the diagnosis of alcoholism disorders but they are plagued with difficulties. I have identified eight sources of error in family studies and will describe them in some detail on the grounds that all or most of the errors are avoidable and should be avoided, whenever possible, in future studies (Goodwin, 1981).

1. *Source of information.* Sources may consist of patient records, questionnaires, and interviews. The problem with records is well known: the information is retrospective, unsystematic, and often comes from different individuals from different backgrounds. When examining such sources, the reader never knows what information has been omitted. If obsessions are not mentioned, it does not mean that the patient does not have obsessions: perhaps he was not asked; perhaps the clinician failed to mention it; perhaps if it was mentioned, the note is illegible.

Questionnaires are as bad as records for other reasons. There is no way to tell (even with "lie" scales) how seriously the subject regarded the questionnaire, or whether he or she understood the question (or even cared to understand). Finally, with mailed questionnaires, there is the inevitable low return rate with its inevitable bias.

What about interviews? When they are unstructured (e.g., seat-of-the-pants), one can never know who was asked what. When the interviews are structured (a format is used), one can never be certain that the questions were asked in the same way. Rarely does one know the experience, training, and biases of the interviewers (who can range from moonlighting housewives to venerable academics). One can never know whether the subject understood the question, listened, lied, or had a faulty memory.

Regarding memory, the question "How well do people remember life changes?" was raised in a study of 416 normal subjects (Jenkins, Hurst, & Rose, 1979). Life events were assessed at two examinations that occurred 9 months apart. At the second examination, subjects were asked to report events during the 6-month period preceding the first examination. Nine months later, subjects "forgot" more than one third of the events reported originally, including such items as being in an automobile accident or the victim of a crime. These authors now believe that their findings raise serious doubts about the validity of retrospective studies.

Also, one rarely knows how much weight to give to an answer. If a man was scolded once by his fundamentalist wife for having a beer at a ballgame, do you score "Family complains about drinking" positive? If he had one blackout at age 19, do you score him positive for blackouts? If he *thinks* he had a blackout but is not sure, what then? Such questions require a judgment by the interviewer, and interviewers differ widely in judgment and in other ways.

Finally, in family studies in which all the information comes from the patients, how much can you trust this secondhand information? If the proband says that his father was an alcoholic, attended Alcoholics Anonymous regularly, took disulfiram, and had a history of "seeing" reptiles, then perhaps this secondhand information can be trusted. Often, however, the patient is not so helpful. If his father, uncle, or brother "drank too much" or "really poured it down but could hold it," then in which diagnostic box do you put these elusively described kin? If your bias favors a genetic basis for alcoholism, very likely an alcoholic's "heavy drinking" father who "never got into trouble" will go in the alcoholic box, whereas if you are trying to make some other point, then he may be placed elsewhere.

The truth is, there is no way to know in which box to put the family member. Probably the honest thing to do is to put the member in no box or in a "maybe" box. In which case, in the final data analysis, when "maybes" are almost always lumped with "definites," it will not make any different anyway.

2. *Conflicting stories.* Few family history studies (perhaps none) deal with the problem of conflicting stories. The proband may say that his father was "a drunk"; the proband's sister may say that her father drank a lot but never had problems; and the proband's paternal uncle may say that his brother drank no more than he did himself, which was modest indeed. How does one recognize such conflicting stories? They are inevitable, given the differing opinions of what constitutes a drinking problem, plus the fact that, among mobile Americans, many know little about their relatives. Still no one mentions conflicts. How they are dealt with is anyone's guess. Again, the investigator's bias probably determines which version is accepted.

3. *Definitional chaos.* The definitions used in alcoholism diagnosis are diverse. They range from such statements as "admission to alcoholism unit" to "drinking in excess of community norms" to "had delirium tremens." Most studies still rely on a clinician's making a diagnosis. Few have operational criteria, and the criteria differ from study to study.

In fact, it is debatable whether operational criteria have improved the art of diagnosis to the extent claimed by proponents. Overall and Hollister (1979a) compared six different research diagnostic criteria in patients who were receiving a clinical diagnosis of schizophrenia. They found that the diagnoses which were based on criteria differed greatly depending on the criteria used and also differed from the clinical diagnosis. Similarly, Kendell, Brockington, and Leff (1979) found a low concordance of the various diagnostic criteria with the clinical diagnosis and also a low concordance between the various diagnostic criteria themselves.

In an exchange of letters discussing the merits of operational criteria, Overall and Hollister (1979b) charged that diagnostic criteria are being widely and uncritically adopted without validation. Spitzer, Endicott, & Williams (1979) wrote that the purpose of the Washington University criteria, the New York criteria, and the DSM-III criteria was to improve clinical practice by incorporating into diagnostic criteria the distinctions that were shown by research studies to have validity in terms of course, response to therapy, familial pattern, and the like. Overall and Hollister (1979b) suggested that there was little documentation for this claim, and cited one study in which "the better of the objective research diagnostic criteria was as good at predicting outcome as were the original clinical criteria" but no better. They pointed out the critical difference that specific wording of diagnostic criteria can make and concluded that

not only are diagnostic criteria being formulated and published without validation, but that continued revision renders existing sets of criteria obsolete before
they can be evaluated: "That appears to be one sure way to keep ahead of the
scientific community, but it fails to provide evidence that change constitutes
improvement."

As long as investigators cannot agree on what something is, obviously they
cannot be trusted to count how many have it. If it were not for the fact that nearly
all papers report high prevalences of alcoholism in families of alcoholics, the
definition problem alone would probably justify the throwing out of all family
studies.

4. *Sample bias.* Alcoholism and alcohol problems are unevenly distributed
in the population. First, drinkers have to be distinguished from alcoholics. Jews,
Catholics, the well educated, young people, and people living in cities more
often are drinkers than are other groups. But these same demographics do not
apply to alcoholics: for example, among the Irish, there are fewer drinkers but
more alcoholics than among the Jews, and alcoholics as a group seem less
educated than drinkers as a group (Goodwin, 1988).

The problem with sample bias, of course, is *generalization.* A good example
is the reported difference in alcoholism rates between men and women. Among
private patients, there are about three male alcoholics for every female alcoholic;
among hospitalized patients, the ratio is 6 to 1; among individuals who are
arrested for alcohol problems, the ratio is 11 to 1. Thus, when people want to
know the "real" difference, you have to ask, "Which men? Which women?" It
rarely is asked.

5. *Observer bias.* The old saying that people find what they expect to find
seems particularly applicable to alcohol studies, where it is unlikely that anyone
begins the study without a prejudice. This "halo" effect (finding what one
expects) could be avoided if family members were interviewed blindly (without
the interviewer knowing the diagnosis of the proband). But few studies take this
precaution.

6. *The age-at-risk problem.* Before counting the noses of alcoholic relatives,
one has to take into consideration how many have entered the age at risk for
alcoholism. To do this, one must know the age at risk. Do we?

Some investigators (Cotton, 1979) have applied the Weinberg abridged
formula to determine the "lifelong expectance" of alcoholism among relatives.
This formula requires knowledge of the age at risk, which is usually taken to
be 20 to 40 years. But is this truly the age at risk? Everyone knows some
alcoholics who seem to become alcoholics after the age of 40. Alcoholism among
teenagers seems to be increasing. Are we justified in saying that 20 and 40 are
the cut-off points?

Age at risk is thus another serious problem. Ideally, one should follow each
family member to the grave and hope that each lives a long life. Unfortunately,
in this publish-or-perish era, with the standard 3-year grant, such ambitious
follow-ups are impossible.

7. *The chicken and egg problem.* In studying psychiatric morbidity both in

patients and in their family members, there is often the problem of which illness came first in those instances where two illnesses seem present. With alcoholism, for example, the differential diagnosis often includes sociopathy and depression.

Does the alcoholic male become depressed because he drinks or was he depressed and then began drinking? Did he start behaving antisocially before he started drinking or were his fighting, truancy, and arrests the consequences of his drinking?

The problem of which illness came first, like the age at risk, may be difficult to reckon with but should not be forgotten, particularly when one reads about depression or sociopathy in the families of alcoholics. If, as has been reported (Winokur, Cadoret, Baker, & Dorzab, 1975), female relatives of alcoholics often suffer from unipolar depression while male relatives suffer from alcoholism, this question has to be asked: Were the female relatives really secret drinkers (as apparently many women are) who get depressed because they drink too much? It is a difficult problem, and the investigator should not be blamed if the answer is elusive.

8. *Assortative mating*. In studying the prevalence of psychiatric morbidity in the families of psychiatric patients, assortative mating must be considered, although it rarely is. *Assortative mating* refers to the fact that most people do not marry randomly: neighbors marry neighbors, Catholics marry Catholics, and drinkers marry drinkers. If the drinker is a heavy drinker and is then hospitalized, he or she quite likely will come in contact with schizophrenics, manic-depressives, and other nonalcoholic patients. Sometimes the alcoholic and the nonalcoholic patients mate and have children. If, as a consequence, they had a mixture of, say, manic-depressives and alcoholics in the family, it does not necessarily mean that alcoholism and manic-depressive illness are expressions of the same genotype. Assortative mating leads to much confusion in making sense of family histories.

These are some of the problems in family studies. There are others, but let us assume for the sake of argument that alcoholism does run in families, which raises the possibility of a genetic factor. However, the nature–nurture studies have been done and they also have problems.

Twin Studies

A classical method for evaluating whether genetic factors predispose individuals to a particular disease is to compare identical twins with fraternal twins, where at least one member of each pair has the disease. As proposed by Francis Galton, this approach assumes that monozygotic and dizygotic twins differ only with respect to genetic makeup and that environment is as similar to members of a monozygotic pair as to a dizygotic pair. Given these assumptions, the prediction is that genetic disorders will more often be concordant among identical twins than among fraternal twins.

The twin approach has been applied to the problem of diagnosing alcoholism in several studies (Goodwin, 1988) with most finding that identical twins were more concordant for alcoholism than were fraternal twins.

Furthermore, twin studies have inherent weaknesses. For example, the assumption that identical and fraternal twins have equally similar environments is dubious. In one study (Partanen, Bruun, & Markkanen, 1966), identical twins differed from fraternal twins in that they lived longer together, were more concordant with respect to marital status, and were more equal in "social, intellectual and physical dominance relationships." Even in rare instances in which monozygotic twins are reared apart, zygosity may influence environmental effects. A person's appearance, for example, influences other people's behavior toward him or her; individuals who look alike may be treated alike. In this and in other ways, the interaction between physical characteristics and the environment tends to reduce intrapair differences in identical twins and to increase differences in fraternal twins.

In addition, generalizing from twin data is hazardous. Twins represent a genetically selected population; they have a higher infant mortality, a lower birth weight, a slightly lower intelligence, and the age of their mother on the average is higher.

Adoption Studies

Perhaps the most productive method for distinguishing nature from nurture is to study individuals who are raised apart from their biological relatives. To do such a study is not easy. In the United States and in many other countries, it is difficult to obtain access to adoption agency records. Most agencies possess little information about the drinking habits of the individuals whose children are being placed for adoption. Finally, in such a highly mobile nation as the United States, dispersion of individuals from coast-to-coast and overseas and the lack of national registries make the task of locating people a formidable undertaking. Probably this is the reason why two of the three major adoption studies of alcoholism have been conducted in Scandinavian countries (Goodwin, 1988). These studies, plus one that was conducted in the United States, all found a high rate of alcoholism in the adopted-out children of alcoholics.

Even though adoption studies pose many difficulties, if their results are to be meaningful, the following requirements must be met: (1) Reliable information must be available about the biological and adoptive parents of two groups of adoptees—those of alcoholic parentage and those of normal parentage—as well as detailed information about the adoptees themselves. (2) The adoptive parents of both groups should be comparable with regard to drinking habits, psychopathology, and socioeconomic other demographic variables. (3) The adoptees should have been separated from their biological parents within a few months or preferably after birth, have had no subsequent contact with them, and be matched for age and sex. (4) The adoptees should have transversed the age of risk for the illness being studied, which, in the case of alcoholism, is estimated to be between 20 to 40 years of age. The latter requirement, to some extent, is less important than the first three, since lifetime morbidity risks can be calculated using various mathematical formulae.

Assuming these requirements are met, the finding that the children of alcoholics had significantly more alcoholism than the children of nonalcoholics would be impressive. It would not necessarily mean that the transmission was *genetic* in the strict sense; for example, rather than originating in DNA molecules, the traits favoring alcoholism would have derived from intrauterine or early neonatal influences. It is even possible (although today considered most unlikely) that heavy drinking by one of the parents would influence germ cells in a way that predisposes the offspring to alcoholism, and hence the transmission has a mutational rather than a Mendelian basis. Nevertheless, finding an increased prevalence of alcoholism among the adopted children of alcoholics strongly suggests that the experiences occurring after the child's birth are not *solely* responsible for the development of alcoholism. Indeed, we cannot dismiss the fact that in the three studies previously mentioned high rates of alcoholism were found in adopted-out children of alcoholics (Bohman, 1978; Cadoret, Cain, & Grove, 1979; Goodwin, 1988).

Genetic Marker Studies

In the search for a genetic basis for medical and psychiatric illnesses, the ultimate goal is to identify a gene or genes that are directly responsible for the illness. When a specific gene or genes cannot be located, another finding that strongly suggests genetic factors is the identification of a so-called *genetic marker*. A marker is a gene or a stretch of DNA that may be completely unrelated to the disease but that lies so close to the disease gene that during the reproductive process it is rarely separated from it. In this situation, the detection of this close neighboring gene suggests with high probability that the disease gene is present as well.

The medical conditions for which there have been a gene identification include cystic fibrosis, hemophilia A and B, and a form of muscular dystrophy. Markers have been identified for Huntington's disease, neurofibromatosis, and sickle-cell anemia. To predict which children in a family that is carrying genes for a particular illness will develop the illness, gene and/or marker analysis is generally reliable. But this procedure introduces the thorny question of genetic counseling that will be touched on later.

In the field of alcoholism studies, there is evidence that certain genes, especially the genes for the MNS blood group (Hill, Aston, & Rabin, 1988) and for esterase-D (Tanna, Wilson, Winokur, & Elston, 1988), may lie close to some gene determinants of alcoholism.

Before DNA analysis was possible, numerous reports of biological markers for alcoholism had been reported (Goodwin, 1988). They included blood group A, nonsecretors of ABH blood group substances, HLA antigens, a higher percentage of nontasters of phenylthiocarbamide (PTC), and color blindness, all known to be inherited. Attempts to confirm these findings have almost always been negative. In the case of color blindness, alcoholism was indeed found to be associated with this condition in other studies, but the color blindness appeared to be caused by toxic effects on the liver and was not of the X-linked genetic type. Most of the marker studies have involved comparisons of alcoholism factors with prevalences that are reported in various populations. Undoubtedly, one reason for the inconsistency arises from the still primitive state of population genetics; genetic factors influencing taste, color vision, blood factors, and the like vary so widely from population to population that deciding what is "normal" becomes highly arbitrary.

Moreover, phenotype is constantly influenced by environment, so that in the case of color blindness, for example, it is virtually impossible to distinguish a sex-linked genetic defect from an acquired impairment *unless* color blindness is studied in family members. In fact, Cruz-Coke and Varela (1966) did study family members of color-blind alcoholics and found a familial pattern of color blindness that is consistent with sex-linked recessive transmission. The study needs replication, however, and if confirmed by other investigators, it would provide strong evidence that certain types of alcoholism are associated with a genetic factor.

As of now, the sex-linkage hypothesis appears to be improbable on clinical grounds. As Winokur (1967) pointed out, if the hypothesis were true, 50% of the brothers of alcoholic probands should be affected, since the mother would distribute her X-linked recessive alcoholism gene and normal gene equally to her sons. If fathers of some of the alcoholic probands also were alcoholics, 50% of the sisters of these probands would also be affected with alcoholism, since this number of sisters would have received a recessive gene for alcoholism from both their fathers and their heterozygous mothers. Clinical data do not conform to either of these expectations. Family studies almost always show a higher prevalence of alcoholism among the fathers of alcoholics than among the mothers.

DNA Studies

Reference has been made to the identification of putative markers for alcoholism in the analysis of DNA. The ultimate goal in DNA research is to locate the chromosomal location of the gene or genes that confer vulnerability to alcoholism and characterize these genes and their protein products. As of this writing, one study has found a putative gene—not a marker—for alcoholism (Blum *et al.*, 1990). Analyzing DNA in the brains of alcoholics and nonalcoholics, a gene was found on chromosome 11 that directs the synthesis of the protein in a particular receptor for the neurotransmitter dopamine. The gene was present in 24 (69%) of 35 brain samples of alcoholics and absent in 28 (80%) of 35 nonalcoholics.

The process for locating the gene was not random, because the investigators knew what they were looking for. They were looking for genes that synthesize dopamine receptors (of which there are two types, D_1 and D_2). The dopamine receptors have been identified with the so-called reward system in the brain and particularly with the actions of cocaine. However, animal studies have indicated that dopamine is also involved in alcohol-seeking behavior. Thus, the gene was a "candidate" gene in that it was believed to be implicated in alcohol-related behaviors.

An editorial in the *Journal of the American Medical Association* accompanied the publication of these new findings that were reported by Gordis, Tabakoff, Goldman, and Berg (1990). The editorial congratulated these investigators on their highly promising research but pointed out certain shortcomings. Among them, (1) the sample was small; (2) no information was given about the subjects other than that half the group was alcoholic and the other half nonalcoholic; and (3) although matched for age and sex, the experimental and control groups may have differed in important ways unrelated to alcoholism. Of course, the editorial writers pointed out that confirmation of the work was of the highest importance.

The latter point has been made about all studies linking a gene or genes to a behavior disorder. For example, gene for bipolar disorder was found on a chromosome 11 (but only in members of the Old Order Amish community); a "susceptibility locus" for schizophrenia was found on chromosome 5. A gene for familial Alzheimer's disease was found on chromosome 21, and among non-Amish subjects, a gene locus on the X chromosome was associated with depression (Goodwin, 1989).

One investigator placed the depression gene close to the gene for color blindness on the long arm of the X chromosome. Other researchers located the gene at the opposite end. One group found no evidence for X-linkage at either end (Goodwin, 1989). As noted earlier, the transmission of alcoholism does not conform to a sex-linkage pattern (Winokur, 1967).

GENETIC COUNSELING

Prenatal and presymptomatic diagnostic tests are now available for a number of medical conditions, including hemophilia, Huntington's disease, and cystic fibrosis. Presumably, similar tests will soon be available for certain psychiatric conditions, although, as noted above, inconsistent findings so far raise doubts about the validity of these tests. In some illnesses, the tests are based on gene identification and others on marker analysis. In either case, some tests are highly reliable, such as that for Huntington's disease, and others are so frequently inaccurate that experts generally agree they do not merit population screening (an example being cystic fibrosis). These tests raise many practical and ethical considerations. It has been pointed out that the science and ethics of DNA diagnostic testing are as intertwined as the two strands of the double helix.

The spotlight has shifted from the tests themselves to applying information provided by the tests. Should the geneticist inform the patient that he or she is a carrier of a particular illness or is in the presymptomatic stages of the disease? Does the patient want to know? Is a carrier obligated to tell a potential spouse? Is a carrier to refrain from having children?

Based on recent experience with Huntington's disease, many people do not want to know whether they are carriers or are in the presymptomatic stages of the disease. Since predictive testing for Huntington's disease became available in 1986, over the next four years, only about 150 people have undergone diagnostic testing at 16 centers around the country. Almost certainly, genetic testing will be expanded to include tests for such common diseases as cardiovascular disease, cancer, mental illness, and Alzheimer's disease. At a 1990 symposium sponsored by the American Medical Association, three questions were presented that will be particularly pressing in the next few years: (1) Who owns genetic information? Do individuals have a right to deny such information to insurers, employers, and public health agencies? Or should such information be released to these agencies much the same way as personal financial data are released to credit companies? (2) Should an individual who has a unique mutation that leads to a new genetic test be allowed to financially exploit that test? (3) In decisions to develop new tests, how important is the profit motive? If a test would have great use in the Third World, such as a test for parasitic infections, should it be developed irrespective of low-profit potential?

In the United States, only about 1,000 genetic counselors are in practice and they have difficult jobs. The precision formerly attributed to Mendelian genetics has been diluted somewhat by new information of mitochondrial DNA, imprinting, mosaicism, and transposable human genetic elements. Pedigree studies, once believed so reliable, are now questioned.

Some professionals feel that genetic counseling is premature with regard to identifying mental illnesses, unless Huntington's disease is considered a mental illness. For one thing, there is a lack of certainty about the reliability of reported findings. There has been a failure to replicate studies associating particular genes or markers with behavioral disorders. Those disorders include schizophrenia, bipolar and unipolar depression, and Alzheimer's disease. So far, only one study has identified a gene with alcoholism. Undoubtedly, by the time this book is published, there will be studies confirming or refuting this original report.

It *is* known that genetic illnesses tend to run in families. Individuals with a family history of either schizophrenia, affective disorder, alcoholism, or other illnesses that run in families should be aware of this familial transmission. However, they should also be aware of the uncertainty of whether the causes are, strictly speaking, genetic or a mixture of genetic and environmental influences. For example, at this point, mathematical precision in predicting how many offspring of alcoholics will develop alcoholism is not possible. Although in this chapter, and in many other sources, specific figures are provided, these *always* consist of averaging a range of findings. Thus, when it is said that about one quarter of the sons of alcoholics become alcoholic, this is an *average* figure derived from many studies. The range is from 10% to 50%!

Possessing the above information, one need not be a genetic counselor or even a physician or a psychologist to apprise possible carriers of a disease of the facts as they are known. Before the situation improves, one badly needs agreement about the "boundaries" of behavioral disorders. With the publication of every new edition of the DSM, diagnostic rules change. The standard and the revised editions of the DSM-III were admirable attempts to achieve diagnostic homogeneity, but the frequent changing of the rules has undermined this worthy objective. In the late 1980s it was clearly easier to analyze a stretch of DNA than it was to agree about the definition of an illness being studied.

In summary, there probably is no great need for full-time professional genetic counselors in the field of mental illness until some of the above deficiencies have been corrected.

SUMMARY

Alcoholism is the model illness that this chapter focused on in a discussion of genetic research. The concept of a familial disorder was discussed and the historical development of alcoholism as a familial disorder was described. The chapter then examined the strategies and methods used in genetic research, including the recent findings and research issues in family studies, twin studies, adoption studies, genetic marker studies, and DNA studies. The chapter concluded with a brief review of the theory and practice of genetic counseling.

REFERENCES

Blum, K., Noble, E. P., Sheridan, P. J., Montgomery, A., Ritchie, T., Jagadeeswaran, P., Nogami, H., Briggs, A. H., & Cohn, J. B. (1990). Allelic association of human dopamine D$_2$ receptor gene in alcoholism. *Journal of the American Medical Association, 263*(15), 2055–2060.

Bohman, M. (1978). Genetic aspects of alcoholism and criminality. *Archives of General Psychiatry, 35,* 269–276.

Cadoret, R. J., Cain, C. A., & Grove, W. M. (1979). Development of alcoholism in adoptees raised apart from alcoholic biologic relatives. *Archives of General Psychiatry, 37,* 561–563.

Cotton, N. S. (1979). The familial incidence of alcoholism: A review. *Journal of Studies on Alcohol, 40,* 89–116.

Cruz-Coke, R., & Varela, A. (1966). Inheritance of alcoholism. *Lancet, 2,* 1282.

Goodwin, D. W. (1979). Alcoholism and heredity: A review and hypothesis. *Archives of General Psychiatry, 36,* 57–61.

Goodwin, D. W. (1981). Family studies of alcoholism. *Journal of Studies on Alcohol, 42*(1), 156–162.

Goodwin, D. W. (1985). Alcoholism and genetics. The sins of the fathers. *Archives of General Psychiatry, 42,* 171–174.

Goodwin, D. W. (1988). *Is alcoholism hereditary?* New York: Ballantine Books.

Goodwin, D. W. (1989). The gene for alcoholism. *Journal of Studies on Alcohol,* 50th anniversary edition, 397–398.

Gordis, E., Tabakoff, B., Goldman, D., & Berg, K. (1990). Finding the gene(s) for alcoholism. *Journal of the American Medical Association, 263*(15), 2094–2095.

Hebb, D. O. (1958). *A textbook of psychology.* Philadelphia: W. B. Saunders.

Hill, S. Y., Aston, C., & Rabin, B. (1988). Suggestive evidence of genetic linkage between alcoholism and the MNS blood group. *Alcoholism: Clinical and Experimental Research, 12*(6), 811–814.

Jenkins, C. D., Hurst, M. W., and Rose, R. M. (1979). Life changes: Do people really remember? *Archives of General Psychiatry, 36,* 379–384.

Kendell, R. E., Brockington, I. F., and Leff, J. P. (1979). Prognostic implications of six alternative definitions of schizophrenia. *Archives of General Psychiatry, 36*, 25–31.

Overall, J. E., & Hollister, L. E. (1979a). Comparative evaluation of research diagnostic criteria for schizophrenia. *Archives of General Psychiatry, 36*, 1198–1205.

Overall, J. E., & Hollister, L. E. (1979b). In reply (to Spitzer *et al.*, Research diagnostic criteria.) *Archives of General Psychiatry, 36*, 1382–1383.

Partanen, J., Bruun, K., & Markkanen, T. (1966). Inheritance of drinking behavior: A study on intelligence, personality, and use of alcohol in adult twins. *Finnish Foundation for Alcohol Studies, 14.*

Spitzer, R. L., Endicott, J., & Williams, J. B. W. (1979). Research diagnostic criteria [Letter to the editor]. *Archives of General Psychiatry, 36*, 1381–1382.

Tanna, V. L., Wilson, A. F., Winokur, G., & Elston, R. C. (1988). Possible linkage between alcoholism and esterase-D. *Journal of Studies on Alcohol, 49*, 472–476.

Thomas, L. (1979). *The medusa and the snail*. New York: Viking Press.

Winokur, G. (1967). X-borne recessive genes in alcoholism [Letter to the editor]. *Lancet, 2*, 466.

Winokur, G., Cadoret, R., Baker, M., & Dorzab, J. (1975). Depression spectrum disease versus pure depressive disease; some further data. *British Journal of Psychiatry, 127*, 75–77.

CHAPTER 15

Behavioral Medicine

KENT F. BURNETT, GAIL H. IRONSON, AND C. BARR TAYLOR

INTRODUCTION

Biomedical and behavioral science research conducted during the latter half of this century has convincingly demonstrated the influence of personal behavior on disease pathophysiology. Furthermore, change in behavior has been shown to reduce disease morbidity and mortality. Two examples of the latter, from the many that will be cited in this chapter, are the changes in life-style that account for as much as 50% of the greater than 30% reduction in cardiovascular mortality that has occurred in the past 20 years (Goldman & Cook, 1984; Taylor, Ironson, & Burnett, 1990), and the changes in sexual behavior among homosexuals that have reduced the incidence of acquired immune deficiency syndrome (AIDS) in the gay community (Stall, Coates, & Hoff, 1988). Research conducted within the field of behavioral medicine has contributed significantly to the progress that has been made toward effective prevention and treatment of these and many other medical disorders.

Behavioral medicine was first defined as a distinct discipline at the Yale Conference in 1977, at which a group of medical and behavioral science researchers met to discuss how the behavioral sciences in general, and psychology in particular, could be better integrated with medicine in an effort to promote

Kent F. Burnett • Counseling Psychology Program and Department of Psychology, University of Miami, Coral Gables, Florida 33124-2040.   Gail H. Ironson • Departments of Psychology and Psychiatry, University of Miami, Coral Gables, Florida 33124-2040.   C. Barr Taylor • Laboratory for the Study of Behavioral Medicine, Department of Psychiatry, Stanford University School of Medicine, Stanford, California 94305.

Research in Psychiatry: Issues, Strategies, and Methods, edited by L. K. George Hsu and Michel Hersen. Plenum Press, New York, 1992.

health and prevent illness. The often cited definition of the new field that emerged from the conference was:

> Behavioral Medicine is the interdisciplinary field concerned with the development and integration of behavioral and biomedical science knowledge and techniques relevant to health and illness and the application of this knowledge and these techniques to prevention, treatment, and rehabilitation. (G. E. Schwartz & Weiss, 1978, p. 250)

The emergence of behavioral medicine as an interdisciplinary specialty within medicine was paralleled in 1978 by the establishment of a Division of Health Psychology (Division 38) within the American Psychological Association. Another field that is closely related to behavioral medicine is psychosomatic medicine. Historically, the field of psychosomatic medicine has been concerned with examining the relationship between physical illness and psychosocial variables. Considerable attention has been directed toward stress-related conditions, such as ulcers, hypertension, migraine headache, and asthma. Although psychoanalytic conceptualizations of the interplay between personality and illness (e.g., Alexander, 1950) clearly dominated most early work in this field, more recently psychosomatic medicine has moved toward identification with the biopsychosocial model of medicine, a much broader theoretical framework that views illness as the result of a complex interaction between diverse biological, psychological, social environmental and physical environmental factors (G. L. Engel, 1980; Weiner, 1982).

Behavioral medicine interventions have tended to be symptom focused, to rely on cognitive/behavioral interventions, and to include measurable outcomes. As a result, a wide array of measurement tools applicable to clinical practice has been developed, together with excellent descriptions of intervention procedures applicable to many behavioral medicine problems (Blumenthal & McKee, 1987; Melamed & Siegel, 1980). On the other hand, particularly in recent years, behavioral medicine has moved somewhat away from its early focus on evaluating and developing interventions to also emphasize the study of mechanisms relating psychological and behavioral processes to diseases. This chapter will emphasize behavioral medicine interventions.

Despite its relatively brief history, behavioral medicine is already firmly established as an important subspecialty in both medicine and psychology, and interest in behavioral medicine continues to grow at a rapid rate. Behavioral medicine sections are included in many departments of Family Medicine and Psychiatry, and behavioral medicine practices have become a routine part of most medical settings. Psychologists have perhaps seized on this change more than have psychiatrists. In 1985, 12.5% of the 50,000 members of the American Psychological Association (APA) were on medical school faculties, compared to only 6% a decade earlier. Funding for behavioral medicine research from the National Institutes of Health has also grown dramatically, rising from approximately $66 million in 1983 to $196 million in 1988 (Krasnegor, 1990).

Behavioral medicine researchers are making contributions in such a wide array of basic and applied research areas that it is impossible in a chapter such as this to address all of the potential topics. Rather, a limited number of topics have been selected in order to provide examples of contemporary research in behavioral medicine. Consistent with the current emphasis in behavioral medicine on the prevention and treatment of chronic illness, major sections of this chapter are devoted to behavioral medicine findings relevant to cardiovascular disease and cancer, the two leading causes of death and disability in the United States today. Also, a major section of this chapter is devoted to the role of behavioral medicine in preventing the spread of AIDS, one of the most important challenges that lies ahead for behavioral medicine and for our society. A series of briefer sections provide overviews of behavioral medicine research on chronic respiratory disorders, gastrointestinal disorders, pain syndromes, and computer applications in behavioral medicine. A concluding section examines a variety of methodological issues that are pertinent to most if not all of the research topics addressed in this chapter.

CARDIOVASCULAR DISORDERS

Although cardiovascular disease has declined by more than 30% in the last 25 years (Jenkins, 1988), it is still the leading cause of mortality in the United States, accounting for approximately 38% of all deaths. The identification and modification of the behavioral correlates of cardiovascular disease have been two of the central themes in the field of behavioral medicine. Based on large-scale, long-term prospective studies, typified by the Framingham study, many risk factors for cardiovascular disease have been identified, including family history, hypertension, serum cholesterol, obesity, and smoking. With the exception of family history, each of these risk factors is either a potentially modifiable behavior or a physiological condition with potentially modifiable behavioral correlates. Since hypertension has been identified as the chief risk factor for cardiovascular disease and has many behavioral correlates, this topic will be covered first and in some depth. This section will also focus on selected research findings relevant to the topics of heart disease prevention, coronary-prone behavior, cardiovascular reactivity, and cardiac rehabilitation. Because of limitations of space, we will not discuss the vast literature that has developed around smoking cessation interventions, but this area has been one of the most important and successful in behavioral medicine (for reviews, see J. L. Schwartz, 1987; Taylor & Killen, 1991).

Hypertension

Hypertension affects up to 30% of the adult population in the United States and is a major risk factor for cardiovascular disease, renal disease, stroke, and arteriosclerosis. "Secondary" forms of hypertension are those that can be attributed to known causes such as kidney disease, tumors of the adrenal glands, narrowing of the aorta, and primary aldosteronism. Less than 20% of the cases of hypertension are classified as secondary; the remainder of cases cannot be attributed to any obvious pathogenic process or physical cause and are classified as "primary" or "essential" hypertension. Recent research has suggested that a subgroup of hypertensive patients may suffer from a disease that involves combined difficulty with weight, blood pressure and glucose regulation. Evidence for this hypothesis comes from the well-known association among these conditions. N. M. Kaplan (1990) suggested that the common problem is one of insulin insensitivity.

The results of major within-population and national cooperative group studies (Inter-Society Commission for Heart Disease Resources, 1970) have shown that the risk of premature mortality is significantly greater in persons whose blood pressure is elevated beyond 140/90 mm Hg, and that morbidity and mortality gradually increase as blood pressure rises beyond this level. Although some forms of secondary hypertension can be surgically corrected, the mainstay of treatment for hypertension is a stepped-care pharmacological approach, in which diuretics, adrenergic inhibiting agents, and vasodilators are sequentially introduced in a manner designed to achieve the desired blood pressure goal with minimum side effects.

The results of the Hypertension Detection and Follow-up Program (HDFP) have clearly demonstrated the effectiveness of the stepped-care approach in reducing blood pressure levels, as well as associated morbidity and mortality (Hypertension Detection and Follow-up Program Cooperative Group, 1979); however, drug therapy is not without its limitations. Many antihypertensive medications have significant physiological and psychological side effects, with up to 10% of patients being highly intolerant of particular drugs (Smith, 1977) and up to 35% of patients, for a variety of reasons, failing to take enough of their medication to maintain adequate blood pressure control. Furthermore, only 50% of hypertensive patients who begin treatment will remain in treatment for more than one year (National Heart, Lung, and Blood Institute Working Group, 1982). Clearly, developing techniques for helping patients to better adhere to drug therapy for hypertension represents an important challenge for behavioral medicine.

Although drug therapy remains the treatment of first choice for most hypertensive patients, many nonpharmacological factors, such as weight, diet, exercise, and stress are also known to influence blood pressure. There is a strong relationship between obesity and hypertension. In one review (Hovell, 1982), an average weight loss of 11.7 kg was associated with an average blood pressure reduction of 21 mm/Hg systolic and 13 mm/Hg diastolic. A major focus of behavioral medicine has been to develop interventions for weight reduction. The status of this area has been extensively reviewed elsewhere (see Brownell & Jeffery, 1987). Even though changes in dietary sodium, potassium, and calcium also may help to reduce blood pressure, there have been few studies addressing issues relating to how such changes can be best introduced and maintained in hypertensive patients.

A number of uncontrolled and controlled investigations have documented blood pressure reductions, independent of weight loss, in hypertension patients who are following exercise training. A review of research on exercise and hypertension by Dubbert, Rappaport, and Martin (1987) concluded that clinically significant reductions in blood pressure have generally been observed only in studies that employed endurance training at 65% to 80% maximum heart rate during training sessions of 30-minutes duration three or more times per week.

Considerable interest in relaxation training, stress management, and related techniques as interventions for hypertension was generated following publication of the research of Benson, Beary, and Carol (1974) describing the "relaxation response." They argued that a variety of relaxation techniques, including progressive muscle relaxation training and diverse forms of meditation, have the ability to reduce sympathetic nervous system activity and to produce beneficial short-term decreases in oxygen consumption, heart rate, and blood pressure. Research on the effects of relaxation training and related techniques (e.g., thermal biofeedback) has since been expanded to include evaluation of multifaceted behavioral and cognitive stress management training programs.

Several recent reviews have summarized the effectiveness of relaxation and stress management procedures in the treatment of hypertension (Agras, 1981; McCaffrey & Blanchard, 1985; Pickering, 1982). With an occasional exception, studies on such techniques have produced decreases in systolic pressure ranging from 5 to 20 mm Hg and decreases in diastolic pressure ranging from 3 to 15 mm Hg. Generally, magnitude of change has been greatest for those with the highest initial blood pressure. Overall, however, there has been no consistent evidence of the superiority of any one relaxation or stress management procedure over any other; however, some researchers have argued (Agras & Jacob, 1979) that progressive muscle relaxation training may have some advantage in terms of cost effectiveness.

Most studies on relaxation procedures have involved short-term demonstrations of change in blood pressure, with follow-ups rarely exceeding 1 year. One exception is a large-scale study by Agras, Taylor, Kraemer, Southam, and Schneider (1987), in which 137 subjects at two worksites were randomized to either relaxation therapy or blood pressure monitoring. At 30-months follow-up, the mean blood pressure reduction for the relaxation group was −9.2/−10.1 mm Hg; however, the blood pressure monitoring group had also reduced their blood pressure by −8.4/−9.8, indicating that blood pressure monitoring alone may possibly be the most cost effective way to help hypertensive patients normalize their blood pressure. The results of a companion study by Chesney, Black, Swan, and Ward (1987) indicated that blood pressure monitoring may be especially useful for patients newly diagnosed as hypertensive. The potential clinical efficacy of blood pressure monitoring is further illustrated by research showing that hypertensive patients can be trained to lower their blood pressure through intensive blood pressure self-monitoring and feedback using a home sphygmomanometer (e.g., B. T. Engel, Glasgow, & Gaarder, 1983).

Combined interventions would seem to be the best approach to treating hypertension, since reductions in salt and alcohol intake (and perhaps increases or reductions in other nutrients), weight reduction, and increases in exercise and the practice of relaxation/stress management and/or blood pressure feedback have independent beneficial effects on lowering blood pressure. At least one combined approach has shown such benefits (Rosen, Kostis, & Brondolo, 1989) and another treatment program combining these treatment elements has been developed and is being evaluated (Blanchard, Martin, & Dubbert, 1988). In 1984, the Joint National Commission on Detection, Evaluation, and Treatment of High Blood Pressure (Joint National Commission, 1984) recommended that nonpharmacologic approaches should be part of a comprehensive approach to hypertension. The commission recommended that:

1. For newly identified hypertensive patients with blood pressures in the mild range, repeated measurement of blood pressure should occur before any therapy is instituted (many newly identified hypertensives turn out to be normotensive on repeated measurement.)
2. Nonpharmacologic approaches should be considered before initiation of antihypertensive medication (except for patients with malignant hypertension who need immediate blood pressure reduction).
3. Nonpharmacologic approaches should be monitored as closely as pharmacologic interventions.
4. Patients who remain hypertensive should be given pharmacologic therapy. Behavioral interventions can help with adherence.
5. Nonpharmacologic interventions should continue even when pharmacologic therapy is introduced.
6. Periodic stepdown or decrease in medication should be considered in controlled hypertensives while nonpharmacologic interventions are practiced.

Clinical trials are now underway to evaluate the effectiveness of nonpharmacologic approaches. The evaluation of nonpharmacologic interventions involves a number of taxing methodological problems. Blood pressure must be measured accurately and blood pressure level must be stable. Because blood pressure levels are influenced by many factors—temperature, time of day, person, specific position, excitement, and exercise—to name but a few, accurate measurement should entail careful training of observers and frequent measurement under uniform conditions. Observer drift over time in blood pressure measurements has been reported, and is related to such factors as rounding measurements up or down, loss of hearing, and degradation of technique.

Higher blood pressure levels are more likely to be affected by intervention, to return toward the mean, and to require pharmacological intervention. However, other factors that influence blood pressure must always be thoroughly examined, including weight, exercise, stress, adherence, and diet. Studies are currently underway that address the multiple determinants of hypertension and that hopefully will shed further light on the role of nonpharmacological interventions.

Coronary Heart Disease (CHD)

Community-Based Heart Disease Prevention

Community-based heart disease prevention programs provide an important illustration of the interface between behavioral medicine and public health (Winett, King, & Altman, 1989). The first large-scale projects of this nature were the Stanford Three-Community Project (TCP) and the North Karelia Project in Finland. Baseline evaluations for the Stanford TCP were begun in 1972 in three Northern California communities, each comprised of approximately 15,000 persons. This was followed by a 2-year mass media educational intervention in two of the communities, while the third community served as a control. In addition, in one of the intervention communities, residents were screened, and those at highest risk for cardiovascular disease were offered more intensive face-to-face behavioral interventions. The outcome data for the TCP indicated an average cardiovascular risk reduction, based on the Cornfield risk index, of 17% for those in the intervention communities compared to an approximate 6% increase in risk in the control community (Farquhar, Maccoby, Wood, Alexander, Breitrose, Brown, Haskell, McAlister, Meyer, & Nash, 1977). The magnitude of risk reduction for high-risk participants who received the intensive face-to-face intervention was even greater, primarily because of a relatively high rate of smoking cessation among these participants.

The North Karelia Project in Finland was also begun in 1972 and involved mass media educational efforts, as well as educational interventions offered through existing health care providers. A 10-year follow-up of participants in the North Karelia Project found a reduction in cardiovascular risk factors, as well as an 11% reduction in cardiovascular disease mortality compared to other residents of Finland (Puska, Nissinen, Tuomilehto, Salonen, Koskela, McAlister, Kottke, Maccoby, & Farquhar, 1985).

Based on the success of the TCP, in 1978 researchers from the Stanford Heart Disease Prevention Program began the Five City Project (FCP), involving slightly over 100,000 residents in two intervention communities and slightly over 200,000 residents in three control communities. The interventions were similar in concept to those of the TCP study, but were considerably more extensive, involving cooperative efforts by many institutions (e.g., governmental agencies, worksites, schools, and restaurants) throughout the community. The results of this intervention were recently reported by Farquhar, Fortmann, Flora, Taylor, Haskell, Williams, Maccoby, and Wood (1990). After 30 to 64 months of education, significant net reductions in community averages favoring treatment occurred in the plasma cholesterol level (2%), blood pressure (4%), resting pulse rate (3%), and smoking rate (13%) of the cohort sample. Furthermore, these risk factor changes resulted in significant decreases in composite total mortality risk scores (15%) and coronary heart disease risk scores (16%). These results provide strong support for the concept of community-based intervention. Farquhar, Maccoby, and Solomon (1984) have provided an excellent conceptual overview of these and other large-scale, community-based health promotion projects. An excellent review of the youth component of most large-scale, community-based health promotion projects can be found in Perry, Knut-Inge, & Shultz (1988).

Coronary Prone Behavior

The modern conceptualization of coronary prone behavior was originated in the late 1950s by cardiologists Meyer Friedman and Ray Rosenman, who observed that a substantial number of their patients with coronary heart disease also appeared to be quite hostile, competitive, achievement oriented, and time urgent. They dubbed these characteristics the Type A behavior pattern and hypothesized that these behavioral and personality tendencies place individuals at greater risk for developing coronary heart disease (CHD) than individuals exhibiting Type B behavior, defined as the bipolar opposite of each of the Type A dimensions. Friedman and Rosenman also developed a Type A Structured Interview (SI) designed to determine an individual's level of Type A behavior.

In California in 1960, the SI was given to approximately 3,200 men, aged 39 to 59, who participated in the prospective Western Collaborative Group Study (WCGS). These men were all free of CHD at the beginning of the study. At 8.5 years follow-up, the risk ratio for total CHD in the Type A men was 2.24 compared to the Type B's (Rosenman, Brand, Jenkins, Friedman, Straus, & Wurm, 1975). Similar results were also found in a subsample of men participating in the WCGS who took the Jenkins Activity Survey (JAS), a brief self-report measure of Type A (Jenkins, Rosenman, & Zyzanski, 1974). Further reinforcing the Type A concept were the findings of the Framingham Heart Study, another large-scale prospective investigation, the results of which showed significantly higher risk ratios for Type A men in white-collar jobs, as well as for working women and housewives identified as Type A (Haynes, Feinleib, & Kannel, 1980). The Framingham Type A scale is also a brief self-report measure.

Many subsequent investigations, however, have failed to show the expected elevated risk for persons identified as Type A (for reviews, see Johnston, 1988; Haynes & Matthews, 1988). The negative findings include the results of the famous Honolulu Heart Study, in which approximately 2,200 men of Japanese descent were administered the JAS and followed for a period of 8 years. Contrary to expectations, Type A scores were unrelated to incidence of total CHD, myocardial infarction, or angina pectoris (Cohen & Reed, 1985). However, the rate of cardiovascular disease in this population was extremely low; therefore, this population may be unrepresentative. Negative findings also were found in the Multiple Risk Factor Intervention Trial (MRFIT), a large-scale prospective investigation in which men at high risk for CHD were randomly assigned to either a special behavioral counseling intervention or to usual medical care. No associations were found between Type A scores (SI or JAS) and total mortality or CHD mortality for either group during the initial 7-year follow-up period (Shekelle, Hulley, Neaton, Billings, Borhani, Gerace, Jacobs, Lasser, Mittlemark, & Stamler, 1985). One investigation of 189 cardiac catheterization patients actually found that Type B behavior, rather than Type A, was most predictive of myocardial infarction, as well as mortality, over the following one-year period (Dimsdale, Block, Gilbert, Hackett, & Hutter, 1981). Although several other prospective studies have also failed to find the predicted relationship between Type A and CHD, the most damaging negative findings are those of the recently reported 22-year follow-up of the WCGS (Ragland & Brand, 1988a, 1988b), which failed to find any higher risk for CHD mortality for Type A subjects. Thus, at present the evidence from population-based studies does not provide strong support for the validity of the Type A concept with respect to CHD.

More consistent evidence is emerging, however, that hostility, one of the major subcomponents of the Type A behavior pattern, may play a role in the development of CHD. For example, a retrospective study by Barefoot, Dahlstrom, and Williams (1983) found a significantly higher CHD mortality rate for physicians who 25 years earlier had taken the Minnesota Multiphasic Personality Inventory (MMPI) and obtained high scores (> 14) on the Hostility (Ho) scale. Similarly, studies examining the degree of coronary artery disease have shown significant associations with hostility (Dembroski, McDougall, Williams, Haney, & Blumenthal, 1985; Williams, Barefoot, Haney, Harrell, Blumenthal, Pryor, & Peterson, 1988). A recent "component" reanalysis of taped Type A interviews from the WCGS sample also revealed a significant relationship between hostility and CHD incidence. Furthermore, the relationship between hostility and CHD was much greater than that found for the global Type A construct (Hecker, Chesney, Black, & Frautschi, 1988). Dembroski and Costa (1988) have provided an excellent overview of research in this area.

Various stress management techniques—in isolation or in combination with other interventions like exercise—have shown that Type A, measured in various ways, can be altered in noncardiac populations (e.g., Schaeffer, Krantz, Weiss, Zoltick, Yaney, Karch, & Bedynek, 1988). (The effects of interventions in patients with cardiac disease are reviewed in the section on Cardiac Rehabilitation.)

This area also is fraught with methodological problems. One major area of concern is that constructs like Type A, coronary-prone, hostility, and anger remain ill-defined from a psychometric standpoint. Uniform instruments have not been used. Such instruments as the Jenkins Activity Survey, Framingham Type A Scale, Thurstone Temperament Scale, and Type A Interview appear to measure significantly different constructs. Likewise, anger-related measures, such as the Cook-Medley Ho Scale and the Speilberger State-Trait Anger Scale, also appear to measure different aspects of hostility.

Cardiovascular Reactivity

A large volume of research has been conducted on the topic of cardiovascular reactivity in response to laboratory stressors. Since the main purpose of this line of research has been to investigate the physiological mechanisms linking

Type A behavior and CHD, it is not surprising that most studies have focused on differences in cardiovascular reactivity between Type A and Type B persons. Even though there have been some negative findings, most studies have shown moderately greater cardiovascular reactivity for Type A persons compared to Type B persons, with the most consistent differences having been found for systolic blood pressure and plasma epinephrine. These findings have been interpreted as evidence that Type A persons have greater sympathetic beta-adrenergic activation in response to stress than Type B persons (Contrada & Krantz, 1988).

Type A/Type B differences appear to be most pronounced in laboratory situations involving high-performance demands or harassment (e.g., Diamond, Schneiderman, Schwartz, Smith, Vorp, & Pasin, 1984). It is noteworthy that these findings have been obtained almost exclusively in studies that employed the Type A Structured Interview as a means of classifying subjects, since the SI has a stronger focus on vigorous speech stylistics and hostility than the JAS (Matthews, Krantz, Dembroski, & MacDougall, 1982). These and related findings are explored in depth in a recent review article on cardiovascular reactivity to stress by Contrada and Krantz (1988).

In view of such findings, it is of interest that a recent meta-analytic review on the relationship between hypertension and cardiovascular reactivity to stress concludes that excessive sympathetic nervous system activity may play an important role in the development of hypertension for some individuals (Fredrikson & Matthews, 1990). Furthermore, with a few notable exceptions (Gatchel, Gaffney, & Smith, 1986), psychological interventions have had limited success in reducing reactivity.

Most of the methodological problems facing the measurement of blood pressure also apply to cardiovascular reactivity; however, measurement of cardiovascular reactivity is even more complex, ideally involving multiple measures of cardiovascular functioning (e.g., electrocardiogram, blood pressure, peripheral resistance). In addition, evidence is accumulating that diverse subject characteristics, such as age, sex, and ethnicity, significantly affect cardiovascular reactivity in response to certain laboratory tasks (e.g., Ironson, Gellman, Spitzer, Llabre, Pasin, Weidler, & Schneiderman, 1989; Tischenkel, Saab, Schneiderman, Nelesen, Pasin, Goldstein, Spitzer, Woo-Ming, & Weidler, 1989). An in depth consideration of research design and measurement considerations in behavioral medicine research on cardiovascular reactivity can be found in Schneiderman, Weiss, and Kaufmann (1989).

Cardiac Rehabilitation

In addition to facilitating surgical and medical treatment, cardiac rehabilitation programs typically provide secondary prevention programs that are aimed at reducing established CHD risk factors. Thus, most programs focus on exercise promotion, smoking cessation, dietary modification for hypercholesterolemia, weight control for the obese, blood pressure normalization for hypertensives, and appropriate behavioral management of diabetes when present. Of course, program goals in many of these discrete areas are often overlapping because obesity, hypertension, hypercholesterolemia, sedentary life-style, and adult-onset diabetes often are found to coexist as well as benefit from similar behavioral treatments. The empirical literature relevant to the efficacy of secondary prevention efforts in each of these areas is thoroughly documented in a recent position paper of the American Association of Cardiovascular and Pulmonary Rehabilitation (Miller, Taylor, Davidson, Hill, & Krantz, 1990).

Although emotional distress is present in almost all patients following a coronary event, the signs and symptoms of psychological difficulties generally subside within several weeks to a month following myocardial infarction (MI) or coronary artery bypass graft (CABG) surgery. However, significant emotional distress continues to be present after this period in as many as 15% of patients (Taylor, Debusk, Davidson, Houston, & Burnett, 1981). Thus, many programs also include general psychological screening, as well as referral for treatment, for depression, anxiety, low self-esteem, sexual difficulties, and other psychological problems (Blumenthal & Emery, 1988; Miller *et al.*, 1990). In fact, in some states, psychological screening has become a mandatory condition for participation in cardiac rehabilitation programs (Blumenthal, 1985).

Cardiac rehabilitation may also facilitate return to work. A study by Dennis, Houston-Miller, Schwartz, Ahn, Kraemer, Gossard, Junea, Taylor, and DeBusk (1988) showed that a symptom-limited treadmill test performed 3 weeks after myocardial infarction and a formal recommendation to the patient and primary physician that the patient return to work within the next 2 weeks reduced the return-to-work time by more than 3 weeks in the treatment compared to the control group. The 32% reduction in the convalescence period was associated with $2,102 of additional earned salary per intervention patient in the 6 months after myocardial infarction.

The merit of stress management training in general, and Type A behavior modification in particular, as part of an overall approach to secondary prevention are relatively controversial issues within cardiac rehabilitation. Particularly disturbing are the results of the 22-year follow-up of the Western Collaborative Group Study, which found lower mortality rates among Type A post-MI patients than among Type B post-MI patients (Ragland & Brand, 1988a). The longer survival of Type A post-MI patients in this sample has resulted in considerable debate over possible mechanisms to explain this paradoxical finding, as well as renewed controversy about the merit of attempting to alter Type A behavior in post-MI patients.

Several small-scale investigations of Type A behavior modification in cardiac patients have obtained promising results (e.g., Roskies, Kearny, Spevack, Surkis, Cohen, & Gilman, 1979; Suinn, 1975); however, the Recurrent Coronary Prevention Project (RCPP) in San Francisco is the only large-scale clinical trial to date to address this issue. In the RCPP, approximately 600 post-MI patients were randomized to a behavioral counseling program designed to reduce Type A behavior, while approximately 300 post-MI patients were randomized to a control condition consisting of traditional cardiologic care. The experimental behavioral counseling program was based on cognitive social learning theory and was administered in a small-group format over a period of 3 years. After 3 years of treatment, Type A behavior had dropped significantly in 44% of the behaviorally counseled patients compared to 25% of the control patients, and the rate of cardiac recurrence in the behaviorally counseled patients was almost half that of patients who received traditional cardiologic care, 7% compared to 13% (Friedman, Thoresen, Gill, Powell, Price, Rabin, Breall, Dixon, Levy, & Bourg, 1984). Reduction in Type A behavior in the RCPP has also been related to reduced CHD mortality (Friedman, Thoresen, Gill, Ulmer, Powell, Rice, Brown, Thompson, Rabin, Breall, Bourg, Levy, & Dixon, 1986). Further research is needed to determine long-term differences in Type A behavior and survival.

Results of recent research also have shown that intensive reduction in serum cholesterol, achieved through a very low fat dietary, exercise, and stress management regimen, can actually lead to a reduction in the size of atherosclerotic lesions in the coronary artery vessels (Ornish, 1990). This research was not designed to determine the individual contribution of the various components for achieving these effects.

CANCER

In the United States in 1990, the American Cancer Society estimated that 1,040,000 new cases of cancer and 510,000 deaths were due to cancer (American Cancer Society, 1990). Although 5-year survival rates are increasing (51% for whites, 38% for blacks), cancer remains the second leading cause of death in the United States (Peterson, 1986). The most common cancers (in descending order) are breast, colon/rectum, lung, uterine/cervical for women, and prostate, lung, colon/rectum, and bladder for men.

Emotional distress often accompanies cancer. The prevalence of DSM-III diagnoses among 215 patients at three cancer centers were found to be 47% (Derogatis, Morrow, Fetting, Penmen, Piasetsky, Schmale, Henrichs, & Carnicke, 1983). In most of these cases (85%), a central feature is anxiety or depression, both considered treatable. In addition to treating anxiety and/or depression, mental health professionals may play an important role in many aspects relevant to cancer. These include: (1) behavior modification aimed at early detection (mammography, pap smears), (2) behavior modification aimed at changing risk factors (smoking, increased fiber intake), (3) education focusing on what to expect after surgery (breast reconstruction, sexual functioning, use of stoma), (4) individual psychotherapy and/or pharmacotherapy, (5) interventions dealing with anticipatory nausea and vomiting, (6) interventions dealing with the treatment of pain, and (7) group interventions providing support, exchange of information, and coping skills. Since coverage of all topics is beyond the scope of this chapter, discussion is limited to the following three: (1) psychological factors and coping strategies related to cancer and its progression, (2) the treatment of anticipatory nausea and vomiting, and (3) group interventions.

Psychological Factors, Coping, and Cancer Progression

Many researchers have investigated the relationship between predisposing psychological factors and the appearance of cancer and between coping responses to cancer and the progression of disease. Although it is difficult to tease apart cause and effect, several patterns have emerged. A high prevalence of loss, repressed emotional conflicts, depression, hopelessness, and an inability to express frustration and anger have been identified as factors related to cancer in a summary by Derogatis (1986).

In one prospective study (Shekelle, Raynor, Ostfeld, Garron, Bieliauskas, Liu, Maliza, & Paul, 1981), depression was associated with a two-fold increased risk of cancer in a 17-year follow-up of 2,020 men. A hopeless/helpless attitude has been related to an unfavorable disease course in studies of breast cancer patients (Greer, Morris, & Pettingale, 1979; Pettingale, Morris, Greer, & Haybittle, 1985), melanoma patients (Diclemente & Temoshok, 1985), and cervical cancer patients (Goodkin, Antoni, & Blaney, 1986).

In terms of coping strategies, those with a fighting spirit were most likely to be alive at 5-year (Greer *et al.*, 1979) and 10-year follow-ups (Pettingale *et al.*, 1985) of breast cancer patients. Although denial appeared to be a less functional coping strategy, associated with poorer progression than fighting spirit in the above study and in a study of melanoma patients (Rogentine, Van Kammen, Fox, Docherty, Rosenblatt, Boyd, & Bunney, 1979), those with denial did better than either the stoic acceptance group or those with a helpless/hopeless attitude (Greer *et al.*, 1979; Pettingale *et al.*, 1985).

Failure to express negative emotions has been related to cancer progression as well (Bahnson & Bahnson, 1966; Blumberg, West, & Ellis, 1954; Schmale & Iker, 1966; Temoshok, Heller, Sagebiel, Blois, Sweet, DiClemente, & Gold, 1985). Temoshok and Heller (1981) have summarized some of the literature by describing a "Type C" or cancer prone individual as one who suppresses negative emotions (including anger), is cooperative and unassertive, and who complies with external authorities. Support for this description was found in a study of melanoma patients (Temoshok *et al.*, 1985). Hostility, another negative emotion, has been identified prospectively as associated with 20-year mortality from malignant neoplasms (Shekelle, Gale, Ostfeld, & Paul, 1983).

It is important to note that some studies do not support a connection between psychosocial factors and cancer (Cassileth, Lusk, Miller, Brown, & Miller, 1985; Jamison, Burish, & Wallston, 1987); however, both of these studies were done with patients who had advanced cancer. No studies have been done attempting to modify these psychosocial factors and then to determine the impact of the intervention on disease progression: This may be a fruitful area for future research.

Anticipatory Nausea and Vomiting (ANV)

Several of the anticancer drugs are associated with high rates of nausea and vomiting; for example, over 90% of those taking cisplatin have ANV (Morrow & Dobkin, 1987). After several sessions of chemotherapy with these agents, a conditioned stimulus, such as the nurse or the smell of alcohol, which has been paired with the chemotherapy, may elicit a response (nausea, vomiting) before the chemotherapy begins. This is called *anticipatory nausea and vomiting*.

ANV can be treated with a variety of techniques including progressive muscle relaxation with guided imagery (Burish & Lyles, 1981; Burish, Carey, Krozely, & Greco, 1987; Carey & Burish, 1987; Lyles, Burish, Krozely, & Oldham, 1982), hypnosis with imagery (Redd, Andersen, & Minagawa, 1982), systematic desensitization (Morrow & Morrell, 1982), biofeedback (Burish, Shartner, & Lyles, 1981), and distraction (Redd, Jacobsen, Die-Trill, Dermatis, McEvoy, & Holland, 1987).

Group Interventions

Group interventions with cancer patients may reduce emotional distress and prolong survival time. A review of the effects of psychosocial interventions in cancer patients is provided by Watson (1983). Several representative interventions are described below.

Spiegel and his colleagues (Spiegel, Bloom, & Yalom, 1981; Spiegel, Bloom, Kraemer, & Gottheil, 1989) compared the results of a group psychosocial intervention to a routine oncology care control group in metastatic cancer patients. The intervention included group discussion of coping with cancer, assertiveness with doctors, extracting meaning from tragedy, and dealing with loss. At the 1-year follow-up, the intervention group had less tension, less depression, less fatigue, and fewer phobias (Spiegel *et al.*, 1981). At the 10-year follow-up (Spiegel *et al.*, 1989), the intervention group showed a significantly longer survival time (36.6 months from entry to the study) than the control group (18.9 months). While several other studies also have found supportive group therapy to be of benefit (Ferlic, Goldman,& Kennedy, 1979; Vachon, Lyall, Rogers, Cochrane, & Freeman, 1981), others have found no particular benefit (Bloom, Ross, & Burnell, 1978; C. Jacobs, Ross, Walker, & Stockdale, 1983).

Some groups have been more skills oriented. One such study (Telch & Telch, 1986) included coping skills training (cognitive, behavioral, and affective). The components focused on (1) relaxation and stress management, (2) communication and assertion training, (3) cognitive restructuring and problem solving, (4) feelings management, and (5) pleasant activity planning. Homework assignments, goal-setting, self-monitoring, behavioral rehearsal, role playing with feedback, and coaching constituted the behavioral part of the skills training. A variety of outcomes, including greater improvement in patients' self-efficacy, mood, independent observer ratings of distress, and decreased severity and intensity of cancer problems, favored the coping skills group over both the supportive therapy group (discussing feelings, thoughts, and concerns) and the no-treatment control group.

Relaxation techniques with imagery have also been included in a number of studies. Gruber, Hall, Hersh, and Dubois (1988) found improvements in immune function in metastatic cancer patients who practiced ritualized relaxation and guided imagery. Stolbach, Brandt, Borysenko, Benson, Maurer, Lessermen, Albright, and Albright (1988) found similar techniques (meditation, breathing techniques, and imagery), in addition to group support and cognitive skills (coping skills, hardiness), to be associated with improved functioning, a fighting spirit, and less dysphoric mood (less anxiety, depression, and hopelessness). In summary, the interventions described appear to have a beneficial effect on mood and health, although health effects documented thus far are small.

CHRONIC RESPIRATORY DISORDERS

Chronic Obstructive Pulmonary Disease

Chronic emphysema, bronchitis, and asthma comprise a category of respiratory disorders known as *chronic obstructive pulmonary disease* (COPD). The common feature of each condition is extreme difficulty in expiring air from the lungs. Recent estimates place COPD as the fourth leading cause of death in the United States, following cardiovascular disease (CHD and stroke), cancer, and accidental death.

Medical management of COPD patients usually involves some combination of (1) chest physical therapy for control of coughing and excessive mucus, (2) antibiotics for control of infections, (3) corticosteroids for control of inflammation, and (4) bronchiodilators for control of airway obstructions that are due to spasms. Oxygen therapy may also be required in severe cases.

Smoking is the major risk factor for emphysema and bronchitis and can also trigger as well as exacerbate asthma. Even though loss of pulmonary function in emphysema and bronchitis is for the most part irreversible, smoking cessation is a necessary component of treatment for all patients who continue to smoke and has been shown to slow progression of the disease. Comprehensive pulmonary disease rehabilitation programs also have begun to play an important part in the treatment of COPD patients. Such programs are multidisciplinary and are designed to provide medical, educational, and psychological support, in addition to their primary focus—exercise training. Although exercise is usually quite difficult for COPD patients, and can exacerbate symptoms, considerable research supports the utility of supervised exercise training as a method of improving pulmonary capacity, physical endurance, and overall quality of life. Psychological and behavioral aspects of COPD patient care are discussed in greater detail in a review by R. M. Kaplan, Reiss, and Atkins (1985).

Asthma

The term *extrinsic asthma* is often used to describe asthma symptoms that can be linked to known environmental irritants, such as allergens or viral infections. By contrast, the term *intrinsic asthma* is often used to describe asthma symptoms that cannot be linked to known environmental irritants. In many such cases, psychosocial factors, including stress reactions, are believed to play an important role. Thus, a significant portion of asthma research has focused on psychosocial factors, both as they relate to the onset as well as to the amelioration of symptoms. Some representative findings are discussed in the following sections.

Psychosocial Factors in Asthma

Numerous studies have focused on the discovery of unique personality characteristics associated with asthma. For example, early research found that asthma patients had elevated scores of MMPI scales 1, 2, and 3 (hypochondriasis, depression, and hysteria, respectively). These results were somewhat confounded, however, by the fact that many of the scale items referred to somatic complaints, including problems with breathing. Significant elevations were also found on the Beck Depression Inventory. Unfortunately, because of the retrospective nature of this type of research, it becomes difficult if not impossible to make any judgments about whether depression is a cause or an effect of asthma. Diverse emotional reactions do appear to play an important role as precipitating events in up to 30% of asthma episodes (Weiner, 1977); however, at this time, there is no compelling evidence to suggest a unique personality type associated with asthma.

On the other hand, scores on objective personality instruments have been helpful with respect to treatment planning. For example, researchers at the National Jewish Hospital in Denver found that high scores on the empirically derived Panic-Fear scale of the MMPI, although uncorrelated with severity of illness, were predictive of "as needed" medication usage, steroid usage, and likelihood of rehospitalization. Interestingly, patients with moderate scores had the most positive outcomes, whereas patients with low scores tended to undermedicate and consequently have more relapses (Dirks, Kinsman, Jones, & Fross, 1978). In addition to personality variables, it is important to note that parent–child relationship issues (M. A. Jacobs, Anderson, Eisman, Muller, & Friedman, 1967), as well as other family dynamics (Liebman, Minuchin, & Baker, 1974), have been implicated in the etiology and maintenance of asthma.

Relaxation, Biofeedback, and Self-Management Training

Because of the demonstrated role of emotional reactions in precipitating asthma, the therapeutic benefits of a wide variety of stress management procedures have been investigated. Interventions in this category include relaxation training, systematic desensitization, self-management training, and frontalis electromyogram (EMG) biofeedback. In addition, several investigations have employed biofeedback of respiratory resistance as a method of enhancing pulmonary function.

In a review, Cluss and Fireman (1985) reported that significant improvements in spirometric measures were obtained in approximately half of the 11 studies examining the effects of relaxation training for asthma patients. Likewise, they reported that two thirds of the studies on biofeedback have demonstrated statistically significant effects. Biofeedback studies have typically involved either biofeedback of respiratory resistance (e.g., Steptoe, Phillips, & Harling, 1981), frontalis EMG biofeedback (e.g, Kotses & Glaus, 1981), or relaxation training augmented with frontalis EMG biofeedback (e.g., Scherr, Crawford, Sergent, & Scherr, 1975). It should be noted, however, that the clinical significance of most of these studies was marginal, since few patients achieved greater than 15% improvement in spirometric measures.

Broad spectrum self-management programs represent another approach to teaching patients to cope with the stress of chronic illness. Approximately a dozen, fairly broad spectrum self-management programs for asthmatic children and their families have been reported, generally with encouraging results (Cluss & Fireman, 1985). Typically, these programs focus on education, compliance with therapeutic regimen, self-esteem enhancement, decision-making skills, and specific behavioral management techniques for coping with stress and illness.

Another important area for future research concerns *panic-dypsnea*, a vicious cycle observed in some asthma and other COPD patients, in which fear leads to shortness of breath, which in turn leads to increased fear and further shortness of breath. R. M. Kaplan *et al.* (1985) have suggested that comprehensive treatment centers attempt to increase patients' self-efficacy regarding exercise and other known irritants, which may provoke the panic-dypsnea cycle, by providing guided mastery experiences in supervised settings, followed by a systematic evaluation of the extent to which these experiences generalize to relevant high-risk situations outside the clinical setting. Under careful supervision and with proper safeguards, many basic tenets and parameters of self-efficacy theory (Bandura, 1977; 1986) could be investigated using this research paradigm.

GASTROINTESTINAL DISORDERS

It has long been believed that psychological and behavioral factors play a role in the onset of gastrointestinal disorders. Overall, the results of recent research lend support to this contention, while also suggesting the treatment efficacy of psychological and behavioral interventions for a number of gastrointestinal disorders.

Upper Gastrointestinal Disorders

Psychological and behavioral factors involved in disorders of the upper gastrointestinal (GI) system have recently been comprehensively reviewed by Young, Richter, Bradley, and Anderson (1987). Disorders in this category include the following: rumination syndrome, psychogenic vomiting, gastrointestinal reflux, abnormal esophageal contraction disorders, peptic ulcer, and nonulcer dyspepsia.

Behavioral interventions appear to show considerable promise in the treatment of several disorders of the upper gastrointestinal system. Both supportive nurturing and aversive conditioning, for example, have proved useful in the treatment of rumination syndrome, a condition in which food is voluntarily chewed, but is then spit out or regurgitated. This disorder may be contrasted with psychogenic vomiting, in which regurgitation is believed to be influenced by psychological factors but is not under voluntary control. Although behavioral interventions for psychogenic vomiting have not been studied extensively, data from a limited number of small-scale investigations suggest that psychogenic vomiting often extinguishes in the absence of social attention related to the vomiting. Systematic desensitization and other procedures designed to lessen sensitivity in high-risk situations have also been found to be useful (Young et al., 1987).

Patients with abnormal esophageal contraction disorder report chest pain that cannot be attributed to either heartburn (gastroesophageal reflux) or cardiac abnormality. In approximately 10% of these patients, diffuse esophageal spasm is implicated as the cause, whereas high-amplitude peristaltic contractions are implicated in approximately 50% of patients (Katz, Dalton, Richter, Wu, & Castell, 1987). This latter condition is sometimes referred to as "nutcracker esophagus." Although it is clear that psychological factors are involved in this disorder and that psychological stress exacerbates symptoms, the exact etiology of the condition is unknown (Clouse & Lustman, 1983; Richter, Obrecht, Bradley, Young, & Anderson, 1986). A small number of case studies have reported successful outcomes associated with the use of progressive muscle relaxation training, employed either along or in concert with esophageal biofeedback, to teach patients to inhibit abnormal esophageal spasms (e.g., Latimer, 1981).

Many studies have documented the fact that psychological stress augments physiological activity related to peptic ulcers, and most patients have been found to have higher than normal levels of stress, anxiety, and depression (Feldman, Walker, Green, & Weingarden, 1986; Young et al., 1987). Since medical intervention for peptic ulcer disease is highly successful for most patients, there has been limited interest in psychological interventions; however, the highly positive results of recent controlled research lend support to the use of broadly focused psychoeducational interventions designed to enhance patient's stress management, assertion, and other social coping skills (e.g., Brooks & Richardson, 1980). Young et al. (1987) suggested that the value of psychological therapies as an adjunct to medical treatment is probably highly underrated, particularly in terms of long-term adjustment.

With few exceptions, research on upper gastrointestinal disorders has consisted of a limited number of small-scale uncontrolled investigations. Comparative group outcome studies, comparing alternative treatment paradigms would be useful. Further, Young et al. (1987) noted that different types of interventions are likely to be most effective with patients from different age groups. For instance, they noted that supportive nurturing or aversive conditioning may prove most effective in treating rumination syndrome in children and institutionalized populations, whereas other types of treatment (eg., biofeedback or relaxation training) may prove most useful in combating rumination syndrome in adults of normal intelligence.

Fecal Incontinence

Biofeedback has been used with success to treat patients who have fecal incontinence. For this condition, biofeedback usually involves the use of three balloons that are inserted rectally. The uppermost balloon is lodged in the rectosigmoid space, the next balloon is positioned in the internal sphincter, and the third balloon is in the external sphincter. Patients are taught to contract the external sphincter in synchrony with internal sphincter relaxation when they sense rectal distension. They can monitor these contractions by observing pressure readings obtained from the balloons. In a study of 50 patients, 36 reported a decreased frequency of incontinence of 90% or more following therapy (Cerulli, Nikoomanesh, & Shuster, 1979). The basic procedure was also used to increase sensitivity to cues for defecation in six of seven incontinent diabetic patients (Wald & Tunuguntla, 1984).

Important methodological issues related to the treatment of fecal incontinence have been identified in a recent review by Wald and Handen (1987). They noted that despite the evidence in support of biofeedback training for fecal incontinence, there have been no controlled investigations. Without controlled investigations, clinical improvements cannot unequivocally be attributed to the biofeedback procedures employed. In the only component analysis to date, Latimer, Campbell, and Kasperski (1984) found that several patients with fecal incontinence responded successfully to sensory discrimination training alone, one to exercise training alone, one to no treatment, and one to contingency management training. Such data reinforce the need for controlled comparative outcome studies, evaluating the clinical effectiveness of biofeedback treatment components, as well as diverse treatment paradigms.

Irritable Bowel Syndrome

Irritable bowel syndrome (IBS) is a functional digestive disorder characterized by abnormal bowel movement and abdominal pain occurring without evidence of organic abnormality (Latimer, 1983). Estimates of the prevalence of this condition range from 8% to 22% (see Blanchard, Schwarz, & Radnitz, 1987; Mitchell & Drossman, 1987).

Patients with IBS may present with a wide range of symptoms, including diarrhea, constipation, bloating, excessive gas, and fecal incontinence (Mitchell & Drossman, 1987). Although not well understood, IBS appears to involve overresponsiveness of the gastrointestinal tract to a wide variety of stimuli, including psychological stress. Lactose intolerance, caffeine, and difficult to digest foods, such as cabbage and beans, may also cause increased symptomatology in some IBS patients (Mitchell & Drossman, 1987). The most common medical treatments include (1) dietary management through increased dietary fiber, (2) prescription of anticholinergic drugs, and (3) prescription of psychoactive medications for depression or anxiety (Blanchard et al., 1987).

The results of controlled psychological research lend tentative support to the efficacy of both short-term psychodynamic therapy (Svedlund, Sjodin, Ottosson, & Dotevall, 1983) and hypnotherapy (Whorwell, Prior, & Faragher, 1984), and also to behavioral relaxation training (progressive muscle relaxation and thermal biofeedback) supplemented with cognitive strategies for coping with stress (Neff & Blanchard, 1987). One year follow-up data for each of these interventions have been quite encouraging. By far, the most systematic controlled research series to date has been conducted by Blanchard and his colleagues at SUNY-Albany, with 58% of IBS patients who were treated using the above described multicomponent behavioral treatment program showing symptom reductions of 50% or greater for 1 year or longer (Blanchard, Schwarz, & Neff, 1988; Blanchard, Schwarz, Neff, & Gerardi, 1988).

In their recent review of IBS research, Mitchell and Drossman (1987) offered a series of methodological guidelines for conducting research on this complex disorder: (1) employ specific diagnostic criteria, (2) develop and use standard methods of measuring gut physiology, (3) use standardized psychological measures, (4) use treatment protocols that assess psychosocial, physiological, symptomatic, and functional effects, and (5) employ multivariate analyses appropriate to the complexity of factors that affect IBS.

Inflammatory Bowel Disease

The term *inflammatory bowel disease* (IBD) usually refers to a number of different conditions of unknown origin that are characterized by inflammation of some portion of the gastrointestinal tract. The two most common disorders in this category are *ulcerative colitis* (UC) and *Crohn's disease* (CD). Usually, both diseases produce diarrhea, abdominal pain, and anorexia. In addition, UC generally involves the appearance of blood and mucus in the stools. Virtually all of the psychological and behavioral research literature on IBD has focused on UC and CD.

Although the etiology of IBD is unknown, its causes almost certainly are primarily physical in nature (as compared to IBS). Nonetheless, many psychological theorists have suggested that psychological factors may also play an important role. The most commonly cited psychological characteristics of CD patients are dependency, depression, anxiety, and introversion (Schwarz & Blanchard, 1990). With few exceptions, research with UC patients has revealed little elevation in psychopathology as compared to other medical patients or normals. On average, both CD and UC patients appear to be less psychologically disturbed than IBS patients. On the other hand, in a 6-month prospective study, Green, Blanchard, and Suls (1989) have shown a moderate-to-high association between symptom severity in IBD and ratings of daily stress.

Controlled research on the psychological treatment of IBD patients has been limited; however, one study by Milne, Joachim, and Niedhardt (1986) examined the effects of stress management training on 80 IBD patients and found significant reductions in measures of psychological and somatic distress compared to controls. Improvements were maintained at 1-year follow-up; however, the study was marred by the fact that the experimental group was significantly higher than the control group at pretreatment on several distress measures. Shaw and Ehrlich (1987) used relaxation training to help UC patients control pain associated with their condition. Compared to controls, at posttreatment and 6-weeks follow-up, treated subjects reported less pain and less use of anti-inflammatory medication. Finally, Schwarz and Blanchard (1990) described their use of a multicomponent behavioral treatment program, similar to that described above for treatment of IBS, for the treatment of 11 IBD patients. Although treated subjects showed significant symptom reductions on several measures, an active control group achieved similar levels of symptom reduction as a result of symptom monitoring alone. Commenting on their findings, Schwarz and Blanchard (1990) stated that it is unlikely that psychological and behavioral interventions can have a "major curative effect on IBD, unlike IBS," (p. 103). They suggested that future research should focus on the effectiveness of interventions designed specifically to aid IBD patients in coping with the stress and pain of a chronic illness, and that such interventions need to be evaluated intensively, over a period of at least 1 year, in comparison to less expensive alternatives, such as membership in self-help support groups.

PAIN SYNDROMES

Some of the earliest and most important work in behavioral medicine has focused on the treatment of *chronic pain* (arbitrarily defined as pain lasting 6 months or longer and where psychological factors significantly contribute to the maintenance of the pain). Behavioral treatments for chronic pain are designed to help the patient: (1) reduce reliance on medication, (2) increase motor activity and capacity for work, (3) improve mood variables, (4) reduce pain complaints, and (5) reduce utilization of health care services (Winters, 1985).

An operant approach to the treatment of chronic pain has been described by Fordyce (1976). The approach can be adapted for use in a wide variety of settings, including both the hospital and home (Sarafino, 1990). In order to reduce reliance on medication, the patient is placed on a fixed, rather than "as needed" schedule for receiving medication. The medication itself is mixed with a flavored syrup to create a "pain cocktail." Then the amount of medication is gradually reduced over a period of weeks or months. Concurrent with medication tapering, significant others in the patient's social environment are trained to reward physical activity and other "well behaviors" and to avoid inadvertently reinforcing "pain behaviors," such as verbal complaints of pain. Significant decreases in medication taking and increases in physical activity have been documented in patients who have completed this type of program (e.g., Fordyce, 1976).

Numerous methods for training pain patients to achieve physical relaxation have been investigated, since it has been observed that physical relaxation often serves to reduce or alleviate the experience of pain. Most of the research in this area has been conducted with chronic headache patients and has employed either progressive muscle relaxation training, EMG biofeedback, or thermal biofeedback. In general, the benefits of progressive muscle relaxation training and biofeedback appear to be about equal, although relaxation training and thermal biofeedback are slightly more effective for migraine headache pain, and biofeedback is slightly more effective for muscle contraction headache. However, relaxation training is often tried first for both types of headaches because of its simplicity and low cost compared to biofeedback (Blanchard & Andrasik, 1985). Although results vary widely from patient to patient, most studies show mean reductions in pain ratings of about 60% for patients who are treated using these procedures. Treatment effects are generally well maintained at 1- to 2-years follow-up, with the exception of EMG biofeedback for muscle-tension headache (Blanchard, 1987).

According to Sarafino (1990), cognitive interventions for the relief of pain can be divided into four categories: (1) active or passive attention-diversion, (2) imagery, (3) redefinition, and (4) hypnosis. *Attention-diversion* involves attending to some real object or event in lieu of focusing on the pain. By contrast, *imagery* involves focusing on some imagined pleasant scenario. *Redefinition*, or cognitive restructuring, involves training the patient to counter maladaptive self-statements related to pain with more adaptive self-statements. Cognitive treatments for depression have also been applied with some success to the treatment of chronic pain. Sarafino suggests that attention-diversion and imagery are the most appropriate and effective cognitive treatments for mild to moderate pain, whereas redefinition is a more useful treatment for severe and chronic pain conditions. *Hypnosis* also seems to provide pain reduction for some types of acute pain, especially when used with highly suggestible individuals.

A number of multifocus or eclectic inpatient programs have also been reported. Generally, such programs include exercise training, relaxation training, and biofeedback as well as personal, family, and/or vocational counseling. A review of behavioral approaches to pain by Winters (1985) concludes that multifocus approaches to chronic pain appear to produce benefits on a diversity of measures; however, further research is needed, as most studies in this area have major methodological limitations.

Goodkin (1989) suggested that clinical research on interventions for chronic pain should include subjective measures of feeling state as well as objective measures such as physical activity, pain behavior, and degree of behavioral impairment. In addition, in clinical trials involving pharmacologic agents for the treatment of chronic pain, drug challenge tests and blood level tests should be employed.

ACQUIRED IMMUNE DEFICIENCY SYNDROME

Perhaps no medical disease in recent times has attracted more attention and more fear than acquired immune deficiency syndrome (AIDS). It strikes people in their prime years, there is no vaccine and no cure, the costs involved are staggering, and most people with the diagnosis die within 2 or 3 years after a devastating downhill course. The only good news is that AIDS is preventable: most new adult cases could be prevented by practicing safe sex and not sharing contaminated needles. Behavioral medicine can and has contributed in the fight against AIDS, both by identification of psychosocial factors associated with the progression of the disease and by prevention and treatment programs targeted at these cofactors and at the emotional sequelae of the disease.

Epidemiology

As of July, 1990, 260,000 cases of AIDS have been reported worldwide (World Health Organization [WHO], 1990). Because of underreporting WHO estimates 800,000 cases of AIDS, with 8 to 10 million people infected with the AIDS virus. Projections made by WHO indicate that some 15 to 20 million people may be infected by the year 2000. In the United States, 135,644 AIDS cases have been reported, with an estimated 1 million infected (Centers for Disease Control [CDC], 1990). The population groups most affected in the United States have been homosexual/bisexual men and intravenous (IV) drug abusers. There has been a marked shift in transmission patterns such that proportionately homosexual men account for fewer cases (from 66% of AIDS cases in 1986 to 57% in 1988), whereas IV drug abusers are accounting for more (from 17% to 24%). Women and teenagers are two groups with growing rates of seropositivity (Chu, Buehler, & Berkelman, 1990; Boyer & Schafer, 1990). In addition, ethnic minorities comprise 41% of AIDS cases (Centers for Disease Control, 1989). The above groups would all be appropriate targets for prevention programs. More details about demographics and the course of the disease may be found in Ironson and Schneiderman (in press).

Changing Behavior

Since there is no cure for AIDS, prevention is the major hope for limiting the spread of the disease. That dramatic change in behavior can occur has been demonstrated in San Francisco, where, in 1985, 37.4% of gay men reported unprotected insertive intercourse and 33.9% reported unprotected receptive intercourse; by 1988, however, these behaviors had changed to 1.7% and 4.2%, respectively (Ekstrand & Coates, 1990).

A recent article by Coates and Greenblatt (1989) has described the central elements of community-based intervention. Their intervention recommendations included the following: (1) establishment of community norms favoring safer sex; (2) provision of informational material including how the AIDS virus can be prevented; (3) coverage of motivational material such as assessment of participants' human immunodeficiency virus (HIV) risk, advice about antibody testing, and anonymous case histories of individuals who have become infected with the AIDS virus; (4) acquisition of skills such as negotiating for safer sex, clean needles, and use of condoms; and finally (5) advocating social policy legislation.

Coates, McKusick, Stites, and Kuno (1989) found that a stress management program focusing on meditation, relaxation, coping, and positive health habits reduced the number of sexual partners. Similarly, an intervention by Kelly, St. Lawrence, and Hood (1989) resulted in decreased unprotected anal intercourse and increased use of condoms. Their 12-week intervention included cognitive-behavioral training to refuse unsafe sex, AIDS risk education, and social support.

Drug and alcohol use may promote AIDS transmission and/or progression by influencing behavior so that people are more likely to engage in unsafe sex or share contaminated needles, and also by direct effects on the immune function (Goodkin, 1990). Alcohol, amyl nitrate, marijuana (Stall, McKusick, Wiley, Coates, & Ostrow, 1986), cocaine, and amphetamine (Martin, 1990) have all been associated with unsafe sexual activities. Conversely, cessation of drug use has been associated with lower rates of risky sexual behavior (Martin, 1990) and slower disease progression (Kaslow, Blackwelder, Ostrow, Yerg, Palinicek, Coulson, & Valdiserri, 1989).

In a review of studies of IV drug users, DesJarlais, Friedman, and Casriel (1990) found AIDS risk reductions among IV drug users who enter drug treatment, and among those who continue to inject, if they are provided with a means for safer injection. The authors suggested separating different groups for intervention: those who want to stop injecting, those who are likely to continue injecting, and those who are at risk for beginning to inject.

More research is needed to determine whether these interventions can be adopted for use in other high-risk groups, such as ethnic minorities, young gay men, and clients at sexually transmitted disease clinics.

Psychological Factors, Stress, and Psychoneuroimmunology

Individuals infected with the HIV virus face a multitude of stressors. First is the anxiety and affective distress associated with notification of HIV-1 status (Ironson, LaPerriere, Antoni, O'Hearn, Schneiderman, Klimas, & Fletcher, 1990). Multiple losses often occur during the course of the disease, including loss of health, loss of income, and loss of independence. Among gay men, loss of a significant other may occur as well. Depression may be present in as many as 80% of patients (Goodkin, 1988) and an increased suicide rate 66 times that of the general population has been found (Marzuk, Tierney, Tardiff, Gross, Morgan, Hsu, & Mann, 1988). Anxiety is also high, especially during the prodromal phase of the illness and at evidence of progression (Atkinson, Grant, Kennedy, Richman, Spector, & McCutchan, 1988; Nichols, 1983).

There is a growing literature that shows an association between poorer immune function and several of these stressors, such as bereavement (Irwin, Daniels, Smith, Bloom, & Weiner, 1987; Irwin, Daniels, Risch, Bloom, & Weiner, 1988), loneliness (Kiecolt-Glaser, Ricker, George, Messicak, Speicher, Garner, & Glaser, 1984), loss of a relationship (Kiecolt-Glaser, Fisher, Ogrocki, Stout, Speicher, & Glaser, 1987), unemployment (Arnetz, Wasserman, Petrini, Brenner, Levi, Eneroth, Salovaara, Hjelm, Salovaara, Theorell, & Petterson, 1987), and uncontrollable events (Baum, McKinnon, & Silvia, 1987). In addition, affective states such as depression (Calabrese, Kling, & Gold, 1987) and anxiety (Linn, Linn, & Jensen, 1981) have been associated with decrements in immune function.

A number of longitudinal studies are currently underway to investigate the association between psychological factors, immune function, and disease progress. Kemeny, Fahey, Schneider, Weiner, Taylor, and Visscher (1989) found depressed mood to be correlated with immune parameters relevant to HIV progression, and chronically depressed HIV seropositive subjects showed steeper declines in CD4 T-cell levels over a 5-year period than nondepressed subjects (Kemeny, Duran, Weiner, Taylor, Visscher, & Fahey, 1990). However, there were no differences between bereaved and nonbereaved men in the seropositive groups on immune parameters. Ironson et al. (1990) found an association between anxiety before receiving one's seropositivity diagnosis and change in natural killer cell functioning after receiving one's diagnosis. Preliminary findings from the longitudinal follow-up suggest that certain coping styles (e.g., openness about being gay) are associated with slower disease progression (Ironson, Simoneau, Friedman, LaPerriere, Antoni, Schneiderman, & Fletcher, 1991). Temoshok and her colleagues (Soloman, Kemeny, & Temoshok, 1990) have preliminary analyses suggesting that improvements in immune function, symptoms, and disease outcome are associated with the following: positive mood states, "upness," not doing unwanted favors, active coping, hardiness, less defensiveness, more openness about being gay, exercise, and anger expression. Although work in this area is just beginning, it provides information that may be useful in developing and testing future interventions.

Thus, there is ample reason to believe that the multitude of stressors facing HIV-infected individuals may adversely affect disease progression. A next logical step then would be to design interventions to buffer any negative impact. Two interventions, exercise (LaPerriere, Antoni, Schneiderman, Ironson, Klimas, Caralis, & Fletcher, 1990) and a cognitive behavioral stress management package consisting of information, cognitive restructuring, assertiveness training, and social support (Antoni, Baggett, Ironson, August, LaPerriere, Klimas, Schneiderman, & Fletcher, 1991) have been shown to have a buffering effect on mood and immune function for seropositives receiving their serostatus notification. Whether these interventions have an impact in the long run remains to be seen. Another stress management intervention (Coates *et al.*, 1989) that included components of safe sex discussion, meditation, and relaxation failed to have an impact on immune function.

COMPUTERS IN BEHAVIORAL MEDICINE

The microcomputer revolution has had a tremendous impact on clinical research and practice in behavioral medicine. In this section, we focus on some of the most notable applications of microcomputer technology in the areas of clinical assessment and intervention.

Computer-Assisted Assessment

Computer-based administration, scoring, and interpretation are currently available for a large number of psychological tests and behavioral performance measures. Although most of these instruments are simply computer-based versions of tests that were originally developed for traditional paper-and-pencil administration, a significant number of recently developed tests have been designed expressly for computerized administration, particularly in the area of clinical neuropsychological assessment. The interested reader is referred to Stoloff and Couch (1988) for a comprehensive listing of available testing software, and to Butcher (1987) for an in depth consideration of practical, ethical, and methodological issues related to computerized psychological testing.

A wide variety of useful computer-based clinical interviews also have been developed. Wilkinson and Markus (1989) have recently described research on the validity of PROQSY, a computerized version of the Clinical Interview Schedule. In addition to validity data, the researchers also collected data on the experience of computerized interviewing from the patients' perspective. Interestingly, though all patients reported that the computer interview was an acceptable experience, the computer interview was rated as preferable to a physician-conducted interview by 73% of those patients who reported an unsatisfactory relationship with their physician.

Other possible advantages of computer-based interviews are discussed in a review article by Erdman (1988). Erdman's review also describes a variety of computer-based "consulting" programs designed to aid clinicians in diagnostic decision-making and treatment planning. Among those program described are computerized consultation programs for the DSM-III-R, depression, suicide, and hyperactivity.

Certainly, one of the most ambitious and interesting computer-based interviews to date is SEXPERT, an expert-systems-based interview designed to help couples diagnose sexual dysfunctions and to recommend treatment (Binik, Servanschreiber, Freiwald, & Hall, 1988). The knowledge base for the SEXPERT interview is quite extensive, containing over 2,200 if-then decision rules for evaluating a couple's responses to the interview and arriving at a tentative diagnosis. SEXPERT is a highly sophisticated program and will likely serve as a model for many future behavioral medicine applications.

Computer-Assisted Intervention

A major methodological problem in behavioral medicine is the standardization of treatment. Computer-assisted intervention is a potentially cost-effective, highly replicable method for disseminating therapeutically effective interventions in behavioral medicine. Interest in computer-assisted intervention has increased considerably in recent years, as the cost of traditional methods of health care service delivery continues to rise.

Behavioral interventions, because of their comparatively high degree of specificity of therapeutic procedures and goals, have proven to be highly amenable to incorporation into interactive computer programs. One early computer-assisted behavioral intervention was the Computer-Assisted Diet and Exercise Training program (CADET) that was developed for use in the behavioral treatment of moderate obesity (Burnett, Taylor, & Agras, 1985). The CADET program operated in a completely portable battery-operated computer, small enough for obese patients to carry around with them throughout their normal daily routine. Patients used the computer to make daily self-reports of all food items consumed and all exercise. In return, the program provided patients with intensive quantitative and qualitative goal-related feedback throughout the day. In addition, the computer, which contained a real-time clock, issued periodic audible prompts ("beeps") to remind patients to make timely self-reports. The most recent versions of the CADET program include an extensive on-line food item database which can be searched almost instantaneously.

Research on the CADET approach has yielded promising treatment results (Burnett *et al.*, 1985; Taylor, Agras, Losch, Plante, & Burnett, 1991), in addition to demonstrating its potential cost effectiveness (Agras, Taylor, Feldman, Losch, & Burnett, 1990). Portable computers have also been used to implement *in situ* treatment of obsessive-compulsive behavior disorder (Baer, Minichiello, Jenike, & Holland, 1988) and to assist in the behavioral and medical management of insulin-dependent diabetes (Surwit, 1990).

Most other computer-assisted interventions of relevance to behavioral medicine have employed desktop microcomputers and have utilized what may be described as a "psychoeducational approach," in which the computer is mainly used to (1) instruct the patient about important aspects of treatment, (2) assign and monitor homework, and (3) assess and reinforce patient progress. Computer-assisted interventions of this type have been evaluated positively in a number of areas, including treatment of moderate depression (Selmi, Klein, Greist, Johnson, & Harris, 1982), training for adherence to tricyclic antidepressants (Sorrell, Greist, Klein, Johnson, & Harris, 1982), training for adherence to medication-taking in the elderly (Leirer, Morrow, Pariante, & Sheikh, 1988), and exposure therapy for agoraphobia (Ghosh & Marks, 1987). Computer-assisted intervention has also been successfully used to promote health-related behavior in large-group settings such as schools and factories, where intensive prevention efforts might otherwise not be feasible (Burnett, Magel, Harrington, & Taylor, 1989).

Based on the initial success of this method of intervention, across such diverse applications, it seems fair to say that computer-assisted intervention represents an important and promising new frontier for behavioral medicine. Further long-term research is needed, however, to determine for whom and under what conditions computer-assisted intervention will prove to be most appropriate and advantageous.

RESEARCH STRATEGIES AND MAJOR METHODOLOGICAL ISSUES

A variety of research strategies are employed in the field of behavioral medicine; however, the most commonly used strategies fall into one of the following categories: (1) behavioral epidemiology, (2) research on basic biological mechanisms that relate behavior to disease, and (3) intervention research. Due to space limitations, this section is focused primarily on intervention research. The section begins by presenting an heuristic framework for viewing the process of scientific advancement in clinical intervention. This is followed by discussion of some important methodological issues that researchers should consider when designing or evaluating intervention research.

Developmental Stages of Intervention Research

Based on successful programs of research in a variety of fields, Agras and Berkowitz (1980) have described a progressive, developmental model of clinical intervention research. In Agras and Berkowitz's model, the generation of new clinical intervention and measurement procedures is viewed as emerging from any of the following sources: (1) clinical observations, (2) theoretical models, (3) basic laboratory studies, and (4) uncontrolled clinical tests. New intervention and measurement procedures are first tested in single-subject research and laboratory analogue studies. Promising new procedures are then refined and evaluated in short-term comparative outcome studies, followed by studies evaluating a diversity of maintenance strategies and by studies designed to determine which treatment components are most effective. Longer-term evaluations of treatment programs with integrated maintenance plans are then undertaken, followed by research on the most effective methods of disseminating treatment and training therapists to deliver it.

Clinical research rarely progresses smoothly through each of these developmental stages. Occasional setbacks are an almost inevitable part of conducting research; however, viewing clinical research within an heuristic framework can facilitate systematic evaluation of the current state of knowledge in a particular area and can aid the researcher in making informed decisions about what types of studies are most likely to make a contribution.

Subject Characteristics

Behavioral medicine research on cardiovascular reactivity serves to highlight the importance of subject characteristics both as predictor and moderator variables. The importance of ethnic background and gender, for example, has been well demonstrated by recent research showing that cardiovascular reactivity is sometimes higher in whites, sometimes in blacks, and sometimes reflects an ethnicity-by-sex interaction, depending upon the specific type of laboratory challenge task, the specific measure of reactivity (e.g., systolic blood pressure, diastolic blood pressure, heart rate, total peripheral resistance, cardiac output), and subject status as hypertensive or normotensive (see Ironson *et al.*, 1989; Tischenkel *et al.*, 1989; Saab, Tischenkel, Spitzer, Gellman, Pasin, & Schneiderman, 1990; Schneiderman, Chesney, & Krantz, 1989). Socioeconomic status and socioecological variables (e.g., residency in a high-stress, high-crime urban area) also appear to play prominent roles as predictors and moderators of main effects (see Durel & Schneiderman, 1991).

Findings such as these suggest that men and women, as well as persons of differing ethnic and sociocultural backgrounds, may require somewhat different intervention strategies. There is a pressing need for further systematic research on the role of subject characteristics as predictor and moderator variables in all areas of behavioral medicine research.

Disease Severity and Disease Progression

Disease severity and disease progression are important methodological issues in many areas of behavioral medicine research. For example, several studies have implicated failure to express negative emotions and hostility as playing critical roles in cancer progression; however, two other studies failed to find any such connection (see the section on cancer in this chapter). Both of the studies with negative findings were carried out in patients who suffered from advanced cancer. This suggests that degree of disease severity and progression are variables that must be included in the design of studies in this area.

Similarly, psychosocial interventions designed to reduce recurrence of cardiac events in cardiac patients may be less effective in those with advanced coronary artery disease or with severe damage from prior acute myocardial infarction (see Powell & Thoresen, 1988). In addition, degree of disease progression appears to be an important factor in research on immune system responsiveness to psychosocial and behavioral interventions in AIDS patients. One might expect, for example, that psychosocial interventions might have more of an impact on the immune system early in the course of a disease when the immune system is still relatively healthy, rather than later when the body is overrun by the virus.

Generalizability

Generalizability is a concept that is closely related to reliability. It is used to describe the degree to which measures obtained in one context or setting are likely to be reliable estimates of that measure in other contexts or settings of interest to the researcher. The example of blood pressure measurement is useful in illustrating certain aspects of generalizability. Research on blood pressure generalizability by Llabre, Ironson, Spitzer, Gellman, Weidler, and Schneiderman (1988) has shown that blood pressure is much more variable in the home and work settings than in the laboratory; therefore, generalizability from measurements made in the laboratory to other settings is somewhat limited. Also, because blood pressure is much more variable at home or work than in the laboratory, many more blood pressure measurements are needed in those settings (6 to 10 readings compared to 1) in order to be representative.

Fortunately, technological advances in ambulatory blood pressure monitoring have now made it possible for researchers to conduct long-term studies of blood pressure reactivity in real-life settings in response to real-life stressful events, as well as throughout the course of the subject's normal daily routine. In addition to ambulatory monitoring of physiological variables, related data, as suggested by the biopsychosocial framework, can be collected by asking research subjects to provide daily self-reports on relevant social, cognitive, and behavioral variables.

Reliability and Validity of Personality-Related Measures

Currently, there is considerable controversy and confusion within behavioral medicine concerning the best method for measuring personality-related constructs such as Type A, anger, hostility, and healthy personality. The search for reliable and valid measures of these constructs must take into account the numerous sociocultural, socioeconomic, and socioecological variables previously described. It seems highly unlikely that any one measure will have predictive validity for all groups. Hence a series of measures, each of which has been shown to have predictive validity for a particular group, setting, or situation may be necessary.

Standardization of Treatment

Many behavioral interventions reported in the research literature are described in such sparse detail that exact replication is not possible. In addition, it is often the case that inadequate information is given regarding the experience and skill of therapists and the methods used to train therapists to deliver specific interventions (Agras, 1982). Behavioral intervention research would be greatly enhanced if more researchers would carefully describe these aspects of their research, thus permitting meaningful comparisons between studies, as well as evaluation of the replicability of the intervention in other settings (another aspect of generalizability). One of the benefits of research using computer-assisted intervention is the strict standardization of treatment.

Maintenance of Treatment Effects

Agras (1982) estimated that the median length of follow-up for studies employing behavioral interventions was 4 weeks, compared to 26 weeks for medical studies. Further, he estimated that only about 2% of studies on behavioral interventions employed long-term outcomes or maintenance procedures. Without adequate follow-up data, it is impossible to adequately determine the clinical utility of intervention procedures. As promising new procedures are first evaluated, the lack of long-term follow-up may be justifiable on practical grounds; however, as research in any particular clinical area matures, long-term follow-up should become a routine part of research designs.

SUMMARY

In the last 20 years, behavioral medicine has become a routine part of the practice of medicine. Behavioral medicine has provided the necessary tools to help persons change long-standing maladaptive patterns, such as overeating, smoking, and a sedentary life-style. For such other problems as chronic respiratory illness and chronic pain, behavioral medicine interventions, although not curative, have helped patients to lead more active lives and to cope more effectively with the consequences of their illness.

Interventions based on behavioral learning principles are now being applied to a variety of medical problems. Although some procedures—like progressive muscle relaxation or hypnosis—have been shown to offer simple help for a variety of problems, most practitioners have come to recognize and appreciate the complexity of behavior change and to utilize more long-term multimodal cognitive/behavioral interventions. Furthermore, the adoption of a healthy "life-style" is key to many interventions. Such a life-style involves regular exercise, consumption of a low-fat, low cholesterol diet, not smoking, maintenance of relatively low body weight, not using illicit drugs, not consuming alcohol or doing so in small amounts, resting, relaxing, laughing, achieving a balance between work and play, and ensuring that psychological demands rarely exceed personal coping resources. The adoption of such a life-style prevents, avoids, postpones, or minimizes many medical problems.

Although the field is still far from recommending specific interventions for specific problems, a few procedures have consistently been shown to be useful. Monitoring, a component of most behavioral interventions, is by itself a useful intervention. For instance, monitoring may help to prevent the development of hypertension in borderline hypertensive patients. Progressive muscle relaxation is also a generally useful procedure. It has been shown to help reduce blood pressure in poorly controlled hypertensives, to control headache and other pains, to reduce muscle tension, and even to reduce the toxicity of Type A behavior. Biofeedback seems to work in ways similar to progressive muscle relaxation and to have no more specific benefit unless physiologic feedback is critical for change, as is the case, for instance, with fecal incontinence. Of course, many patients prefer biofeedback to other behavioral interventions.

Where is behavioral medicine going? Behavioral medicine will continue to become a routine part of medical care. A major focus of behavioral medicine in the 1990s will be on developing and evaluating long-term, multicomponent, cost-effective, life-style-related interventions. Environmental and institutional interactions will probably achieve as much importance as personal change. At the same time, behavioral medicine research will focus on mechanisms, particularly on mechanisms involving the interactions among genetic, behavioral, and attitudinal factors that affect disease processes.

REFERENCES

Agras, W. S. (1981). Behavioral approaches to the treatment of essential hypertension. *International Journal of Obesity, 5,* 59–71.

Agras, W. S. (1982). Behavioral medicine in the 1980s. *Journal of Consulting and Clinical Psychology, 50,* 797–803.

Agras W. S., & Berkowitz, R. (1980). Clinical research in behavior therapy: Halfway there? *Behavior Therapy, 11,* 472–487.

Agras, W. S., & Jacob, R. G. (1979). Hypertension. In O. F. Pomerleau & J. P. Brady (Eds.), *Behavioral medicine: Theory and practice* (pp. 205–232). Baltimore: Williams & Wilkins.

Agras, W. S., Taylor, C. B., Kraemer, H. C., Southam, M. A., & Schneider, J. A. (1987). Relaxation training for essential hypertension at the worksite: II. The poorly controlled hypertensive. *Psychosomatic Medicine, 49,* 264–273.

Agras, W. S., Taylor, C. B., Feldman, D. E., Losch, M., & Burnett, K. F. (1990). Developing computer-assisted therapy for the treatment of obesity. *Behavior Therapy, 21,* 99–109.

Alexander, F. (1950). *Psychosomatic medicine.* New York: W. W. Norton.

American Cancer Society. (1990). *Cancer facts and figures 1990.* New York.

Antoni, M. H., Baggett, L., Ironson, G., August, S., LaPerriere, A., Klimas, N., Schneiderman, N., & Fletcher, M. A. (1991). Cognitive behavioral stress management intervention buffers distress responses and elevates immunological markers following notification of HIV-1 seropositivity. *Journal of Consulting and Clinical Psychology, 59,* 906–915.

Arnetz, B. B., Wasserman, J., Petrini, B., Brenner, S. O., Levi, L., Eneroth, P., Salovaara, H. K., Hjelm, R., Salovaara, L., Theorell, T., & Petterson, I. L. (1987). Immune function in unemployed women. *Psychosomatic Medicine, 49,* 3–12.

Atkinson, J. H., Jr., Grant, I., Kennedy, C. J., Richman, D. D., Spector, S. A., & McCutchan, J. A. (1988). Prevalence of psychiatric disorders among men infected with human immunodeficiency virus. A controlled study. *Archives of General Psychiatry, 45,* 859–864.

Baer, L., Minichiello, W. E., Jenike, M. A., & Holland, A. (1988). Use of a portable computer program to assist behavioral treatment in a case of obsessive-compulsive disorder. *Journal of Behavior Therapy and Experimental Psychiatry, 19,* 237–240.

Bahnson, C. B., & Bahnson, M. B. (1966). Role of the ego defenses: Denial and repression in the etiology of malignant neoplasm. *Annals of the New York Academy of Sciences, 123,* 827–845.

Bandura, A. (1977). Self-efficacy: Toward a unifying theory of behavioral change. *Psychological Review, 84,* 191–215.

Bandura, A. (1986). *Social foundations of thought and action.* Englewood Cliffs, NJ: Prentice-Hall.

Barefoot, J. C., Dahlstrom, W. G., & Williams, R. B. (1983). Hostility, CHD, incidence, and total mortality: A 25-year follow-up study of 255 physicians. *Psychosomatic Medicine, 45,* 59–63.

Baum, A., McKinnon, Q., & Silvia, C. (1987, March). *Chronic stress and the immune system.* Paper presented at the meeting of the Society of Behavioral Medicine, Washington, DC.

Benson, H., Beary, J. F., & Carol, M. P. (1974). The relaxation response. *Psychiatry, 37,* 37–46.

Binik, Y. M., Servanschreiber, D., Freiwald, S., & Hall, K. S. K. (1988). Intelligent computer-based assessment and psychotherapy—an expert system for sexual dysfunction. *Journal of Nervous and Mental Disease, 176,* 387–400.

Blanchard, E. B. (1987). Long-term effects of behavioral treatment of chronic headache. *Behavior Therapy, 18,* 375–385.

Blanchard, E. B., & Andrasik, F. (1985). *Management of chronic headache: A psychological approach.* New York: Pergamon Press.

Blanchard, E. B., Schwarz, S. P., & Radnitz, C. R. (1987). Psychological assessment and treatment of irritable bowel syndrome. *Behavior Modification, 11,* 348–372.

Blanchard, E. B., Martin, J. E., & Dubbert, P. M. (1988). *Non-drug treatments for essential hypertension.* New York: Pergamon Press.

Blanchard, E. B., Schwarz, S. P., & Neff, D. F. (1988). Two-year follow-up of behavioral treatment for irritable bowel syndrome. *Behavior Therapy, 19,* 67–73.

Blanchard, E. B., Schwarz, S. P., Neff, D. F., & Gerardi, M. A. (1988). Prediction of outcome from the self-regulatory treatment of irritable bowel syndrome. *Behavior Research and Therapy, 26,* 187–190.

Bloom, J. R., Ross, R. D., & Burnell, G. (1978). The effect of social support on patient adjustment after breast surgery. *Patient Counseling and Health Education, Autumn,* 50–59.

Blumberg, E. M., West, P. M., & Ellis, F. W. (1954). A possible relationship between psychological factors and human cancer. *Psychosomatic Medicine, 16,* 277–286.

Blumenthal, J. A. (1985). Psychologic assessment in cardiac rehabilitation. *Journal of Cardiopulmonary Rehabilitation, 5,* 208–215.

Blumenthal, J. A., & Emery, C. F. (1988). Rehabilitation of patients following myocardial infarction. *Journal of Consulting and Clinical Psychology, 56,* 374–381.

Blumenthal, J. A., & McKee, D. C. (Eds.). (1987). *Applications in behavioral medicine and health psychology: A clinician's source book.* Sarasota, FL: Professional Resource Exchange.

Boyer, C., & Schafer, R. (1990, August). *Symposium on adolescent attitudes toward condom use.* Paper presented at the scientific meetings of the American Psychological Association, Boston, MA.

Brooks, G. R., & Richardson, F. C. (1980). Emotional skills training: A treatment program for duodenal ulcer. *Behavior Therapy, 11,* 198–207.

Brownell, K. D., & Jeffery, R. W. (1987). Improving long-term weight loss: Pushing the limits of treatment. *Behavior Therapy, 18,* 353–374.

Burish, T. G., & Lyles, J. N. (1981). Effectiveness of relaxation training in reducing adverse reactions to cancer chemotherapy. *Journal of Behavioral Medicine, 4,* 65–78.

Burish, T. G., Shartner, C. D., & Lyles, J. N. (1981). Effectiveness of multiple-site EMG biofeedback and relaxation training in reducing the aversiveness of cancer chemotherapy. *Biofeedback and Self-Regulation, 6,* 523–535.

Burish, T. G., Carey, M. P., Krozely, M. G., & Greco, F. A. (1987). Conditioned side effects induced by cancer chemotherapy: Prevention through behavioral treatment. *Journal of Consulting and Clinical Psychology, 55,* 42–48.

Burnett, K. F., Taylor, C. B., & Agras, W. S. (1985). Ambulatory computer-assisted therapy for obesity. *Journal of Consulting and Clinical Psychology, 53,* 698–703.

Burnett, K. F., Magel, P. M., Harrington, S., & Taylor, C. B. (1989). Computer-assisted behavioral health counseling for high school students. *Journal of Counseling Psychology, 36,* 63–67.

Butcher, J. N. (1987). *Computerized psychological assessment.* New York: Basic Books.

Calabrese, J., Kling, M., & Gold, P. (1987). Alterations in immunocompetence during stress, bereavement, and depression: Focus on neuroendocrine regulation. *American Journal of Psychiatry, 144*(9), 1123–1134.

Carey, M., & Burish, T. G. (1987). Providing relaxation training to cancer chemotherapy patients: A comparison of three delivery techniques. *Journal of Consulting and Clinical Psychology, 55,* 732–737.

Cassileth, B. R., Lusk, E. J., Miller, D. S., Brown, L. L., & Miller, C. (1985). Psychosocial correlates of survival in advanced malignant disease. *New England Journal of Medicine, 312,* 1551–1555.

Centers for Disease Control (1989, March). *HIV/AIDS surveillance report,* 1–18. Atlanta, GA.

Centers for Disease Control (1990, July). *HIV/AIDS surveillance report,* 1–18. Atlanta, GA.

Cerulli, M. A., Nikoomanesh, P., & Shuster, M. M. (1979). Progress in biofeedback conditioning for fecal incontinence. *Gastroenterology, 76,* 742–746.

Chesney, M. A., Black, G. W., Swan, G. E., & Ward, M. M. (1987). Relaxation training for essential hypertension at the worksite: I. The untreated mild hypertensive. *Psychosomatic Medicine, 49,* 250–263.

Chu, S., Buehler, J., & Berkelman, R. (1990). Impact of the human immunodeficiency virus epidemic on mortality in women of reproductive age, United States. *Journal of the American Medical Association, 264,* 225–229.

Clouse, R. E., & Lustman, P. J. (1983). Psychiatric illness and contraction abnormalities of the esophagus. *New England Journal of Medicine, 309,* 1337–1342.

Cluss, P. A., & Fireman, P. (1985). Recent trends in asthma research. *Annals of Behavioral Medicine, 7,* 11–16.

Coates, T. J., & Greenblatt, R. M. (1989). Behavioral change using community level interventions. In K. Holmes (Ed.), *Sexually transmitted diseases* (pp. 1075–1080). New York: McGraw-Hill.

Coates, T. J., McKusick, L., Stites, D. P., & Kuno, R. (1989). Stress management training reduced number of sexual partners but did not improve immune function in men infected with HIV. *American Journal of Public Health, 79,* 885–887.

Cohen, J. B., & Reed, D. (1985). Type A behavior and coronary heart disease among Japanese men in Hawaii. *Journal of Behavioral Medicine, 8,* 343–352.

Contrada, R. J., & Krantz, D. S. (1988). Stress, reactivity, and Type A behavior: Current status and future directions. *Annals of Behavioral Medicine, 10,* 64–70.

Dembroski, T. M., & Costa, P. T. (1988). Assessment of coronary-prone behavior: A current overview. *Annals of Behavioral Medicine, 10,* 60–63.

Dembroski, T. M., McDougall, J. M., Williams, R. B., Haney, T. L., & Blumenthal, J. A. (1985). Components of Type A, hostility, and anger-in: Relationship to angiographic findings. *Psychosomatic Medicine, 247,* 219–233.

Dennis, D. C., Houston-Miller, N., Schwartz, R. G., Ahn, D. K., Kraemer, H. C., Gossard, D., Junea, M., Taylor, C. B., & DeBusk, R. F. (1988). Early return to work after uncomplicated myocardial infarction. *Journal of the American Medical Association, 260,* 214–220.

Derogatis, L. R. (1986). Psychology in cancer medicine: A perspective and overview. *Journal of Consulting and Clinical Psychology, 54,* 632–638.

Derogatis, L. R., Morrow, G. R., Fetting, J., Penmen, D., Piasetsky, S., Schmale, A. M., Henrichs, M., & Carnicke, C. L. (1983). The prevalence of psychiatric disorders among cancer patients. *Journal of the American Medical Association, 249,* 751–757.

DesJarlais, D. C., Friedman, S. R., & Casriel, C. (1990). Target groups for preventing AIDS among intravenous drug users: 2. The "hard" data studies. *Journal of Consulting and Clinical Psychology, 58,* 50–56.

Diamond, E. L., Schneiderman, N., Schwartz, D., Smith, J. C., Vorp, R., & Pasin, R. D. (1984). Harassment, hostility, and Type A as determinants of cardiovascular reactivity during competition. *Journal of Behavioral Medicine, 7,* 171–189.

DiClemente, R. J., & Temoshok, L. (1985). Psychological adjustment to having cutaneous malignant melanoma as a predictor of follow-up clinical status. *Psychosomatic Medicine, 47,* 81 (Abstract).

Dimsdale, J. E., Block, P. C., Gilbert, J., Hackett, T. P., & Hutter, A. M. (1981). Predicting cardiac morbidity based on risk factors and coronary angiographic findings. *American Journal of Cardiology, 47,* 73–76.

Dirks, J. F., Kinsman, R. A., Jones, N. F., & Fross, K. H. (1978). New developments in panic-fear research in asthma: Validity and stability of the MMPI panic-fear scale. *British Journal of Medical Psychology, 51,* 119–126.

Dubbert, P. M., Rappaport, N. B., & Martin, J. E. (1987). Exercise in cardiovascular disease. *Behavior Modification*, 11, 329–347.

Durel, L., & Schneiderman, N. (1991). Biobehavioral bases of hypertension in blacks. In P. M. McCabe, N. Schneiderman, T. F. Field, & J. S. Skyler (Eds.), *Stress, coping, and disease* (pp. 3–34). Hillsdale, NJ: Lawrence Erlbaum.

Ekstrand, M. L., & Coates, T. J. (1990). Maintenance of safer sexual behaviors and predictors of risky sex: The San Francisco Men's Health Study. *American Journal of Public Health*, 80, 973–977.

Engel, B. T., Glasgow, M. S., & Gaarder, K. R. (1983). Behavioral treatment of high blood pressure: III. Follow-up results and recommendations. *Psychosomatic Medicine*, 45, 23–29.

Engel, G. L. (1980). The clinical application of the biopsychosocial model. *American Journal of Psychiatry*, 137, 535–544.

Erdman, H. P. (1988). Computer consultation in psychiatry. *Psychiatric Annals*, 18, 209–216.

Farquhar, J. W., Maccoby, N., Wood, P. D., Alexander, J. K., Breitrose, H., Brown, B. W., Jr., Haskell, W. L., McAlister, A. L., Meyer, A. J., & Nash, J. D. (1977). Community education for cardiovascular health. *Lancet (1)*, 1192–1195.

Farquhar, J. W., Maccoby, N., & Solomon, D. (1984). Community applications of behavioral medicine. In W. D. Gentry (Ed.), *Handbook of behavioral medicine* (pp. 437–478). New York: Guilford Press.

Farquhar, J. W., Fortmann, S. P., Flora, J. A., Taylor, C. B., Haskell, W. L., Williams, P. T., Maccoby, N., & Wood, P. D. (1990). Effects of communitywide education on cardiovascular disease risk factors. *Journal of the American Medical Association*, 264, 359–365.

Feldman, M., Walker, P., Green, J. L., & Weingarden, K. (1986). Life events stress and psychosocial factors in men with peptic ulcer disease. *Gastroenterology*, 91, 1370–1379.

Ferlic, M., Goldman, A., & Kennedy, B. J. (1979). Group counseling in adult patients with advanced cancer. *Cancer*, 43, 760–766.

Fordyce, W. E. (1976). *Behavioral methods for chronic pain and illness*. St. Louis: C. V. Mosby.

Fredrikson, M., & Matthews, K. A. (1990). Cardiovascular responses to behavioral stress and hypertension. *Annals of Behavioral Medicine*, 12, 30–39.

Friedman, M., Thoresen, C. E., Gill, J. J., Powell, L., Price, V. A., Rabin, D. D., Breall, W. S., Dixon, T., Levy, R., & Bourg, E. (1984). Alteration of Type A behavior and reduction in cardiac recurrences in post-myocardial infarction patients. *American Heart Journal*, 108, 237–248.

Friedman, M., Thoresen, C., Gill, J., Ulmer, D., Powell, L., Rice, V., Brown, B., Thompson, L., Rabin, D., Breall, W., Bourg, E., Levy, R., & Dixon, T. (1986). Alteration of Type A behavior and its effects on cardiac recurrences in post-myocardial infarction patients. Summary results of the recurrent coronary prevention project. *American Heart Journal*, 112, 653–665.

Gatchel, R. J., Gaffney, F. A., & Smith, J. E. (1986). Comparative efficacy of behavioral stress management versus propranolol in reducing psychophysiological reactivity in post-myocardial infarction patients. *Journal of Behavioral Medicine*, 9, 503–513.

Ghosh, A., & Marks, I. M. (1987). Self-treatment of agoraphobia by exposure. *Behavior Therapy*, 18, 3–16.

Goldman, L., & Cook, G. F. (1984). The decline in ischemic heart disease mortality rates. *Annals of Internal Medicine*, 101, 825–836.

Goodkin, K. (1988). Psychiatric disorders in HIV-spectrum illness. *Texas Medicine*, 84, 55–61.

Goodkin, K. (1989). Antidepressants for the relief of chronic pain: Do they work? *Annals of Behavioral Medicine*, 11, 83–101.

Goodkin, K. (1990). Deterring the progression of HIV infection. *Comprehensive Therapy*, 16, 17–23.

Goodkin, K., Antoni, M. H., & Blaney, P. H. (1986). Stress and hopelessness in the promotion of cervical intraepithelial neoplasia to invasive squamous cell carcinoma of the cervix. *Journal of Psychosomatic Research*, 30, 67–76.

Green, B., Blanchard, E. B., & Suls, J. B. (1989, November). *Long-term monitoring of psychosocial stress and inflammatory bowel disease symptoms in patients with inflammatory bowel disease*. Paper presented at the twenty-third annual meeting of the Association for the Advancement of Behavior Therapy. Washington, DC.

Greer, S., Morris, T., & Pettingale, K. W. (1979). Psychological response to breast cancer: Effect on outcome. *Lancet*, 2, 785–787.

Gruber, B. L., Hall, N. R., Hersh, S. P., & Dubois, P. (1988). Immune system and psychologic changes in metastatic cancer patients while using ritualized relaxation and guided imagery: A pilot study. *Scandinavian Journal of Behavior Therapy, 17,* 25–46.

Haynes, S. G., & Matthews, K. A. (1988). Review and methodologic critique of recent studies on Type A behavior and cardiovascular disease. *Annals of Behavior Medicine, 10,* 47–60.

Haynes, S. G., Feinleib, M., & Kannel, W. B. (1980). The relationship of psychosocial factors to coronary heart disease in the Framingham study: III. Eight-year incidence of coronary heart disease. *American Journal of Epidemiology, 111,* 37–58.

Hecker, M. H. L., Chesney, M. A., Black, G. W., & Frautschi, N. (1988). Coronary-prone behaviors in the Western Collaborative Group Study. *Psychosomatic Medicine, 50,* 153–164.

Hovell, M. F. (1982). The experimental evidence for weight-loss treatment of essential hypertension: A critical review. *American Journal of Public Health, 72,* 359–368.

Hypertension Detection and Follow-up Program Cooperative Group. (1979). Five year findings of the hypertension detection and follow-up program. *Journal of the American Medical Association, 242,* 2562–2571.

Inter-Society Commission for Heart Disease Resources. Atherosclerosis Study Group and Epidemiology Study Group (1970). Primary prevention of the atherosclerotic diseases. *Circulation, 42,* A55.

Ironson, G., & Schneiderman, N. (in press). Psychoneuroimmunology and HIV-1: Scope of the problem. In N. Schneiderman (Ed.), *Psychoneuroimmunology and HIV-1.* Geneva, Switzerland: World Health Organization.

Ironson, G. H., Gellman, M. D., Spitzer, S. B., Llabre, M. M., Pasin, R. D., Weidler, D. J., & Schneiderman, N. (1989). Predicting home and work blood pressure measurements from resting baselines and laboratory reactivity in black and white Americans. *Psychophysiology, 26,* 201–207.

Ironson, G., LaPerriere, A., Antoni, M, O'Hearn, P., Schneiderman, N., Klimas, N., & Fletcher, M. A. (1990). Changes in immune and psychological measures as a function of anticipation and reaction to news of HIV-1 antibody status. *Psychosomatic Medicine, 52,* 247–270.

Ironson, G. H., Simoneau, J., Friedman, A., LaPerriere, A., Antoni, M., Schneiderman, N., & Fletcher, M. A. (1991). *Psychosocial predictors of disease progression in seropositive gay men.* Paper presented at the annual meeting of the American Psychological Association, San Francisco, CA.

Irwin, M., Daniels, M., Smith, T., Bloom, E., & Weiner, H. (1987). Impaired natural killer cell activity during bereavement. *Brain, Behavior, and Immunity, 1,* 98–104.

Irwin, M., Daniels, M., Risch, S., Bloom, E., & Weiner, H., (1988). Plasma cortisol and natural killer cell activity during bereavement. *Biological Psychiatry, 24,* 173–178.

Jacobs, C., Ross, R. D., Walker, I. M., & Stockdale, F. E. (1983). Behavior of cancer patients: A randomized study of the effects of education and peer support groups. *Journal of Clinical Oncology, 6,* 347–350.

Jacobs, M. A., Anderson, L. S., Eisman, H. D., Muller, J. J., & Friedman, S. (1967). Interaction of psychologic and biologic predisposing factors in allergic disorders. *Psychosomatic Medicine, 29,* 572–585.

Jamison, R. N., Burish, T. G., & Wallston, K. A. (1987). Psychogenic factors in predicting survival of breast cancer patients. *Journal of Clinical Oncology, 5,* 768–772.

Jenkins, C. D. (1988). Epidemiology of cardiovascular diseases. *Journal of Consulting and Clinical Psychology, 56,* 324–332.

Jenkins, C. D., Rosenman, R. H., & Zyzanski, S. J. (1974). Prediction of clinical coronary heart disease by a test for the coronary prone behavior pattern. *New England Journal of Medicine, 290,* 1271–1275.

Johnston, D. W. (1988). Psychological risk factors for disease: Nature, importance, and modification. *Current Opinion in Psychiatry, 1,* 734–739.

Joint National Commission (1984). The 1984 report of the Joint National Committee on Detection, Evaluation, and Treatment of High Blood Pressure. *Archives of Internal Medicine, 144,* 1045–1057.

Kaplan, N. M. (1990). *Clinical hypertension* (5th ed.). Baltimore: Williams & Wilkins.

Kaplan, R. M., Reiss, A., & Atkins, C. J. (1985). Behavioral issues in the management of chronic obstructive pulmonary disease. *Annals of Behavioral Medicine, 7,* 5–10.

Kaslow, R. A., Blackwelder, W. C., Ostrow, D. G., Yerg, D., Palinicek, J., Coulson, A. H., & Valdiserri, R. O. (1989). No evidence for a role of alcohol or other psychoactive drugs in accelerating immunodeficiency in HIV-1 positive individual. *Journal of the American Medical Association, 261,* 3424–3429.

Katz, P. O., Dalton, C. B., Richter, J. E., Wu, W. C., & Castell, D. O. (1987). Esophageal testing of patients with non-cardiac chest pain and/or dysphagia. *Annals of Internal Medicine, 106,* 593–597.

Kelly, J. A, St. Lawrence, J. S., & Hood, H. V. (1989). Behavioral interventions to reduce AIDS risk activities. *Journal of Consulting and Clinical Psychology, 57,* 60–67.

Kemeny, M. E., Fahey, J. L., Schneider, S., Weiner, H., Taylor, S., & Visscher, B. (1989). Psychosocial co-factors in HIV infection: Bereavement, depression and immune status in HIV seropositive homosexual men. *Psychosomatic Medicine, 51,* 255.

Kemeny, M. E., Duran, R., Weiner, H., Taylor, S. E., Visscher, B., & Fahey, J. L. (1990). Chronic depression precedes a decline in CD4 helper/inducer T cells in HIV positive men. Unpublished manuscript.

Kiecolt-Glaser, J., Ricker, D., George, J., Messicak, G., Speicher, C., Garner, W., & Glaser, R. (1984). Urinary cortisol levels, cellular immunocompetency, and loneliness in psychiatric inpatients. *Psychosomatic Medicine, 46,* 15–23.

Kiecolt-Glaser, J., Fisher, L., Ogrocki, P., Stout, J., Speicher, C., & Glaser, R. (1987). Marital quality, martial disruption, and immune function. *Psychosomatic Medicine, 49,* 13–34.

Kotses, H., & Glaus, K. (1981). Application of biofeedback to the treatment of asthma: A critical review. *Biofeedback and Self-Regulation, 6,* 573–590.

Krasnegor, N. A. (1990). Health and behavior: A perspective on research supported by the National Institutes of Health. *Annals of Behavioral Medicine, 12,* 72–78.

LaPerriere, A. R., Antoni, M. H., Schneiderman, N., Ironson, G., Klimas, N., Caralis, P., & Fletcher, M. A. (1990). Exercise intervention attenuates emotional distress and natural killer cell decrements following notification of positive serologic status for HIV-1. *Biofeedback and Self-Regulation, 15,* 229–241.

Latimer, P. R. (1981). Biofeedback and self-regulation in the treatment of diffuse esophageal spasm: A single case study. *Biofeedback and Self-Regulation, 6,* 181–189.

Latimer, P. R. (1983). *Functional gastrointestinal disorders: A behavioral medicine approach.* New York: Springer.

Latimer, P. R., Campbell, D., & Kasperski, J. (1984). A component analysis of biofeedback conditioning of fecal incontinence. *Biofeedback and Self-Regulation, 9,* 311–324.

Leirer, V. O., Morrow, D. G., Pariante, G. M., & Sheikh, J. I. (1988). Elder's nonadherence, its assessment, and computer-assisted instruction for medication recall training. *Journal of the American Geriatric Association, 36,* 877–884.

Liebman, R., Minuchin, S., & Baker, L. (1974). The use of structural family therapy in the treatment of intractable asthma. *American Journal of Psychiatry, 131,* 535–540.

Linn, B. S., Linn, M. W., & Jensen, J. (1981). Anxiety and immune responsiveness. *Psychological Reports, 49,* 969–970.

Llabre, M. M., Ironson, G. H., Spitzer, S. B., Gellman, M. D., Weidler, D. J., & Schneiderman, N. (1988). How many blood pressure measurements are enough?: An application of generalizability theory to the study of blood pressure reliability. *Psychophysiology, 25,* 97–106.

Lyles, J. N., Burish, T. G., Krozely, M. G., & Oldham, R. K. (1982). Efficacy of relaxation training and guided imagery in reducing the aversiveness of cancer chemotherapy. *Journal of Consulting and Clinical Psychology, 50,* 509–524.

Martin, J. L. (1990). Drug use and unprotected anal intercourse among gay men. *Health Psychology, 9,* 450–465.

Marzuk, P. M., Tierney, H. K., Tardiff, K., Gross, E. M., Morgan, E. G., Hsu, M. A., & Mann, J. (1988). Increased risk of suicide in persons with AIDS. *Journal of the American Medical Association, 259,* 1333–1337.

Matthews, K. A., Krantz, D. S., Dembroski, T. M., & MacDougall, J. M. (1982). Unique and common variance in structured interview and Jenkins Activity Survey measures of the Type A behavior pattern. *Journal of Personality and Social Psychology, 42,* 303–313.

McCaffrey, R. J., & Blanchard, E. B. (1985). Stress management approaches to the treatment of essential hypertension. *Annals of Behavioral Medicine, 7*, 5–12.

Melamed, B. G., & Siegel, L. J. (1980). *Behavioral medicine: Practical applications in health care.* New York: Springer Publishing.

Miller, N. H., Taylor, C. B., Davidson, D. M., Hill, M. N., & Krantz, D. S. (1990). Position paper of the American Association of Cardiovascular and Pulmonary Rehabilitation: The efficacy of risk factor intervention and psychosocial aspects of cardiac rehabilitation. *Journal of Cardiopulmonary Rehabilitation, 10*, 198–209.

Milne, B., Joachim, G., & Niedhardt, J. (1986). A stress management program for inflammatory bowel disease patients. *Journal of Advanced Nursing, 11*, 561–567.

Mitchell, C. M., & Drossman, D. A. (1987). The irritable bowel syndrome: Understanding and treating a biopsychosocial disorder. *Annals of Behavioral Medicine, 9*, 13–18.

Morrow, G. R., & Morrell, C. (1982). Behavioral treatment for the anticipatory nausea and vomiting induced by cancer chemotherapy. *New England Journal of Medicine, 307*, 1476–1480.

Morrow, G. R., & Dobkin, P. L. (1987). Behavioral approaches for the management of aversive side effects of cancer treatment. *Psychiatric Medicine, 5*, 299–314.

National Heart, Lung, and Blood Institute Working Group. (1982). Management of patient compliance in the treatment of hypertension. *Hypertension, 4*, 415–423.

Neff, D. F., & Blanchard, E. B. (1987). A multi-component treatment for irritable bowel syndrome. *Behavior Therapy, 18*, 70–83.

Nichols, S. E. (1983). Psychiatric aspects of AIDS. *Psychosomatics, 24*, 1083–1089.

Ornish, D. (1990). *Dr. Dean Ornish's program for reversing heart disease.* New York: Random House.

Perry, C. L., Knut-Inge, K., & Shultz, J. M. (1988). Primary prevention of cardiovascular disease: Communitywide strategies for youth. *Journal of Consulting and Clinical Psychology, 56*, 358–364.

Peterson, L. (1986). Introduction to the special series. *Journal of Consulting and Clinical Psychology, 54*, 591–592.

Pettingale, K. W., Morris, T., Greer, S., & Haybittle, J. L. (1985). Mental attitudes to cancer: An additional prognostic factor. *Lancet, 1*, 750.

Pickering, T. G. (1982). Non-pharmacologic methods of treatment of hypertension: Promising but unproved.. *Cardiovascular Reviews and Reports, 3*, 82–88.

Powell, L. H., & Thoresen, C. E. (1988). Effects of Type A behavioral counseling and severity of prior acute myocardial infarction on survival. *American Journal of Cardiology, 62*, 1159–1163.

Puska, P., Nissinen, A., Tuomilehto, J., Salonen, J. T., Koskela, K., McAlister, A., Kottke, T. E., Maccoby, N., & Farquhar, J. W. (1985). The community-based strategy to prevent coronary heart disease: Conclusions from the ten years of the North Karelia Project. In L. Breslow, I. B. Lave, & J. E. Fielding (Eds.), *Annual review of public health* (pp. 147–193). Palo Alto, CA: Annual Reviews.

Ragland, D. R., & Brand, R. J. (1988a). Type A behavior and mortality from coronary heart disease. *New England Journal of Medicine, 318*, 65–69.

Ragland, D. R, & Brand, R. J. (1988b). Coronary heart disease and mortality in the Western Collaborative Group Study. *American Journal of Epidemiology, 127*, 462–475.

Redd, W. H., Andersen, G. V., & Minagawa, R. Y. (1982). Hypnotic control of anticipatory emesis in patients receiving cancer chemotherapy. *Journal of Consulting and Clinical Psychology, 50*, 14–19.

Redd, W. H., Jacobsen, P. B., Die-Trill, M., Dermatis, H., McEvoy, M., & Holland, J. C. (1987). Cognitive/attentional distraction in the control of conditioned nausea in pediatric cancer patients receiving chemotherapy. *Journal of Consulting and Clinical Psychology, 55*, 391–395.

Richter, J. E., Obrecht, W. F., Bradley, L. A., Young, L. D, & Anderson, K. O. (1986). Psychological comparison of patients with nutcracker esophagus and irritable bowel syndrome. *Digestive Diseases and Sciences, 31*, 131–138.

Rogentine, G. N., Van Kammen, D. P., Fox, B. H., Docherty, J. P., Rosenblatt, J. E., Boyd, S. C., & Bunney, W. E. (1979). Psychological factors in the prognosis of malignant melanoma: A prospective study. *Psychosomatic Medicine, 41*, 647–655.

Rosen, R. C., Kostis, J. B., & Brondolo, E. (1989). Nondrug treatment approaches for hypertension. *Clinics in Geriatric Medicine, 5*, 791–802.

Rosenman, R. H., Brand, R. J., Jenkins, C. D., Friedman, M., Straus, R., & Wurm, M. (1975). Coronary heart disease in the Western Collaborative Group Study: Final follow-up 8.5 years. *Journal of the American Medical Association, 233,* 872–877.

Roskies, E., Kearny,H., Spevack, M., Surkis, A., Cohen, C., & Gilman, S. (1979). Generalizability and durability of treatment effects in an intervention program for coronary-prone (Type A) managers. *Journal of Behavioral Medicine, 2,* 195–207.

Saab, P., Tischenkel, N., Spitzer, S. B., Gellman, M. D., Pasin, R. D., & Schneiderman, N. (1991). Race and blood pressure status influences cardiovascular responses to challenge. *Journal of Hypertension, 9,* 249–258.

Sarafino, E. P. (1990). *Health psychology: Biopsychosocial interactions.* New York: Wiley.

Schaeffer, M. A., Krantz, D. S., Weiss, S. M., Zoltick, J. M., Yaney, S. F, Karch, R., & Bedynek, J. L. (1988). Effects of occupational behavioral counseling and exercise interventions on Type A components and cardiovascular reactivity. *Journal of Cardiopulmonary Rehabilitation, 10,* 371–377.

Scherr, M., Crawford, P., Sergent, C., & Scherr, C. (1975). Effect of biofeedback techniques on chronic asthma in a summer camp environment. *Annals of Allergy, 35,* 289–295.

Schmale, A. H., Jr., & Iker, H. P. (1966). The psychological setting of uterine cancer. *Annals of the New York Academy of Sciences, 125,* 807–813.

Schneiderman, N., Chesney, M. A., & Krantz, D. S. (1989). Biobehavioral aspects of cardiovascular disease: Progress and prospects. *Health Psychology, 8,* 649–676.

Schneiderman, N., Weiss, S. M., & Kaufman, P. G. (Eds.). (1989). *Handbook of research methods in cardiovascular behavioral medicine.* New York: Plenum Press.

Schwartz, G. E., & Weiss, S. M. (1978). Behavioral medicine revisited: An amended definition. *Journal of Behavioral Medicine, 1,* 249–251.

Schwartz, J. L. (1987). *Review and evaluation of smoking cessation methods: The United States and Canada 1978–1985.* Bethesda, MD: Division of Cancer Prevention and Control, National Cancer Institute No. (NIH) 87–2940.

Schwartz, S. P., & Blanchard, E. B. (1990). Inflammatory bowel disease: A review of the psychological assessment and treatment literature. *Annals of Behavioral Medicine, 12,* 95–105.

Selmi, P. M., Klein, M. H., Greist, J. H., Johnson, J. H., & Harris, W. G. (1982). An investigation of computer-assisted cognitive behavior therapy in the treatment of depression. *Behavior Research Methods and Instrumentation, 14,* 181–185.

Shaw, L., & Ehrlich, A. (1987). Relaxation training as a treatment for chronic pain caused by ulcerative colitis. *Pain, 29,* 287–293.

Shekelle, R. B., Raynor, W. J., Ostfeld, A. M., Garron, D. C., Bieliauskas, L. A., Liu, S. C., Maliza, C., & Paul, O. (1981). Psychological depression and 17-year risk of death from cancer. *Psychosomatic Medicine, 43,* 117–125.

Shekelle, R. B., Gale, M., Ostfeld, A. M., & Paul, O. (1983). Hostility, risk of coronary heart disease and mortality. *Psychosomatic Medicine, 45,* 109–114.

Shekelle, R. B., Hulley, S. B., Neaton, J. D., Billings, J. H., Borhani, N. O., Gerace, T. A., Jacobs, D. R., Lasser, N. L., Mittlemark, M. B., & Stamler, J. for the Multiple Risk Factor Intervention Trial Research Group. (1985). The MRFIT behavior pattern study: II. Type A behavior and incidence of coronary heart disease. *American Journal of Epidemiology, 122,* 559–570.

Smith, W. M. (1977). Treatment of mild hypertension: Results of a ten-year intervention trial. *Circulation Research, 17,* 286–308.

Soloman, G. F., Kemeny, M. E., & Temoshok, L. (1990). Psychoneuroimmunologic aspects of immunodeficiency virus infection. In R. Ader (Ed.), *Psychoneuroimmunology* (2nd ed., pp. 1081–1106). San Diego: Academic Press.

Sorrell, S. P., Greist, J. H., Klein, M. H., Johnson, J. H., & Harris, W. G. (1982). Enhancement of adherence to tricyclic antidepressants by computerized supervision. *Behavior Research Methods and Instrumentation, 14,* 176–180.

Spiegel, D., Bloom, J., & Yalom, I. (1981). Group support for patients with metastatic cancer. *Archives of General Psychiatry, 38,* 527–533.

Spiegel, D., Bloom, J. R., Kraemer, H., & Gottheil, E. (1989). Psychological support for cancer patients. *Lancet (2),* 1447.

Stall, R. D., McKusick, L., Wiley, J., Coates, T., & Ostrow, D. (1986). Alcohol and drug use during sexual activity and compliance with safe sex guidelines for AIDS: The AIDS Behavioral Research Project. *Health Education Quarterly*, 13, 359–371.

Stall, R. D., Coates, T. J., & Hoff, C. (1988). Behavioral risk reduction for HIV infection among gay and bisexual men. *American Psychologist*, 43, 878–885.

Steptoe, A., Phillips, J., & Harling, J. (1981). Biofeedback and instructions in the modification of respiratory resistance: An experimental study of asthmatic and non-asthmatic volunteers. *Journal of Psychosomatic Research*, 25, 541–551.

Stolbach, L. L., Brandt, U. C., Borysenko, J. Z., Benson, H., Maurer, S. N., Lessermen, J., Albright, T. E., & Albright, N. L. (1988, April). *Benefits of a mind/body group program for cancer patients*. Paper and poster presented at the annual meeting of the Society of Behavioral Medicine, Boston.

Stoloff, M. L., & Couch, J. V. (1988). *Computer use in psychology: A directory of software* (2nd ed.). Washington, DC: American Psychological Association.

Suinn, R. M. (1975). The cardiac stress management program for Type A patients. *Cardiovascular Rehabilitation*, 5, 13–15.

Surwit, R. S. (1990, April). Computer-assisted clinical management of intensive insulin therapy in diabetes. In K. F. Burnett (Chair), *Computer-assisted intervention in behavioral medicine*. Symposium conducted at the annual meeting of the Society of Behavioral Medicine. Chicago.

Svedlund, J., Sjodin, I., Ottosson, J., & Dotevall, G. (1983). Controlled study of psychotherapy in irritable bowel syndrome. *Lancet (2)*, 589–592.

Taylor, C. B., Agras, W. S., Losch, M., Plante, T. G., & Burnett, K. F. (1991). Improving the effectiveness of computer-assisted weight loss. *Behavior Therapy*, 22, 229–236.

Taylor, C. B., & Killen, J. D. (1991). *The facts about smoking: What it does to you and how you can stop*. New York: Consumer Reports Press.

Taylor, C. B., Debusk, R. F., Davidson, M. D., Houston, N., & Burnett, K. (1981). Optimal methods for identifying depression following hospitalization for myocardial infarction. *Journal of Chronic Diseases*, 34, 127–133.

Taylor, C. B., Ironson, G., & Burnett, K. F. (1990). Adult medical disorders. In A. S. Bellack, M. Hersen, & A. E. Kazdin (Eds.), *International handbook of behavior modification and therapy* (2nd ed., pp. 371–397). New York: Plenum Press.

Telch, C. F., & Telch, M. J. (1986). Group coping skills instruction and supportive group therapy for cancer patients: A comparison of strategies. *Journal of Consulting and Clinical Psychology*, 54, 802–808.

Temoshok, L., & Heller, B. (1981). *Stress and "Type C" versus epidemiological risk factors in melanoma*. Paper presented at the 89th annual convention of the American Psychological Association, Los Angeles.

Temoshok, L., Heller, B., Sagebiel, R. W., Blois, M. S., Sweet, D. M., DiClemente, R. J., & Gold, M. L. (1985). The relationship of psychosocial factors to prognostic indicators in cutaneous malignant melanoma. *Journal of Psychosomatic Research*, 29, 139–153.

Tischenkel, N. J., Saab, P., Schneiderman, N., Nelesen, R. A., Pasin, R. D., Goldstein, D. A., Spitzer, S. B., Woo-Ming, R., & Weidler, D. J. (1989). Cardiovascular and neurohumoral responses to behavioral challenge as a function of race and sex. *Health Psychology*, 8, 503–524.

Vachon, M. L., Lyall, W. A., Rogers, J., Cochrane, J., & Freeman, S. J. (1981). The effectiveness of psychosocial support during post-surgical treatment of breast cancer. *International Journal of Psychiatry in Medicine*, 11, 365–372.

Wald, A., & Handen, B. L. (1987). Behavioral aspects of disorders of defecation and fecal continence. *Annals of Behavioral Medicine*, 9, 19–23.

Wald, A., & Tunuguntla, A. K. (1984). Anorectal sensorimotor dysfunction in fecal incontinence and diabetes mellitus. *New England Journal of Medicine*, 310, 1282–1287.

Watson, M. (1983). Psychosocial intervention with cancer patients: A review. *Psychological Medicine*, 13, 839–846.

Weiner, H. (1977). *Psychobiology and human disease*. New York: Elsevier.

Weiner, H. (1982). Psychobiological factors in bodily disease. In T. Millon, C. Green, & R. Meagher (Eds.), *Handbook of clinical health psychology* (pp. 31–52). New York: Plenum Press.

Whorwell, P. J., Prior, A., & Faragher, E. B. (1984). Controlled trial of hypnotherapy in the treatment of severe refractory irritable-bowel syndrome. *Lancet (2)*, 1232–1234.

Wilkinson, G., & Markus, A. C. (1989). PROQSY: A computerized technique for psychiatric case identification in general practice. *British Journal of Psychiatry, 154,* 378–382.

Williams, R. B., Barefoot, J. C., Haney, T. L., Harrell, F. E., Blumenthal, J. A., Pryor, D. B., & Peterson, B. (1988). Type A behavior and angiographically documented coronary atherosclerosis in a sample of 2,289 patients. *Psychosomatic Medicine, 50,* 139–152.

Winett, R. A., King, A. C., & Altman, D. G. (1989). *Health psychology and public health: An integrative approach.* New York: Pergamon Press.

Winters, R. (1985). Behavioral approaches to pain. In N. Schneiderman & J. T. Tapp (Eds.), *Behavioral medicine: A biopsychosocial approach* (pp. 565–588). Hillsdale, NJ: Lawrence Erlbaum.

World Health Organization (1990, July). *Current and future dimensions of the HIV/AIDS pandemic a capsule summary.* Geneva, Switzerland.

Young, L. D., Richter, J. E., Bradley, L. A., & Anderson, K. O. (1987). Disorders of the upper gastrointestinal system: An overview. *Annals of Behavioral Medicine, 9,* 7–12.

PART V

SPECIAL POPULATIONS

CHAPTER 16

Research in Child and Adolescent Psychiatry

DENNIS P. CANTWELL

INTRODUCTION

In this chapter, I present an overview of current issues concerning research in child and adolescent psychiatry. First, I will review some issues as to why child psychiatry as a discipline has not had as much research as other academic specialties. Then I will discuss newer developments, such as the National Plan for Research on Child and Adolescent Mental Disorders and the Institute of Medicine Report on *Research on Children and Adolescents with Mental, Behavioral, Developmental Disorders*. Following this, I will review the importance of research for clinical practice, teaching, individual growth, and advancement in the field in general. Research training will also be discussed. Finally, I will present a brief description of an empirical model for the study of child and adolescent psychopathology that can be a template to guide future studies.

IN THE PAST

Among medical subspecialties, child psychiatry has the reputation for having a lack of empirical research compared to other medical specialties,

Dennis P. Cantwell • Department of Psychiatry, University of California at Los Angeles, Los Angeles, California 90024.

Research in Psychiatry: Issues, Strategies, and Methods, edited by L. K. George Hsu and Michel Hersen. Plenum Press, New York, 1992.

including adult psychiatry. Some of the reasons for this lack of research are historical. In 1959, the American Board of Psychiatry and Neurology established child psychiatry as a board certifiable medical specialty. Prior to this, child psychiatry did not have strong developmental roots in medicine or pediatrics, but rather grew up independent of other medical specialties and even independent of adult psychiatry. Child psychiatry is not as much an offspring of adult psychiatry as an independent outgrowth.

In 1992, the Commonwealth Fund spurred the development of Commonwealth Child Guidance Clinics. In these community clinics, service was often the overriding concern. Children were seen by a multidisciplinary team comprising a child psychiatrist, a psychologist, and a social worker. Those who provided service did not promote an empirical approach to the study of the problems of the children they were treating.

The American Association of Psychiatric Clinics for Children was formally established in 1946. This association used the Commonwealth Child Guidance Clinics as its base, and these clinics became to a large extent the training grounds for future child psychiatrists. These clinics did not have medical roots, and many lacked medical and general psychiatric input in their operation.

Although it is true that service demands played a large role in inhibiting research development in these clinics, it also must be pointed out that there was a lack of contact with other academic disciplines which could have instilled models for research. Other medical specialties that developed primarily within medical school settings and hospitals had their faculty and trainees exposed to colleagues from other disciplines, who were also involved in academic work.

However, there is more than a historical base for a lack of research in child and adolescent psychiatry up to the present time. There are difficulties which are specific to the field. I have pointed out elsewhere (Cantwell, 1979) that attitudes that tend to inhibit research activity may be more prevalent in child psychiatry, at least in the past, then in other specialties. A tendency to cling tenaciously to certain clinical beliefs, whether or not they are supported by research evidence, and the implicit attitude that we know all the answers and we only need to apply the answers we know, are not attitudes which are likely to spur research.

Jones (1965) has summarized the process whereby the "argument-from-authority" approach seems to carry more weight in child psychiatry than it does in a discipline such as internal medicine or pediatrics. The practicing clinical child psychiatrist has the richest observational experience and theoretically would be the one most likely to make a valuable contribution, at least to clinical research. In practice, however, in the past and even somewhat today, clinicians are often isolated from the researchers in medical centers and, as a consequence, strain may develop between the two. Practitioners are concerned about the care of their patients. They have to provide the best available treatment for each patient at one particular point in time. They cannot wait for the definitive proof of each treatment from controlled research studies. There are a myriad of conflicting viewpoints about the etiology of various forms of child psychopathology. Likewise, there is a myriad of viewpoints as to how to best treat particular individual patients with various types of disorders. We still have individual schools of therapeutic intervention—individual psychodynamic psychotherapy, psychoanalysis, various schools of family therapy, various schools of behavioral and cognitive-behavioral intervention, and psychopharmacologic management. It must be admitted that most of the interventions in child psychiatry (and these include both psychosocial and biological interventions) remain geared toward symptomatic treatment, not tied to underlying knowledge about the pathogenesis of a particular disease process. Time and time again we see that newer forms of therapeutic intervention are often promoted by charismatic individuals of both a popular and a professional audience. This takes the place of testing the new therapeutic intervention through the empirical scientific method and the publication of results in a peer-reviewed scientific journal.

Thus, in choosing among conflicting viewpoints, clinicians very often have little in the way of hard research data to serve as a guide. They can fall back on their own clinical judgement and/or the opinions of senior figures in the field with whom they find themselves in agreement. With the approach of seniority, then, the healthy skepticism and the youthful humility of young clinicians may give way to overconfidence and dogmatism. Respect for a newly proposed theory of etiology or a newly proposed intervention technique may often rest on the reputation of the person who proposes it rather than on the empirical scientific evidence that the etiologic factor is indeed a valid one, and/or that the therapeutic intervention is an effective and safe one.

Moreover, there are certain research difficulties that are inherent in the study of child and adolescent psychopathology. As has been discussed elsewhere (Cantwell, 1979), the child and adolescent patient is a growing organism during the time that research is being done. Children and adolescents actively develop in many spheres. Thus, longitudinal observations, such as in follow-up studies or response-to-treatment studies, actually have the investigator seeing a different child at a different time. The child lives in a complex family environment and in a larger psychosocial environment that continually affects his or her development in many areas. In most types of investigations, these variables that are multiple and complex in nature cannot be manipulated experimentally. Obviously, family involvement is much greater in studies with children than it is in studies with adults. Families may be reluctant to involve their children in research studies because they may see that as a process of using their children as guinea pigs. Clinicians may also not wish to involve patients in studies because of an overprotective attitude toward their patients. Moreover, clinicians may be more suited to take part in certain studies themselves, such as studies of psychotherapy of children in multiple centers, but may be reluctant to do so for a variety of reasons. Child and adolescent patients' rights issues are much more complex than is the case with adults. Human use issues are much more complicated when dealing with child and adolescent subjects than when dealing with adult subjects. Many of the methods used in adult psychiatric research have had to be significantly modified for use with children because of developmental issues. Indeed, this area itself has become a separate division of research.

Given all of the above reasons, it is not surprising then to see that research in child and adolescent psychiatry is somewhat behind that of adult psychiatry and far behind other medical subspecialties. However, lack of a research component during clinical child fellowship training and lack of the ability to obtain postfellowship research training may also be cited as reasons for the absence of significant research in the field.

The amount of time for clinical training in child psychiatry has remained at 2 years since child psychiatry became a board certifiable specialty more than 30 years ago. However, the field has grown tremendously and the "required" aspects of training as demanded by the Residency Review Committee have likewise expanded, leaving little time for research training during the 2 years of a clinical fellowship. Research training is not a mandated part of clinical fellowship training. Indeed, in some programs, there may be a lack of genuine interest in research.

THE PRESENT

The last decade has seen a number of events that have improved the likelihood that significant child and adolescent research is likely to be done. In 1983, a consortium of agencies produced a document entitled, *Child Psychiatry: A Plan for the Coming Decades* (American Academy of Child Psychiatry, 1983). This document detailed recommendations for all aspects of child and adolescent psychiatry but emphasized the importance of the need for more research being done in child and adolescent psychiatry.

In 1989, the Institute of Medicine produced a document entitled, "Research on Children and Adolescents with Mental, Behavioral, and Developmental Disorders" (Institute of Medicine, 1989). This publication was the outcome of the multiple committees which met to study issues that were related to child psychiatry research. The document deals with research progress and promising opportunities as well as the barriers to research. It detailed a national plan which was sponsored by the National Institute of Mental Health (NIMH) for research in child and adolescent mental disorders. In its conclusions, there are recommendations concerned with prevalence, costs, causes and determinants, intervention, overcoming the barriers to a research project, and a national plan for child and adolescent research.

The NIMH raised child and adolescent psychiatry to the branch level within the institute and fostered research in child and adolescent psychiatry. More recently, the NIMH produced a national plan for research on child and adolescent mental disorders which was published in 1990. The NIMH has also stimulated further research by funding training programs in child and adolescent psychiatry at a number of leading centers in the United States; but more programs obviously are necessary.

In the modern clinical practice of child psychiatry, the therapist requires detailed assessments of the patients and their families, as well as reports of the psychosocial environment of their patients. There are a number of questions that must be answered in any diagnostic evaluation. These include what types of psychiatric disorders the child may be presenting with and what are the likely etiologic factors. Based on answers to these questions, the most efficient and effective treatment intervention for that disorder must be applied for that particular patient.

Clinical practice of this type can occur only if there is a continued striving to improve both diagnostic methods and treatment methods. Improvement will occur if significant clinical research in these areas is undertaken and if the individual clinical practitioner is competent to match the most effective treatment with an individual patient with a specific disorder. The clinical practitioner who leaves a standard 2-year clinical fellowship program in child psychiatry must be, at the very least a sophisticated consumer of research. To do this, he or she must be able to keep up with current knowledge in the field about etiology and treatment issues. After this period of training, the practitioner is likely to practice for some 40 years. The exponential growth over the last 40 years and the push to further growth mentioned above make it likely that there will be a continued exponential growth in the field of child and adolescent psychiatry in the next 40 years.

In 1989, the American Academy of Child and Adolescent Psychiatry received a report from the Work Group on Scientific Issues (Report of the Work Group on Scientific Issues, 1989). This group sought to address the current status of scientific research in child and adolescent psychiatry. A full discussion of that report is beyond the scope of this chapter, but some points made in that report bear repeating. The authors of the report suggested that there were 4,500 child and adolescent psychiatrists in the United States at the time the report was written. Of these, somewhat more than 600 psychiatrists were working full time in academic medical centers. Of this group, only a small proportion were devoting much of their time to research. Moreover, there were nearly 100 funded child psychiatry academic positions available in 1988.

In reviewing the years since *Child Psychiatry: A Plan for the Coming Decade* (American Academy of Child Psychiatry, 1983) was published, the authors of the report did suggest that progress had been made. There were strong suggestions that child psychiatry was producing more scientific information than prior to 1983 and providing more opportunities for research. They made several recommendations that they felt would improve the likelihood of more research being done in child and adolescent psychiatry in the future.

Several years ago (Cantwell, 1989), I put forth an empirical model for the study of disorders of childhood and adolescence. This model presupposes that the *disorders* that children and adolescents present with are the main focus of research interest. Furthermore, the model is conceptualized as consisting of several domains for investigation. These would include: clinical phenomenology; psychosocial factors; demographic factors; biological laboratory studies; family genetic studies; family interaction studies; outcome studies; and intervention studies. Obviously, these domains of investigation overlap with one another and this can cause refinement in one domain after the overlap is noted. Currently, investigations are underway with the majority of the psychiatric disorders of childhood and adolescence in almost all of these domains, but much more research is needed (Rutter, 1986).

From the standpoint of clinical phenomenology, we still need a considerable amount of work that will define the inclusion and exclusion criteria for specific disorders. We have examined the diagnostic systems in the DSM-III and in the DSM-III-R; and soon there will be a DSM-IV. The approach used in the creation of the DSM-IV has been more empirical than that used in the development of its predecessors. It is hoped that this will result in an improved nosological and classification system.

Subtyping of disorders is an important issue for differential pathogenesis, outcome, and intervention. Also, co-morbidity is recognized as an increasingly difficult issue which may also affect outcome, intervention, and any type of biological or psychological laboratory study. A large number of children and adolescents with psychiatric disorders present with mixtures of problems rather than with disorders "in pure culture." This makes research in a variety of areas much more difficult.

The clinical phenomenology of disorders can be more precisely defined by the use of standardized instruments which have been developed in child psychiatric research in the last 10 to 15 years. These include structured and semistructured parent and child interviews, parent- and teacher-rating scales, self-rating scales, and others. Work on the development of these instruments is an important research endeavor in itself and is forming a major focus of the future child Epidemiologic Catchment Area (ECA) study. The child ECA study promises to be the first major epidemiological study of childhood disorders on a national basis in the United States.

Once the clinical phenomenology of a disorder has been defined and subtyped in some meaningful fashion, studies in other domains of this model can be undertaken. Such demographic factors as epidemiologic rates of incidence and prevalence, lifetime expectancy, and morbid risk rates can be undertaken. The impact of age, sex, social class, and ethnicity on the phenomenologic picture of various disorders needs to be investigated. For example, we still do not know if the clinical phenomenologic picture of depression and mania is exactly the same in infants, preschoolers, grade schoolers, early adolescents, and late adolescents as it is in adults. There is some suggestion that some of the core symptoms do cut across age levels, but that other symptoms vary with age and developmental level and may also vary with gender. However, much more work needs to be done to refine this issue.

It is true that biological laboratory studies are lacking for many disorders in adult psychiatry, but they are sorely lacking for the psychiatric disorders of children and adolescents. Neurophysiologic studies, neuroendocrine studies, biochemical studies, neuropharmacologic studies, receptor studies and brain-imaging studies all hold promise for elucidating the biological underpinnings of some disorders of childhood and adolescence. Family genetic studies in child and adolescent psychiatry have mostly been limited to those of family aggregation studies, and some adoption and twin studies. There are few linkage, segregation, and gene-mapping studies. However, as indicated in Rutter's recent review (Rutter, Bolton, Harrington, Le Couteura, MacDonald, & Simonoff, 1990), this is an area of very promising research in the near future in the study of child and adolescent child psychopathology.

Because the children who are seen in research studies are generally living in their home of origin, family interaction studies, such as the analysis of parenting styles or the assessment of the amount of expressed emotion on the development of certain types of psychiatric disorder, will most likely prove to be fruitful areas of research.

Child psychiatry has the opportunity of also using "high-risk" methodology, in studying children of parents with defined disorders, such as bipolar and unipolar mood disorder or schizophrenia, and also in studying development of psychopathology in children who are at risk for reasons other than their parents' having a defined psychiatric disorder. For example, Cantwell and Baker (1991) have concentrated on children with communication disorders, whom they predicted would be at risk for the development of psychiatric and learning disorders. This group of children has been followed now for almost 10 years, and the predictions have turned out to be true. This is a high-risk group for the development of both learning and psychiatric disorders and the two types of disorders are intimately intertwined. That is, if these children with communication disorders develop a learning disorder, then they are much more likely to develop a psychiatric disorder than the children with speech and language disorders who do not develop learning problems.

From the standpoint of clinical child psychiatry, outcome and intervention studies are most likely the two important domains that need to be investigated in the areas that have been outlined above in the empirical model. Child psychiatrists must be interested in what happens to children who present with different types of disorders. What is the natural history without treatment? Who gets well? Who remains ill? And who develops an adult picture that looks somewhat different than the picture they presented with in childhood? We need to know much more about the prognostic factors that relate to complete resolution of the disorder versus continuing manifestations of the disorder in unmodified form. Outcome studies also include the issue of developmental psychopathology, that is, the continuities and discontinuities between infancy, childhood, adolescence, and adult life, and the mechanisms by which these continuities and discontinuities occur. By looking at the continuities and discontinuities and by elucidating pathophysiological mechanisms, the practitioner can hope to define and describe more effective intervention strategies that are both psychosocial and biological.

In the area of intervention, aside from psychopharmacologic studies and some studies in the behavioral area, there is little in the way of systematic studies of the comparative efficacy of various types of interventions with different disorders. Which children with what types of disorder will respond to what types of intervention and with what type of an outcome are questions that need answering for almost all child and adolescent psychopathology.

All of the needed studies in the field in all these areas of the model proposed above are not being undertaken at the present time. We still need much more work on nosology, the classification of psychiatric disorders of childhood and adolescence, epidemiological, longitudinal, and treatment studies, all of which have a clinical orientation, as well as more basic research about the biological as well as the psychosocial underpinnings of the disorders. Methodological research is basic to all of the aforementioned studies—that is, the development of better research methods and instruments of assessment and outcome in the field of child and adolescent psychiatry. Existing methods for evaluating parenting skills, for assessing the effects of various types of family interaction, and for determining the effects of psychosocial factors on the child's development are still rather rudimentary. Improvement in any one or all of the above areas is likely to have a major impact on child and adolescent mental health.

Of course, there are many other areas that could be discussed in detail, but the overall conclusion remains the same. Much more research is needed in almost all areas of child and adolescent psychiatry. There is a reawakening of interest in and funding for child and adolescent research at the national level. Whether this interest can be carried into the future given the dwindling base of full-time academic child psychiatrists is questionable.

SUMMARY

In this chapter, I have presented an overview of the issues of research in child and adolescent psychiatry and discussed the obstacles to research that have occurred in the past. I have proposed recommendations for overcoming those obstacles and also mentioned some areas in which vital research is occurring at the present time. As has been discussed before, research is necessary for improvement in clinical practice, for the instruction of future child psychiatrists, for the professional improvement of the individual practitioner, as well as for the growth of the field in general. In all areas of medicine, yesterday's answers must become today's questions. In child and adolescent psychiatry, for too long the answers given in yesteryear often remain the answers that are given today. Although the field may not be confronted with new questions, there is evidence that in the last 10 years this situation is beginning to change.

REFERENCES

American Academy of Child Psychiatry. (1983). *Child psychiatry: A plan for the coming decades.* Washington, DC: Author.

Cantwell, D. P. (1979). Implications of research in child psychiatry. In J. D. Noshpitz (Ed.), *Basic handbook of child psychiatry* (pp. 458–465). New York: Basic Books.

Cantwell, D. P. (1989). *Scientific status of child psychiatry.* Burlingame Award Lecture, Institute of the Living, Hartford, CT.

Cantwell, D. P., & Baker, L. (1991). *Psychiatric and developmental disorders in children with communication disorder.* Washington, DC: American Psychiatric Association Press.

Institute of Medicine. (1989). *Research on children and adolescents with mental, behavioral and developmental disorders.* Washington, DC: National Academy Press.

Jones, H. G. (1965). Research methodology in child psychiatry. In J. G. Howell (Ed.), *Modern perspectives in child psychiatry* (pp.3–21). Springfield, IL: Charles C Thomas.

Report of the Work Group on Scientific Issues. (1989). T. Shapiro, *American academy of child and adolescent psychiatry.*

Rutter, M. (1986). Child psychiatry looking thirty years ahead. *Journal of Child Psychology and Psychiatry, 27,* 803–840.

Rutter, M., Bolton, P., Harrington, R., Le Couteura, R., MacDonald, H., & Simonoff, E. (1990). Genetic factors in child psychiatric disorders: I. In review of research findings. II. Empirical research strategies. III. Empirical findings. *Journal of Child Psychology and Psychiatry, 31,* 3–84.

CHAPTER 17

Issues in Geriatric Research

DAVID A. LOEWENSTEIN AND CARL EISDORFER

INTRODUCTION

With the increasing number and proportion of the population growing older, more emphasis has been placed upon addressing the issues that are related to aging. This rapid growth of the elderly sector of our population has also prompted concerns about spiraling health care costs and the necessity for substantial research advances in the prevention and treatment of disease. It is remarkable that until recent years, the special characteristics and needs of elderly patients were largely neglected.

In psychiatry, the enthusiasm and interest which have surrounded these emerging areas, such as the study of dementia, geriatric psychopharmacology, psychopathology in later life, and psychotherapeutic interventions, have thus far outpaced the development of research paradigms and assessment instruments that are appropriate for use with an older adult population. Indeed, the study of aged individuals presents a challenge to investigators who must contend with such issues as medical co-morbidity, decreased perceptual thresholds, diverse educational and cultural backgrounds, as well as motivation and competence. These issues tend to increase between subject variability. To further complicate matters, researchers must also cope with the relative paucity of measures that have been validated with older adults and the special issues that are pertinent to longitudinal studies with the elderly, such as increased likelihood of subject attrition through illness and death. All of this reinforces the

David A. Loewenstein and Carl Eisdorfer • Department of Psychiatry and Center for Adult Development and Aging, University of Miami School of Medicine, Miami, Florida 33136.

Research in Psychiatry: Issues, Strategies, and Methods, edited by L. K. George Hsu and Michel Hersen. Plenum Press, New York, 1992.

contention that a broad knowledge of methodological issues is essential to the scientist who is conducting research with geriatric populations as well as the practitioner who needs to be informed about the newly emerging data. In the next decade, the burgeoning research in geriatric psychiatry will demand a special appreciation of such fundamental issues as reliability and validity, as well as appropriate research design and methodology if the clinician is to evaluate and to choose wisely among the different interventions and therapeutic modalities when they become available.

In this chapter, we will outline a broad array of issues that must be considered in conducting research as well as in interpreting findings based upon work with older adults. Measurement and the establishment of reliability and validity of specific procedures utilized with the elderly will also be discussed. Finally, examples of research paradigms and methodological approaches to the collection and analysis of data will be illustrated to demonstrate how special considerations of geriatric populations can be incorporated into prospective research designs to yield data that are both accurate and meaningful.

In order to gain a true appreciation of the pertinent issues specific to research with geriatric populations, it is important to consider some fundamental aspects of research design and methodology. A crucial aspect of any study centers around measurement. Whether we propose to examine reaction times, electrophysiological response, cerebral metabolic rates, or change in mood associated with a particular pharmacologic agent, it is essential that we have the means to observe and quantify these phenomena in such a way that the resultant measure can be shared and replicated. We become dependent upon the instrument of measurement that determines the extent to which we can obtain and interpret the information that we seek.

SCALES OF MEASUREMENT

For most biological, psychological, or social research, the end product of measurement is quantified on the basis of either nominal, ordinal, interval, or ratio level scales. The type of measure employed will determine in large part how data are collected and will, of necessity, influence the acceptable modes of statistical analyses and ultimately the interpretation of these data. Scales of measurement determine what questions can be asked of the data and are a limiting factor in determining which conclusions can subsequently be drawn.

A *nominal scale* is one in which the measures are differentiated by virtue of being different rather than being quantitatively related. Here the number is used as a name. For example, the numbers on football jerseys distinguish between players but do not rank or distinguish them as being more or less important than each other. In a research study, one might want to determine whether older and younger men differ in terms of their frequency of *yes, no,* or *maybe* responses to a particular question. Each of these three responses is qualitatively different, but one response does not have more value or is assigned more weight than another one. As a result, statistical treatment of these data might include a technique such as a chi-square analysis to determine whether these groups differ as to their distribution or expected frequencies for these types of responses.

An *ordinal scale* of measurement encompasses those values that can be ranked relative to each other but only indicates magnitude. For example, in a beauty contest, where finalists are ranked from first to tenth place, a 1 would be superior to a 2 and a 9 would be superior to a 10. However, the difference between 1 and 2 would not necessarily be the same as the difference between 9 and 10. Therefore, a number has no relationship to another number other than with its magnitude and degree of primacy.

An *interval scale* of measurement, on the other hand, assumes an equal interval between numbers. For example, if one were to rate social desirability on a 7-point Likert scale, the difference between 1 and 2 should hypothetically equal the distance between 6 and 7.

Finally, a *ratio scale* has all the characteristics of an interval level scale, with the addition of an absolute zero point (such as certain thermometers or a scale for measuring height or weight).

To sum up, the following are examples of different scales of measurement: (1) the *Nominal Scale*—Yes, no, or maybe responses; (2) the *Ordinal Scale*—finish of the horses in the Kentucky Derby; (3) the *Interval Scale*—the responses on a 1–7 Likert scale; and (4) the *Ratio Scale*—A Kelvin thermometer.

Data from an interval or ratio level scale would be analyzed differently from those of ordinal level scales. For example, an interval measure based on observations of the members of two independent groups would be analyzed using statistics, such as a student's *t*-test, whereas more than two groups would be analyzed utilizing an analysis of variance (ANOVA) procedure. For ordinal level data, analogous tests would be the Mann-Whitney U and the Kruskal-Wallis which are based upon a comparison of ranks.

RELIABILITY AND VALIDITY

Measurement is prone to errors of different types. The inability to obtain accurate readings of that which is under investigation can lead to experimenter misjudgments and thus to serious errors of inference. Therefore, the *reliability* of measures utilized in a particular investigation is important to ensure accuracy. Although reliability is assessed in a variety of ways, the most common types that investigators wish to establish include the following: (1) *Interrater reliability*—to determine whether different independent raters' scores record and quantify a series of identical observations in a similar manner; (2) *Test–retest reliability*—to determine the consistency or stability of a test score over time. For example, a person who is given an IQ test should obtain a similar score when the same test is administered a short time later; (3) *Internal consistency*—to determine whether items that tap a particular construct within a test are endorsed in a similar manner. One way to accomplish this is to divide the test in half and to correlate performance on one half of the test with another. Sophisticated statistical techniques utilizing coefficient alpha, Spearman-Brown, and Kuder-Richardson formulas are all means of assessing the internal consistency of a test (Allen & Yen, 1979).

While reliability (i.e., the extent to which the evaluation consistently measures the same thing) is important, equally important is the concept of *validity*. Validity reflects whether a certain test measures what it purports to measure. Although they are distinct entities, reliability and validity are related. For example, if we were to develop an interviewer-based scale for cognitive impairment, it first would be important to determine whether the cognitive impairment measure was reliable. One way to ascertain reliability would be to determine whether raters who utilized the instrument would rate a patient's cognitive impairment in a similar manner. Another type of reliability or stability of the measure could be established by determining whether the same person tested a day later under similar circumstances had a similar degree of cognitive impairment. In other words, it would be important to determine whether this technique for assessment of cognitive impairment was *consistent* over time. In approaching the concept of validity, however, it would be important to determine whether this new measure of global cognitive impairment truly measured cognitive impairment in a particular individual.

Validity can be established in a number of ways: (1) *Face validity* represents the weakest argument as a measure. It is based on a common sense approach to whether a test *seems* to measure what the investigator purports it to measure. (2) *Content validity* is established by the recorded experience of knowledgeable individuals in a particular field who are evaluating the content of a test to be certain that it is indeed tapping a particular domain. (3) *Concurrent or convergent validity* is determined by correlating or establishing the correspondence of the particular measure of interest and a separate measure which is widely recognized (ideally through research findings) as tapping into the targeted construct. (4) *Discriminative validity* involves establishing that a measure distinguishes between groups that it should differentiate. (5) *Factorial validity* is established by determining whether the constructs that theoretically underlie the measure are supported by factor analysis of the derived data.

Since reliability and validity are interrelated, the validity of a particular measure for example, can never exceed the square root of its reliability. Although this can be demonstrated mathematically, of interest for this discussion is that the accuracy of measurement has a sort of a rate-limiting influence on the validity of a specific measure.

RESEARCH WITH OLDER ADULT POPULATIONS

Whether one is a research investigator or a clinical consumer of research findings, it is important to gain an understanding of the techniques or procedures used (i.e., how reliable or how valid is a certain measure for use with older adults). One of the difficulties with many currently available instruments is that they have not been utilized or validated with geriatric populations (Kane & Kane, 1981; La Rue, 1987; Loewenstein, Amigo, Duara, Guterman, Hurwitz, Berkowitz, Wilkie, Weinberg, Black, Gittelman, & Eisdorfer, 1989). As a result, obtained measures are often prone to error because certain mediating variables or factors associated with aging may influence performance. Furthermore, though certain instruments may have been established as valid for younger groups, it is not clear that these measures reflect the same underlying processes for older adults. For example, it has been speculated that depression in younger adults, in whom there is often more expressed dysphoria and guilt, may be expressed differently than depression in older adults, in whom there is more generalized malaise, somatic concerns and preoccupations (Olsen, Guterman, Loewenstein, & Mintzer, 1988) and, indeed, a greater likelihood of physical dysfunction. It is therefore important that investigators who work with older individuals carefully assess the appropriateness of their testing measures in terms of their reliability and validity and that those reviewing such research be sensitive to the problem.

Factors to Consider in Research with Geriatric Populations

The following factors may influence the reliability and/or the validity of specific measures that are employed with older adults.

Sensory Input

One of the most common pitfalls in working with older adults is the failure to consider their potential difficulties with sensory input. As men and women grow older, there is an enhanced probability that difficulties with auditory and visual acuity may confound the interpretation of certain measures. For example, in neuropsychological investigations that are designed to examine brain–behavior relationships, written arithmetic is often administered to assess calculation ability. This is a useful and an appropriate measure for younger adult populations. However, among older adults, the written arithmetic may be difficult for the individual to discern because of the size of the print. As a result, determination as to whether poor performance is related to deficits in impaired arithmetic skills or visual acuity is often problematic. Similarly, psychological measures of expressive and receptive language skills or of memory can be confounded by the presence of an undetected auditory acuity deficit. In light of these difficulties, investigators need to design their studies carefully and may need to conduct pilot investigations prior to the actual investigation to determine whether any subtle sensory or memory loss will adversely affect performance on specific measures. Although some researchers routinely exclude those individuals with hearing and/or visual loss, this decision does not address the problem of individuals with undetected, albeit significant underlying problems. Pilot testing and appropriate modification of test stimuli are both important means with which to minimize potential difficulties with sensory impairment.

Mental Status

With advancing age, there is an enhanced probability that adults may suffer from cognitive impairment secondary to medical or neurological conditions (Kane & Kane, 1981). It had been estimated that 3 to 4 million people in the United States suffer from Alzheimer's disease and other forms of dementia (Cohen & Eisdorfer, 1986). But recent estimates suggest that more than 4 million individuals over the age of 65 years are affected by Alzheimer's disease alone (Evans, Funkenstein, Albert, Scherr, Cook, Chown, Herberty, Hennekens, & Taylor, 1989). Because many research investigations require intact cognitive function on the part of study participants, neuropsychological impairment or dementia may confound test results. One method of screening out those individuals with possible dementia is to conduct a diagnostic interview utilizing the DSM-III criteria for a dementia syndrome. One of the most widely utilized screening instruments for detection of cognitive impairment is the Folstein Mini-Mental State Examination (MMSE) (Folstein, Folstein, & McHugh, 1975), a 30-point scale tapping different aspects of memory, language, and visuoconstructive function. It is generally accepted that those patients with scores of 24 or above have normal cognition, whereas those individuals with scores of 23 or below may evidence cognitive impairment. Since this test is sensitive to educational and cultural factors, it should be utilized judiciously with any individual with a limited education or a cultural background significantly different from individuals who reside in the United States. Test results may also be influenced by the subject's command of the English language, particularly with regard to performance on measures tapping semantic memory and language skills. Tests, such as proverbs, that require a reasonable knowledge of idiomatic English may be impaired not as a function of deficits in abstraction but in communication.

It is probably judicious to utilize the MMSE in addition to a screening interview to determine eligibility for a study in which the cognitive status of participants may play an important role. In borderline cases, more extensive neuropsychological measures may be employed to determine a person's eligibility for a particular study.

Educational and Cultural Background

Performance on many measures is often influenced by degree of premorbid educational attainment. For example, many questionnaires require a certain level of reading comprehension. Other measures may require a certain level of arithmetic skills or exposure to specific types of prior knowledge.

Since a number of older adults come from different countries and backgrounds (where they have received only a limited amount of formal education), this variable should also be considered. In some cases, this factor has little bearing on a subject's performance or the investigator's interpretation of test results. In other instances, deficiencies in acquired academic skills may severely affect the subject's understanding of a particular task and severely confound performance. Once again, it may be advisable to conduct pilot testing before a study commences to determine the level of educational and/or other premorbid skills required to complete test material. Such pretesting will allow for the formulation of suitable inclusion/exclusion criteria to be utilized in the formal investigation.

Reaction Times and Response Tendency

Many investigators make the common error of not allowing suitable time limits for completion of test materials by older adults. This may present difficulties for older adults who are unnecessarily penalized for slower psycho-motor speed/reaction times. The problem can be minimized by judicious pilot testing before a study is conducted. Unless a study is specifically concerned with the measurement of reaction time *per se*, the issue of response latency can confound experimental results. A number of studies have indicated that some older persons, particularly men, may hold back responses if they are uncertain of the correct answer. Thus, control of such variables should be factored into experimental designs where results could be confounded by these issues.

Saliency and Familiarity of Test Material

The saliency of test material is often an important determinant of an individual's performance. For example, a memory test which contains elements that pertain to situations or concepts that are more familiar to younger people will be better remembered by those who are younger. Similarly, test items that are culturally bound will elicit a different response depending on an individual's cultural background. Older individuals who have never seen a computer may have difficulties in utilizing a computer terminal to make responses unless they are well practiced and familiarized with test equipment and materials. Pilot testing and careful construction of test items will help the investigator to avoid such difficulties. Some tests require complex performance. Thus, working with dotted lines and geometric figures may be familiar to those who have been more recently educated. However, this kind of test procedure may slow down the older novice. Similarly, the style of the question, such as a complex multiple-choice format which requires "test-taking experience," should be carefully screened for its value in assessing what is being evaluated.

Physical Health

With investigations that focus on the cognitive, psychological, or physiological functioning of normal adults, it is generally assumed that subjects are healthy and that measures are not confounded as a function of a particular disease state. In older adults, the increased probability of underlying disease and/or use of different medications requires a careful medical screening in studies where poor health or certain medication regimens could affect obtained results. For example, in studies involving the study of cognitive processes in healthy elderly individuals, the investigator must take into account the greater risk of cerebrovascular disease and neuropsychiatric conditions that might affect cognition.

In our cognitive/neuropsychological studies of normal elderly adults, all participants receive a comprehensive medical, neurological, and psychiatric evaluation, as well as psychometric screening to ensure that there are no underlying conditions which would adversely affect cognitive performance. In many of our studies, we obtain Magnetic Resonance Imaging (MRI) of the brain to rule out ischemic lesions or other abnormalities that may not be identified upon routine examination (Duara, Barker, Loewenstein, Pascal, & Bowen, 1989). A thorough evaluation of normal elderly volunteers is essential in many of our projects which demand that participants be "truly healthy." In actual practice, it is often difficult and cost prohibitive to conduct extensive medical evaluations on those individuals who are study participants. Depending on the research question, medical questionnaires or a brief medical screening are often adequate to exclude certain individuals with specific health problems or to account for spurious factors in subsequent statistical analysis of particular sets of data.

Motivation

One cannot automatically assume that older adults are motivated to participate in all investigations or to comply with study directives in the same manner as younger adults. For example, we have experienced difficulties recruiting normal elderly controls for neuropsychological normative studies, since many older adults are anxious about taking any test that might reveal a memory deficit. Younger participants rarely exhibit such anxiety. Furthermore, younger participants may be much more exposed to or familiar with participating in research investigations, whereas older adults may not possess such familiarity. Special attention must be paid to such issues as length of task, potential for patient fatigue, adequate debriefing, and clarity of test instructions/ materials when working with older study patients. Moreover, reinforcements for younger and older volunteers may differ. College students may be required to "volunteer" to gain experience, whereas some older volunteers may wish to obtain free examinations, have early access to new medications, or simply relieve boredom. Attention to motivational issues is often minimal, yet they can affect the data significantly.

External Validity

Thus far, we have focused our attention on threats to experimental or internal validity when conducting research with older adults. Another potential difficulty with research utilizing older adult populations is the lack of generalizability or external validity. Simply put, *external validity* relates to the extent to which the results of a particular investigation can be applied to a specific population. Neugarten (1974) divided the older population into three categories. The young-old, who are 55 to 65 years old, are often working and are at the peak of their social and vocational status. On the other hand, the middle-old, aged 65 to 75, make up the majority of the retired population. The old-old, who are over age 75, are generally thought of as the poorest and frailest of elderly adults (Rogers, 1982). Although other classification systems exist, suffice it to say that older people are certainly not a homogeneous group. As such, it is quite important that results from a particular investigation not be automatically generalized or applied to all older adults. For example, certain medications may be very effective for individuals in their 50s and 60s. To assume that this treatment regimen would necessarily be effective for persons in their 70s, 80s, and 90s may be erroneous. The general age of a study population has a direct bearing on health status, work status, marital status, perceptual changes (particularly vision and hearing), cognitive impairment, certain attitudes, financial resources, physiological responses, and reactions to certain pharmacologic agents. As such, the results of a particular study should only be generalized to the appropriate age groups. In studies where a wide range of older adults are utilized, covariate analyses should be employed to statistically determine if treatment effects are associated with chronological age. Even when groups are randomly selected from an older population, the relatively small numbers of subjects employed by most investigators does not always ensure that groups will be equivalent relative to age. Covariate analysis statistically determines the effect of age on the outcome variable(s) of interest and statistically allows for corrections so that any differences in age are adjusted for.

In the study of older adults, it is important for the researcher to consider the limits of generalizing from results that are based on a particular sample. For example, a study that examines patterns of behavioral disturbance among agitated Alzheimer disease (AD) patients by definition utilizes subjects who are self-selected, since they are those persons who have been *identified* as having AD and those who have agreed (or their families have agreed for them) to be studied. Patients in one section of the country may have different interpersonal behavioral presentations simply because they have different living arrangements. Patterns of interactions with family members or access to particular resources may vary by region and culture. Certainly, patients who are nursing home residents may have different patterns of agitation from those patients who live at home, and the degree of agitation may be related to such factors as degree of cognitive impairment, co-morbid psychiatric disease, and the social setting and sensory stimulation within the environment. As such, it is important that the researcher be prudent in generalizing results from a particular study to any other population than that represented by the sample. A main consideration in maintaining external validity is to ensure that the study sample reflects a representative subset of the larger population to which the researcher wishes to generalize. Research findings can be applied only to the larger population for which the subjects were representative.

In summary, a concern with internal validity identifies the methodological flaws and confounds that may render the results of a particular study uninterpretable and meaningless. On the other hand, external validity applies to the correct generalization of the results of the study to the population that is represented by the study sample.

Illustrations

The concepts of reliability and validity can be examined by using as a model a study (Loewenstein et al., 1989) that described, developed, and validated functional assessment instruments for older adults. A functional assessment scale allows trained raters to behaviorally assess such functional capacities as telling time, using the telephone, preparing a letter for mailing, counting currency, writing a check, balancing a checkbook, shopping for groceries, as well as eating and dressing/grooming subskills. After two years of pilot testing and test construction/modification, the next step involved a determination as to whether the test was reliable (accurate) and valid (measuring what was intended to be measured). To establish reliability, a group of patients with dementia and a group of normal healthy elderly controls were assembled and required to perform those tasks that were part of the newly developed Direct Assessment of Functional Status scale (DAFS). Two trained raters independently rated the functional performance of individuals within each of the two study groups so that the *interrater reliability* of each functional subscale could be established. Interrater reliabilities for each functional subscale for both cognitively impaired patients and normal controls were established by examining rater concordance utilizing Cohen's *kappa*, a procedure designed to measure interrater reliability while accounting for chance agreement. The high interrater reliabilities obtained by Loewenstein et al. (1989) ensured that the DAFS instrument could be scored and interpreted in a *similar* manner by different raters.

Test–retest reliability was established by reevaluating both patients and controls several weeks after their initial assessment to determine the *consistency* or *stability* of performance on the DAFS functional scale. If subjects obtained very different scores on different administrations of a test, the researcher should certainly question the reliability of that measure. In this instance, we contrasted the total scores on each functional subscale at Testing 1 and compared these to the performance on these scales at Testing 2 for both cognitively impaired and neurologically normal participants. Performance on a particular subscale was evaluated for consistency across Time 1 and Time 2 using the Spearman rank-order correlation coefficient. This ensured that the total subscale scores from Time 1 to Time 2 were related to one another (e.g., reliable). Of course, the correlation of Time 1 and Time 2 scores only means that they are related. It does not necessarily mean that the scores for any person are identical or that the same total scores were derived from an endorsement of similar items from Time 1 to Time 2. In this case, it would have been beneficial to examine patterns of *internal consistency* across the two testing sessions. Coefficient alpha, Spearman-Brown, and Kuder-Richardson formulas can all be utilized to determine internal consistency (Allen & Yen, 1979).

Validity was also a necessary consideration in the Loewenstein *et al.* (1989) study. Convergent validity was established by comparing patient's total score on the newly developed DAFS functional scale with a well-established measure designed to measure reported functional status at home. We utilized the Blessed Dementia Rating Scale (BDRS) (Blessed, Tomlinson, & Roth, 1968), which has been established as a measure of general functional status in both research and clinical settings. In our investigation, the correlation between the total BDRS score and the DAFS functional measure was −.588. The correlation between a modified BDRS score (which excluded items related to affect and mood and only tapped specific behaviors related to functional performance within the home) and the DAFS score was −.673, indicating a moderately strong relation between the two measures. Subsequently, convergent validity was also established for individual subscales comprising the DAFS instrument by comparing them to other functional indices that tap the patient's functional behavior within the home environment.

In a study (Loewenstein *et al.*, 1989) designed to establish discriminative validity, the performance of Alzheimer's disease (AD) patients was contrasted to that of elderly patients with a primary depression and with healthy elderly controls. There were no statistically significant differences between depressives and normal controls on any of the functional subscales. However, relative to normal controls, the AD group scored lower on scales tapping such abilities as using the telephone, preparing a letter for mailing, identifying road signs, counting currency, writing a check, balancing a checkbook, and shopping with a written list. AD patients did not score lower on their ability to tell time, to identify currency, or to employ basic eating and dressing/grooming skills. Presumably, these functions do not deteriorate until the later stages of the disease process.

In summary, the DAFS functional scale was found to have excellent inter-rater and test–retest reliabilities for patients presenting to a memory disorders clinic with cognitive impairment and for normal elderly controls. Furthermore, the instrument evidenced both convergent and discriminative validity. Face and content validity were established during the pilot-testing phase of the project. Since control subjects were observed and rated on tasks that they were required to perform in their home environment, it is highly unlikely that the patients would have derived any significant advantage through the use of environmental cues. Indeed, the strong convergent validity evidenced by the DAFS scale indicates that the instrument taps functional skills utilized in the patient's everyday life.

In a second study, the investigators wished to determine whether the administration of a certain medication would affect learning in the elderly. They selected 30 subjects from a nursing home and randomly assigned each one to one of three treatment groups. The subjects were then administered either Drug A, Drug B, or Drug C. Each subject in one of the three groups received 100 mg of the drug per day for 4 weeks. Measures of learning in the subjects were obtained at weekly intervals over the course of the study. At the end of the investigation, statistical analysis revealed that there was no difference between the drugs as to learning at Week 1, Week 2, and Week 3. However, all groups showed an improvement over their poor 1 to 3 performances at Week 4. It was then concluded that none of these drugs had an effect on learning in the elderly after 3 weeks, but at Week 4, all three drugs seemed to facilitate learning.

However, there are a number of problems with the aforementioned study. First, the investigators did not establish baseline performance on the learning measure for the three groups. Specifically, it is possible that the study groups may not have started out with the same degree of learning proficiency on the test. If one group actually had superior performance on the task prior to the administration of the drug, then the fact that performance of the three groups were equivalent at Weeks 1 to 3 indicates that the other two drugs may indeed have had an effect. Some investigators erroneously assume that because subjects are randomly assigned to treatment groups, their baseline learning performance should be relatively equivalent. In fact, this probably would occur only in studies with extremely large sample sizes. However, in clinical research, investigators rarely have the luxury of such large groups of individuals. Therefore, it is clear that initial baseline performance should be ascertained. Subsequently, any initial differences in age or learning performance could be corrected for by covariate analyses that can statistically equate groups and can correct for initial group differences. Were the subjects matched for gender and were other factors that may have been different between the two groups (e.g., anxiety) sufficiently controlled for? What was the breakdown of study participants in terms of educational attainment, gender, and cultural background? Another concern with this type of investigation stems from the nature of the dependent measure employed. Has this measure of learning been shown to be reliable and valid for older adults in the age ranges examined in this study? Are there demonstrable practice effects associated with the measure, and did the results obtained at Week 4 merely reflect increasing familiarity with the test (e.g., practice effects)? Inclusion of a placebo control group that was tested with the learning measure at Weeks 1 to 4 and a baseline learning measure obtained for all groups before administration of a particular drug or placebo would have provided the necessary information to draw valid inferences and to address some of the aforementioned concerns. As the study stands, there is no way of determining whether any of the drugs truly had an effect and, if so, at what point a specific effect was evident.

In this hypothetical investigation, there was no mention of ages or age ranges, so that the generalizability of this experiment, had it been internally valid, is unknown. Furthermore, the use of nursing home residents raises the possibility of co-morbid physical disease, perceptual difficulties, or cognitive impairment, which may have confounded the results. What was the motivation for subjects to participate in the study? Was the learning test too simple (ceiling effects) or too difficult (floor effects)? Many of these questions could have been put to rest if the investigators had conducted appropriate pilot testing prior to the administration of the formal study. The investigators utilized 100 mg of each drug, but each class of medication may have optimal doses for a desired effect, and these may well be different for the elderly than with younger individuals. Perhaps the administration of the investigational drugs should have been individually titrated for each individual or blood levels with the drug should have been assessed rather than the dose. Indeed, this could have been included as part of the analyses. Would the research design have been more powerful if after Week 4 a particular drug were replaced with placebo and later readministered to determine whether withdrawal and subsequent readministration of the drug supported the notion of efficacy? Finally, could the lack of group differences during Weeks 1 to 3 be attributed to the small sample sizes utilized and the resultant lack of statistical power?

Power is the ability of a statistical test to detect true group differences when indeed they do exist or in rejecting the null hypothesis when the assumption of no differences between groups is false. When small numbers of subjects are utilized, it takes a substantial difference between groups on a particular measure to achieve statistical significance. Conversely, with very large numbers of subjects, small or even trivial differences can be statistically significant. (A statistician friend of ours once commented that if one expected a substantially large difference between groups, one would need relatively few subjects per group since it is possible to catch large bass in a net with a large mesh. If one's desire is to catch minnows or to look for small effects, then one needs many little holes (i.e, a fine mesh) or large numbers of subjects so that the minnows or the small effects will not slip out undetected.) Thus, an important part of any research investigation is to determine what differences between groups would be clinically meaningful and then to calculate the number of subjects required to obtain an adequate degree of power. A discussion of statistical power and power analysis can be found in Cohen (1987).

In a hypothetical third study, investigators wanted to determine whether Alzheimer's Disease (AD) patients who were depressed evidence more functional impairment than AD patients who are not depressed. The investigators matched AD patients on age and a measure of global cognitive impairment and utilized caregivers' reports of functional status as the dependent measure. Results indicated that depressed AD patients actually evidenced lower scores on the functional measure than their nondepressed counterparts. It was concluded, therefore, that depression further impairs an AD patient's ability to perform essential activities of daily living and that treatment of depression may improve a patient's functional performance.

There are a number of limitations associated with this hypothetical investigation. First, we are not informed how a diagnosis of either AD or depression is being rendered. Is the diagnosis of depression scaled as present versus absent or can the actual magnitude of depression be quantified? Ultimately, severity of depression may be more important than merely a knowledge of whether depression exists. For example, it may be possible that specific functional impairments are associated only with severe depression or that the effects of depression on functional status is dependent on level of cognitive function. This, of course, would argue for obtaining both measures of the severity of depressive symptomatology and cognitive deterioration, preferably utilizing an interval or ratio level scale of measurement. Any measure of cognition or depression would have to be reliable and valid for this sample of subjects. Assuming that qualified professionals were utilized in the current investigation and were able to accurately diagnose depression in the study group, we are still left with the question about the functional status measure. A fundamental question is whether this functional assessment instrument is reliable for this particular sample of AD patients. Furthermore, it is possible that functional performance as assessed by the judgments of caregivers may be biased relative to the informants' relation to the patient, the extent of time they spend with the patient, their denial of patient deficits, or, conversely, their oversensitivity to the patient's suspected impairments. Do the caregivers' levels of distress and their own affective states influence their assessment of the patients' levels of function and, if so, is their affective state related to the affective states of the patients? One possible explanation for these results is that depressed patients *appeared* to have decreased functional capacity only because they were more withdrawn and *unwilling* to engage in their activities of daily living. If this were the case, the inference that depression further diminishes the functional capacities of AD patients would certainly be questionable. Finally, we are not given any information about patients' and caregivers' characteristics, such as age and gender. Furthermore, caregiver variables, such as relation to a patient (e.g., spouse versus daughter), living arrangements (home versus Adult Congregate Living Facility), and degree of daily contact may all be extremely important mediating variables as to how functional performance is assessed. In this particular study, it would have been more beneficial to utilize a standardized instrument directly measuring function that is not reliant on caregivers' judgments and that has been validated with cognitively impaired and nonimpaired elderly adults (which also can be employed with depressed and nondepressed AD patients).

One further methodologic issue of consequence that can influence studies of adult life and aging and actually affect all longitudinal research relates to cross-sectional versus longitudinal designs. If a researcher were in a rush to complete a study on the effects of aging on some psychiatric or psychological variable within a year or so, it obviously would be impossible to conduct the study in real time. Real-time studies involve the identification of a population and then subsequently following it longitudinally. Such a procedure could help the researcher to understand the effect of aging or of a life event (e.g., retirement, the loss of a spouse, or a disease). Difficulties with real-time studies include that of the cohort effect. Specifically, how does a group of 65-year-old individuals differ from previous and future age cohorts at 65 years of age? For example, those individuals who are reaching age 65 in 1991 may have very different characteristics from those who became 65 in 1981 or in 1971. Educational attainment, childhood-rearing practices, widespread social events (e.g., a world war), and exposure to illnesses are examples of crucial variables which may influence a particular cohort of individuals, thus confounding any simple attribution of a finding to an age *per se*. As such, it is potentially risky to attribute certain features to 65-year-old individuals without evaluating the potential impact of specific cohort effects.

Still another difficulty with longitudinal analyses is that investigators may be limited in the length of time that a cohort can be followed.

Methods that employ overlapping groups of individuals over time (i.e., the cross-sequential study model) attempt to compensate for some of the problems inherent in longitudinal studies by abbreviating the time required for certain analyses. Thus, groups of persons who are 50 to 55, 55 to 60, 60 to 65, and 65 to 70 can be followed for 10 years to extrapolate to a study of 50- to 80-year-old individuals in 10 rather than in 30 years. This, then, represents a cross-sequential model. In addition, more sophisticated models enable investigators to study overlap between groups to explore possible cohort effects.

In studying the aging process or the natural history of a disease, a simple cross-sectional design is best used as a pilot in order to generate hypotheses that are then tested utilizing more sophisticated longitudinal models.

One final issue refers to that of homogeneity versus heterogeneity of different constellations of patient presentations and behaviors. In recognition of the great heterogeneity found in studies of later life, Eisdorfer (1984) proposed a number of postulates that may be used to disaggregate diseases of later life which may appear as a final entity. For example, dementia has a number of established etiologies. On the other hand, Alzheimer's disease (where less is known) may, in the end, represent *several conditions* with a final similar presentation. A model of such heterogeneity exists in pneumonia, now recognized as a heterogeneous condition, with each case having its own differential diagnosis.

The postulates for heterogeneity proposed by Eisdorfer (1984) are as follows:

1. More than one etiology is found for what appears to be a phenomenologically similar state.
2. Risk factors differ for different groups (e.g., one subgroup is shown to have a particular genetic predisposition).
3. A given treatment is only effective in one subgroup of patients.
4. There are differences in the physical and behavioral manifestations of the disease.
5. The clinical course may be different between groups. For example, one group may show specific changes in function or tends to die earlier.

Consideration of heterogeneity among different disorders and disease states among the elderly can enhance our understanding of particular disease processes. Such consideration can also serve to facilitate more powerful research studies by avoiding the indiscriminate lumping of all older adult subjects into a particular group. Indeed, these subjects are probably heterogeneous and, if they are considered uniformly, important differences could be masked.

SUMMARY

In this chapter, we have examined those factors that are important to assess when conducting research with geriatric populations. Sensory and physiological thresholds, physical health, psychomotor speed/reaction times, educational and cultural background, as well as motivation all represent important mediating variables. If not accounted or controlled for, they can threaten the internal and external validity of a particular study. When using assessment measures with the elderly, it is important that they be both reliable and valid *for that population*. In the absence of complete reliability/validity data for instruments in a particular area, investigators must decide whether to develop and validate their own existing measures or to select those instruments that currently have the most extensive validation data and that have been widely used with geriatric populations. Whatever type of dependent measure is ultimately selected, pilot testing is an important aspect of any research investigation. The results of preliminary work prior to a formal study can help to identify potential difficulties and suggest appropriate modifications in the research paradigm. External validity or generalizability is important in any study and often is problematic in investigations with older subjects. It is important to view a sample of subjects as a subset of a larger population. As such, the results of a particular investigation can only be applied to the population actually represented by the study participants. For example, results obtained by young-old subjects cannot necessarily be applied to the old-old. Finally, researchers are obligated to review carefully the methodological and statistical aspects of a particular investigation to evaluate the meaning of obtained results and their applicability to specific elderly clinical and research populations.

REFERENCES

Allen, M. J., & Yen, W. M. (1979). *Introduction to measurement theory*. Belmont, CA: Wadsworth.

Blessed, G., Tomlinson, B. E., & Roth, M. (1968). Association between quantitative measures of dementing and senile change in the cerebral grey matter of elderly subjects. *British Journal of Psychiatry, 114*, 197–211.

Bowen, B., Barker, W. W., Loewenstein, D. A., Sheldon, J., & Duara, R. (1990). MR signal abnormalities in memory disorder and dementia. *American Journal of Neuroradiology, 11*, 283–290.

Cohen, J. (1987). *Statistical power analysis for the behavioral sciences*. Hillsdale, NJ: Lawrence Erlbaum.

Cohen, D., & Eisdorfer, C. (1986). *The loss of self*. New York: W. W. Norton.

Duara, R., Barker, W. W., Loewenstein, D., Pascal, S., & Bowen, B. (1989). Sensitivity and specificity of positron emission tomography (PET) in aging and dementia. *European Neurology, 29*, 9–15.

Eisdorfer, C. (1984). *On heterogeneity of Alzheimer's disease*. Paper presented to the Albert Einstein College of Medicine Symposium on Aging.

Evans, D. A., Funkenstein, H. H., Albert, M. S., Scherr, P. A., Cook, N. R., Chown, M. J., Herberty, L. E., Hennekens, C. H., & Taylor, J. O. (1989). Prevalence of Alzheimer's disease in a community population of older persons: Higher than previously reported. *Journal of the American Medical Association, 262*, 2551–2556.

Folstein, M. F., Folstein, S., & McHugh, P. R. (1975). Minimental state: A practical method for grading the cognitive state of patients for the clinician. *Journal of Psychiatric Research, 12*, 289–298.

Kane, R. A., & Kane, R. L. (1981). *Assessing the elderly: A practical guide to measurement*. Lexington, MA: Heath.

La Rue, A. (1987). Methodological concerns: Longitudinal studies of dementia. *Alzheimer's Disease and Associated Disorders, 1*, 180–192.

Loewenstein, D. A., Amigo, E., Duara, R., Guterman, A., Hurwitz, D., Berkowitz, N., Wilkie, F., Weinberg, G., Black, B., Gittelman, G., & Eisdorfer, C. (1989). A new scale for the assessment of functional status in Alzheimer's disease and related disorders. *Journal of Gerontology, 44*, 114–121.

Neugarten, B. L. (1974, September). Age groups in American society and the rise of the young-old. *Annals of the American Academy*, 187–198.

Olsen, E., Guterman, A., Loewenstein, D. A. M., & Mintzer, J. (1988). Depression in the older patient: Common but complex. *The Older Patient, 2*, 12–18.

Rogers, D. (1982). *The adult years: An introduction to aging*. Englewood Cliffs, NJ: Prentice-Hall.

CHAPTER 18

The Chronically Mentally Ill

SHIRLEY M. GLYNN

INTRODUCTION

In working with the chronically mentally ill, empirical investigations and clinical treatments share many similarities. Both require a commitment to interacting with relatively impaired patients whose gains can typically be measured best after months or years of intervention, rather than days or weeks. Both involve working with patients who frequently have limited resources, lead impoverished lives, and require as much aid in the "nuts and bolts" of living as they do symptom relief. Finally, at least at our present level of knowledge, both researchers and clinicians who are working with the chronically mentally ill must be prepared to be confronted with the limits of their efforts. Whether they work in academic research settings or in public mental health clinics, psychiatrists and other mental health professionals must anticipate that, regardless of the intervention, the majority of chronically mentally ill patients are unable to return to their highest level of premorbid functioning (Stephens, 1978) and that some minority of patients appear to achieve very limited benefits from either psychopharmacologic and/or psychosocial treatments (Davis, Schaffer, Killian, Kinard, & Chan, 1980).

Even in light of the time required to do research with the chronically mentally ill, the difficulty in working with severely impaired patients, and the continual need to recognize (although not necessarily to submit to) treatment

Shirley M. Glynn • Veterans Administration Medical Center of West Los Angeles, Los Angeles, California 90073.

Research in Psychiatry: Issues, Strategies, and Methods, edited by L. K. George Hsu and Michel Hersen. Plenum Press, New York, 1992.

limitations, investigators committed to research with the seriously psychi-atrically ill have a unique opportunity to develop assessment and intervention techniques which may have a profound effect on their subjects' lives. This endeavor is especially important because the chronically mentally ill have long been an underserved population who have critical need of the benefits and positive outcomes of research investigations. Over the long haul, the challenges of research with the chronically mentally ill can be more than offset by the rewards to both the investigator and the subject.

Research is, of course, an exacting pursuit which requires careful attention to a myriad of details that distinguish a major contribution to knowledge from a worthless expenditure of time and resources. Because the other chapters in this volume focus on more general issues concerning research design, data analysis, and interpretation of results, this chapter will highlight those topics which are most critical in pursuing research with the chronically mentally ill. Since some of the issues addressed here (e.g., assessment) are also covered in other chapters, the reader is encouraged to consider all of the information in the volume before designing an empirical investigation. However, the topics dis-cussed in this chapter are those requiring the most careful attention when conducting research with the chronically mentally ill.

First, I will begin by discussing issues pertaining to subject selection and description. Although this topic may seem rather obvious, many researchers fail to address this area adequately, making it difficult for others to interpret their findings. Second, I will discuss issues relevant to the conceptualization and operationalization of the *independent variables*. The independent variable is the variable manipulated by the investigator in the experiment. In psychiatry research, the independent variable is often a particular treatment intervention (e.g., a specific medication or a type of psychotherapy). I will follow with a discussion of the critical considerations concerning *dependent variables*. In a true experiment, the dependent variables can be understood as those characteristics which might be expected to change as a result of the variable under the investigators' control. For example, an experimenter may hypothesize that administration of a specific pharmacologic agent (the independent variable) should relieve depressive symptoms (the dependent variable). However, depres-sion can be measured in many different ways (e..g, by self-report, through behavioral observation, by clinical interview, by reports of significant others) using a number of different scales, and the researcher must be alert to the benefits and costs of each measurement strategy and tool. Poor choice of a dependent measure has ruined many otherwise well-conceptualized experi-ments; therefore, the common pitfalls in the selection of dependent variables when working with the chronically mentally ill will be highlighted in this section.

Some research designs do not include actual experimental manipulation of variables, but instead examine the relationship of variables which occur natu-rally (e.g., IQ, family history of mental illness, etc.) and, thus, cannot be controlled by the experimenter. These are called *quasi-experiments* or *correlational studies*. Most of the discussion of independent and dependent variables will also pertain to the predictor and predicted variables in these alternative research designs.

A final introductory statement is in order. Thus far, I have written as if there were a widely accepted, consensual definition of the term the *chronically mentally ill*. However, a recent review of the definition of chronic mental illness used by the 50 states in allocating services and resources found marked disparities in conceptualization of this term (Schinnar, Rothbard, Kanter, & Adams, 1990). For example, all states used diagnoses of schizophrenia or affective disorders for inclusion in this category, but there was variability in whether such diagnoses as organic psychoses, personality disorders, and neuroses were also included.

In her excellent article on the conceptualization of chronic mental illness, Bachrach (1988) suggested that diagnosis, duration of illness, and ensuing functioning disability are all critical, but somewhat independent, aspects of chronic mental illness. Importantly, in recognition of the increasing prominence of community-based treatment, Bachrach did not consider prior or current psychiatric hospitalization as a defining characteristic of this population. In this chapter, I shall observe the recommendations made by Bachrach and explicitly define the overall population of interest using the criteria of diagnosis, duration of illness, and functional disability. In the following discussion of research issues, I am highlighting those that particularly apply to adult persons with diagnoses in the DSM-III-R (American Psychiatric Association, 1987) 295-301 series (which includes schizophrenic, affective, anxiety, and personality disorders), who have evidenced or might be expected to evidence long-term (greater than 6 months) psychiatric symptoms in support of the diagnosis and/ or impairments in multiple domains of functioning (e.g., occupationally, socially, personal care, etc.). This definition specifically excludes those subjects whose primary diagnosis is mental retardation, organic brain syndrome, or substance abuse.

SUBJECT SELECTION AND DESCRIPTION

One of the most critical issues facing a researcher in the field of chronic mental illness is deciding on the necessary characteristics of the population required to answer the experimental question of interest. An equally pressing issue involves locating persons who possess these characteristics and then persuading them (or their legal representatives) to participate in the investigation. Although both of these endeavors may sound quite straightforward, they require careful thought and a high energy level. In many ways, the experimental question helps to define the necessary features of the potential subject pool. For example, a new antipsychotic medication might be developed for persons with schizophrenia, or a new psychosocial treatment to cope with anxiety associated with depression might be tested. Obviously, only persons meeting the diag nosis for the relevant disorder would be accepted into the protocol. However, there are at least three issues which merit additional consideration in the development and implementation of a research protocol: (1) subject demographics, (2) subject clinical characteristics (concurrent psychiatric diagnoses, current clinical status, and phase of illness), and (3) locating and recruiting participants.

Subject Demographics

Demographics can play a pivotal role in subject selection and interpretation of the results of research investigations. Consider, for example, the issue of subject gender. It has been well documented that males predominate in most psychiatric (as well as general medical) subject samples (Wahl, 1977). Reasons for this overrepresentation of males in psychiatric research include the disproportionate number of men found in inpatient settings (Seeman, 1986) in which much research is conducted, and fears of the potential teratogenic effects of many novel psychopharmacologic compounds (Mogul, 1985).

However, gender may be a critical issue in interpreting the results of psychiatric studies, and this omission may have detrimental results. Consider, for example, a recent study by Haas, Glick, Clarkin, Spencer, and Lewis (1990) on the differential response of male and female patients to inpatient family intervention. These investigators randomly assigned patients to participate in a multifaceted inpatient program alone or *in conjunction with* psychoeducational family therapy. At 18-months follow-up, they found that female patients appeared to benefit from the addition of family therapy to their other treatment, whereas males appeared to do worse in the combined condition. These results suggest that gender may be a critical variable in explaining the positive outcomes of family-based interventions, yet a number of recent family intervention studies on schizophrenic patients failed to even report statistical analyses of sex effects (e.g., Falloon, Boyd, McGill, Razani, Moss, & Gilderman, 1982; Hogarty, Anderson, Reiss, Kornblith, Greenwald, Javna, & Madonia, 1986). Given the findings of Haas *et al.* (1990), an examination of gender effects in these other studies might have been very revealing. Investigators who fail to examine gender differences in their results or who omit females from their samples without justification limit the usefulness of their results.

Similarly, ethnic differences may play an important role in explaining empirical results and must thus be carefully evaluated. For example, it has now been documented that Asians display a unique sensitivity to neuroleptic medication, and thus frequently require lower dosages to achieve a therapeutic effect (Lin, Poland, Nuccio, Matsuda, Hathuc, Su, & Fu, 1989). Investigators wishing to pursue research with these pharmacologic agents need to make informed decisions about how best to design their studies to be certain that the differential responses to a medication which are seen in an ethnic group do not obscure any other relevant experimental findings.

Clinical Characteristics

Diagnostic Issues

Careful thought must be paid to issues pertaining more specifically to the characteristics of the illness itself. Accurate diagnosis is, of course, a critical prerequisite in most psychiatric research. Typically, investigators must ensure that the subjects in their studies have been diagnosed reliably using a widely accepted diagnostic system, such as the DSM-III-R or the ICD-9-CM (World Health Organization, 1980). Under most circumstances, these diagnoses must be based on comprehensive interviews of patients using such structured formats as the Present State Exam (PSE) (Wing, Cooper, & Sartorius, 1974) or the Structured Clinical Interview System (SCID) (Spitzer & Williams, 1985).

With our advancing refinements of nosology in psychiatry, even greater attention will need to be paid to the issue of accurate diagnosis, especially as this pertains to assessment of *subtypes* of various disorders as well as to the presence of other concurrent psychiatric diagnoses in a research subject. For example, in the field of schizophrenia, there is currently great emphasis being placed on the subtyping of schizophrenic patients into those who experience predominantly positive symptoms (e.g., hallucinations, delusions) versus those who experience predominantly negative symptoms (e.g., poverty of speech, affective flattening). Much of this interest in subtyping based on symptoms is sparked by the hypothesis of Crow (1980, 1985) that these different symptoms may have different etiologies, and thus different courses and remedies. Needless to say, most researchers in schizophrenia would be wise to assess both positive and negative symptoms in their sample in order to examine any effects related to schizophrenic subtype.

Just as identifying subtypes of psychiatric illnesses is attracting more research interest, so is the examination of the impact of concurrent psychiatric diagnoses. For example, a recent large-scale depression study contrasted two psychotherapeutic interventions—interpersonal problem-solving therapy (Klerman, Weissman, Rounsaville, & Chevron, 1984) and cognitive therapy (Beck, Rush, Shaw, & Emery, 1979)—with imipramine and a placebo clinical management control (Elkin, Shea, Watkins, Imber, Sotsky, Collins, Glass, Pilkonis, Leber, Docherty, Fiester, & Parloff, 1989). There was a significant improvement in depression for most patients over the duration of the study. Generally, subjects in the imipramine condition showed the most improvement, those in the placebo clinical management condition showed the least, and subjects in the psychotherapeutic conditions were in between. Not surprisingly, a subsequent analysis revealed that these treatment effects were attenuated in depressed patients with concurrent personality disorders (Shea, Pilkonis, Beckham, Collins, Elkin, Sotsky, & Docherty, 1990). In addition, although statistical significance was not achieved, the authors interpreted their data as suggesting that patients with concurrent personality disorders benefitted more from the cognitive therapy, whereas the patients without concurrent personality disorders did better in the other treatment conditions. The primary result was best understood by seeing the patient in the context of his or her other psychopathology. This finding highlights the importance of evaluating a broad range of symptoms and of considering the possible impact of concurrent diagnoses when designing studies and interpreting results.

No discussion of diagnostic issues in research on the chronically mentally ill would be complete without mention of complications that are due to substance abuse. Just as in the general population, substance abuse and dependence is becoming a more prominent problem among the chronically mentally ill (Brown, Ridgely, Pepper, Levine, & Ryglewicz, 1989). Subject substance use can raise two especially problematic issues for the researcher. First, substance use can sometimes compromise the accurate diagnosis of a potential research participant. For example, consider the case of a 30-year-old patient who has been experiencing paranoid delusions and auditory hallucinations consistent with a diagnosis of schizophrenia intermittently for the past 8 years, but who also reports heavy alcohol consumption and cocaine use around the time the symptoms began and continuing through to the present. In such a case, the patient's inability to recall accurately the exact circumstances surrounding the initial exacerbation of symptoms coupled with the continued substance abuse which prohibits the evaluation of symptoms when the patient is substance free probably precludes making a diagnosis with enough certainty to merit inclusion in a research protocol.

Second, even when a clear diagnosis can be made, continued substance abuse may adversely affect the patient's symptomatology, which can be especially troubling in an intervention study in which symptom severity serves as the dependent measure. Ideally, substance abusing patients would probably be excluded from research protocols that do not specifically examine the substance abuse issue. Unfortunately, in many settings, such a policy would seriously diminish the number of subjects available for research. In addition, excluding these subjects would greatly reduce the generalizability of findings to the large population of patients with concurrent substance abuse. In many cases, the only option available to the researcher is to allow recruitment of substance-abusing patients who have met other inclusion and exclusion criteria for the study, to monitor subsequent substance use through toxicology screens and clinical interviews, and to examine the influence of substance use on the dependent variables of interest.

Current Clinical Status

Diagnosis is only one of a number of critical research issues pertaining to subject's clinical condition, however. An equally important topic concerns the severity and stability of the subject's symptoms at the initiation of the research. Consider, for example, an investigation of a new antidepressant agent. If it is given to 30 persons with diagnoses of recurrent major depressive disorder who are currently hospitalized in a symptomatic state, and 20 of them show little or no depression 3 weeks later, it might be concluded that the medication holds promise. On the other hand, if it is given to 30 persons with the same diagnosis, but who are stable outpatients exhibiting few symptoms, the significance of the finding that 20 of them show little or no depression 3 weeks later is much more limited. Thus, most intervention research in chronic mental illness requires a documented recent exacerbation of illness in order to assure that the subject has an increased probability of imminent relapse and that any intervention mitigates against that likelihood.

Although many research protocols require a recent symptom *exacerbation* as part of their subject inclusion criteria, they also frequently demand a subsequent symptom *stabilization*; that is, the potential subject's symptoms recently worsened, but now are beginning to improve. This requirement for stabilization is particularly important in tests of psychosocial interventions and low-dose medication strategies. For example, the National Institute of Mental Health is currently funding a five-site collaborative study examining the impact of three medication strategies (high, low, and targeted dose) and two family interventions (behavioral family management vs. monthly supportive family meetings) on relapse in schizophrenia (Schooler & Keith, 1983). Although the protocol requires that subjects have had a recent increase in schizophrenic symptoms, it excludes most subjects whose symptoms do not remit to at least a moderate level, as measured on the Brief Psychiatric Rating Scale (BPRS) (Overall & Gorham, 1962). Presumably, unremitting symptoms would make the patients poor candidates for low doses of strategies and/or unable to tolerate family therapy sessions thus resulting in high attrition. In addition, the concept of relapse can be ambiguous when applied to patients who evidence high levels of persisting symptoms at the beginning of a study (Falloon, 1984); thus, initially highly symptomatic patients should not be included in a relapse prevention study.

Phase of Illness

Finally, the subject's phase of illness can be an important, although a frequently underattended to, variable. A number of reports now indicate that long-term prognosis in schizophrenia is much better than had been originally thought (Ciompi, 1980a; Harding, Brooks, Ashikaga, Strauss, & Breier, 1987a,b). One implication of these findings is that an outcome study which includes subjects with long duration of schizophrenia may report more favorable findings than one which focused on recent-onset patients. Many extraneous variables (related to phase of illness rather than to a particular intervention of interest) may affect the outcome findings. For example, patients with a relatively recent onset of illness may be less inclined to accept medication and continued psychiatric care. Any investigator conducting research in this area would be advised to take this issue into account (Carpenter, Kirkpatrick, & Buchanan, 1990).

Subject Recruitment

Research of the chronically mentally ill involves locating individuals who meet predetermined research criteria and persuading them to participate in the study. Consider, for example, a study of a new antipsychotic agent. In the typical protocol, a subject must agree to being closely monitored during the "drug wash-out" period, as well as during the period in which he or she is randomly assigned to receive either the new agent or a placebo. Needless to say, many potential subjects are not receptive to such a plan; they may fear the side effects of the new medication; they may be unwilling to risk being unmedicated during a drug-free period; or they may consider the extra visits to the clinic for physical examinations and symptom evaluation to be a waste of their time.

Psychosocial intervention studies face similar recruitment difficulties. Consider a recent study reported by Hogarty et al. (1986) which set out to determine the efficacy of psychoeducational family therapy versus individual social skills training in reducing relapse in schizophrenia. These authors lost 22% of their identified sample before the intervention ever began; the primary reason for the loss of subjects was their withdrawal of consent or their refusal of the protocol upon discharge. Another 13 subjects (10% of the initial sample) either relapsed while they were being engaged in the study or failed to meet the minimal treatment-exposure criteria. These numbers highlight the challenges of recruiting and maintaining chronically ill patients in a research protocol.

INDEPENDENT VARIABLES

Probably the most frequently studied independent variable in research on the chronically mentally ill is some type of biomedical or psychosocial intervention. The general topics of research in pharmacology therapy and psychotherapy have been discussed elsewhere in this volume. Designing intervention studies in a chronically mentally ill sample involves three specific issues: (1) potential pharmacotherapy/psychotherapy interactions, (2) the need for long-term interventions (Schatzberg & Cole, 1986), and (3) implementation of the research protocol within a larger, preexisting service delivery system. Each of these will be discussed.

Pharmacotherapy/Psychotherapy Interaction Issues

By definition, the chronically mentally ill are among the most impaired psychiatric patients. Psychotropic medications in conjunction with supportive counseling or psychotherapy typically offer these patients the greatest likelihood of successful community adjustment and symptom control. Therefore, research may specifically be designed to the efficacy of a combination of treatments: for example, in a sample of depressed patients, does the addition of cognitive therapy offer any additional benefits over the administration of antidepressants alone (e.g., Simons, Murphy, Levine, & Wetzel, 1986)? In such a study, both medication and psychotherapy can be administered in a standardized manner, using random assignment of subjects to both the individual and combined treatment conditions. The relative improvements obtained with each of the individual and the combined treatments can then be compared.

However, when one treatment is administered in a standardized manner whereas the other is not, often the results may become difficult to interpret. Consider, for example, a recent study on the use of the behavioral technique known as *implosion therapy* with war veterans with chronic posttraumatic stress disorder (PTSD). Implosion therapy involves the repeated vivid recollection of a traumatic memory in a supportive clinical environment in order to extinguish anxiety and reduce avoidance responses associated with the memory of the trauma (Boudewyns, & Shipley, 1983). In their investigation, Keane, Fairbank, Caddell, and Zimering (1989) randomly assigned 24 Vietnam veterans with chronic PTSD to either implosion therapy or a waiting-list control group. They found that subjects receiving the implosion therapy achieved significantly greater improvement in their PTSD symptoms at the end of treatment and at 6-months follow-up than those in the control condition. However, during the treatment, 55% of the implosion patients and 77% of their control patients were also administered by physicians not involved in the study either anxiolytic, sleep, or pain medications. This nonstandardization of medication across the two groups makes it difficult to interpret the overall positive findings. For example, if most of the patients in the implosion group were receiving anti-anxiety agents, whereas most of the control group were not, these pharmacologic differences might have contributed to the significant findings; this issue was not fully explored in this particular study. Because chronic patients are often given combination treatments, the effect of the treatment under study being confounded by those of treatments not under control of the investigators can become a particularly difficult methodological issue in the research of this population.

The simplest way to avoid this problem is to eliminate the use of medication in psychotherapy studies and to prohibit the use of psychotherapy in medication studies. Obviously, such a recommendation can rarely be followed in a study of the chronically mentally ill. As an alternative, the researcher can standardize in advance the medication to be used in a psychotherapy study or can standardize the psychotherapy to be used in a drug study. Standardization minimizes the possible confounding of the medication and psychotherapy effects. If standardization is not possible, then the next best strategy is for the researcher to collect and record information on all additional uncontrolled interventions given in the study. Subsequent data analyses may be able to determine if these uncontrolled additional treatments had any effect on the treatment outcome.

The Need for Long-Term Intervention

Unlike acute patients, chronic patients suffer multiple impairments over extended periods of time. One consequence of this prolonged and extensive impairment is that it may take longer for the patients to benefit from treatment.

The importance of extended treatment is especially apparent in investigations on psychosocial interventions. For example, Woods, Higson, and Tannahill (1984) monitored the progress of six treatment-refractory schizophrenic female patients who were participating in a 5-year comprehensive token-economy behavioral skills training program. Patients were given a specified number of tokens for adequate self-care and mealtime behaviors; tokens could be used to purchase a variety of back-up reinforcers, including consumable items and special privileges. All staff were trained to high rates of reliability in identifying appropriate behaviors, awarding tokens accurately, and recording data in order to monitor patient progress. Although token reinforcement generally increased hygiene and table manners, the rate of improvement differed dramatically from patient to patient. Three patients appeared very responsive to the token reinforcement and had achieved high levels of skill in the various personal care areas within 6 months of the introduction of the program; two additional patients were responsive to the token payments but demonstrated much more gradual levels of improvement and, in fact, their performance did not stabilize until after at least 2 years of token payments; the final patient was not consistently responsive to token reinforcement. As these results suggest, research outcomes with chronically mentally ill patients often require years of treatment.

Interfacing with Other Service Providers

Many of the chronically mentally ill are served by a variety of different services and agencies. A typical adult male veteran with a diagnosis of schizophrenia who is living in a residential facility may have at least eight professionals assuming responsibility for his care: a psychiatrist, an internist, a psychotherapist, an occupational therapist or skills group leader, a social worker/case manager at the local Veterans Administration (VA) medical center, a social worker and the owner or supervisor at the residential care facility, and a case worker at the social security office or the VA disability claims office. Add in a couple of concerned family members in addition to representatives of one or two other involved agencies, such as probation officers for patients also in the legal system, a child care specialist for patients who require supervision for their offspring, or a public conservator, and it becomes clear just how complicated the support and service systems for these patients can be.

It is helpful (and exceedingly realistic) for any researcher who is working with the chronically mentally ill to conceptualize his or her study as being embedded in a complex service-delivery system and that the assessment and intervention procedures being shared are only a small part of this large system. The investigator must be prepared to facilitate working relationships with a variety of other professionals and to anticipate and plan for circumstances in which the requirements of the research conflict with the demands of the other services. For example, consider the case of a bipolar patient residing in a residential facility who is reasonably well stabilized on lithium but is being recruited as a candidate for the study of a new medication with fewer side effects. If the protocol calls for a drug washout phase and random assignment to a placebo condition, the investigator, the patient, and the residential facility staff must jointly contemplate the possibility that the patient's condition might deteriorate during the medication-free period. Detailed plans must therefore be set up to allow for early detection and treatment of worsening symptoms and behavior, so that the patient's condition does not deteriorate to the extent that his or her stay at the residential facility becomes jeopardized. It is incumbent upon any investigator who is conducting research with the chronically mentally ill to anticipate what detrimental consequences may ensue from their participation in a study and to work diligently to keep these to an absolute minimum.

DEPENDENT VARIABLES

In most psychiatric research, the dependent variables are some aspects of the patient's symptoms or behavior that are appropriately quantified. Often the assessment of these variables constitutes an assessment of outcome of a particular intervention. In research with the chronically mentally ill, two issues relating to outcome deserve special attention: (1) the need for multidimensional assessment and long-term follow-up, and (2) the measurement constraints that are due to extreme scores.

The Need for Multidimensional Assessment and Long-Term Follow-up

Let us consider a general question often posed in treatment/outcome research: has this patient improved as a result of this medication (or psychological treatment)? The simplicity of this question is deceptive, however, because it implies that there is a generally accepted, unidimensional definition of improvement which can be accurately and reliably measured. In reality, of course, psychiatric symptoms even in a single patient tend to be diverse, and an intervention may reduce one set of symptoms while worsening another. For example, alcoholic patients may experience a temporary increase of depression and anxiety when they stop drinking. In evaluating the efficacy of an intervention designed to reduce drinking, the investigator must therefore monitor both alcohol consumption *and* mood.

Among chronically mentally ill patients, the need for assessment of multiple domains of psychopathology is even more imperative (Schwartz, Myers, & Astrachan, 1975). By definition, these patients typically experience a wide array of symptoms. For example, a schizophrenic patient may be delusional, depressed, anxious, and agitated, and, furthermore, may exhibit impaired concentration. Any researcher trying to understand the impact of an intervention on such a patient must examine potential changes on each one of these symptoms. In addition to utilizing measurement scales designed to assess the variable of most critical interest, use of a broader instrument, such as the Brief Psychiatric

Rating Scale (BPRS) or the Symptom Checklist 90 (SCL-90) (Derogatis, 1977) may facilitate assessment of multiple symptom domains.

Furthermore, patients are more than just the sum of their symptoms. For instance, they are individuals that function in a variety of social roles—as spouses, friends, members of extended families, wage earners, and the like. Taken together, level of functioning in these various roles is typically referred to as "social adjustment." Although psychopathology and social adjustment are statistically correlated (Casey, Tyrer, & Platt, 1985; Strauss & Carpenter, 1972), they exert independent effects on the patients' lives. For example, among a group of psychiatric patients, Case et al. (1985) found that social adjustment deficits were much more strongly associated with referrals for psychiatric care than were the severity of their psychiatric symptoms.

Needless to say, most chronically mentally ill patients have relatively poor social adjustment. They are often unemployed (Goldstrom & Manderscheid, 1982) and socially isolated (Tolsodorf, 1976). An intervention may successfully reduce symptoms but it may not improve social adjustment. It is therefore incumbent on any researcher in this field to pay attention to the effect of any intervention on social functioning, and to design interventions which are targeted specifically at improving social adjustment.

Presently, there are a number of different social adjustment measures available to researchers, including the Social Adjustment Scale (Weissman & Paykel, 1974), the Katz Adjustment Scale (Katz & Lyerly, 1963), the Quality of Life Scale (Heinrichs, Hanlon, & Carpenter, 1984) and the Social Behavior Assessment Schedule (Platt, Weyman, Hirsch, & Hewett, 1980) (see Weissman, 1975, for a review). Although these scales may be used to assess the social functioning of chronically mentally ill patients, they may be problematic to use. Most of the scales require an extended face-to-face interview with the patient as well as with a significant other; this process can therefore be costly and time consuming. In addition, functioning in some social roles is particularly difficult to quantify (e.g., adequacy as a son; appropriate breadth of leisure pursuits), so that rigorous interviewer training is therefore necessary to ensure reliable data collection, adding further to the complexity and cost of the task.

The importance of long-term follow-up in the chronically mentally ill is also becoming increasing clear. A series of studies now indicate that long-term prognosis in schizophrenia is better than originally proposed by Kraepelin (1915). For example, Harding et al. (1987b) found that, 20 to 30 years after their earlier psychiatric hospitalization, close to half of a sample of schizophrenic patients in Vermont were free of psychotic symptoms and most had been able to attain at least some level of independent social and vocational functioning in the community. Similar findings on the long-term course of schizophrenic illness in Europe (Ciompi 1980a,b) highlighted the need to take a "long-haul" view of outcome with this patient population. Importantly, McGlashan (1986) recently compared predictors of outcomes during first, second, and third decade post-discharge from the Chestnut Lodge. He found that the outcomes during the different decades were correlated with different variables. For example, a family history of psychiatric illness predicted a poorer outcome during the third, but not during the first, decade postdischarge. These findings suggest that a different set of research questions may have to be formulated in the study of the outcome of schizophrenia. I have already mentioned that selecting the appropriate variable to measure is one of the most crucial tasks in conducting outcome research in the chronically mentally ill. Equally important is finding the right scale or metric with which to evaluate the variable. By definition, chronically mentally ill patients have severe symptoms and very impaired social functioning. Any scales used in research with this population must therefore permit measurement of change even in the extreme ranges.

Consider, for example, a study we conducted on the use of the serotonin depletor fenfluramine on symptoms in chronic schizophrenia (Marshall, Glynn, Midha, Hubbard, Bowen, Banzett, Mintz, & Liberman, 1989). Our subjects were floridly psychotic schizophrenic patients who had been specifically admitted to a unit for treatment-refractory patients at Camarillo (California) State Hospital. Based on previous positive findings with autistic (Geller, Ritvo, & Freeman, 1982; Ritvo, Freeman, & Yuwiler, 1986) and schizophrenic (Shore, Korpi, & Bigelow, 1985) patients, we hypothesized that fenfluramine may be beneficial for chronic schizophrenic symptoms. Instead, in a double-blind trial, we found that fenfluramine led to an increase in depression and paranoia, as measured on the BPRS. If these findings indicated an across-the-board worsening of symptoms, we might also have found increases on the BPRS items that were thought to reflect psychotic processes (e.g., hallucinatory behavior, unusual thought content, and conceptual disorganization). However, we did not find evidence of a global worsening of psychotic symptoms on the BPRS. In examining our data, however, it became clear that the initial severity of our patients' psychosis was rated so highly that there was little or no room left in the scale to indicate worsening, even if this occurred. This measurement constraint at the maximum score on a scale is termed a *ceiling effect*; and our experience indicates that it can create major evaluation difficulties in research with the chronically mentally ill. Given the severity of symptoms that many of the chronically mentally ill experience, researchers who anticipate potential ceiling effects on their assessment instruments may be advised to revise the anchor points of the scale or to select other assessment instruments which are more specifically designed for rating highly symptomatic patients.

SUMMARY

Parallel to treatment strategies, research with the chronically mentally ill requires careful thought and an intensive commitment of resources. With each passing year, research funding becomes more competitive as other populations of need are identified, making it even more difficult to conduct empirical research with this patient group. Of course, I believe that our most troubled and disabled patients merit our professional expertise at least as much as, if not more than, any other patient population.

Professional expertise entails a knowledge of the subtleties of the challenge confronting us, however. For researchers in the field of chronic mental illness, the first challenge involves finding subjects who meet the requirements of the protocol, and then recruiting them into the project. The second challenge involves designing an independent variable that is not confounded by other variables, is intensive and extended enough to impact on patients, and that can be embedded in the patient's current network of services. The final challenge involves assuring that the many domains of patient functioning and symptoms are adequately measured, using instruments appropriately scaled for the patients and designed to assess the variables of interest.

The complexities of research with the chronically mentally ill make the task particularly challenging, and the potential for alleviating the suffering of millions of mentally ill patients around the world makes it worthwhile and rewarding.

REFERENCES

American Psychiatric Association. (1987). *Diagnostic and statistical manual of mental disorders* (3rd ed., rev.). Washington, DC: Author.

Bachrach, L. (1988). Defining chronic mental illness: A concept paper. *Hospital and Community Psychiatry, 39,* 383–388.

Beck, A., Rush, A., Shaw, B., & Emery, G. (1979). *Cognitive therapy of depression.* New York: Guilford Press.

Boudewyns, P. A., & Shipley, R. H. (1983). *Flooding and implosive therapy: Direct therapeutic exposure in clinical practice.* New York: Plenum Press.

Brown, V., Ridgely S., Pepper, B., Levine, I., & Ryglewicz, H. (1989). The dual crisis: Mental illness and substance abuse. *American Psychologist, 44,* 565–569.

Carpenter, W., Kirkpatrick, B., & Buchanan, R. (1990). Conceptual approaches to the study of schizophrenia. In A. Kales, C. Stefanis, & J. Talbott (Eds.), *Recent advances in schizophrenia* (pp. 95–113). New York: Springer-Verlag.

Casey, P., Tyrer, P., & Platt, S. (1985). The relationship between social functioning and psychiatric symptomatology in primary care. *Social Psychiatry, 20,* 5–9.

Ciompi, L. (1980a). Catamnestic long-term study on the course of life and aging of schizophrenics. *Schizophrenia Bulletin, 6,* 606–618.

Ciompi, L. (1980b). Three lectures on schizophrenia. *British Journal of Psychiatry, 136,* 413–420.

Crow, T. (1980). Molecular pathology of schizophrenia: More than one dimension of pathology? *British Medical Journal, 280,* 66–68.

Crow, T. (1985). The two-syndrome concept: Origins and current status. *Schizophrenia Bulletin, 11,* 471–486.

Davis, J., Schaffer, C., Killian, G., Kinard, C., & Chan, C. (1980). Important issues in the drug treatment of schizophrenia. *Schizophrenia Bulletin, 5,* 109–126.

Derogatis, L. (1977). *The SCL-90 Manual: Administration, and procedure for the SCL-90.* Baltimore: Johns Hopkins University, School of Medicine.

Elkin, I., Shea, T., Watkins, J., Imber, S., Sotsky, S., Collins, J., Glass, D., Pilkonis, P., Leber, W., Docherty, J., Fiester, S., & Parloff, M. (1989). National Institute of Mental Health treatment of depression collaborative research program. *Archives of General Psychiatry, 46,* 971–983.

Falloon, I. (1984). Relapse: A reappraisal of assessment of outcome in schizophrenia. *Schizophrenia Bulletin, 10,* 293–299.

Falloon, I., Boyd, J., McGill, C., Razani, J., Moss, H., & Gilderman, A. (1982). Family management in the prevention of exacerbations of schizophrenia. *New England Journal of Medicine, 306,* 1437–1440.

Geller, E., Ritvo, E., & Freeman, B. (1982). Preliminary observations on the effects of fenfluramine on blood serotonin and symptoms in three autistic boys. *New England Journal of Medicine, 307,* 165–169.

Goldstrom, I., & Manderscheid, R. (1982). The chronically mentally ill: A descriptive analysis from the uniform client data instrument. *Community Support Services Journal, 2,* 4–9.

Haas, G., Glick, I., Clarkin, J., Spencer, J., & Lewis, A. (1990). Gender and schizophrenia outcome: A clinical trial of an inpatient family intervention. *Schizophrenia Bulletin, 16,* 277–292.

Harding, C., Brooks, G., Ashikaga, T., Strauss, J., & Breier, A. (1987a). The Vermont longitudinal study of persons with severe mental illness: I. Methodology, study sample, and overall status 32 years later. *American Journal of Psychiatry, 144,* 718–726.

Harding, C., Brooks, G., Ashikaga, T., Strauss, J., & Breier, A. (1987b). The Vermont longitudinal study of persons with severe mental illness: II. Long-term outcome of subjects who retrospectively met DSM-III criteria for schizophrenia. *American Journal of Psychiatry, 144,* 727–735.

Heinrichs, D., Hanlon, T., & Carpenter, W. (1984). The Quality of Life Scale: An instrument for rating the schizophrenic deficit syndrome. *Schizophrenia Bulletin, 3,* 388–398.

Hogarty, G., Anderson, C., Reiss, D., Kornblith, S., Greenwald, D., Javna, C., & Madonia, M. (1986). Family psychoeducation, social skills training, and maintenance chemotherapy in the aftercare treatment of schizophrenia. *Archives of General Psychiatry, 43,* 633–642.

Katz, M., & Lyerly, S. (1963). Methods for measuring adjustment and social behavior in the community: I. Rationale, description, discriminative validity and scale development. *Psychological Reports, 13,* 503–535.

Keane, T., Fairbank, J., Caddell, J., & Zimering, R. (1989). Implosive (flooding) therapy reduces symptoms of PTSD in Vietnam combat veterans. *Behavior Therapy, 20,* 245–260.

Klerman, G., Weissman, W., Rounsaville, B., & Chevron, E. (1984). *Interpersonal psychotherapy of depression.* New York: Basic Books.

Kraepelin, E. (1915). *Lehrbuch der Psychiatrie [Clinical psychiatry].* (Translated from the 7th German edition by A. R. Diefendorf.) New York: Scholars' Facsimiles and Reprints.

Lin, K., Poland, R., Nuccio, I., Matsuda, K., Hathuc, N., Su, T., & Fu, P. (1989). A longitudinal assessment of haloperidol doses and serum concentrations in Asian and Caucasian schizophrenic patients. *American Journal of Psychiatry, 146,* 1307–1311.

Marshall, B., Glynn, S., Midha, K., Hubbard, J., Bowen, L., Banzett, L., Mintz, J., & Liberman, R. (1989). Adverse effects of fenfluramine in treatment refractory schizophrenia. *Journal of Clinical Psychopharmacology, 9,* 110–115.

McGlashan, T. (1986). Predictors of shorter-, medium-, and longer-term outcome in schizophrenia. *American Journal of Psychiatry, 143,* 50–55.

Mogul, K. (1985). Psychological considerations in the use of psychotropic drugs with women patients. *Hospital and Community Psychiatry, 36,* 1080–1085.

Overall, J., & Gorham, D. (1962). The Brief Psychiatric Rating Scale. *Psychological Reports, 10,* 799–812.

Platt, S., Weyman, A., Hirsch, S., & Hewett, S. (1980). The Social Behaviour Assessment Schedule (SBAS): Rationale, contents, scoring and reliability of a new interview schedule. *Social Psychiatry, 15,* 43–55.

Ritvo, E., Freeman, B., & Yuwiler, A. (1986). Fenfluramine treatment of autism: UCLA collaborative study of 810 patients at nine medical centers. *Psychopharmacology Bulletin, 22,* 133–140.

Schatzberg, A., & Cole, J. (Eds.). (1986). *Manual of clinical psychopharmacology.* Washington, DC: American Psychiatric Press.

Schinnar, A., Rothbard, A., Kanter, R., & Adams, K. (1990). Crossing state lines of mental illness. *Hospital and Community Psychiatry, 41,* 756–760.

Schooler, N., & Keith, S. (1983). *National Institute of Mental Health cooperative agreement program protocol for treatment strategies in schizophrenia study.* Unpublished manuscript.

Schwartz, C., Myers, J., & Astrachan, B. (1975). Concordance of multiple assessments of the outcome of schizophrenia. *Archives of Psychiatry, 32,* 1221–1227.

Seeman, M. (1986). Current outcome in schizophrenia: Women versus men. *Acta Psychiatrica Scandinavica, 73,* 609–617.

Shea, M., Pilkonis, P., Beckham, E., Collins, J., Elkin, I., Sotsky, S., & Docherty, J. (1990). Personality disorders and treatment outcome in the NIMH treatment of depression collaborative research program. *American Journal of Psychiatry, 147,* 711–718.

Shore, D., Korpi, E., & Bigelow, L. (1985). Fenfluramine and chronic schizophrenia. *Biological Psychiatry, 20,* 329–352.

Simons, A., Murphy, G., Levine, J., & Wetzel, R. (1986). Cognitive therapy and pharmacotherapy for depression. *Archives of General Psychiatry, 43,* 43–48.

Spitzer, R., & Williams, J. (1985). *Structured Clinical Interview for DSM-III-R, Patient version.* New York: New York State Psychiatric Institute, Biometrics Research Department.

Stephens, J. (1978). Long-term prognosis and follow-up in schizophrenia. *Schizophrenia Bulletin, 4,* 25–47.

Strauss, J., & Carpenter, W. (1972). The prediction of outcome in schizophrenia. *Archives of General Psychiatry, 27,* 739–746.

Tolsodorf, C. (1976). Social networks, support and coping. *Family Process, 15,* 407–418.

Wahl, O. (1977). Sex bias in schizophrenia research: A short report. *Journal of Abnormal Psychology, 86,* 195–198.

Weissman, M. (1975). The assessment of social adjustment. *Archives of General Psychiatry, 32,* 357–365.

Weissman, M., & Paykel, E. (1974). Social adjustment scale. In Weissman, M., & Paykel. E. (Eds.), *The depressed woman* (pp. 236–264). Chicago: University of Chicago Press.

Wing, J., Cooper, J., & Sartorius, N. (1974). *The measurement and classification of psychiatric symptoms.* London: Cambridge University Press.

Woods, P., Higson, P., & Tannahill, M. (1984). Token-economy programmes with chronic psychotic patients: The importance of direct measurement and objective evaluation for long-term maintenance. *Behaviour Research and Therapy, 22,* 41–51.

World Health Organization. (1980). *ICD-9-CM: International classification of diseases, 9th revision, clinical modification.* Ann Arbor: Commission on Professional and Hospital Activities.

PART VI

EPILOGUE

CHAPTER 19

The Future of Psychiatric Research

The Need for a Conceptual Agenda

MARK D. SULLIVAN AND GARY J. TUCKER

INTRODUCTION

The psychiatrist and philosopher Karl Jaspers has described four types of science:

> the physical, biological, psychological, and mind sciences—as exhausting the content of all existents . . . in each of the four realms, actuality has a different mode of objectiveness; and the actualities mesh. Physics (together with chemistry) is relatively an internally coherent field of study. So is biology, although the coherence is due to its relation to the exact natural sciences, on which it draws at each step while its own roots remain obscure. Psychology is far more questionable; in fact, it strays into the realms of life and the mind, or else it poses as a universal science. Mind science, finally, is actual only as a multiplicity resulting from research into the documents, works, deeds or institutions of Man; by no means has it produced a kind of unity we see in physics and biology. It is the arena for the battles of differing world views, battles which decide, radically and without appeal, about the meaning and value of proposed inquiries and modes of research. (Jaspers cited in Ehrlich, Ehrlich, & Pepper, 1986, p. 360)

Currently, psychiatric research encompasses all four of these types of science. These types designate both areas of interest and methods of inquiry.

Mark D. Sullivan and Gary J. Tucker • Department of Psychiatry, University of Washington, Seattle, Washington 98195.

Research in Psychiatry: Issues, Strategies, and Methods, edited by L. K. George Hsu and Michel Hersen. Plenum Press, New York, 1992.

Each is characterized by different assumptions concerning its object of study and the proper approach to it. Psychiatric residents embarking upon a research career often delve into a research program that exists within one of these types of science and forget how their project relates to the mission of psychiatric research as a whole. It is easy to ignore the theoretical assumptions behind an empirical research method; but the correlations produced by any research which is ignorant of its assumptions are frequently of dubious meaning and importance. The purpose of this chapter, then, is to explore some of the basic assumptions that underlie psychiatric research in order to better understand its overall direction and purpose.

Perhaps what is most confusing to this research field is the desire to apply standards of proof of one scientific endeavor to the subjective data of psychiatric or experiential issues. In any major psychiatric department that has a large research effort, there are frequently warring camps of those who are doing "real science" (or who just use the word *science* by itself), and those who are seen as "just fussing around." Usually, the former refers to a field that can be objectified and studied, such as the study of a neurotransmitter level or a receptor that can be cloned. Although the latter often refers to epidemiological or phenomenological studies—again, the hierarchical status is based primarily on the ability to objectify the data. As long as we ignore the fact that often we are dealing with different types of data with varied criteria, then what is being discussed will never be clear. In part, what we are looking for is a "transducer" that will convert the power of experiential information into some types of physical and quantifiable event. Until we have this, most of our reasoning is by analogy and, perhaps, by anthropomorphic measures.

Psychiatric research is stretched between the mind and the brain. The tension between these two extremely different objects of study constantly threatens to destroy any bridge that can be built between them. On the one hand, the predominance of psychiatric subject matter is based on the patient's reported symptoms. After all, we have few signs in psychiatric illnesses which are reliable: only some abnormalities in thought process, some disturbances in memory function, or some degree of psychomotor retardation. On the other hand, there is the brain itself, immensely complex but available to objective study. Thus, we are left with a dilemma that has faced clinical medicine and psychiatry since their origins: the distinction between subjective evidence that can only be reported to someone else (any attempt to quantify or verify such evidence ultimately depends on the subject's self-reporting), and objective evidence that can be independently quantified or verified.

The great appeal of a thoroughly biological psychiatry is its stabilization of inquiry through its substitution of the brain for the mind as the object of study. Such substitution seems to offer to psychiatric research an independent objectivity otherwise unavailable to it. Inspired by this hope for a thoroughly objective behavioral science, the National Institute of Mental Health has declared the 1990s as "the decade of the brain." We will argue, however, that attention to the brain alone cannot provide the categories necessary for clinically relevant psychiatric research. Psychiatry cannot be reduced to biology. As we proceed with the elucidation of neural mechanisms behind psychiatric illnesses, we must properly define and categorize these illnesses. The articulation of taxonomy must guide the articulation of mechanism. Although attempts have been made to derive this taxonomy from biology by means of sociobiological theory, we will argue that this attempt cannot succeed. Psychiatry will continue to be characterized by the creative tension between biology and psychology. Psychiatric research must be directed toward the difficult but exciting project of building a bridge between the brain and the mind.

THE CHALLENGE FROM MEDICINE

Because it lacks a common theoretical base, psychiatric research is fragmented along ideological lines. Debates about the etiology and appropriate therapy of psychiatric disorders have become at times fractious and divisive as, for example, in the Osheroff case (cf. Klerman, 1990, and Stone, 1990). If we are unable to reach a consensus about the standard of care in our field, the courts may force one upon us. If we cannot unify the body of knowledge that defines us as a profession, then government and market forces may carve us into pieces of their own liking.

Recently, Paul McHugh (1987) has challenged psychiatry to follow medicine's path out of sectarianism. Psychiatry remains divided primarily by allegiances to various treatments and thereby various conceptions of etiology. When introduced to a psychiatrist, McHugh noted that we are inclined to ask: What is your philosophy? Such a question indicates that psychiatry is divided into "religious groups." It is not unified by common education and method as are other medial specialties. Although tenaciously held, these philosophies are almost always derived from therapeutic encounter with patients. Thus, they are generally based upon treatment experiences discovered by accident which may be entirely idiosyncratic.

McHugh pointed toward the transformation in American medicine that was wrought by William Osler as a model for contemporary psychiatry. Prior to Osler and his political avatar, Abraham Flexner, medicine was beset by a similar proliferation of therapeutic ideologies. There was no consensus about the proper way to test therapies or how to determine the cause of medical disorders. The unity found within medicine today with respect to methods of inquiry and theories of disease etiology was achieved, according to McHugh, through Oslerian efforts at "building rational therapeutics upon comprehensive biological medicine." McHugh summarized what we can expect from such a path:

> eventually an appreciation of the varieties of etiology and mechanism found in different psychiatric disorders . . . [W]e can anticipate the emergence of a psychiatry identified by its subject matter, unified in its conceptual base, and no longer subdivided into camps with different "orientations." . . . Psychiatry will bind itself more and more closely to medicine and will free itself from the politics of interpretive communities arguing with each other. (McHugh, 1987, p. 918)

The fragmentation of psychiatry is thus seen as a temporary, developmental phase already completed by the rest of medicine. It is not permanent or insurmountable, but requires a disciplined return to the basics of scientific biological medicine. A rigorous and unified method based in biology will allow psychiatry, like medicine before it, to define its diseases and their mechanisms.

PSYCHIATRY'S BASIC SCIENCES: THE NEUROSCIENCES?

Although McHugh does not restrict the basic sciences of psychiatry to the neurosciences, other researchers have done so. Detre (1987), for example, asked that the specialties of psychiatry and neurology be combined into a field which he labels "clinical neuroscience" that will allow us to "relinquish our role as social pseudoscientists on semipermanent vacation from medicine." He argued:

> The source of the confusion is that while the "mind" and mental functions constitute a legitimate and convenient conceptual framework to describe certain phenomena about psychiatric illness, it is not an avenue for the further generation of biological theories by which we can deduce from the nature of mental defect its etiology and pathogenesis. (Detre, 1987, p. 622)

The appeal of a neuroscientifically based psychiatry is easy to see. At the very least, anchoring psychiatry to the neurosciences may provide us with a conceptually different diagnostic framework. Despite improvements in diagnostic reliability brought about by the DSM-III (American Psychiatric Association, 1980) and the DSM-III-R (American Psychiatric Association, 1987), there remain intractable problems within a polythetic, phenomenologically based diagnostic system. For example, Bannister (1968) noted that "schizophrenia" is a disjunctive category. For a diagnosis of the disorder to be made, only a selection of clinical symptoms is necessary. Two patients could meet diagnostic criteria with completely different sets of symptoms. How are we to argue that these patients belong in the same diagnostic category instead of in different ones? Although there have been improvements upon previous diagnostic systems, the DSM-III or the DSM-III-R has not circumvented these basic conceptual difficulties.

If the DSM-III-R is not the final answer, where do we look to get our diagnostic categories right? What can provide a common ground for all the diverse abnormalities of behavior and experience encompassed by psychiatric diagnosis? In medicine, pathology has provided an objective and universal groundwork for diagnosis. Osler's clinical diagnosis, which was based on bedside examination, could always be confirmed or disconfirmed at autopsy by a pathological diagnosis. Pathology allows diseases which present similarly to be distinguished and diverse manifestations of the same disease to be unified. By the same token, insofar as neurophysiological processes are associated with all behavior and experience, neuropathology may provide objective evidence of the disruption of these processes. Perhaps, therefore, neuropathology can offer psychiatry an objective and universal diagnostic system. After all, only if mental disorders are categorized on the basis of neuropathology can they fully qualify as medical diseases, and only for diseases where the causes are known can there be a distinction between curative and palliative therapy. Unfortunately, careful examination of this line of argument indicates that neuropathology alone cannot lead psychiatry out of its existential dilemma, wedged between the biomedical sciences on the one hand and the psychosocial sciences on the other. Descriptive neuropathology can only discover brain differences (i.e., deviations from a statistical norm). By itself, it cannot tell us what these differences mean. Good (e.g., genius) and bad (e.g., schizophrenia) brain differences can be distinguished only through reference to their associated products: experience and behavior. For brain differences to be meaningful, they must be correlated with differences in behavior. That is, neuropathology must rely on psycho-pathology to interpret the meaning of its findings. The neuropathologist must be told which behavior needs to be explained and which brain difference is pathological.

If psychopathology cannot obtain objectivity without neuropathology, and if neuropathology cannot be made clinically meaningful without psychopathology, how can the two disciplines be connected in a systematic and nonarbitrary way? Where should we look for the "transducer" that will allow us to link neuropathology and psychopathology? The first task in this regard is to find the proper psychopathological system (if there is one proper system) for categorizing abnormalities in behavior and experience which would then allow for the correlation with neuropathological findings.

To decrease the level of arbitrariness inherent in our diagnostic system, some researchers have proposed that we look for anatomical correlates of symptoms rather than syndromes (e..g, Bannister, 1968). Symptoms are simpler and more homogeneous than syndromes. We might expect that individual symptoms would correspond to individual abnormalities within a single neuro-logical structure or system. In this respect, some studies have found that specific symptoms and experiences of patients are better indicators of prognosis than their respective diagnostic categories. For instance, the number of hallu-cinations and delusions of a patient with schizophrenia was more predictive of the course of the illness than the diagnosis of schizophrenia (Cloninger, Martin, Guze, & Clayton, 1985). However, seeking correlates of symptoms rather than syndromes may simply disguise but not solve the problem of neuropsycho-pathological correlation. Just as we must define and demarcate syndromes, so must symptoms be distinguished from each other and from nonsymptomatic experience and behavior. When does an elevated mood become a symptom? If after his father's death, a son experiences a vision of his father speaking to him, is this one symptom (i.e, a symptom of acute grief) or two symptoms (i.e., a visual hallucination and an auditory hallucination). If ideas of reference come from both newspapers and TV programs, does that qualify as one symptom or two? The task of assigning meaning to a psychopathological event cannot be circumvented by focusing on individual symptoms rather than syndromes. Furthermore, apparently identical symptoms may occur in two apparently different disorders. As such, they may well be correlated with different neuro-pathological events (e.g., hallucinations occurring in seizure disorders versus those occurring after taking psychedelic drugs).

We have made it clear that it is not possible to make inferences about behavior if we only examine the brain. We must *first* identify and describe the behavior to be explained and then seek to find its neuropathological correlate. Refinements of our behavioral categories can be made through reference to commonalities in neural mechanisms, but only our behavioral categories can tell us which areas of the brain to look at and which brain differences are meaning-ful. Finding the appropriate behavioral taxonomy, furthermore, is not a simple task. How are we to be sure that our psychopathology is the correct one to guide research in neurophysiology and neuropathology? We need some natural order-ing of behavior, a natural psychopathology, which would allow for direct correlation with neuropathology. Where might we find a potential Linnaeus of the psyche for inspiration? What source could provide the universal, biolog-ically relevant taxonomy of behavior that we seek? Samuel Guze (1989) has argued that, since "psychopathology is the manifestation of disordered pro-cesses in various brain systems," it can be derived through a better understand-ing of brain biology. In short, he argued that biology can provide all the categories necessary for the description and explanation of behavior.

Nevertheless, while cellular/molecular biology may provide answers to questions of proximate causation (How are these symptoms produced?), it cannot provide answers to questions of ultimate causation (Why do these symptoms occur at all?) or of meaning (Is this a normal or pathological event?). Having shed any reference to a divine intent, modern biological science gener-ally relies upon evolutionary theory to provide answers to these "why" ques-tions. Both the brain and the behavior produced by it have evolved under the pressures of natural selection. Only by promoting survival could these organs and functions themselves have survived. The basic assumption here is that survival is the "ultimate good," an arguable proposition in itself. Be that as it may, it seems plausible to look toward evolutionary biology for behavioral categories that might directly correspond to brain structures, as many re-searchers already have. A detailed exploration of this option will demonstrate the immense problems of this reductionist biological approach, as well as highlight the conceptual assumptions, widely held but seldom questioned, on which psychiatric research is based.

SOCIOBIOLOGY: THE EXPLANATION
FOR HUMAN BEHAVIORS?

Sociobiology, the study of the genetic basis for social behavior, has been proposed as the most rational source for a scheme of behavior classification (McGuire & Essock-Vitale, 1981). A given behavior, such as grooming, has many different meanings depending upon the context within which it occurs. Grooming could be intended to please or enrage parents; it could serve to make or break bonds of friendship. This multiplicity of meanings provides for the possibility of many alternative modes for categorizing behavior, none of which is entirely satisfactory. Sociobiology radically simplifies the categorization of social behavior by defining the purpose of a behavior in terms of its evolutionary significance. Through sociobiological eyes, we would look through signs, symptoms, and behaviors to their ultimate *biological* function (i.e., their ability to increase one's inclusive fitness or to maximize the propagation of one's genes in future generations). These biological functions, as revealed through evolutionary history, could serve as the basis for a specieswide classification of behaviors. Grooming would therefore be understood and classified in terms of its impact upon genetic propagation.

The power of sociobiology as a discipline or perspective lies in its promise of an external position for the understanding of human behaviors. The social sciences are forever trapped within the cultures that they study and critique. Since acquired characters are not inherited, our genetic endowment is prior to its expression in culture. If sociobiology can describe how that genetic endowment underlies and shapes culture, it will grant us a truly novel and powerful tool for self-understanding. If it allows us to determine what is given or innate in our behavior, it might also allow us to develop the most appropriate social norms (i.e, an evolutionarily "correct" ethics or culture). According to E.O. Wilson (1975), "scientists and humanists should consider the possibility that the time has come for ethics to be removed temporarily from the hands of the philosophers and biologicized" (p. 562).

We will argue, however, that sociobiology cannot provide novel explanations for human behavior because it cannot conquer the problems inherent in the attempt to describe the biological purpose of human behavior, problems that have plagued the social sciences since their inception. Before the evolutionary origins of a behavior can be found, the behavior must be defined and categorized. Yet sociobiology offers no novel method to get beneath the cultural purposes of behavior to its purely biological purposes. Sociobiology has no stance independent of culture from which it can derive a typology of social behavior. Without a clear sense of the *nature* of human social behavior, sociobiology cannot offer a definite answer concerning the origin of that behavior. Furthermore, as a result of its focus upon the innate and genetic aspects of behavior, sociobiology is at risk of construing culturally contingent social forms as being biologically determined.

SOCIOBIOLOGY ON HUMAN NATURE

Finding the appropriate unit of behavior to examine is another problem we encounter is a study of human behavior from a sociobiological perspective. However, even in anatomy, there is not *a priori* a correct typology of description. Where, then, shall we find "the natural suture lines along which the phenotype of the individual is to be divided from the purposes of evolutionary theory?" (Lewontin, Rose, & Kamin, 1984, p. 247). It makes little sense to speak of the evolution of the hand or foot *per se*. In order to determine what constitutes an appropriate evolutionary unit, we must understand, for instance, how hand development is genetically tied to other related development and how the hand phenotypically interacts with the environment. Therefore, an apparently prominent anatomical structure the hand might be simply a byproduct of the evolution of other structures (as appears to be the case with the chin). However, to use function as a delineating unit may also be problematic since the function of a structure may be different depending on the context within which the structure operates; for example, the function of body hair differs in our natural environment from that in our social environment.

The crucial contextual role played by the social environment in the case of behavior adds tremendously to this already great difficulty. Because there is no evidence for direct genetic determination of specific human behaviors, sociobiology must look for indirect evidence to determine whether a behavior is genetically determined. One heavily used strategy is to look for behaviors that are present universally in humans and *assume* that a similar expression in such varied cultural environments points toward genetic determination (i.e., the behavior is a part of human nature). Similar behavior in closely related species is used to corroborate these inferences. Unfortunately, there are very few, if any, behaviors that are truly universal among humans. Inferences are therefore made on the basis of near universals or putative universals found in primitive societies. The result is that many possible inferences about human nature can be drawn. For instance, our concept of human nature is very different if we use the gentle !Kung San bushmen and the social chimpanzee as models, than if we use the violent Yanomamo tribesmen and the isolative baboon as models (Voorzanger, 1987). The limitation of this approach is therefore obvious.

Sociobiology claims not just that human society has developed as a result of biological forces, but that social arrangements are also the manifestations of specific actions of genes. However, to claim that genes provide a "possible range" for behavior or that genes hold culture "on a leash" have little meaning. Through the use of such hedging terms as "incomplete penetrance" and "variable expressivity," it is possible to make the theory fit any data. The claim by Wilson (1975) that "genes promoting flexibility in social behavior are strongly selected" (p. 549) has such wide ramifications that it becomes scientifically untestable and therefore meaningless.

The real problem with such terms as *predisposition* and *inclination*, according to Lewontin *et al.* (1984, p. 252), is not so much their vagueness but their tendency to camouflage invalid genetic reasoning. They make it appear as if the genome is the source of all tendencies found in the organism and that the environment only serves to permit or limit the expression of these tendencies. However, phenotype is itself a product of the gene–environment interaction. A phenotype emerges into its environment with tendencies already shaped by that environment. Given what is known about the prolonged postnatal plasticity of the nervous system, the interaction of genes and environment must play a central role in the development of both brain structure and behavioral phenotypes.

SOCIOBIOLOGY AND THE HUMAN ENVIRONMENT

Our discussion now brings us to the crucial issue of the nature of the human environment. This environment is itself composed of natural and social components. Having begun with insect societies, sociobiology tends to look at (without other independently verifiable reasons) the social environment as a derivative of the natural environment. If social structure is genetically determined, as appears to be the case with ants, then the social environment is simply an expression of a species's biological endowment. Since the shape of society is genetically determined, social forces exert no effect independent of natural forces upon behavior. Sociobiology thus looks to the biological individual for the origin of all behavior. Social behavior is understood as the agglomeration of individual biological and behavioral tendencies.

This perspective radically simplifies understanding of social behavior. Because sociobiology sees society growing simply and directly out of individual behavioral phenotypes that are themselves not essentially altered by that society, all the traditionally vexing problems of social theory are bypassed. The relation between the individual and society becomes a unidirectional, linear one rather than a bidirectional, dialectical one. A century of sociology notwithstanding, this model seems unable to account for many common social phenomena. For example, political aggression cannot be understood as a simple summation of individual aggression. Individual aggression might be channeled politically, but in so doing it is shaped by historical, religious, and cultural forces that may not be significant for individual aggression. The individual frustrations of the Romanians became unified politically overnight, but may have remained diffuse and impotent for years longer if social conditions had been different.

In summary then, two main conclusions can be drawn about the capacity of sociobiology to provide a general, unifying account of human social behavior. First, sociobiology has no special method or strategy for describing human behavior that would allow it to correctly define human nature and its origin. Without direct access to the heritable aspects of human behavior, sociobiology is left to seek conventional universals such as social stratification or male dominance as innate. Without further evidence, it is assumed that such traits are heritable and have been selected because they are adaptive. According to Lewontin *et al.* (1984),

> sociobiologists begin with the trait and invent an origin for it which assumes that the trait itself is the efficient case of its evolution. There is no hint in sociobiological theory that evolutionary geneticists are in serious doubt about what fraction of evolutionary change is the result of natural selection for specific characters. (p. 252)

Sociobiology can therefore offer us no guidance in determining which behaviors are true evolutionary products and which are byproducts. The central problem is that sociobiology must be based on and cannot itself provide a theory of human nature. The search for evolutionary causes must begin with an understanding of which trait has been caused or selected. The biologist Bart Voorzanger (1987) succinctly stated: "Instead of using evolutionary biology to get to learn ourselves, we have to know ourselves in order to give an evolutionary reconstruction of our behavior. There is no other way" (p. 265).

Second, sociobiology is unable to show that social behavior can be adequately understood in purely biological terms or that such behavior serves an ultimately biological purpose. Kinship (Sahlins, 1976), language (Sahlins, 1976), and ethics (Ayala, 1987) are three areas that rest upon a biological capacity but are determined in their specifics by social forces. Undoubtedly, evolutionary pressures have impacted upon the nature of these biological capacities, but are likely to have accounted for a small, and as yet unknown, amount of the variance in these cultural practices.

SOCIOBIOLOGY AND PSYCHIATRIC DISORDERS

We now return to the issue of what contribution sociobiology can make to the vexing issues of psychiatry that we have earlier identified. In discussing the relationship of sociobiology and psychiatry, it is important first to understand that sociobiology is not equivalent to behavioral genetics. Sociobiology is concerned with questions of purpose and function and not questions of mechanism. It is therefore focused upon ultimate causation (e.g., "why" questions) rather than proximate causation (e.g., "how" questions). The means according to which chromosomal abnormalities are translated into behavioral abnormalities is not its concern. Furthermore, sociobiology is interested in the normal genetic control of behavior, not with the aberrations in behavior that are produced when genetic material is damaged or altered.

In contrast, behavioral genetics is concerned with proximate causation. In schizophrenia or Alzheimer's disease, molecular geneticists search for the defective genes that produce the defective neuromechanisms. This inquiry does not determine why these defects exist or why schizophrenia has persisted at a prevalence of 1% among different cultures despite its apparent evolutionary disadvantage.

It is also important to distinguish sociobiology from ethology. Although the study of animal behavior can be a valuable source for hypotheses on human behavior, we seek to provide a critique of the general idea that biology alone can provide the tools we need for a clinically adequate categorization of behavior. It is a critique of the notion that psychology can be reduced to evolutionary biology.

We will now offer a brief review of some recently proposed sociobiological psychiatric theories. Such theories represent attempts to understand the evolutionary history and ground of psychiatric disorders: Why have they persisted? What are their functional origins? What is their relation to more normal or adaptive behavior? Most psychobiological theories in this area fall into one of two types. The first sees psychiatric symptoms as covertly or ultimately adaptive. Lewis (1934), for example, discussed the adaptive aspect of depression. He argued that depression may be a way in which a suffering individual can provide cues to others so as to predictably elicit empathy and care-taking behavior. The second type of theory sees psychiatric symptoms as evidence of regression from adaptive behavior. McGuire (1981), for example, understood psychiatric syndromes as essentially reductions in the capacity for "species-typical" behavior. Physiological dysregulation produces impaired behavioral plasticity which, in turn, increases the production of species-typical behavior.

These are intriguing ideas, but their similarity to psychoanalytic "functional" theories cannot go unnoticed. Psychoanalysts have often proposed that unpleasant symptoms are adaptive since they serve as defenses against a far worse fate. Furthermore, maladaptive behaviors are thought to have occurred as a result of developmental arrest. Of course, there are differences. Sociobiologists understand the word *adaptive* in terms of genetic propagation or inclusive fitness rather than psychic integrity, and they conceptualize developmental regression in phylogenetic rather than in ontogenetic terms.

Unfortunately, sociobiological theories are as difficult to verify as psychoanalytic ones. Sociobiological psychiatrists admit that there is no way to measure directly the effects of psychiatric disorders on inclusive fitness. They therefore substitute impact upon social functioning as the criterion of adaptiveness. As McGuire (1981) explained:

> actual measures of inclusive fitness are next to impossible to obtain in human behavioral research, primarily because the life span of the subject is approximately the life span of the researcher. Thus we shall use the influences of behaviors on daily functioning as an approximation of the effect of the behavior on inclusive fitness. (p. 689)

It is essential to note that this "approximation," in fact, annuls the difference between behavior understood sociobiologically (i.e., in terms of its biological function) and behavior understood sociologically (i.e., in terms of its social function). This approximation is necessary, not simply because the patients live about as long as the investigators (thus making changes between generations difficult to study), but also because the biological functions of human behavior, such as kinship, ethics, and language, cannot be disentangled from their social functions. Human beings survive by means of social relations that are transmitted between generations. Biological survival is therefore dependent upon social survival.

Mind Science and Biological Science in Psychiatric Research

Biological mechanisms have an objectivity that tempts the researcher to use these mechanisms to define mental illness. For instance, there may be a temptation to *define* schizophrenia as an abnormality of the dopamine system, or obsessive-compulsive disorder as an abnormality of the serotonin system. However, such efforts may be premature and could sometimes lead to the inappropriate classification of diseases. For instance, efforts to categorize mental illness by response to medication is particularly problematic (Baldessarini, 1990). The major issue here is that a single medication may exert its effects through several different mechanisms (e.g., amantadine is effective for both influenza and akathisia).

Rather than settling for simple correlations between psychopathology and neurotransmitter systems, it may be time for psychiatric research to enter a more ambitious phase in which pharmacological and pathological mechanisms are placed within the context of the overall biological *and* social functioning of the human organisms. Mechanisms can be organized and sorted only if the functions they serve for the organisms can be determined. Ultimately, abnormal behavior can be understood only within the context of normal behavior. Only through a renewed interest in the purpose and taxonomy of behavior will psychiatric research move beyond the era when its most important discoveries are accidents.

We have already discussed the reasons for our doubt that sociobiology can provide a comprehensive theory of the purpose of human behavior. Instead, we believe that descriptive and taxonomic work in psychiatry will continue to require reference to disciplines other than biology. Psychiatry will continue to study actualities with "different modes of objectiveness," as was described by Jaspers (Ehrlich *et al.*, 1986) at the outset of this chapter. This will preclude the theoretical and methodological unity sought for psychiatric research by McHugh (1987), Detre (1987), and Guze (1989).

This finding need not be cause for concern or discouragement, however. The tension created by having both the brain and the mind as objects of study defines the unique character of psychiatric research. It sets our research apart from nonmedical mental health research and from neurological research. Our clinical work requires that we alternate between empathic and objective observation, between the first and the third person perspectives, and between attention to the patient's experience and to the patient's behavior. It is probably not reasonable to assume that our research enterprise can escape this tension. Yet it is a tension that may yield many insights. The late physicist, Heinz Pagels (1988) stated:

> Monism, by collapsing the material and mental worlds into one world, has deprived itself of an internal challenge that might have given it greater philosophical life. Dualism, by contrast, maintains a tension between the material and the mental and hence motive for transformation and change. (p. 690)

Where does this leave us with respect to the challenge from Paul McHugh (1987) to build a "rational therapeutics based upon comprehensive biological medicine?" We have learned that biology, even when including evolutionary biology, cannot encompass all that is necessary for psychiatric research. Inquiries into the purpose of human behavior, normal or abnormal, *necessarily* point beyond the biological sciences. We propose that psychiatric research not be defined by its basis in biology or in neuroscience, but by its essential involvement with brain–mind relation. No doubt, some researchers will continue to study brain physiology without direct reference to experience or behavior; others will study experience and behavior without direct reference to the brain. But such efforts will *qualify* as psychiatric research insofar as they are relevant to the understanding of the brain–mind relation and the care of patients suffering from mental illness.

Finally, let us remind ourselves that even medicine is moving beyond the goals set by McHugh (1987) for psychiatry. In chronic and primary care, medicine is questioning the relation between pathology, symptoms, and disability. Although medicine has long defined itself in terms of its attention to objective pathology, the importance of addressing pathology in terms of its impact upon function (biological and social) is now increasingly acknowledged. For medicine, recognition of the functional context within which biological disorder becomes significant does not negate the importance of clinical and research attention to biology. It does highlight that attention to biology alone does not exhaust the responsibility of the physician—either as clinician or researcher. For psychiatry, the search for a better conceptual agenda for research will continue. And although the task may be easier for our study of the brain than of the mind, it is unlikely that it will ever be fully completed. Nor may a single definitive system of brain–mind correlation be derived. Finally, in our care of mentally ill patients, the therapeutic interaction involves so much more than what a scientific (let alone a biological) approach can offer, that we will perhaps forever have to borrow from nonscientific disciplines (in a sense this is true for all of medicine, whatever the specialty, but perhaps will always be particularly true for psychiatry). These considerations, however, do not absolve us from our research efforts, nor do they justify a retreat into psychodynamic semantics on the one hand, or molecular biology on the other.

SUMMARY

At this time, psychiatric research is characterized by a variety of philosophies and research methods that appear incompatible with each other. This diversity of approach means that attention to the conceptual presuppositions of research is essential if its overall direction and purpose are not to be lost. Some psychiatrists have responded to this diversity with a call for unification of psychiatric research around biological methods and theories. Molecular biology is to provide an understanding of the mechanism and evolutionary biology an understanding of purpose of human behavior. We argue, however, that evolutionary theory itself as expressed in sociobiology cannot provide a definitive account of the purpose of human social behavior nor can it provide a definitive psychopathological taxonomy. For human beings, the biological purposes of behavior are enclosed within its social purposes just as the human biological environment is enclosed within the human social environment. Nevertheless, renewed attention to the overall taxonomy and purpose of behavior is necessary if psychiatric research is to move beyond the era when its most important discoveries were just accidents. This will require reference to scientific disciplines other than biology, and careful application of scientific methodology to the research topics, whether they are biomedical or psychosocial. Psychiatric research will be defined by its attention to the brain–mind link. Thus, the placement of biological disorder within a broader functional context situates psychiatry at the forefront of current medical research.

REFERENCES

American Psychiatric Association. (1980). *Diagnostic and statistical manual of mental disorders* (3rd ed.). Washington, DC: Author.
American Psychiatric Association. (1987). *Diagnostic and statistical manual of mental disorders* (3rd ed., rev.). Washington, DC: Author.
Ayala, F. J. (1987). The biological roots of morality. *Biology and Philosophy, 2*, 235–252.
Baldessarini, R. J. (1990). The future of psychiatric research and academic psychiatry. *McLean Hospital Journal, 15*, 57.
Bannister, D. (1968). The logical requirements of research into schizophrenia. *British Journal of Psychiatry, 114*, 181–188.
Cloninger, C. R., Martin, R. L., Guze, S. B., & Clayton, P. J. (1985). Diagnosis and prognosis in schizophrenia. *Archives of General Psychiatry, 42*, 15–25.
Detre, T. (1987). The future of psychiatry. *American Journal of Psychiatry, 144*, 621–624.
Ehrlich, L., Ehrlich, E., & Pepper, G. (1986). Philosophy and science. In K. Jaspers (Ed.), *Basic philosophical writings, selections*. Athens: Ohio University Press.
Guze, S. B. (1989). Biological psychiatry: Is there any other kind? *Psychological Medicine, 19*, 315–323.
Klerman, G. C. (1990). The psychiatric patient's right to effective treatment: Implications of Osheroff vs. Chestnut Lodge. *American Journal of Psychiatry, 147*, 409–418.
Lewis, A. J. (1934). Melancholia. *Journal of Mental Science, 80*, 271–381.
Lewontin, R. C., Rose, S., & Kamin, L. J. (1984). *Not in our genes*. New York: Pantheon Books.
McGuire, M. T. (1981). Psychiatric disorders in the context of evolutionary biology: An ethological model of behavioral changes associated with psychiatric disorders. *Journal of Nervous and Mental Disease, 169*, 689.
McGuire, M. T., & Essock-Vitale, S. M. (1981). Psychiatric disorders in the context of evolutionary biology: A functional classification of behavior. *Journal of Nervous and Mental Disease, 169*, 672–686.
McHugh, P. (1987). William Osler and the new psychiatry. *Annals of Internal Medicine, 107*, 914–918.
Pagels, H. (1988). *The dreams of reason*. New York: Simon & Schuster.
Sahlins, M. (1976). *The use and abuse of biology*. Ann Arbor: University of Michigan Press.
Stone, A. A. (1990). Law, science and psychiatric malpractice: A response to Klerman's indictment of psychoanalytic psychiatry. *American Journal of Psychiatry, 147*, 419–427.
Voorzanger, B. (1987). No norms and no nature: The moral relevance of evolutionary biology. *Biology and Philosophy, 2*, 265.
Wilson, E. O. (1975). *Sociobiology*. Cambridge: Harvard University Press.

Index